—— Second Edition ——

SPORTS NUTRITION

Vitamins and Trace Elements

NUTRITION in EXERCISE and SPORT

Published Titles

Exercise and Disease,
Ronald R. Watson and Marianne Eisinger

Nutrients as Ergogenic Aids for Sports and Exercise,
Luke Bucci

Nutrition in Exercise and Sport, Second Edition,
Ira Wolinsky and James F. Hickson, Jr.

Nutrition Applied to Injury Rehabilitation and Sports Medicine,
Luke Bucci

Nutrition for the Recreational Athlete,
Catherine G. Ratzin Jackson

Sports Nutrition: Minerals and Electrolytes,
Constance V. Kies and Judy A. Driskell

Nutrition, Physical Activity, and Health in Early Life:
Studies in Preschool Children,
Jana Pařízková

Exercise and Immune Function,
Laurie Hoffman-Goetz

Body Fluid Balance: Exercise and Sport,
E.R. Buskirk and S. Puhl

Nutrition and the Female Athlete,
Jaime S. Ruud

Sports Nutrition: Vitamins and Trace Elements,
Ira Wolinsky and Judy A. Driskell

Amino Acids and Proteins for the Athlete—The Anabolic Edge,
Mauro G. DiPasquale

Nutrition in Exercise and Sport, Third Edition,
Ira Wolinsky

Gender Differences in Metabolism: Practical and Nutritional Implications,
Mark Tarnopolsky

Macroelements, Water, and Electrolytes in Sports Nutrition,
Judy A. Driskell and Ira Wolinsky

Sports Nutrition,
Judy A. Driskell

Energy-Yielding Macronutrients and Energy Metabolism in
Sports Nutrition,
Judy A. Driskell and Ira Wolinsky

Published Titles Continued

Nutrition and Exercise Immunology,
David C. Nieman and Bente Klarlund Pedersen

Sports Drinks: Basic Science and Practical Aspects,
Ronald Maughan and Robert Murray

Nutritional Applications in Exercise and Sport,
Ira Wolinsky and Judy Driskell

Nutrition and the Strength Athlete,
Catherine G. Ratzin Jackson

Nutritional Assessment of Athletes,
Judy A. Driskell and Ira Wolinsky

Sports Nutrition: Vitamins and Trace Elements, Second Edition,
Judy A. Driskell and Ira Wolinsky

NUTRITION in EXERCISE and SPORT Series

Second Edition

SPORTS NUTRITION

Vitamins and Trace Elements

Edited by

Judy A. Driskell & Ira Wolinsky

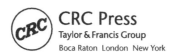

CRC Press
Taylor & Francis Group
Boca Raton London New York

CRC Press is an imprint of the
Taylor & Francis Group, an **informa** business

A TAYLOR & FRANCIS BOOK

First published 2006 by Taylor & Francis

Published 2019 by CRC Press
Taylor & Francis Group
6000 Broken Sound Parkway NW, Suite 300
Boca Raton, FL 33487-2742

© 2006 by Taylor & Francis Group, LLC
CRC Press is an imprint of Taylor & Francis Group, an Informa business

First issued in paperback 2019

No claim to original U.S. Government works

ISBN 13: 978-0-367-45398-5 (pbk)
ISBN 13: 978-0-8493-3022-3 (hbk)

This book contains information obtained from authentic and highly regarded sources. Reasonable efforts have been made to publish reliable data and information, but the author and publisher cannot assume responsibility for the validity of all materials or the consequences of their use. The authors and publishers have attempted to trace the copyright holders of all material reproduced in this publication and apologize to copyright holders if permission to publish in this form has not been obtained. If any copyright material has not been acknowledged please write and let us know so we may rectify in any future reprint.

Except as permitted under U.S. Copyright Law, no part of this book may be reprinted, reproduced, transmitted, or utilized in any form by any electronic, mechanical, or other means, now known or hereafter invented, including photocopying, microfilming, and recording, or in any information storage or retrieval system, without written permission from the publishers.

For permission to photocopy or use material electronically from this work, please access www.copyright.com (http://www.copyright.com/) or contact the Copyright Clearance Center, Inc. (CCC), 222 Rosewood Drive, Danvers, MA 01923, 978-750-8400. CCC is a not-for-profit organization that provides licenses and registration for a variety of users. For organizations that have been granted a photocopy license by the CCC, a separate system of payment has been arranged.

Trademark Notice: Product or corporate names may be trademarks or registered trademarks, and are used only for identification and explanation without intent to infringe.

Visit the Taylor & Francis Web site at
http://www.taylorandfrancis.com

and the CRC Press Web site at
http://www.crcpress.com

Library of Congress Cataloging-in-Publication Data

Sports nutrition : vitamins and trace elements / edited by Judy A. Driskell, Ira Wolinsky.-- 2nd ed.
    p. cm. -- (Nutrition in exercise and sport)
    Wolinsky's name appears first in the statement of resp. on the earlier edition
  ISBN 0-8493-3022-X (alk. paper)
    1. Vitamins in human nutrition. 2. Trace elements in nutrition. 3. Athletes--Nutrition. I. Driskell, Judy A. (Judy Anne) II. Wolinsky, Ira. III. Series.

QP771.S68 2005
613.2'86--dc22   2005048557

Dedication

We appreciate the opportunity to have worked with the chapter authors, experts all, on this book and on our other books in the area of sports nutrition. We learned from them and dedicate this book to them.

Preface

This book addresses vitamin and trace element needs as they relate to exercise and sports. A growing body of research indicates that work capacity, oxygen consumption and other measures of physical performance of individuals, including athletes, are affected by deficiency or borderline deficiency of specific vitamins or essential trace elements. Athletes, as well as the public in general, often have low dietary intakes of many of the vitamins and essential trace elements. The findings of some researchers indicate that large doses of certain vitamins and trace elements given to individuals who had adequate status of that vitamin or trace element improved various measures of physical performance. Other researchers have reported conflicting findings. A critical review of these reports is included in this book.

This volume includes a collection of chapters written by scientists from several academic disciplines who have expertise in an area of vitamin or trace element nutrition as it relates to exercise and sports. Following an introduction are reviews of exercise and sports as they relate to the vitamins (ascorbic acid, thiamin, riboflavin, niacin, vitamin B_6, folate, vitamin B_{12}, pantothenic acid and biotin, choline [an essential nutrient], vitamin A, vitamins D and K, vitamin E), the essential trace elements (iron, zinc, iodine, chromium, selenium), as well as a chapter on boron, manganese, molybdenum, nickel, silicon, and vanadium, and ending in a summary chapter. Sports nutritionists, sports medicine and fitness professionals, researchers, students, health practitioners and the well informed layman will find this book timely and informative.

This book is part of a miniseries we edited that deals with nutrition in exercise and sport. Other books in this miniseries are: *Sports Nutrition: Vitamins and Trace Elements* (first edition); *Macroelements, Water and Electrolytes in Sports Nutrition*; *Energy-Yielding Macronutrients and Energy Metabolism in Sports Nutrition*; *Nutritional Applications in Exercise and Sport*; *Nutritional Assessment of Athletes* and *Nutritional Ergogenic Aids*. Additionally useful will be *Nutrition in Exercise and Sport*, 3rd edition, edited by Ira Wolinsky, and *Sports Nutrition*, authored by Judy Driskell.

Judy A. Driskell, Ph.D., R.D.
University of Nebraska

Ira Wolinsky, Ph.D.
University of Houston

The Editors

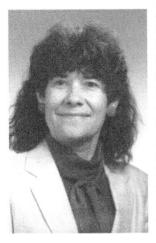

Judy Anne Driskell, Ph.D., R.D. is Professor of Nutrition and Health Sciences at the University of Nebraska. She received her B.S. degree in Biology from the University of Southern Mississippi in Hattiesburg. Her M.S. and Ph.D. degrees were obtained from Purdue University. She has served in research and teaching positions at Auburn University, Florida State University, Virginia Polytechnic Institute and State University, and the University of Nebraska. She has also served as the Nutrition Scientist for the U.S. Department of Agriculture/Cooperative State Research Service and as a Professor of Nutrition and Food Science at Gadjah Mada and Bogor Universities in Indonesia.

Dr. Driskell is a member of numerous professional organizations including the American Society of Nutritional Sciences, the American College of Sports Medicine, the International Society of Sports Nutrition, the Institute of Food Technologists and the American Dietetic Association. In 1993, she received the Professional Scientist Award of the Food Science and Human Nutrition Section of the Southern Association of Agricultural Scientists. In addition, she was the 1987 recipient of the Borden Award for Research in Applied Fundamental Knowledge of Human Nutrition. She is listed as an expert in B-Complex Vitamins by the Vitamin Nutrition Information Service.

Dr. Driskell co-edited the CRC Press books *Sports Nutrition: Minerals and Electrolytes* with Constance V. Kies. In addition, she authored the textbook *Sports Nutrition* and co-authored an advanced nutrition book, *Nutrition: Chemistry and Biology*, both published by CRC Press. She co-edited *Sports Nutrition: Vitamins and Trace Elements* (first edition); *Macroelements; Water, and Electrolytes in Sports Nutrition; Energy-Yielding Macronutrients and Energy Metabolism in Sports Nutrition; Nutritional Applications in Exercise and Sport, Nutritional Assessment of Athletes, Nutritional Ergogenic Aids,* and the current book, *Sports Nutrition: Vitamins and Trace Elements,* 2nd edition, all with Ira Wolinsky. She has published more than 130 refereed research articles and 12 book chapters, as well as several publications intended for lay audiences, and has given numerous presentations to professional and lay groups. Her current research interests center around vitamin metabolism and requirements, including the interrelationships between exercise and water-soluble vitamin requirements.

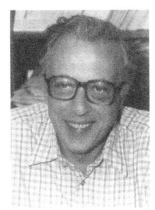

Ira Wolinsky, Ph.D., is Professor Emeritus of Nutrition at the University of Houston. He received his B.S. degree in Chemistry from the City College of New York and his M.S. and Ph.D. degrees in Biochemistry from the University of Kansas. He has served in research and teaching positions at the Hebrew University, the University of Missouri, and The Pennsylvania State University, as well as conducted basic research in NASA life sciences facilities and abroad.

Dr. Wolinsky is a member of the American Society of Nutritional Sciences, among other honorary and scientific organizations. He has contributed numerous nutrition research papers in the open literature. His major research interests relate to the nutrition of bone and calcium and trace elements, and to sports nutrition. He has been the recipient of research grants from both public and private sources. He has received several international research fellowships and consultantships to the former Soviet Union, Bulgaria, Hungary and India. He merited a Fulbright Senior Scholar Fellowship to Greece in 1999.

Dr. Wolinsky has co-authored a book on the history of the science of nutrition, *Nutrition and Nutritional Diseases*. He co-edited *Sports Nutrition: Vitamins and Trace Elements Macroelements* (first edition)*; Water, and Electrolytes in Sports Nutrition; Energy-Yielding Macronutrients and Energy Metabolism in Sports Nutrition*; *Nutritional Applications in Exercise and Sport, Nutritional Assessment of Athletes, Nutritional Ergogenic Aids*, and the current book, *Sports Nutrition: Vitamins and Trace Elements*, 2nd edition, all with Judy Driskell. Additionally, he co-edited *Nutritional Concerns of Women*, two editions, with Dorothy Klimis-Zacas, *The Mediterranean Diet: Constituents and Health Promotion*, with his Greek colleagues, and *Nutrition in Pharmacy Practice*, with Louis Williams. He edited three editions of *Nutrition in Exercise and Sport*. He served also as the editor, or co-editor, for the CRC Series on *Nutrition in Exercise and Sport*, the CRC Series on *Modern Nutrition*, the CRC Series on *Methods in Nutrition Research*, and the CRC Series on *Exercise Physiology*.

Contributors

Enas K. Al-Tamimi, M.S.
Department of Human Nutrition
Kansas State University
Manhattan, KS

Debra A. Bemben, Ph.D.
Department of Health and Exercise Science
University of Oklahoma
Norman, OK

Michael G. Bemben, Ph.D.
Department of Health and Exercise Science
University of Oklahoma
Norman, OK

Wayne E. Billon, Ph.D., R.D.
Department of Health Sciences
Western Carolina University
Cullowhee, NC

Gayatri Borthakur, Ph.D.
Department of Human Nutrition
University of Illinois at Chicago
Chicago, IL

L. Mallory Boylan, Ph.D., R.D.
Nutrition Section
Texas Tech University
Lubbock, Texas

Luke R. Bucci, Ph.D., C.C.N.C. (A.S.C.P.), C.N.S.
Weider Nutrition International
Salt Lake City, UT

Gabriela Camporeale, M.S.
Department of Nutrition and Health Sciences
University of Nebraska
Lincoln, NE

Jamie A. Cooper, M.S.
Department of Military and Emergency Medicine
Uniformed Services University of the Health Sciences
Bethesda, MD

Patricia A. Deuster, Ph.D., M.P.H.
Department of Military and Emergency Medicine
Uniformed Services University of the Health Sciences
Bethesda, MD

Judy A. Driskell, Ph.D., R.D.
Department of Nutrition and Health Sciences
University of Nebraska
Lincoln, NE

Christine M. Hansen, Ph.D.
Department of Food Science and Human Nutrition
Iowa State University
Ames, IA

Michael J. Hartman, M.S.
Department of Health and Exercise Science
University of Oklahoma
Norman, OK

Emily M. Haymes, Ph.D.
Department of Nutrition, Food and Exercise Sciences
Florida State University
Tallahassee, FL

Mark D. Haub, Ph.D.
Department of Human Nutrition
Kansas State University
Manhattan, KS

Edward M. Heath, Ph.D., F.A.C.S.M.
Department of Health, Physical Education and Recreation
Utah State University
Logan, UT

W. Thomas Johnson, Ph.D.
U.S. Department of Agriculture, Agricultural Research Service
Grand Forks Human Nutrition Research Center
Grand Forks, ND

B. STUDIES BEFORE 1960

Seminal data generated during the 1940s influenced subsequent conclusions and research on multiple vitamin-minerals and physical performance. Clearly, supplementation of single or multiple B vitamins (and doses of vitamin C below 1000 mg daily) did not significantly affect physiological parameters or physical exercise performance in well-controlled studies (see Table 1.1).[19] However, only incomplete mixtures of B vitamins were studied (pantothenate, folate and vitamin B_{12} had yet to be characterized), and most of the trace minerals now known to be essential were thought to be coincidental contamination or toxic, and therefore, completely overlooked. Thus, all of these studies were incomplete in terms of nutrients examined, they lacked dose-response data and were usually of very short duration. It is possible that a deficiency of an essential nutrient not recognized as such at the time could have affected results, negating effects of the studied nutrient. However, the prevailing attitude among researchers in exercise physiology was (and still is) that vitamins in general had no effect on physical performance in absence of a prolonged or severe deficiency. Thereafter, newly discovered vitamins and trace minerals were infrequently examined for possible effects on exercise performance. Relatively few multiple combinations were subsequently examined in studies that were frequently incomplete with regard to containing amounts of all known essential micronutrients at doses known or shown to improve status (see comparison of doses to current DVs in Table 1.2). Thus, there were no studies on what today would be considered a complete multiple vitamin-mineral mixture (100% DV of all essential vitamins and minerals) until the 1980s. In other words, the opinions carried over from early research that vitamin and mineral supplements had little, if any, effects on exercise performance were based on weak experimental data.

C. B COMPLEX MIXTURES

Since the known roles of B vitamins emphasized cellular energy metabolism, it was only natural that B vitamins were studied for effects on physical performance. Previous scrutiny of human exercise performance trials after supplementation with one or more B complex vitamins has found apparent dose–response and time effects.[35] For some vitamins (thiamin and pantothenate) more does seem to be better. Since some individual B vitamins will be covered in subsequent chapters, Table 1.1 lists the doses and results for combinations of B vitamins from several studies.[23,30,36–44] Obviously, potential thresholds of effect for enhancement of physical performance by increased B complex vitamin intake are not clearly known and may not be consistent between populations, and multiple dose ranges have been studied in only a few experiments. Notice that there are no studies that have examined a full complement of all eight B vitamins and choline, and only two studies examined six B vitamins. Thus, every study listed is incomplete. Nevertheless, scrutiny of available, but limited, data on mixtures of B complex vitamins given to exercising individuals has found a pattern of higher doses and longer durations associated with greater effects. Human clinical studies comparing placebo, low-dose and high-dose B vitamin mixtures with short and long durations and specific performance endpoints are needed to clarify potential ergogenic benefits of B complex vitamins.

D. MULTIPLE VITAMIN-MINERAL COMBINATIONS

Table 1.2 lists human clinical studies concerning multiple vitamin-mineral supplementation in exercising individuals and performance measurements.[45–60] First, it is immediately apparent that, excluding the macrominerals calcium, magnesium, phosphorus and potassium, no combination tested contained all essential vitamins and minerals. However, considering that there is little or no rationale or evidence for an ergogenic effect from vitamin D, vitamin K, iodine, fluorine and molybdenum, exclusion of these nutrients is not thought to influence findings. Taking these exclusions into account, only the report by Colgan in 1986[52] studied a complete set of essential vitamins and minerals. Usual exclusions were biotin, chromium and selenium, although each formula tested exhibited lack of one or more other essential micronutrients.

TABLE 1.1
Correlation of Dose and Ergogenic Effects of Controlled Human Studies on B Vitamin Combinations

Investigators (year)	Ref.	Length of admin.	Thiamin (mg)	Riboflavin (mg)	Niacin Equiv. (mg)	B_6 (mg)	B_{12} (mcg)	Folate (mg)	Panto-thenate (mg)	Biotin (mg)	Other Nutrients (mg)	Ergogenic Results[a]
Keys and Henschel (1941)	36	4 wks	5		100						C (100)	—
Simonson et al. (1942)	37	15 wks	6	8	80	0.3					80 units filtrate	—[b]
Foltz et al. (1942)	38	Acute iv[c]	3–15	0.3–1.6	10–50	1–5						+
Keys and Henschel (1942)	39	4–6 wks	5–17	0–10	100	0–10			0–20		C (100–200)	—
Frankau (1943)	40	4 d	5	5	50						C (100)	+
Henschel et al. (1944)	41	3 d	5	10	100							—
Early and Carlson (1969)	42	6 d	100	8	100	5	25000		30			+
Buzina et al. (1982)[d]	23	3 mo	5	2		2						+
Read and McGuffin (1983)	43	6 wks	5	5	25	2	0.5		12.5		C (70)	—
Boncke and Nickel (1989)	44	8 wks	90			60	120					+
Boncke and Nickel (1989)	44	8 wks	300			600	600					+

[a] — indicates no significant effect on physiological or performance measurements. + indicates a significant improvement in physiological or performance measurements.
[b] No effects on physical performance, but significant improvement of mental fatigue and subjective feelings.
[c] Vitamins were administered by intravenous means.
[d] Large percentage of subjects exhibited clinical and biochemical signs of vitamin deficiencies.

TABLE 1.2
Comparison of Multiple Vitamin-Mineral Formulas Studied for Effects on Exercise Performance and Metabolism

Author	DV[a]	McCollum 1960	Nelson 1960	Keul 1974	Haralambie 1975	Van Dam 1978	Keul 1979	van der Beek 1981[b]	Barnett 1984	Colgan 1986	Weight 1988
Ref.		45	46	47	48	49	50	30	51	52	53
Total n		82		12	14	40	14	77	20	8	30
Subjects		College students — poor fitness		German fencers	German fencers	German fencers	German cross-country skiers	Dutch sports students	American competitive runners	American marathon runners	South African competitive runners
Duration (weeks)		8	12			3		16	4	24	12
Vitamin A (IU)	5000	25000	NR[f]					5000	6000	5000–45000	3000
Vitamin D (IU)	400	1000						400	600	200–2480	400
Vitamin E (IU)	30			100	50	50	50	150	15	200–1600	516
Vitamin K (mcg)	80										
Ascorbate (mg)	60	300		1000	500	500	500	500	135	2000–16000	850
Thiamin (mg)	1.5	10		20	10	10	10	12	15	40–600	60
Riboflavin (mg)	1.7	10		30	15	15	15	20	15	30–250	60
Niacin Equiv. (mg)	20	100		40	20	20	20	210	75	100–1000	70
Vitamin B_6 (mg)	2.0	2		50	25	25	25	20	21	10–300	60
Vitamin B_{12} (mcg)	6.0	4						30	15	100–300	60

Folate (mcg)	400	1500					4000	400	2000–3000	500
Pantothenate (mg)	10	20	40	20	20	20	100	18	50–1000	70
Biotin (mcg)	300						2000		2000–10000	
Potassium (mg)			200	100	100	100		37.5	198–5000	32
Phosphorus (mg)	1000		2160 (PO_4)	1080	1080 (PO_4)	1080			200–2000	116
Calcium (mg)	1000		500	250	250	250			1000–3500	230
Magnesium (mg)	400		340	170	170	170	100	52.5	1000–2000	116
Iron (mg)	18						100	37.5	30–60	13.4
Zinc (mg)	15							15	50–150	5.2
Copper (mg)	2.0							3	0–5	0.6
Manganese (mg)	2.0							3	20–100	300?
Iodine (mg)	0.15							0.15	0.15–1.0	0.15
Selenium (mg)	0.07								0.2–1.0	0.05
Chromium (mg)	0.12								0.3–1.0	
Molybdenum (mg)	0.075								0.05–5	
Choline (mg)								97.5	200–2000	

(Continued)

TABLE 1.2 (Continued)
Comparison of Multiple Vitamin-Mineral Formulas Studied for Effects on Exercise Performance and Metabolism

Author	DV[a]	McCollum 1960	Nelson 1960	Keul 1974	Haralambie 1975	Van Dam 1978	Keul 1979	van der Beek 1981[b]	Barnett 1984	Colgan 1986	Weight 1988
Other Nutrients		Cerofort ± Lysine	Contents not reported	Beneroc® 3.5 g sucrose, Phosphorus reported as phosphate	Beneroc® 3.5 g sucrose, Phosphorus reported as phosphate	Beneroc® 3.5 g sucrose, Phosphorus reported as phosphate	Beneroc® 3.5 g sucrose, Phosphorus reported as phosphate		Betaine HCL, Inositol, Lecithin, Liver, PABA, Pancreatin, Rice bran extract, Safflower oil, Soya bean extract, Wheat germ extract	Inositol, PABA	
Results		Physical fitness index, cable-tension strength test, Army physical fitness test scores not different from placebo group	No effects on sprints, vertical jump, ergometer test	Ratio of work load to heart rate increased 3%	Improved reflex responses	Improved status, hits, reaction times, muscular irritability	4.3% increase in cross-country ski speed	No effect on aerobic power	No effects on physiological measurements during exercise	Improved marathon times (by 11 min), physiological parameters, 81% fewer infections, 35% fewer injuries	B2, B6 status improved; other nutrient status unchanged, no effects on physiological parameters, peak treadmill speed or 15 km race times

Author	DV[a]	Dragan 1991[c]	Dragan 1991[c]	Colgan 1991	Colgan 1991	Singh 1992[d]	Telford 1992[e]	Savino 1999	Roberts 2001	Cavas 2004
Ref.		54	54	55	55	56	57	58	59	60
Total n		20	20	23	23	22	82	20	8	30
Subjects		Roumanian junior cyclists	Roumanian junior cyclists	American marathon runners	American marathon runners	American regular exercisers	Australian basketball, gymnasts, rowers, swimmers	Italian soccer team children	English endurance athletes	Turkish swimmers
Duration (weeks)		4	4	12	12	12	28–32	4	4	4
Vitamin A (IU)	5000	1000	7.5	5000	5000	(2600)	4500		15000	5000
Vitamin D (IU)	400	3200	400	400	400	400	400	400	400	400
Vitamin E (IU)	30	60	200	15	15	(51)	151		300	30
Vitamin K (mcg)	80		10			500			40	
Ascorbate (mg)	60	120	300	60	500	(169)	550		500	60
Thiamin (mg)	1.5	3.0	79	1.5	1.5	(54)	75		3	1.5
Riboflavin (mg)	1.7	3.0	100	1.7	1.7	(25)	25		3.4	1.7
Niacin Equiv. (mg)	20	36	100	20	20	100	100	9	40	20
Vitamin B_6 (mg)	2.0	10	82	2.0	152	(135)	100		10	2
Vitamin B_{12} (mcg)	6.0	10	100	12	112	(48)	100	1.3	30	6
Folate (mcg)	400		400	400	2400	(288)	200		600	400

(Continued)

TABLE 1.2 (Continued)
Comparison of Multiple Vitamin–Mineral Formulas Studied for Effects on Exercise Performance and Metabolism

Author	DV[a]	Dragan 1991[c]	Dragan 1991[c]	Colgan 1991	Colgan 1991	Singh 1992[d]	Telford 1992[e]	Savino 1999	Roberts 2001	Cavas 2004
Pantothenate (mg)	10		100			(62)	100	3	30	40
Biotin (mcg)	300		100			(400)	100		300	10
Potassium (mg)						99	33			
Phosphorus (mg)	1000									100
Calcium (mg)	1000		121			(57)	115		500	100
Magnesium (mg)	400		40			(57)	7		250	20
Iron (mg)	18		2.5	18	48		1		3	18
Zinc (mg)	15		7.5	15	60	(14.6)	3		15	2
Copper (mg)	2.0		0.3						2	
Manganese (mg)	2.0					15	0.01		3.6	
Iodine (mg)	0.15		0.224	0.15	0.15				0.075	
Selenium (mg)	0.07		0.01			0.05			0.1	0.15

Nutrient	Polivitaminizant S	Cantamega 2000	Perque 2		LifePak®	One A Day Junior
Chromium (mg)	0.12	0.04	0.2			0.2
Molybdenum (mg)	0.075		0.1	0.01		0.075
Choline (mg)		37		75		
Other Nutrients		Betaine hydrochloride, bioflavonoids, glutamic acid, inositol, lecithin, PABA, rutin, soya protein	Aspartate, citrate, fumarate, malate, PABA, quercetin, succinate, trimethylglycine, vanadium, vanilla	Betaine HCL, Bioflavonoids, Glutamic acid, Inositol, Kelp, Lecithin, PABA; 400 kcal carbohydrates, citrate, fluoride, pollen, rose hips	Alpha-carotene, boron, broccoli, cabbage, citrus bioflavonoids, curcumin, grape seed extract, lipoic acid, lutein, lycopene, quercetin, silicon, soy isoflavones, vanadium	

(Continued)

TABLE 1.2 (Continued)
Comparison of Multiple Vitamin-Mineral Formulas Studied for Effects on Exercise Performance and Metabolism

Author	DV[a]	Dragan 1991[c]	Dragan 1991[c]	Colgan 1991	Colgan 1991	Singh 1992[d]	Telford 1992[e]	Savino 1999	Roberts 2001	Cavas 2004
Results		Improved mineral status (calcium, iron, magnesium), fatigue ratings after training and biomarkers of recovery (urine mucoproteins, serum total protein)	No changes in status or biomarkers of recovery	DV amounts had no effect on status or performance	DV plus hematinics improved status and time to exhaustion on cycle ergometer	Vitamin status improved, no performance changes for run to exhaustion, peak torque, power, work	Increased skinfolds, female basketball players increased jumping ability, some increases in vitamin status, no changes in mineral status, no performance changes in other sports (gymnastics, rowing, swimming)	Vitamin status improved, but no effect on body mass or strength	VO$_2$max unchanged	Biomarkers of cardiac and muscle damage reduced

[a] DV = Daily Value for essential vitamins and minerals from 1989 Guidelines[8] (this is the DV most commonly used on labels of dietary supplements). DV has been known formerly as DRI, RDA and RDI.

[b] Reported as unpublished work in van der Beek, 1991.[30]

[c] Nutrient contents of Cantamega 2000 and Polyvitaminizant S products used by Dragan in 1991 differ from current formulas in 2004. The table reflects the formulas used in 1991.

[d] Nutrients indicated by parentheses were analyzed for actual content in the product. Amounts of other nutrients were from the product's label claim. Analyzed amounts were frequently different from label claim.

[e] Amounts for minerals were calculated based on percentage of elemental mineral for each compound described.

[f] NR = Not Reported.

1. Study Quality

The Kleijnen score is a rating of methodological quality of clinical trials, originally used to assess human trials with *Ginkgo biloba* preparations.[61] Maximum score is 100, and seven weighted criteria (patient characteristics, subject number, randomization, intervention description, double-blinding, effect measurements and results accountability) were considered. Studies in Table 1.2 on effects of multiple vitamin-mineral combinations on exercise performance after 1960 ranged from 50–75, indicating that no studies were of high quality (score >80). The most common deficiencies were low subject numbers and under-detailed randomization practices.

Each study in Table 1.2 exhibited serious flaws. Nelson did not report the ingredients or amounts of micronutrients administered.[46] The series of studies using the European product Beneroc® contained small amounts of sugars that should not have been enough to consistently affect exercise performance.[47–50] However, carbohydrate content was not controlled, and order of administration was not randomized, leading to potential order effects. Barnett and others discussed "performance," but actually measured physiological parameters during submaximal exercise under laboratory conditions, and not actual physical performance.[51] Colgan studied the largest doses of micronutrient supplementation, but doses were individualized and statistical analysis not performed, although very large changes in exercise performance were reported.[52] Both Colgan and Dragan used relatively low doses (~100% DV) of multiple vitamin-mineral products as control groups, and did not examine untreated placebo control subjects.[54,55] Van der Beek reported results from an unpublished study performed ten years earlier, with the usual lack of experimental details.[30]

The study by Telford and others contained errors in reporting of micronutrient units, confusing micrograms and milligrams for several nutrients.[57] Furthermore, compliance was very low — the majority of subjects consumed less than half of the required doses. In addition, performance measurements were mostly different for each group of athletes and analyzed separately for each sport, yielding an average subject number per group of 5.25. Iron supplements were given to any subject in either group who exhibited low serum ferritin levels, thus masking any chance for an effect of iron (only 1 mg daily) from the multiple vitamin-mineral group, and making some placebo subjects supplemented. McCollum, Nelson and Singh studied regular exercisers or students, not athletes engaged in supervised training or competitive events, unlike the other studies listed in Table 1.2.[45,46,56] The multiple vitamin-mineral formula used by Singh[56] (and effectively, Telford[57]) did not contain iron or copper, and thus was deficient in the most common and important micronutrient deficiency in exercising individuals.

Thus, each study in Table 1.2 exhibited confounding factors in experimental design and conduct that make interpretation and extrapolation of results problematic. Careful attention to the following list of experimental factors would improve quality of future research:

- Adequate subject numbers to provide necessary statistical power given normal biological variability
- Doses that improve micronutrient status
- Multiple dose ranges per study to explore dose–response relationships
- Subject compliance
- Verification of micronutrient content of dietary supplements
- Multiple measures of micronutrient status and intake, including functional assays
- Bioavailability of supplement studied
- Proper length of study
- Simultaneous measurement of performance, physiological, metabolic, psychological, immunological, neurological and mental parameters
- Complete profile of all known essential vitamins and minerals
- Possible investigator bias in study design, execution, analysis and presentation
- Thorough, nonselective literature reviews for discussion in publications

2. Exercise Performance

Twelve studies listed in Table 1.2 reported actual performance results.[45,46,48–50,52–58] Six studies found improvements in various measurements of physical performance:

1. Improved reaction times in fencers[48,49]
2. Improved speed in cross-country skiers[50]
3. Improved times in time trials or increased poundage lifted[52]
4. Increased time to exhaustion in cycle ergometry[55]
5. Increased jumping ability of female basketball players[57]

Seven studies did not find improvements in various performance measurements:

1. 15-km run times or treadmill speed[53,55]
2. Treadmill run to exhaustion, peak torque, total work or power[56]
3. Jumping ability of male basketball players, swimmers, gymnasts[57]
4. Race times, sprint times, vertical jump or cycle ergometer tests[45,46,57]
5. Strength[58]

Five studies in Table 1.2 did not report actual physical performance measures.[30,47,53, 59,60]

3. Physiological Parameters during Exercise

One study found improved work efficiency[47] and two others found decreased indicators of muscle damage,[54,60] but other studies did not find changes in physiological measurements during different types of exercise.[30,51,53,56,57,59] Parameters measured included blood lactate, glucose, fatty acids, ACTH response, oxygen consumption, heart rate, rectal temperatures, aerobic power and muscle glycogen depletion during exercise under laboratory conditions.

4. Micronutrient Status

From the studies in Table 1.2, micronutrient status was not altered after supplementation in three studies.[53–55] These studies also found no significant effect from multiple vitamin-mineral supplementation on physiological or performance parameters, and two[54,55] were near 100% DV for most nutrients. Status of certain minerals and hemoglobin was improved by a higher-potency supplement, compared with a lower-potency supplement.[54,55] B vitamin status was improved in three other studies, but status of fat-soluble vitamins and minerals were unchanged.[53,56,57,62,63]

Similarly, other studies not listed in Table 1.2 examining the effect of multiple vitamin-mineral combinations (usually lacking minerals) most often found improvements in the status of one or more B vitamins (B_1, B_2 or B_6), but usually not ascorbate or fat-soluble vitamins, unless deficiencies were previously documented.[18,23,64–70] Status usually took six weeks to show an improvement, suggesting studies lasting less than this interval may have missed an effect.[36,38,39,41,51,58–60]

E. MULTIPLE VITAMINS AND MINERALS WITH OTHER NUTRIENTS

Many dietary supplements that contain essential vitamins and trace minerals along with other potentially active agents for physical performance are available, and a few have been studied in exercising individuals. Most common are herbs combined with multiple vitamin-mineral formulas, especially ginseng (*Panax ginseng*) extracts. A recent review listed three studies of healthy exercising adults (but not athletes) given ginseng-multiple-vitamin-mineral combination products.[71] Similarly, 14 studies on mental performance parameters using ginseng-multiple-vitamin-mineral combinations were reported in adults, but not athletes.[71] The products contained a standardized ginseng extract, itself studied extensively for mental and performance effects in athletes,[71] with 100% DV for vitamins and some trace minerals, and also dimethylaminoethanol in one product

(Gericomplex®, Gerimax® and Geriatric Pharmaton®). These studies did show performance or physiological improvements during exercise, and most studies showed improved mental performance, but since the amount of ginseng in these products was equivalent to that of other studies that showed similar improvements, it is difficult to ascribe the changes to the vitamins or minerals.[71]

A study by Ushakov[72] in 1978 reported improved work capacity in seven subjects after 20 days of supplementation with "nutrition correction supplements," an undescribed mixture of "...glutamic and aspartic acids, methionine, group B vitamins, ascorbic acid, vitamin A, rutin, nicotinamide, nucleic acids, organic K, Ca, Mg, and Ph salts." However, administration was not randomized, allowing for possible training effects. Objective measurements of amino acid composition were reportedly improved after supplementation. Again, low subject number and poor study design preclude trustworthy data.

Studies using multiple vitamin-mineral combinations with other nutrients or herbal extracts have not added reliable information on any potential effects on physical performance in exercising individuals.

F. MULTIPLE VITAMIN AND TRACE MINERAL ANTIOXIDANT COMBINATIONS

Several essential vitamins and minerals possess antioxidant activity. These are primarily: (1) vitamin A (as beta carotene, not retinyl esters); (2) vitamin C; (3) vitamin E; and (4) selenium. Other vitamins and minerals do not possess inherent antioxidant activity. Zinc, copper, manganese and iron are essential cofactors for metalloenzyme antioxidants (superoxide dismutases, catalase, peroxidases), and can be considered as antioxidants. However, since these minerals possess many other roles, and because they possess pro-oxidant activities under certain conditions, their roles as antioxidants will not be considered in this chapter. Like the other minerals, selenium (as selenocysteine) is required for glutathione peroxidase (GPx) activity, but since there are only a few other non-antioxidant roles for selenium in GPx, its inclusion instead of zinc, copper, manganese and iron is justified.

While there have been a prodigious number of human studies concerning supplementation of essential micronutrient antioxidant combinations in exercising individuals, very few have actually measured physical performance. In keeping with the theme of this chapter, this review will focus only on physical performance results from studies using combinations of essential vitamins or trace minerals. Table 1.3 shows that performance-related measures in four controlled studies were not affected by antioxidant combinations, except for better lung function immediately after exercise in conditions of high ozone concentrations.[73–76] There are still no reports on the effects of exercise performance (such as time to exhaustion) from combinations of essential vitamin and trace mineral antioxidants without other nutrients. There is insufficient data on hand to determine whether supplementation with only combinations of essential vitamin and trace mineral antioxidants affects physical performance.

IV. EFFECT OF VITAMINS AND MINERALS ON CONDITIONS INDIRECTLY AFFECTING PERFORMANCE

Because a product or nutrient does not alter VO_2max or exercise time to exhaustion does not mean it has no effect on sports performance. Effects of deficiencies and supplementation for essential vitamins and trace minerals on non-performance or non-metabolic actions have relevance for sports nutrition. These conditions include:

- Mental fitness (subjective feelings of well-being, perception of fatigue, coordination, reaction times, decision making, neuromuscular control, neurological parameters)
- Immune system function (resistance to infections and overtraining)
- Prevention and healing of musculoskeletal injuries

The effects of mood, mental effort, sick time and downtime from injuries on physical performance can be indirect and include loss of training time resulting in poorer adaptation to exercise training. These issues are extremely difficult to study under controlled conditions, and may show

TABLE 1.3
Effects of Combinations of Essential Vitamin and Trace Mineral Antioxidant Combinations on Physical Performance

Author	Reference	Daily Dosage	Subjects & Duration	Performance parameters	Results
Kankaanpaa, et al., 1994	73	Beta carotene — 45 mg (75000 IU) Vitamin C — 600 mg Vitamin E — 300 mg Selenium — 150 mcg	20 total male recreational soccer players for 4 weeks	Three 30 sec maximal isokinetic knee flexion-extension tests	Peak torque, work, thigh surface EMG unaffected by supplementation
Grievink, et al., 1998	74	Beta carotene — 15 mg (25000 IU0 Vitamin C — 650 mg Vitamin E — 75 mg	26 total heavily exercising amateur cyclists (16–41 years) for 10 weeks	Lung function with ozone (Forced Vital Capacity, Forced Expiratory Volume in one second, Peak Expiratory Flow, Maximal Mid-expiratory Flow)	Acute effects of ozone on lung function after exercise reversed
Bryant, et al., 2003	75	Vitamin C — 1000 mg Vitamin E — 200 IU	7 total trained male cyclists (21–25 years) for 3 week periods	Cycle ergometry @ 70% VO$_2$ max for 60 min, then 30 min performance ride	Total work during performance ride not different between groups
Bloomer, et al., 2004	76	Vitamin C — 1000 mg Vitamin E — 268 mg (400 IU) Selenium — 90 mcg	18 total healthy, untrained women (19–31 years) for 18 days	Eccentric elbow flexion	Maximal isometric force not different between groups for 96 hours after exercise

large changes only after extended periods. Thus, studies on the effects of combinations of essential vitamins and trace minerals on mental, immune and injury variables are sparse.

A. Mental Performance

In keeping with the theme of this chapter to focus on exercising persons, the rather large background of information on mental effects of deficiencies or supplements of essential vitamins and trace minerals will not be reviewed; rather, the results from human studies listed in Tables 1.1 and 1.2 will be examined. Combinations of essential vitamins and trace minerals have led to improvements in neuromuscular performance in four studies,[37,44,48,49] and less fatigue in two studies.[52,54] Otherwise, there have been no systematic scientific appraisals of subjective feelings in studies on exercising athletes with combinations of essential vitamins and trace minerals. Given the availability of validated assessment tools for mental parameters (quality of life, mood, feelings of well-being questionnaires; reaction times, coordination, mental acuity tests, cognition), and given the large role for physical performance played by how each individual feels, and given the established literature on subjective effects of essential vitamins and trace minerals on these parameters in nonathletes, it is surprising that more investigations have not been performed. Indeed, the connection between mind and body and essential vitamin and trace mineral combinations may account for why roughly half of the U.S. population (and exercising individuals) regularly consumes such products.

B. Immunity

A consensus in the literature indicates that acute exhaustive exercise bouts (overexercise) or heavy chronic exercise (overtraining) are associated with immune function changes consistent with increased risk of upper respiratory tract infections.[77–92] While the exact mechanisms are under investigation, inadequate status of essential vitamins and trace minerals is one suspected culprit.[77–92]

Effects of supplementation with single essential vitamins and trace minerals has been the subject of recent reviews and elsewhere in this volume.[77–92] With regard to combinations of essential vitamins and trace minerals, relatively few studies in exercising persons are available. Table 1.4 lists some of these studies, six of which have found that various combinations of essential vitamins and trace minerals have reduced upper respiratory infection rates and improved specific functions of leukocytes.[52,93–97] The only common theme among these studies was the relatively high intakes of vitamin C and vitamin E, although some results were similar to either vitamin C or vitamin E supplementation alone. Obviously, the field of affecting immune function, infection rate, training status and eventually physical performance with combinations of essential vitamins and trace elements is virtually unstudied in athletes. Nevertheless, the results to date suggest potential for large, real-life impacts on ability to train or perform.

C. Injury and Recuperation

Again, little research has been applied to the role of essential micronutrient deficiencies or supplementation to prevention or recovery from musculoskeletal injuries in athletes.[98] If deficiencies of micronutrients exist, it is possible that healing or tissue repair can be delayed. An extensive review of the available literature has found that large doses of vitamin A, vitamin C or zinc salts may accelerate healing of skin wounds in healthy persons.[98] However, no prospective trials of supplementation with a complete and potent multiple vitamin-mineral formula on injured athletes can be found. Colgan found that his subjects reported 35% fewer injuries after long-term use of individualized combinations of essential vitamins and trace minerals.[52] Animal and human data suggest that provision of large doses of thiamin and pantothenate to healing tissues may accelerate connective tissue repair.[98] Since injuries reduce training time and prevent participation in events, any reduction in healing time and return to active training would greatly aid athletic endeavors.

TABLE 1.4
Effects of Combinations of Essential Vitamin and Trace Mineral Combinations on Immune Function in Exercising Persons

Author	Reference	Daily Dosage	Subjects and Duration	Results
Ismail, et al., 1983	93	Vitamin C — 500 mg Vitamin E — 400 mg	Fit and sedentary persons for 6 months	Lymphocytes responses improved more in fit persons than in sedentary persons
Colgan, 1986	52	See Table 1.2	8 total American marathon runners	81% fewer infections reported compared to unsupplemented periods
Peters et al., 1996	94	Beta-carotene — 18 mg (30000 IU) Vitamin C — 300 mg Vitamin E — 270 mg (400 IU)	total marathon runners, starting after run for 2 weeks	Upper respiratory infections reduced by half (from 40% to 20%) compared to placebo group (results similar to Vitamin C alone)
Petersen et al., 2001	95	Vitamin C — 500 mg Vitamin E — 400 mg	20 total male recreational runners for 21 days	Cytokine release, lymphocyte subpopulations after downhill treadmill running bout not different Plasma vitamin concentrations increased after supplementation
Tauler et al., 2002	96	Beta-carotene — 50000 IU Vitamin C — 1000 mg (last 15 d only) Vitamin E — 500 mg	20 well-trained sportsmen (23 ± 2 years) for 90 days	Increased neutrophil antioxidant enzyme activities Increased neutrophil superoxide dismutase protein concentration Prevented decrease in total & reduced glutathione levels, GSH/GSSG ratio in blood and neutrophils
Robson et al., 2003	97	Baseline supplementation with multiple vitamin-mineral product plus extra antioxidants: Beta-carotene — 18 mg (30000 IU) Vitamin C — 900 mg Vitamin E — 90 mg	12 total healthy endurance subjects (30 ± 6 years) for 7 weeks of baseline with 7 days of extra antioxidants	Neutrophil oxidative burst at rest higher from baseline supplementation Neutrophil oxidative burst after exercise higher after extra antioxidants RPE, HR not different Circulating leucocyte, neutrophil, lymphocyte counts and percentage of oxidizing neutrophils not different

V. SUMMARY AND CONCLUSIONS

The goal of this chapter was to identify essential vitamins and trace minerals, review studies of supplementation with combinations of vitamins and trace minerals, and point out some largely unexplored areas in sports nutrition that affect physical performance.

At this point, what is known about the most commonly used dietary supplement — multiple vitamin-mineral products — and their effects on physical performance? Consumers of multiple vitamin-mineral products want to know whether the pills they are popping keep them healthy and performing at peak efficiency. Consumers want to know if multiple vitamin-mineral products are a waste of money that creates expensive sewage, as many health care professionals claim. Consumers want to know whether these products are safe and contain the amounts of nutrients listed on the label. The following points are based on the evidence to date, along with a familiarity of research from non-exercise fields:

- Deficiencies of water-soluble vitamins, antioxidant vitamins, and key trace minerals (iron, zinc) can decrease physical performance.
- Exercising individuals most at risk are those who do not consume sufficient foods, who ingest mostly refined carbohydrates, who overtrain and who exercise in extreme manners or conditions.
- Multiple vitamin-mineral products with DV amounts of essential vitamins and trace minerals are not associated with improvement in performance and cannot be relied upon to prevent deficiencies of key micronutrients (antioxidants, iron) or favorably affect micronutrient status.
- Multiple vitamin-mineral products containing more than the DV of essential water-soluble vitamins, vitamin E and trace minerals may be associated with improved micro-nutrient status, maintaining physical performance or improving performance if nutrient deficiencies were pre-existing.
- Multiple vitamin-mineral products containing more than the DV of essential water-soluble vitamins, vitamin E and trace minerals do not appear to enhance physical performance for a majority of users.
- Indirect effects (mental effects, fewer illnesses, fewer injuries, better recovery) may account for perceived benefits to performance.
- Apparent exercise intensity or workload effects (i.e., more exercise means more need for supplementation larger than the DV).
- Apparent duration of supplementation effects (longer use brings more and/or larger results).
- More micronutrients (more complete formulas) are associated with better results than incomplete formulas.
- Toxicity from multiple vitamin-mineral products in exercising individuals appears to be extremely uncommon; however, care must be taken to limit intakes of vitamin A (retinols) and minerals, which have lower upper limits of safety than water-soluble vitamins.

In conclusion, the recommendation from a review article by investigators from Harvard Medical School published in the *Journal of the American Medical Association* that it appears prudent for all adults to take vitamin supplements[17] is also appropriate for adults who exercise regularly. The evidence also suggests that regular exercisers who do not perform optimally should consider a trial of increased intakes of antioxidant vitamins and B vitamins along with a multiple vitamin-mineral product with DV amounts of micronutrients (see amounts listed in Tables 1.2, 1.3 and 1.4) — the easiest, least expensive and most trustworthy way to assess utility of essential vitamins and trace minerals.

ACKNOWLEDGMENTS

The authors wish to thank Christina Beer, Jeff Feliciano, Janet Sorenson and Trudy Day for their excellent skills in obtaining, translating and discussing information used in this chapter.

REFERENCES

1. Bender, D.A., *Nutritional Biochemistry of the Vitamins*, 2nd ed., Cambridge University Press, Cambridge, U.K., 2003.
2. Combs, G.F., *The Vitamins. Fundamental Aspects in Nutrition and Health*, 2nd ed., Academic Press, San Diego, 1998.
3. Institute of Medicine, *Dietary Reference Intakes for Thiamin, Riboflavin, Niacin, Vitamin B_6, Folate, Vitamin B_{12}, Pantothenic Acid, Biotin, and Choline*, National Academy Press, Washington, D.C., 1998.
4. Rucker, R.B., Suttie, J.W., McCormick, D.B., and Machlin, L.J., Eds., *Handbook of Vitamins*. Third Edition, Revised and Expanded, Marcel Dekker, New York, 2001.
5. Bowman, B.A. and Russell, R.M., Eds., *Present Knowledge in Nutrition*, 8th ed., International Life Sciences Foundation, Washington, D.C., 2002.
6. Institute of Medicine, *Dietary Reference Intakes for Vitamin C, Vitamin E, Selenium, and Carotenoids*, National Academy Press, Washington, D.C., 2000.
7. Institute of Medicine, *Dietary Reference Intakes for Vitamin A, Vitamin K, Arsenic, Boron, Chromium, Copper, Iodine, Iron, Manganese, Molybdenum, Nickel, Silicon, Vanadium, and Zinc*, National Academy Press, Washington, D.C., 2001.
8. National Research Council, *Recommended Dietary Allowances*, 10th ed., National Academy Press, Washington, D.C., 1989.
9. Shils, M.E., Olson, J.A., Shike, M., Ross, A.C., Eds., *Modern Nutrition in Health and Disease*, 9th ed., Lea & Febiger, Philadelphia, 1999.
10. Kies, C.V. and Driskell, J.A., Eds., *Sports Nutrition. Minerals and Electrolytes*, CRC Press, Boca Raton, FL, 1995.
11. Bogden, J.D. and Klevay, L.M., Eds., *Clinical Nutrition of the Essential Trace Elements and Minerals. The Guide for Health Professionals*, Humana Press, Totowa, N.J., 2000.
12. O'Dell, B.L. and Sunde, R.A., Eds., *Handbook of Nutritionally Essential Mineral Elements*, Marcel Dekker, New York, NY, 1997.
13. American Dietetic Association, Position of the American Dietetic Association: Food fortification and dietary supplements, *J. Am. Diet. Assoc.*, 101, 115, 2001.
14. Department of Agriculture, Department of Health and Human Services, Nutrition and Your Health: Dietary Guidelines for Americans, 5th ed., Government Printing Office, Washington, D.C., 2000.
15. Willett, W.C. and Stampfer, M.J., What vitamins should I be taking, doctor? *N. Engl. J. Med.*, 345, 1819, 2001.
16. Fairfield, K.M. and Fletcher, R.H., Vitamins for chronic disease prevention in adults: Scientific review, *J. Am. Med. Assoc.*, 287, 3116, 2002.
17. Fletcher, R.H. and Fairfield, K.M., Vitamins for chronic disease prevention in adults: Clinical applications, *J. Am. Med. Assoc.*, 287, 3127, 2002.
18. Fogelholm, M., Vitamin and Mineral Status in Physically Active People. Dietary Intake and Blood Chemistry in Athletes and Young Adults, Social Insurance Institution, Turku, Finland, 1992.
19. Keys, A., Physical performance in relation to diet, *Fed. Proc.*, 2, 164, 1943.
20. Barborka, C.J., Foltz, E.E. and Ivy, A.C., Relationship between vitamin B-complex intake and work output in trained subjects, *J. Am. Med. Assoc.*, 122, 717, 1943.
21. Keys, A., Henschel, A., Taylor, H.L., Mickelsen, O. and Brozek, J., Experimental studies on man with a restricted intake of the B vitamins, *Am. J. Physiol.*, 144, 5, 1945.
22. Viteri, F.E. and Torun, B., Anemia and physiological work capacity, *Clin. Haematol.*, 3, 609, 1974.
23. Buzina, R., Grgić, Z., Jusic, M., Sapunar, J., Milanovic, N. and Brubacher, G., Nutritional status and physical working capacity, *Hum. Nutr. Clin. Nutr.*, 36C, 429, 1982.
24. Van der Beek, E.J., van Dokkum, W., Schrijver, J., Wesstra, J.A. and Hermus, R.J.J., Effect of marginal vitamin intake on physical performance of man, *Int. J. Sports Med.*, 5S, 28, 1984.

25. Van der Beek, E.J., van Dokkum, W., Schrijver, J., Wedel, M., Gaillard, A.W.K., Wesstra, A., van der Weerd, H. and Hermus, R.J.J., Thiamin, riboflavin, and vitamins B-6 and C: Impact of combined restricted intake on functional performance in man, *Am. J. Clin. Nutr.*, 48, 1451, 1988.

26. Clarkson, P.M., Exercise and the B vitamins, Ch. 7 in *Nutrition in Exercise and Sport*, 3rd ed., Wolinsky, I., Ed., CRC Press, Boca Raton, FL, 1998, 179.

27. Williams, M.H., Vitamin supplementation and athletic performance, *Int. J. Vit. Nutr. Res.*, S30, 163, 1989.

28. Haymes, E.M., Vitamin and mineral supplementation to athletes, *Int. J. Sport Nutr.*, 1, 146, 1991.

29. Clarkson, P.M., Minerals: exercise performance and supplementation in athletes, *J. Sports Sci.*, 9, 91, 1991.

30. Van der Beek, E.J., Vitamin supplementation and physical exercise performance, *J. Sports Sci.*, 9, 77, 1991.

31. Van der Beek, E.J., van Dokkum, W., Wedel, M., Schrijver, J. and van den Berg, A., Thiamin, riboflavin and vitamin B-6: Impact of restricted intake on physical performance in man, *J. Am. Coll. Nutr.*, 13, 629, 1994.

32. Haymes, E.M., Trace minerals and exercise, Ch. 8 in *Nutrition in Exercise and Sport*, 3rd ed., Wolinsky, I., Ed., CRC Press, Boca Raton, FL, 1998, 197.

33. Weaver, C.M. and Rajaram, S., Exercise and iron status, *J. Nutr.*, 122, 782, 1992.

34. American Dietetic Association, Position of the American Dietetic Association and the Canadian Dietetic Association: Nutrition for physical fitness and athletic performance for adults, *J. Am. Diet. Assoc.*, 93, 691, 1993.

35. Bucci, L.R., Nutritional ergogenic aids, Ch. 14 in *Nutrition in Exercise and Sport*, 2nd ed., Wolinsky, I. and Hickson, J.F., Eds., CRC Press, Boca Raton, 1994, FL, 330.

36. Keys, A. and Henschel, A.F., High vitamin supplementation (B_1, nicotinic acid and C) and the response to intensive exercise in U.S. Army infantryman, *Am. J. Physiol.*, 133, 350, 1941.

37. Simonson, E., Enzer, N., Baer, A. and Braun, R., The influence of vitamin B (complex) surplus on the capacity for muscular and mental work, *J. Indust. Hyg. Toxicol.*, 24, 83, 1942.

38. Foltz, E.E., Ivy, A.C. and Barborka, C.J., Influence of components of the vitamin B complex on recovery from fatigue, *J. Lab Clin. Med.*, 27, 1396, 1942.

39. Keys, A. and Henschel, A.F., Vitamin supplementation of U.S. Army rations in relation to fatigue and the ability to do muscular work, *J. Nutr.*, 23, 259, 1942.

40. Frankau, I.M., Acceleration of coordinated muscular effort by nicotinamide, *Br. Med. J.*, 13, 601, 1943.

41. Henschel, A., Taylor, H.L., Mickelsen, O., Brozek, J.M. and Keys, A., The effect of high vitamin C and B vitamin intakes on the ability of man to work in hot environments, *Fed. Proc.*, 3, 18, 1944.

42. Early, R.G. and Carlson, R.B., Water-soluble vitamin therapy in the delay of fatigue from physical activity in hot climatic conditions, *Int. Z. Angew. Physiol.*, 27, 43, 1969.

43. Read, M.H. and McGuffin, S.L., The effect of B-complex supplementation on endurance performance, *J. Sports Med.*, 23, 178, 1983.

44. Boncke, D. and Nickel, B., Improvement of fine motoric movement control by elevated dosages of vitamin B_1, B_6, and B_{12} in target shooting, *Int. J. Vit. Nutr. Res.*, 30S, 198, 1989.

45. McCollum, R.H., Effect of lysine and a vitamin compound upon the physical performance of subpar college men, Ed.D. thesis, University of Oregon, Corvallis, OR, 1960.

46. Nelson, D.O., Effect of food supplements on the performance of selected gross motor tests, *Res. Q.*, 31, 315, 1960.

47. Keul, J., Haralambie, G., Winker, K.H., Baumgartner, A. and Bauer, G., Die Wirkung eines Multivitamin-Elektrolytgranulats auf Kreislauf und Stoffwechsel bei langwährender Körperarbeit, *Schweiz. Z. Sportmed.*, 22, 169, 1974.

48. Haralambie, G., Keul, J., Baumgartner, A., Winker, K.H. and Bauer, G., Die Wirkung eines Multivitamin-Elektrolytpräparates auf Elektrodermalreflex une neuromuskuläre Erregbarkeit bei langwährender Körperarbeit, *Schweiz. Z. Sportmed.*, 23, 113, 1975.

49. Van Dam, B., Vitamins and sport, *Br. J. Sports Med.*, 12, 74, 1978.

50. Keul, J., Huber, G., Schmitt, M., Spielberger, B. and Zöllner, G., Die Veränderungen von Krieslauf-und Stoffwechselgrössen während eines Skilanglaufes unter einem Multivitamin-Elektrolyt-Granulat, *Dtsch. Z. Sportsmed.*, 30, 65, 1979.

51. Barnett, D.W. and Conlee, R.K., The effects of a commercial dietary supplement on human performance, *Am. J. Clin. Nutr.*, 40, 586, 1984.

52. Colgan, M., Effects of multinutrient supplementation on athletic performance, Ch. 3 in *Sport, Health, and Nutrition*, Katch, F.I., Ed., Human Kinetics Publishers, Champaign, 1986.

53. Weight, L.M., Noakes, T.D., Labadarios, D., Graves, J., Jacobs, P. and Berman, P.A., Vitamin and mineral status of trained athletes including the effects of supplementation, *Am. J. Clin. Nutr.*, 47, 186, 1988.

54. Dragan, G.I., Ploesteanu, E. and Selejan, V., Studies concerning the ergogenic value of Cantamega-2000 supply in top junior cyclists, *Rev. Rhoum. Physiol.*, 28, 13, 1991.

55. Colgan, M., Micronutrient status of endurance athletes affects hematology and performance, *J. Appl. Nutr.*, 43, 16, 1991.

56. Singh, A., Moses, F.M. and Deuster, P.A., Chronic multivitamin-mineral supplementation does not enhance physical performance, *Med. Sci. Sports Exer.*, 24, 726, 1992.

57. Telford, R.D., Catchpole, E.A., Deakin, V., Hahn, A.G. and Plank, A.W., The effect of 7 to 8 month vitamin-mineral supplementation on athletic performance, *Int. J. Sport Nutr.*, 2, 135, 1992.

58. Savino, F., Bonfante, G. and Madon, E., Impiego di integratori vitaminici naturali in bambini durante periodi di convalescenzae in bambini che praticano attivita sportive, *Minerva Pediatr.*, 51, 1, 1999.

59. Roberts, J.D., Buchanan, A.R., Jones, N. and Smales, T., Aerobic adaptations following supplementation of a multinutrient (Lifepak®), *Can. J. Appl. Physiol.*, 26, S264, 2001.

60. Cavas, L. and Tarhan, L., Effects of vitamin-mineral supplementation on cardiac marker and radical scavenging enzymes, and MDA levels in young swimmers, *Int. J. Sport Nutr. Exer. Metab.*, 14, 133, 2004.

61. Kleijnen, J. and Knipschild, P., Ginkgo biloba for cerebral insufficiency, *Br. J. Clin. Pharmacol.*, 34, 352, 1992.

62. Singh, A., Moses, F.M. and Deuster, P.A., Vitamin and mineral status in physically active men: effects of a high-potency supplement, *Am. J. Clin. Nutr.*, 55, 1, 1992.

63. Telford, R.D., Catchpole, E.A., Deakin, V., McLeay, A.C. and Plank, A.W., The effect of 7 to 8 months of vitamin-mineral supplementation on the vitamin and mineral status of athletes, *Int. J. Sport Nutr.*, 2, 123, 1992.

64. Buzina, R. and Suboticanec, K., Significance of vitamins in child health, *Int. J. Vit. Nutr. Res.*, 26 (Suppl.), 9, 1984.

65. Powers, H.J., Bates, C.J., Lamb, W.H., Singh, J., Gelman, W. and Webb, E., Effects of a multivitamin and iron supplement on running performance in Gambian children, *Hum. Nutr. Clin. Nutr.*, 39, 427, 1985.

66. Bates, C.J., Powers, H.J. and Thurnham, D.I., Vitamins, iron, and physical work, *Lancet*, 2, 313, 1989.

67. Guilland, J.C., Penaranda, T., Gallet, C., Boggio, V., Fuchs, F. and Klepping, J., Vitamin status of young athletes including the effects of supplementation, *Med. Sci. Sports Exer.*, 21, 441, 1989.

68. Fogelholm, M., Ruokonen, I., Laakso, J.T., Vuorimaa, T. and Himberg, J.J., Lack of association between indices of vitamin B1, B2, and B6 status and exercise-induced blood lactate in young adults, *Int. J. Sport Nutr.*, 3, 165, 1993.

69. Fogelholm, M., Indicators of vitamin and mineral status in athletes' blood: a review, *Int. J. Sport Nutr.*, 5, 267, 1995.

70. Hofman, Z., Ronsen, O., Sjodin, A. and Laakso, J., Micro-nutrient supplementation in the Olympic cross country ski team (ONCCST), *Med. Sci. Sports Exer.*, 31(Suppl 5), S162, 1999, abstract #701.

71. Bucci, L.R., Turpin, A.A., Beer, C. and Feliciano, J., Ginseng, Ch. 20 in *Nutritional Ergogenic Aids*, Wolinsky, I. and Driskell, J.A., Eds., CRC Press, Boca Raton, FL, 2004, 379.

72. Ushakov, A.S., Myasnikov, V.I., Shestkov, B.P., Agureev, A.N., Belakovsky, M.S. and Rumyantseva, M.P., Effect of vitamin and amino acid supplements on human performance during heavy mental and physical work, *Aviat. Space Environ. Med.*, 49, 1184, 1978.

73. Kankaanpaa, M.J., Marin, E., Ristonmaa, U., Airaksinen, O., Hänninen, O. and Bray, T.M., Effect of vitamin C, vitamin E, β-carotene and selenium supplementation on exercise performance in humans, *Med. Sci. Sports Exer.*, 26, S67, 1994. (abstract #375)

74. Grievink, L., Jansen, S.M., van't Veer, P. and Brunekreef, B., Acute effects of ozone on pulmonary function of cyclists receiving antioxidant supplements, *Occup. Environ. Med.*, 55, 13, 1998.

75. Bryant, R.J., Ryder, J., Martino, P., Kim, J. and Craig, B.W., Effects of vitamin E and C supplementation either alone or in combination on exercise-induced lipid peroxidation in trained cyclists, *J. Strength Cond. Res.*, 17, 792, 2003.

76. Bloomer, R.J., Goldfarb, A.H., McKenzie, M.J., You, T. and Nguyen, L. Effects of antioxidant therapy in women exposed to eccentric exercise, *Int. J. Sport Nutr. Exerc. Metab.*, 14, 377, 2004.

77. Peters, E.M., Exercise, immunology and upper respiratory tract infections, *Int. J. Sports Med.*, 18, S69, 1997.

78. Nieman, D.C., Exercise and resistance to infection, *Can. J. Physiol. Pharmacol.*, 76, 573, 1998.

79. Shephard, R.J. and Shek, P.N., Immunological hazards from nutritional imbalances in athletes, *Exerc. Immunol. Rev.*, 4, 22, 1998.

80. Nieman, D.C. and Pedersen, B.K., Exercise and immune function. Recent developments, *Sports Med.*, 27, 73, 1999.

81. Pedersen, B.K., Bruunsgaard, H., Jensen, M., Krzywkowski, K. and Ostrowski, K., Exercise and immune function: effect of ageing and nutrition, *Proc. Nutr. Soc.*, 58, 733, 1999.

82. Bishop, N.C., Blannin, A.K., Walsh, N.P., Robson, P.J. and Gleeson, M., Nutritional aspects of immunosuppression in athletes, *Sports Med.*, 28, 151, 1999.

83. Gleeson, M. and Bishop, N.C., Elite athlete immunology: importance of nutrition, *Int. J. Sports Med.*, 21, S44, 2000.

84. Mackinnon, L.T., Chronic exercise training effects on immune function, *Med. Sci. Sports Exer.*, 32, S369, 2000.

85. Nieman, D.C., Is infection linked to exercise workload? *Med. Sci. Sports Exer.*, 32, S406, 2000.

86. Gleeson, M., The scientific basis of practical strategies to maintain immunocompetence in elite athletes, *Exerc. Immunol. Rev.*, 6, 75, 2000.

87. Peters, E.M., Vitamins, immunity, and infection risk in athletes, Ch. 6 in *Nutrition and Exercise Immunology*, Nieman, D.C. and Pedersen, B.K., Eds., CRC Press, Boca Raton, FL, 2000, 109.

88. Pedersen, B.K. and Nieman, D.C., Exercise, immune function, and nutrition: summary and future perspectives, Ch. 9 in *Nutrition and Exercise Immunology*, Nieman, D.C. and Pedersen, B.K., Eds., CRC Press, Boca Raton, FL, 2000, 175.

89. Gleeson, M., Lancaster, G.I. and Bishop, N.C., Nutritional strategies to minimise exercise-induced immunosuppression in athletes, *Can. J. Appl. Physiol.*, 26, S23, 2001.

90. Nieman, D.C., Exercise immunology: nutritional countermeasures, *Can. J. Appl. Physiol.*, 26, S45, 2001.

91. Venkatraman, J.T. and Pendergast, D.R., Effect of dietary intake on immune function in athletes, *Sports Med.*, 32, 323, 2002.

92. Nieman, D.C., Current perspective on exercise immunology, *Curr. Sports Med. Rep.*, 2, 239, 2003.

93. Ismail, A.H., Petro, T.M. and Watson, R.R., Dietary supplementation with vitamin E and C in fit and nonfit adults: Biochemical and immunological changes, *Fed. Proc.*, 42, 335, 1983.

94. Peters, E.M., Goetzsche, J.M., Joseph, L.E. and Noakes, T.D., Vitamin C as effective as combination of anti-oxidant nutrients in reducing symptoms of URTI in ultramarathon runners, *S. Afr. J. Sports Med.*, 4, 16, 1996.

95. Petersen, E.W., Ostrowski, K., Ibfelt, T., Richelle, M., Offord, E., Halkjaer-Kristensen, J. and Pedersen, B.K., Effect of vitamin supplementation on cytokine response and on muscle damage after strenuous exercise, *Am. J. Physiol.*, 280, C1570, 2001.

96. Tauler, P., Aguilo, A., Fuentespina, E., Tur, J.A. and Pons, A., Diet supplementation with vitamin E, vitamin C and beta-carotene cocktail enhances basal neutrophil antioxidant enzymes in athletes, *Pflugers Arch.*, 443, 791, 2002.

97. Robson, P.J., Bouic, P.J. and Myburgh, K.H., Antioxidant supplementation enhances neutrophil oxidative burst in trained runners following prolonged exercise, *Int. J. Sport Nutr. Exerc. Metab.*, 13, 369, 2003.

98. Bucci, L.R., *Nutrition Applied to Injury Rehabilitation and Sports Medicine*, CRC Press, Boca Raton, FL, 1994.

Section Two

Vitamins

2 Ascorbic Acid

Robert E. Keith

CONTENTS

I. INTRODUCTION

The relationship between ascorbic acid and exercise has been studied for a number of years, with several review articles having been written covering this topic.[1-5] This chapter will further address the knowledge base concerning vitamin C and exercise. Such topics as the basic functions and deficiency symptoms of ascorbic acid as related to exercise will be covered. In addition, articles related to exercise and vitamin C requirements; immune function; cortisol secretion and stress; muscle soreness; supplementation and sports performance and intakes/needs of physically active persons for the vitamin will be reviewed.

A. HISTORY

While the existence of vitamin C has been known for only a relatively short time, the fact that a vitamin C deficiency could adversely affect physical performance has been documented for centuries.[1,4] There are reports from the British Navy of the late 1700s concerning sailors with scurvy (vitamin C deficiency).[4] These reports describe sailors who had good appetites and were cheerful, yet collapsed and died on deck upon the initiation of physical activity. During the Crimean War (1854–6) and the American Civil War, scurvy was reported among the soldiers. Those having scurvy were reported to have shortness of breath upon exertion and greatly reduced energy and powers of endurance.[4] These are just a couple of examples of how ascorbic acid deficiency has adversely affected the physical ability of sailors and soldiers in the last several centuries, and other stories of scurvy's effects on physical performance exist.[4] Thus, while the study of vitamin C and physical performance is a relatively new area, the fact that scurvy has caused decreases in physical performance has existed for centuries.

B. GENERAL PROPERTIES AND STRUCTURE

Vitamin C is a water-soluble vitamin for humans, primates and guinea pigs. Most other animal species can make ascorbic acid from the sugar glucose, but humans lack an enzyme necessary to convert glucose to ascorbic acid. Vitamin C exists in humans in two biologically active forms, ascorbic acid and dehydroascorbic acid. It is the ability to interconvert between these two forms that gives vitamin C antioxidant capabilities.[6-10]

Dietary intakes of vitamin C are absorbed in the upper small intestines by active transport mechanisms at physiological intakes (50–200 mg/day). Large intakes (gram doses) of the vitamin may be absorbed by passive diffusion. Most (80–90%) of a physiological dose will be absorbed. However, this absorbance value may drop to 10–20% for megadoses. Vitamin C is found in high concentrations in the adrenal glands, pituitary gland, white blood cells, the lens of the eye and brain tissue.[6-10]

C. FUNCTIONS

Ascorbic acid has several important functions as related to physical activity. The vitamin has long been known to be necessary for normal collagen synthesis. Collagen, one of the most abundant proteins in the body, is a vital component of cartilage, ligaments, tendons and other connective tissue. Vitamin C is needed for the formation of the vitamin-like compound carnitine, which is necessary for the transport of long-chain fatty acids into the mitochondria. The fatty acids can then be used as an energy source. The neurotransmitters, norepinephrine and epinephrine also require vitamin C for their synthesis. Ascorbic acid seems to be needed for the proper transport of nonheme iron, the reduction of folic acid intermediates and for the proper metabolism of the stress hormone cortisol. Finally, vitamin C acts as a powerful water-soluble antioxidant. The vitamin seems to exert antioxidant functions in plasma and probably interfaces at the lipid membrane level with vitamin E to regenerate vitamin E from the vitamin E radical. Table 2.1 describes some of these functions in more detail.[6-10]

Through these various functions vitamin C can interface with physical activity at several levels. For example, poor development of connective tissue could result in increased numbers of ligament and tendon injuries and poor healing of these injuries. Inadequate production of carnitine would decrease a person's ability to utilize fatty acids as an energy source. This would force increased use on glycogen stores, exhausting these stores earlier during exercise and causing fatigue and decreased performance. With decreased production of norepinephrine and epinephrine, an athlete might not be able to properly stimulate the neural and metabolic systems necessary for optimal performance. Poor iron and folate metabolism would result in anemia's impairing the transport of oxygen to tissues. This would be a

---

TABLE 2.1
Selected Functions of Vitamin C That Would Affect Physical Performance

Chemical Reaction Requiring Vitamin C	Body Function
1) lysine → hydroxylysine proline → hydroxyproline	Needed for normal collagen (cartilage, connective tissue, ligaments, tendons)
2) lysine → carnitine (liver, kidney)	Necessary for normal fat oxidation in muscle cell mitochondria
3) phenylalanine → dopamine, norepinephrine, epinephrine	Needed for normal neurotransmitter formation
4) ascorbic acid ↔ dehydroascorbic acid	normal antioxidant function

TABLE 2.2
Vitamin C Deficiency Symptoms and Physical Performance

Deficiency Symptom	Effect on Performance
Poor connective tissue development, poor injury healing, swelling, bleeding in joints	Strains, sprains may increase, heal poorly. Poor range of motion
Subcutaneous hemorrhages, increased bruising	Hemorrhages due to contact would be worse, more extensive
Anemia	Decreased aerobic performance
Fatigue	Decreased aerobic and anaerobic performance due to decreased fatty acid use and neurotransmitter function
Muscular weakness, pain	Decreased force production, decreased performance due to pain when moving
Anorexia	Decreased performance due to low energy intake

definite hindrance to optimal performance in aerobic endeavors. Through its various functions, vitamin C has ample opportunity to interface with physical performance at several metabolic sites.

D. DEFICIENCY AND PHYSICAL PERFORMANCE

It should be apparent from the previous section that a vitamin C deficiency (scurvy) would cause a decrease in physical performance. This point is not controversial. Table 2.2 lists the major symptoms of vitamin C deficiency and how each symptom could decrease a certain aspect of physical activity.

Marginal status for ascorbic acid probably also exerts some detrimental effects on performance. For example, Lemmel[11] studied 110 children receiving a diet low in ascorbic acid. The addition of 100 mg daily of ascorbic acid over a 4-month period improved the work capacity and liveliness of 48% of the children as compared with 12% in a control group. Babadzanjan et al.[12] studied 40 train engine drivers and crew. These individuals initially had low vitamin C status. The administration of 200 mg of vitamin C per day normalized blood concentrations and reduced fatigue in these subjects. Buzina and Suboticanec[13] reported that VO_2max values were improved in young adolescents having low plasma concentrations of vitamin C when these adolescents were supplemented with vitamin C. The improvement in the VO_2max stopped when plasma C concentrations were normalized. Van der Beek et al.[14,15] produced marginal vitamin C status in subjects by feeding them 32.5–50% of the Dutch RDA for vitamin C for 3 to 8 weeks. In one study[15], an increased heart rate was seen at the "onset of blood lactate" level during the time of reduced vitamin C intake. In addition, reduced vitamin C status may have been partly responsible for a significant reduction in aerobic power seen in the other study.[14] More recently, Johnston et al.[16] studied the effects of vitamin C supplementation on nine vitamin C-depleted male and female subjects who were apparently healthy and unaware of their low serum vitamin C concentrations. The subjects were given 500 mg of vitamin C a day for 2 weeks. Compared with pre-supplementation values, work performed by the subjects on a graded walking protocol and gross work efficiency increased significantly by 10 and 15%, respectively.

E. RECOMMENDED INTAKES AND FOOD SOURCES

The current adult Dietary Reference Intake/Recommended Dietary Allowance (RDA) for vitamin C is 75 mg/day for women and 90 mg/day for men.[10] This level of intake is known to maintain adequate tissue levels of the vitamin and prevent signs of scurvy in most individuals. However, these guidelines were developed for light to moderately active people, not specifically for athletes or persons engaged in strenuous or prolonged physical activity.

TABLE 2.3
Vitamin C Content (mg) of Selected Fruits and Vegetables

Fruits	Vitamin C	Vegetables	Vitamin C
Kiwi (1)	74	Kale (1/2 C)	27
Strawberries (1/2 C)*	42	Bell Pepper (1)	95
Oranges (1)	70	Turnip Greens (1/2 C)	20
Orange juice (1/2 C)	62	Brussels sprouts (1/2 C)	36
Tangerine (1 fruit)	26	Sweet potato (1)	28
Pineapple (3 slices)	12	Broccoli (1/2 C)	37
Cantaloupe (1/2 C)	113	Spinach (1/2 C)	16
Grapefruit (1/2 C)	41	Cauliflower (1/2 C)	35
Mango (1)	57	Cabbage (1/2 C)	18
Papaya (1/2 C)	46	Potato (1 med)	26
Watermelon (1 slice)	46	Okra (8 pods)	14
		Tomatoes (1 med)	22

*C = cup(s); 1C=240ml

Various forms of physiological stress are known to increase the need for vitamin C. These include infections,[6] cigarette smoking,[17,18] extreme environmental temperature[19,20] and altitude,[20] among others. Strenuous or prolonged exercise is a form of physiological stress[21] and could possibly increase requirements and, thus, recommended intakes of the vitamin in physically active individuals. This point will be further explored later in this chapter. However, to date, no official recommendations for vitamin C intake for physically active individuals have been made.

Vitamin C is found naturally, and almost exclusively, in fruits and vegetables. Some vitamin C can be found in milk and liver, but these values are minimal.[8] In addition to natural sources of the vitamin, many foods such as breakfast cereals, some sports drinks and various nutrition bars, for example, are now fortified with the vitamin. Thus, it is more likely today than ever before that significant vitamin C intake could be obtained from foods other than fruits and vegetables. Nonetheless, vitamin C can be different in terms of intake as compared with many other vitamins, particularly the B complex vitamins. B complex vitamin intake tends to correlate well with total energy intake of an athlete. Thus, if athletes are consuming sufficient energy, it is reasonably likely that their dietary intake for B complex vitamins such as thiamin and niacin is also sufficient. However, because ascorbic acid is found principally in some fruits and vegetables, the possibility exists that athletes could have an otherwise adequate diet but one that is low in vitamin C. This would occur if the athletes did not consume sufficient servings of fruits and vegetables or other vitamin C fortified foods. The vitamin C content of selected fruits and vegetables can be found in Table 2.3.

II.   EXERCISE AND ASCORBIC ACID REQUIREMENTS

One question that researchers have asked is, "What effects does the stress of physical activity have on the requirements for vitamin C?" A possible answer to this question can be evaluated by looking at direct changes in tissue concentrations of blood/plasma, white blood cells and urine. Indirect answers to this question can be obtained by looking in areas such as heat acclimation, muscle soreness or damage, respiratory infection rates and the levels of the stress hormone, cortisol.

A.   DIRECT EFFECTS: BODY TISSUES, BLOOD/PLASMA, WHITE BLOOD CELLS, URINE

Several animal studies[22-27] have been performed that addressed the exercise/vitamin C requirement question. These studies are in general agreement that exercise reduces the vitamin C content of various tissues such as the adrenal glands, spleen, liver and brain. This would seem to indicate that exercise increased the need for vitamin C in these animals.

Studies evaluating the effect of exercise on ascorbic acid needs in humans are greater in number and more diverse in their approach as compared with animal studies. Human studies have addressed the relationship between exercise and vitamin C for blood/plasma and leukocyte concentrations of the vitamin, excretion in the urine, immune function, hormonal status, muscle soreness or damage and heat stress adaptation.

Several papers have evaluated blood/plasma vitamin C changes with exercise or in athletes at rest. Namyslowski and Desperak-Secomska[28] found decreased blood vitamin C levels in a group of physical culture students. Although the diets of the students might not have been adequate in vitamin C, the authors concluded that strenuous exercise had caused an additional decrease in these blood concentrations. Namyslowski[29] followed the first research project with a second study. This study found that blood vitamin C levels decreased in athletes ingesting 100 mg of vitamin C/day. Dietary intakes of 300 mg/day were required to maintain or increase blood concentrations of ascorbic acid in the athletes. Recently, Schroder et al.[30] reported that the plasma vitamin C concentrations of a group of professional basketball players decreased significantly over a 32-day competitive season, with the final plasma value (15.4 µmol/L) falling below the minimum acceptable concentration.

However, several other studies[31–39] have reported normal mean vitamin C concentrations in the plasma of athletes and physically active individuals; although at least one study[37] reported 12% of its subjects with low plasma vitamin C concentrations, while another[33] had mean ascorbic acid concentrations for its subjects at the low end of normal range. Plasma vitamin C concentrations above 23 µmol/L are often considered adequate.[5,40] Mean plasma vitamin C concentrations in active, mostly male subjects have been reported to range from a low of 35 to a high of 86 µmol/L. One study with female ballet dancers reported a plasma vitamin C concentration of 46 µmol/L.[34] Thus, for the most part, resting plasma concentrations in physically active individuals appear to be normal. However, some care must be taken in interpreting these values as compared with a sedentary population. Several papers have reported that recent physical activity can increase plasma vitamin C concentrations for up to 24 hours.[31–33,41] Thus, plasma values for vitamin C in some of the reported studies could possibly be falsely elevated if they were obtained within 24 hours of strenuous exercise. This could be a mitigating factor in evaluating plasma vitamin C in athletes. Furthermore, plasma vitamin C values have been recorded mostly in runners. Data are not available for plasma vitamin C concentrations in other groups such as weightlifters, swimmers and cyclists. Plasma vitamin C values in various athletic groups can be seen in Table 2.4.

TABLE 2.4
Resting or Baseline Plasma Ascorbic Acid Concentrations (µmol/L) in Various Athletic Groups

Athletic group	No. of Subjects	Ascorbic Acid Value	Reference
Various athletes	50 M, 36 F	56	37
Runners	4 M	79	31
Runners	7 M	35	33
Runners	9 M	53	32
Runners	30 M	58	35
Various athletes	55 M	74	36
Ballet dancers	10 M, 12 F	59 M, 46 F	34
Trained runners	6 M, 6 F	72	38
Ultramarathoners	15 M	83	39

Normal plasma ascorbic acid concentration range = 23–114.0 µmol/L[5,40]

Several studies[42–45] have examined the relationship between white blood cell/leukocyte ascorbic acid concentrations and exercise. One study evaluated changes in white blood cell ascorbic acid concentrations in 31 professional soccer players before and after a strenuous 2-hour training session.[42] The white blood cell ascorbic acid content decreased following the training session. The authors likened this fall with the fall in white blood cell vitamin C seen following other stressful events such as myocardial infarction and the common cold. Ferrandez et al.[43] reported on the leukocyte ascorbic acid concentrations in a group of Olympic cyclists in the third year of their 4-year training program. These authors reported that lymphocyte and neutrophil vitamin C concentrations declined significantly over the length of the study. In addition, the authors further reported that lymphocyte and neutrophil ascorbic acid levels declined from a pre-Olympic to a post-Olympic games test. However, two other studies[44,45] do not support an increased vitamin C requirement in athletes based on leukocyte evidence. Robertson et al.[44] reported on the lymphocyte ascorbic acid concentrations in a group of six highly trained runners compared with an equal number of sedentary control subjects. The runners had significantly greater lymphocyte ascorbic acid levels. Krause et al.[45] measured neutrophil function in two groups of biathletes following a strenuous competition. One group received vitamin C at 2 grams per day for a week while the other group received a placebo. Neutrophil function decreased following the competition in both groups with no significant differences between the groups.

Two studies have reported decreased urinary excretion of vitamin C with increased physical activity.[29,46] Bacinskij[46] studied 30 young sedentary male medical students and 33 physical-culture students who participated in various forms of exercise on a daily basis. The physical-culture students excreted only about 50% of the vitamin C excreted by the medical students. The author concluded that persons engaged in physical activity need extra vitamin C. Namyslowski[29] also reported decreased urine vitamin C in a group of skiers. The author suggested that the skiers needed 200–250 mg of vitamin C each day. However, two other studies[31,47] reported no significant differences in urine excretion of vitamin C between runners and male athletes and their sedentary controls.

B. INDIRECT EFFECTS: HEAT ACCLIMATION, MUSCLE SORENESS/DAMAGE, RESPIRATORY INFECTIONS, CORTISOL

Several papers have examined the relationships among exercise, vitamin C needs and adaptation to heat stress in humans.[48–52] An early study[48] found no effect of 500 mg of vitamin C on rectal temperature, sweat rate, recovery heart rate or strength in subjects working in a hot environment. However, studies since then have found some improvement in the ability of humans to exercise in a hot environment when they were given additional vitamin C.[49–52]

Strydom et al.[51] studied the effects of vitamin C ingestion (250 or 500 mg/day for 21 days vs. placebo) in a group of 60 mining recruits undergoing climatic room acclimatization. Subjects were not exposed to heat for at least 6 months prior to the study. Exercise consisted of a 4-hour step test in a comfortable environment (20–22°C) versus repeated testing in a hot environment (32.2°C wet bulb and 33.9°C dry bulb). Results indicated no differences among groups for heart rate or total sweat rate. However, rectal temperatures were significantly lower in the groups receiving vitamin C. The authors concluded that the rate and degree of heat acclimatization was enhanced by vitamin C supplementation.

Kotze et al.[52] also investigated heat acclimation in 13 male volunteers. Subjects exercised 4 hours each day for 10 days in a manner and under conditions previously described by Strydom et al.[51] Volunteers were placed into diet groups receiving 250 or 500 mg vitamin C daily or a placebo. Groups receiving vitamin C had a reduction in total sweat output and rectal temperature. The authors concluded that vitamin C may be effective in reducing heat strain in unacclimatized persons.

Four papers[53–56] outlined below have reported on vitamin C and muscle soreness or damage. Two of the papers[53,54] reported that vitamin C had no effects on muscle soreness. However, two other studies[55,56] did find that vitamin C supplementation above RDA levels improved muscle soreness or damage markers.

An early study by Staton[53] showed no differences in delayed muscle soreness as measured after a sit-up test between subjects receiving 100 mg of vitamin C and those receiving a placebo. Thompson et al.[54] gave 1,000 mg of ascorbic acid 2 hours prior to exercise to nine active males. These same subjects also received a placebo treatment on another trial. Subjects underwent a 90-minute shuttle running test that mimicked multiple sprints. Measurements were taken for muscle damage (creatine kinase) and lipid peroxidation (malondialdehyde) as well as muscle soreness. No differences were noted between treatment and placebo trials. The authors concluded that acute supplementation of vitamin C had no beneficial effects on muscle soreness. However, the authors stated that short-term ascorbic acid supplementation might have been ineffective because the timing of the supplement was incorrect. However, in a study by Jakeman and Maxwell[55] post-exercise maximal voluntary isometric contraction of an eccentrically exercised leg was determined over a 7-day period of time. In general, retention of force production was better in a group of subjects receiving 400 mg of vitamin C a day for 21 days prior to exercise as compared with a group receiving vitamin E. The authors concluded that vitamin C may offer some protection from eccentric exercise-induced muscle damage.

In a second study, Thompson et al.[56] measured muscle soreness and muscle function in 16 (eight vitamin C, eight placebo) regularly training male subjects. The vitamin C group received 400 mg of the vitamin a day for 2 weeks prior to testing. Subjects undertook a 90-minute strenuous intermittent shuttle run. Muscle soreness was assessed using a 10-point scale and muscle function was assessed on the flexors and extensors of both legs using an isokinetic dynamometer. Vitamin C had beneficial effects on muscle soreness and muscle function. In addition, plasma malondialdehyde and interleukin-6 concentrations were lower at certain post-exercise time periods in the vitamin C group.

Research has previously documented that strenuous or prolonged exercise can compromise the immune system.[38,57] This compromised immune system may then allow for an increased incidence of infections, particularly upper respiratory tract infections (URTI), in athletes. Several studies[58–61] have investigated the relationship between ascorbic acid and URTI.

Peters et al.[58] evaluated the effects of a vitamin C supplement (600 mg/day for 21 days or a placebo) on the incidence of URTI in a group of ultramarathoners following a race. Runners were monitored for 14 days following the race. A total of 68% of the runners in the placebo group had symptoms of URTI following the race. Only 33% of the vitamin C-supplemented subjects had symptoms. This difference was significant. Peters et al.[59] followed up their initial research with another study involving ultramarathoners, vitamin C and URTI. Results were similar to the first study. Runners received either 500 mg of vitamin C a day or a placebo for 21 days prior to a 90-kilometer race. URTI was monitored for 14 days post-race. URTI occurred in 16% of the vitamin C runners and 40% of the placebo runners. Again, this difference was significant. Peters et al.[58] concluded that vitamin C supplementation may enhance resistance to post-race URTI. Other studies[60] have looked at vitamin C supplementation and URTI in school children undergoing training at a ski camp and military troops undergoing strenuous training. Vitamin C was given at levels of 600–1000 mg/day and placebo groups were included. Vitamin C supplementation reduced URTI symptoms in these studies approximately 50%. In contrast to the four previous studies, Himmelstein et al.[61] did not find a significant difference in URTI between vitamin C-treated and placebo marathon runners. In this study,[61] 44 marathon runners were given either 1,000 mg of vitamin C a day or a placebo for 2 months prior to their marathon. They were then followed for 1 month post-marathon. URTI incidence in the vitamin C runners was 33% and for the placebo runners 43%.

The secretion of the hormone cortisol also has been studied in relation to exercise and vitamin C. Cortisol is released from the adrenal gland in response to physiological and psychological stress.[5,62] Cortisol is generally thought of as a catabolic hormone, resulting in, among other functions, a loss of lean body mass. Increased secretion of cortisol may indicate a higher level of stress on the organism. Ascorbic acid is required for the synthesis of cortisol and may have a dampening effect on plasma cortisol concentrations in response to stress. This could indicate a lower level of stress in relation to the stressor. Peake[5] has reviewed the relationships between ascorbic acid and cortisol metabolism.

Five recent studies[38,57–59,63] have attempted to elucidate the relationship among cortisol, exercise and ascorbic acid. Nieman et al.[57] gave 12 experienced marathon runners either a vitamin C supplement (1000 mg/day for 8 days) or a placebo. Subjects then ran on a treadmill at 75–80% VO_2max for 2.5 hours. Five blood samples were taken before and up to 6 hours following exercise. These investigators found no significant differences in plasma cortisol concentrations between the vitamin C and placebo groups. However, mean cortisol concentrations were lower at four of the five time points in the vitamin C group. Robson et al.[38] gave 900 mg of vitamin C a day or a placebo for 7 days to 12 endurance athletes. There were no between-group differences in post-exercise plasma cortisol concentrations following a 2-hour treadmill run at 65% VO_2max. In contrast to the findings by Robson et al.[38] and Nieman et al.,[57] three other studies[58,59,63] have reported decreases in plasma cortisol concentrations following exercise in vitamin C-supplemented groups. Nieman et al.,[63] in a second study, reported that supplemental vitamin C reduced post-race cortisol concentrations in a group of ultramarathoners. In addition, Peters et al.[58,59] reported that supplemental vitamin C (1000–1500 mg/day) for 7 days prior to racing, on race day, and 2 days following competition significantly reduced post-race plasma cortisol concentrations compared with placebo subjects in two groups of 15–16 ultramarathoners. However, while cortisol was reduced, plasma markers of tissue inflammation were significantly elevated.

In summary, vitamin C requirements have been shown to be increased with various forms of stress such as smoking, illness and injury. It seems likely that strenuous or prolonged exercise also creates sufficient stress to increase vitamin C requirements. While not always clear, the overall data reviewed in this section would tend to indicate such. All animal studies indicated decreased tissue vitamin C levels with exercise. In humans, three papers reported decreased plasma ascorbic acid concentrations with training, two of three papers reported decreased leukocyte concentrations with training and two of four papers reported decreased urine excretion. In addition, four out five papers reported improved heat acclimation with additional vitamin C, four out five papers reported decreased URTI incidence while two (out of four) papers reported improvement in muscle soreness markers and three (out of five) reported reduced plasma cortisol concentrations with additional vitamin C. These results, coupled with the knowledge that ascorbic acid is needed for such functions as epinephrine, carnitine and collagen synthesis as well as normal iron metabolism, would give support to the concept that strenuous or prolonged exercise and training would increase vitamin C requirements. On the other hand, it is not likely that light to moderate levels of exercise and training would significantly increase vitamin C requirements.

III. EFFECTS OF SUPPLEMENTAL ASCORBIC ACID ON VARIOUS ASPECTS OF PHYSICAL PERFORMANCE

Numerous studies have been performed over the last 50–60 years concerning the relationship between ascorbic acid intake and improvement of physical performance. Many of these studies have found positive effects and an equal number have found no effects. It should be noted that many positive studies were performed early in the study of this vitamin. These studies suffer from poor control and dubious statistical analyses. In addition, the initial vitamin C status of the subjects was usually not ascertained and could have been low. However, several "no effect" articles could be criticized for giving ascorbic acid doses that were probably too low to have possible ergogenic effects.

A. POSITIVE FINDINGS

Studies finding positive effects of vitamin C on performance have been reported for both animal[65–68] and human subject groups. Several early human studies (prior to 1950) did report positive effects of vitamin C in the diet on physical performance including such findings as delayed muscular fatigue and an increase in the amount of work performed.[69–73]

Several studies performed since 1960 also have reported positive performance changes in subjects given additional ascorbic acid. Hoogerwerf and Hoitink[74] worked 33 untrained male students on a cycle ergometer at 120 watts for 10 minutes. The study was performed in a double-blind manner with 15 students receiving 1,000 mg of ascorbic a day for 5 days while the rest of the students received a placebo. Blood ascorbate concentrations in the subjects were within normal range at the beginning of the study. The researchers found that excess metabolism due to work decreased and mechanical efficiency increased significantly in the group receiving ascorbic acid as compared with the placebo group. Margolis[75] studied 40 adult male workers; half of the subjects received a vitamin C supplement of 100 mg while the other subjects served as controls. The authors concluded that the vitamin C supplement was helpful in reducing fatigue and in increasing or preventing a decrease in muscular endurance. Spioch et al.[76] gave 30 healthy men 500 mg of ascorbic acid intravenously prior to a 5-minute step test. Oxygen consumption was reduced by 12%, oxygen debt by 40%, total energy output by 18% and pulse rate by 11% compared with the same test without ascorbic acid. Mechanical efficiency also improved in the subjects when they received the ascorbic acid. Meyer et al.[77] investigated the effect of a predominately fruit diet containing 500–1000 mg of vitamin C on the athletic performance of six male and three female university and high school students. All students performed 1 hour of exercise and a 20-km run each day. Measurements were taken before, during and after the diet, which was continued for 14 days. Running times of the students were reduced following the diet but no changes were noted for resting heart rate. Howald et al.[78] studied 13 athletes undergoing a moderately intense continuous training program. The athletes were initially given a placebo for 14 days. This was followed by a vitamin C supplement of 1,000 mg/day for the next 14 days. Exercise tests were performed at the end of each dietary period. The exercise test was a progressive cycle ergometer test starting at a workload of 30 watts and increasing in 40-watt increments every 4 minutes until the subject reached exhaustion. Subjects exhibited a significantly greater physical working capacity at a heart rate of 170 beats/minute. In addition, heart rates were consistently lower at each workload throughout the progressive test when the subjects were receiving the vitamin C. Finally, the addition of vitamin C to the diets of a group of trained Indian university women also resulted in an improvement in their VO_2max and work efficiency in the Harvard step test.[79]

B. STUDIES SHOWING NO EFFECT

While many studies do report an ergogenic effect of ascorbic acid, an almost equal number have found no effect of supplementing the vitamin on performance.

Several studies conducted prior to 1960,[80–85] as well as a number of newer studies, found no effect of vitamin C on performance. Rasch[86] found no differences in performance of cross-country runners receiving either 500 mg of vitamin C/day or a placebo. The experiment lasted one cross-country season, and diets during this time were not controlled. Margaria et al.[87] administered 240 mg of vitamin C to subjects 90 minutes before exercise. These authors found no effects of the vitamin on treadmill run time to exhaustion or VO_2max as compared with control conditions. Snigur[88] studied school children for a period of 2 years. Half of the children were given an ascorbic acid supplement of 100 mg a day and the rest of them acted as controls. Normal dietary vitamin C intake of the children was calculated at 40 mg/day. No differences between groups were seen for fatigability as estimated by strength of the wrist muscles or vital capacity of the lungs. Another investigator[89] gave subjects a vitamin C supplement or a placebo in a double-blind protocol and exercised them on a motor-driven treadmill. No differences were noted for oxygen consumption, respiratory quotient, pulse or respiratory rate. Gey et al.[90] used 286 soldiers as subjects in an experiment that lasted for 12 weeks. Subjects were administered 1,000 mg of vitamin C or a placebo in a double-blind manner. No differences were seen for endurance performance or overall improvement as measured by the mean distance covered on a 12-minute walk/run test. Bailey et al. conducted two studies[91,92] in which young male subjects were exercised on a level motor-driven treadmill at various speeds. The experiments were conducted in a double-blind manner with subjects receiving either 2,000 mg of ascorbic acid or a placebo for 5 days. No differences were noted for minute ventilation, oxygen uptake, oxygen pulse or respiratory variables. In yet another study,[93] the effects of giving 250–1,000 mg of ascorbic acid, either as a supplemental tablet or by drinking orange juice, was evaluated in normal athletic subjects. A placebo and untreated control group were included. No differences were noted among groups for sprint times, long-distance running or work efficiency as measured by the Harvard step test. Horak and Zenisek[94] gave two groups of well-trained athletes either 200 mg of ascorbic acid daily as a supplement or a diet high in vitamin C foods. These authors reported no significant relationship between resting vitamin C concentrations and work efficiency.

Keren and Epstein[95] reported on the effects of a vitamin C supplement on both anaerobic and aerobic performance. Ascorbic acid at 1,000 mg/day or a placebo were given in a double-blind manner for 21 days to a group of male subjects undergoing training. No differences were noted for VO_2max or anaerobic performance. Keith and Merrill[96] reported no differences in maximum grip strength or in muscular endurance in 15 male subjects receiving either a single dose of 600 mg of vitamin C or a placebo given 4 hours prior to exercise. Mean muscular endurance values were actually worse on the vitamin C supplement, although this value was not significantly different. The experiment was performed using a double-blind crossover protocol. Normal vitamin C intake of the subjects was calculated to be 140 mg/day. Keith and Driskell[97] found no differences in forced expiratory volume, vital capacity, treadmill workload, resting heart rate or post-exercise lactic acid in a group of male subjects receiving 300 mg of ascorbic acid versus a group receiving a placebo for 21 days. The study was conducted in a double-blind crossover manner with a 3-week washout period between treatments. Subjects had normal plasma ascorbic acid concentrations at the beginning of the study. In a final study for this section, Driskell and Herbert[98] administered 1,000 mg of ascorbic acid daily or a placebo to male subjects undergoing treadmill testing. The experiment lasted 6 weeks. No significant differences were noted for a variety of performance measures.

Summarizing the data on ascorbic acid as a possible ergogenic aid is difficult. Several studies report an ergogenic effect while just as many studies cite no effect. Weaknesses can be found in studies taking both points of view. However, several of the later studies, in which initial vitamin C status was apparently adequate and supplemental vitamin C was given at 200–1000 mg, seemed to show no ergogenic effects of additional vitamin C. While exceptions may be found, supplemental vitamin C, when given to well-nourished subjects, would seem to have no pronounced or consistent ergogenic effects.

IV. DIETARY INTAKES OF ASCORBIC ACID IN PHYSICALLY ACTIVE PERSONS

Numerous studies have reported on the vitamin C intake of different types of male and female athletes.[33,36,99–125] These studies are summarized in Table 2.5. Generally, mean vitamin intakes in these groups were above the DRI/RDA. The range of mean vitamin C intakes for males was 94 to 600 mg/day, while female athletes had intakes of 55 to 847 mg/day. Almost all studies reported mean vitamin C intakes in athletes to be above the RDA and at levels that would probably be considered adequate or good for athletes under most conditions.

However, while mean intakes for the athletic groups were generally adequate, several studies did report that a portion of their athletic population consumed ascorbic acid in suboptimal amounts. In male athletes, Steen and McKinney[118] reported that 23% of their wrestlers consumed less than two thirds of the RDA for vitamin C. Other papers have indicated similar figures:

- Hickson et al.,[101] 12–20% of football players below 2/3 RDA.
- Guilland et al.,[36] 25% with low intakes.
- Cohen et al.,[34] 10% of dancers below the RDA.
- DeBolt et al.[112] reported that 10% of Navy SEALS were below the RDA.

TABLE 2.5
**Mean Dietary Intakes (mg/day) of Vitamin C in Various
Athletic Groups**

Athletic Group	Subject Number	Vitamin C Intake	Reference
Males			
Endurance runners	15	219	99
Marathon runners	291	147	100
High school footballers	134	180	101
Competitive runners	30	109	35
Basketball players	16	184	102
Elite triathletes	20	275	103
Compet. bodybuilders	13	272	104
Various athletes	55	95	36
Cross country runners	12	262	105
Swimmers	22	186	106
Ice hockey players	48	161	107
Elite Nordic skiers	5	282	108
Elite ballet dancers	10	170	34
Ultramarathoners	82	520	58
Elite Nordic skiers	13	232–371 (R)	109
College athletes	—	97–433 (R)	110
College soccer	18	252,529	111
Navy SEALS	267	353	112
Gaelic footballers	25	73	120
Professional soccer	21	94	121
Elite soccer	8	520	122
Elite alpine ski racers	12	600	123
Females			
Marathon runners	56	115	100
University dancers	21	148	113
College basketball	10	55	102
High school gymnasts	13	84	114
College basketball	13	106	115
College gymnasts	9	207	115
Compet. bodybuilders	11	196	104
Swimmers	21	188	106
Adolescent gymnasts	42	112	107
Trained cyclists	8	80	116
Elite Nordic skiers	7	234	108
Elite ballet dancers	12	162	34
Adolescent ballerinas	92	148	117
Elite Nordic skiers	14	173–210 (R)	109
Various college athletes	—	84–223 (R)	110
Adolescent volleyball	65	93	124
Artistic gymnasts	29	847	125
Elite heptathletes	19	151	126

Note: R = range, instead of mean.

Female athletes show similar figures:

- Nowak et al.[102] reported mean intakes of a group of basketball players to be below the RDA.
- Hickson et al.[115] found 13–22% of basketball players and gymnasts to be below 2/3 RDA.
- Keith et al.[116] showed that 25% of the cyclists in their study consumed less than 2/3 RDA.
- Loosli et al.[119] found 10% of gymnasts to be below 2/3 RDA.
- Cohen et al.[34] and Benson et al.[117] found 8–25% of surveyed dancers to be consuming vitamin C at less than the RDA.

Thus, while group means for intake of vitamin C appear to be acceptable, anywhere from 10 to 25% of an athletic group may be consuming suboptimal levels of the vitamin as compared with the RDA. Improved dietary intakes would be needed in these athletes to assure adequate physical performance. It also should be noted that the above listed percentages were based on the previous RDA for vitamin C of 60 milligrams a day. The current RDA for vitamin C has been increased to 75 milligrams for women and 90 milligrams for men. Thus, the percentage of athletes consuming low amounts of vitamin C may actually be greater than the numbers listed in the various studies.

V. SUMMARY AND RECOMMENDATIONS

Historical and scientific evidence demonstrate that vitamin C deficiency or even marginal vitamin C status can adversely affect physical performance. Ascorbic acid can adversely affect physical functioning at several different metabolic sites such as: impaired collagen formation leading to increased ligament and tendon problems; decreased synthesis of carnitine ,which would impair the use of fatty acids as an energy source; decreased synthesis of epinephrine and norepinephrine resulting in improper metabolic responses to exercise; as well as improper iron metabolism possibly resulting in anemia and fatigue with consequential decreases in aerobic performance. Thus, all physically active persons should strive to maintain optimal vitamin C status through intake of generous servings of fruits and vegetables high in ascorbic acid, or if this is not possible, through proper supplementation with the vitamin through pills or with foods that have had vitamin C added. The RDA for vitamin C is 75 mg for adult women and 90 mg for adult men. These values may not be sufficient for athletes engaged in strenuous, prolonged physical activity events and training. Appropriate intakes for these athletes may range from 100 to 1000 mg each day.

Numerous studies have investigated both the effects that exercise has on vitamin C needs and the effect that supplemental vitamin C has on subsequent athletic performance. Several animal and human studies do seem to indicate that strenuous or prolonged exercise or physical training, in all likelihood, increases the need for vitamin C. It is less likely that light or moderate levels of activity and training increase vitamin C requirements. Animal studies consistently show reduced tissue levels of ascorbic acid with exercise. Several human studies have shown reduced plasma and leukocyte concentrations and reduced urinary excretion of the vitamin with exercise. In addition, supplemental dietary vitamin C has been shown to increase adaptation to exercise in the heat and reduce upper respiratory tract infections in individuals undergoing strenuous exercise. Supplemental vitamin C also has been shown, in some studies, to reduce plasma cortisol concentrations and muscle soreness markers following exercise. Vitamin C intake in these studies generally ranged from 100 to 1500 mg/day. Numerous other data from dietary intake studies with athletes show mean vitamin C intakes of most athletic groups to be in the 55 to 850 mg/day range; intakes that are generally above RDA values. However, several of these studies report that up to 25% (or perhaps more) of the athletes consumed vitamin C at less than RDA levels. Thus, while mean ascorbic acid intakes appear to be adequate, a large percentage of athletes could be consuming suboptimal intakes of the vitamin.

Numerous studies have been conducted in an attempt to find possible ergogenic effects of ascorbic acid. The results of these studies are mixed. Many report possible ergogenic effects of vitamin C, while just as many studies find no effect of ascorbic acid supplementation on subsequent performance. Most of the more recent, and generally better controlled studies do not seem to indicate an ergogenic effect of vitamin C. At the present time, the data do not seem to support a clear or consistent ergogenic effect of vitamin C.

While a wealth of knowledge does exist concerning ascorbic acid and exercise, many areas remain understudied. The relationship between exercise and vitamin C requirements is still one such area. Most of the work done in this area has been performed with runners. Little or no work has been done that has reported on the relationships between vitamin C requirements and exercise for strength-power athletes, swimmers (who undergo large training volumes) and cyclists. Studies on plasma and leuko-cyte ascorbic acid concentrations and changes, as well as urine excretion values, cortisol concentration changes and upper respiratory tract infections in these groups have not been performed. Little, if any, work has been performed evaluating how exercise might alter ratios of ascorbic acid and dehydroascor-bic acid in tissues. This ratio has been shown to be altered in some disease states. Newer studies looking at the effects of ascorbic acid on heat acclimation need to be done. Heat stress and dehydration are extremely important concerns for many athletes. No studies have investigated the relationship between heat stress and vitamin C for more than 25 years. All of these subjects need to be explored in the future to further our understanding of vitamin C and physical activity.

REFERENCES

1. Gerster, G., Review: The role of vitamin C in athletic performance, *J. Am. Coll. Nutr.,* 8, 636, 1989.
2. Clarkson, P.M., Vitamins and trace minerals, in *Ergogenics: Enhancement of Performance in Exercise and Sport,* Lamb, D.R. and Williams, M.H., Eds., Perspectives in Exercise Science and Sports Medicine, Vol. 4, Wm. C. Brown, 1991, 123.
3. Keith, R.E., Vitamins and physical activity, in *Nutrition in Exercise and Sport,* Wolinsky, I. and Hickson, J.F., Eds., 2nd ed., CRC Press, Boca Raton, Fl., 1993, 159.
4. Carpenter, K.J., *The History of Scurvy & Vitamin C,* Cambridge University Press, 1986.
5. Peake, J.M., Vitamin C: Effects of exercise and requirements with training, *Int. J. Sport Nutr. Ex. Metab.,* 13, 125, 2003.
6. Basu, T.K. and Schorah, C.J., *Vitamin C in Health and Disease,* AVI Pub. Co., Westport, Conn., 1982.
7. Davies, M.B., Austin, J. and Partridge, D.A., *Vitamin C: Its Chemistry and Biochemistry,* The Royal Society of Chemistry, Cambridge, England, 1991.
8. Moser, U. and Bendich, A., Vitamin C, in *Handbook of Vitamins,* Machlin, L.J., Ed., 2nd ed., Marcel Dekker, Inc., New York, 1991, 195.
9. Mahan, L.K. and Escott-Stump, S., *Krause's Food, Nutrition and Diet Therapy,* 9th ed., W.B. Saunders Co., Philadelphia, 1996.
10. Gropper, S.S., Smith, J.L. and Groff, J.L., *Advanced Nutrition and Human Metabolism,* 4th ed., Thomson Wadsworth Pub., Belmont, Calif., 2005, 262.
11. Lemmel, G., Vitamin C deficiency and general capacity for work, *Munch. Med. Wochenschr.,* 85, 1381, 1938.
12. Babadzanjan, M.G., Kalnyn, V.R., Koslynn, S.A. and Kostina, E.I., Effect of vitamin supplements on some physiological functions of workers in electric locomotive teams, *Vopr. Pitan.,* 19, 18, 1960.
13. Buzina, R. and Suboticanec, K., Vitamin C and physical working capacity, *Int. J. Vit. Nutr. Res.,* S27, 157, 1985.
14. Van der Beek, E.J., van Dokkum, W., Schrijver, J., Wesstra, J.A., van der Weerd, H. and Hermus, R.J.J., Effect of marginal vitamin intake on physical performance of man, *Int. J. Sports Med.,* 5, 28, 1984.
15. Van der Beek, E.J., van Dokkum, W., Schrijver, J., Wesstra, A., Kistemaker, C. and Hermus, R.J.J., Controlled vitamin C restriction and physical performance in volunteers, *J. Am. Coll. Nutr.,* 9, 332, 1990.
16. Johnston, C.S., Swan, P.D. and Corte, C., Substrate utilization and work efficiency during submaximal exercise in vitamin C depleted-repleted adults, *Int. J. Vit. Nutr. Res.,* 69, 41, 1999.

17. Keith, R.E. and Mossholder, S.B., Ascorbic acid status of smoking and nonsmoking adolescent females, *Int. J. Vit. Nutr. Res.,* 56, 363, 1986.
18. Schectman, G., Byrd, J.C. and Gruchow, H.W., The influence of smoking on vitamin C status in adults, *Am. J. Pub. Health,* 79, 158, 1989.
19. Thaxton, J.P. and Pardue, S.L., Ascorbic acid and physiological stress, in *Ascorbic Acid in Domestic Animals,* Wegger, I., Tagwerker, F.J. and Moustgaard, J., Eds., The Royal Danish Ag. Soc., Copenhagen, 1984, 25.
20. Askew, W.A., Environmental and physical stress and nutrient requirements, *Am. J. Clin. Nutr.,* 61(supp), 631, 1995.
21. Stone, M.H., Keith, R.E., Kearney, J.T., Fleck, S.J., Wilson, G.D. and Triplett, N.T., Overtraining: A review of the signs and symptoms and possible causes, *J. App. Sport Sci. Res.,* 5, 35, 1991.
22. Stojan, B., Pfefferkorn, B. and Schmieder, J., Studies on the ascorbic acid content of the adrenals of the rat after muscular work under normal and lowered oxygen partial pressure, *Acta Biol. Med. Ger.,* 18, 369, 1967.
23. Hughes, R.E., Jones, P.R., Williams, R.S. and Weight, P.F., Effect of prolonged swimming on the distribution of ascorbic acid and cholesterol in the tissues of the guinea pig, *Life Sci.,* 10, 661, 1971.
24. Akamatsu, A., Whan, Y.W., Yamada, K. and Hosoya, N., The effect of high environmental temperature and exercise on the metabolism of ascorbic acid in rats, *Vitamins* (Jpn.), 60, 199, 1986.
25. Keith, R.E. and Lee, S., Effects of dietary ascorbic acid and exercise on tissue ascorbic acid, lactate dehydrogenase and thiobarituric acid reactive substances in guinea pigs, *FASEB J.,* 7, A611, 1993.
26. Keith, R.E. and Pomerance, G.M., Exercise and tissue ascorbic acid content in guinea pigs, *Nutr. Res.,* 15, 423, 1995.
27. Altenburger, E., Relationship of ascorbic acid to the glycogen metabolism of the liver, *Klin. Wochenschr.,* 15, 1129, 1936.
28. Namyslowski, L. and Desperak-Secomska, B., The vitamin C content of the blood in a selected group of students during 1952 and 1953, *Rocz. Panstw. Zakl. Hig.,* 6, 289, 1955.
29. Namyslowski, L., Investigations of the vitamin C requirements of athletes during physical exertion, *Rocz. Panstw. Zakl. Hig.,* 7, 97, 1956.
30. Schroder, H., Navarro, E., Tramullas, A., Mora, J. and Galiano, D., Nutrition antioxidant status and oxidative stress in professional basketball players: Effects of a three compound antioxidative supplement, *Int. J. Sports Med.,* 21, 146, 2000.
31. Fishbaine, B. and Butterfield, G., Ascorbic acid status of running and sedentary men, *Int. J. Vitam. Nutr. Res.,* 54, 273, 1984.
32. Gleeson, M., Robertson, J.D. and Maughn, R.J., Influence of exercise on ascorbic acid status in man, *Clin. Sci.,* 73, 501, 1987.
33. Duthie, G.G., Robertson, J.D., Maughn, R.J. and Morrice, P.C., Blood antioxidant status and erythrocyte lipid peroxidation following distance running, *Arch. Biochem. Biophys.,* 282, 78, 1990.
34. Cohen, J.L., Potosnak, L., Frank, O. and Baker, H., A nutritional and hematologic assessment of elite ballet dancers, *Phys. Sportsmed.,* 5, 43, 1985.
35. Weight, L.M., Noakes, T.D., Labadarios, D., Graves, J., Jacobs, P. and Berman, P.A., Vitamin and mineral status of trained athletes including the effects of supplementation, *Am. J. Clin. Nutr.,* 47, 186, 1988.
36. Guilland, J-C., Penaranda, T, Gallet, C., Boggio, V., Fuchs, F. and Klepping, J., Vitamin status of young athletes including the effects of supplementation, *Med. Sci. Sport Ex.,* 21, 441, 1989.
37. Telford, R.D., Catchpole, E.A., Deakin, V. McLeay, A.C. and Plank, A.W., The effect of 7 to 8 months of vitamin/mineral supplementation on the vitamin and mineral status of athletes, *Int. J. Sport Nutr.,* 2, 123, 1992.
38. Robson, P.J., Bouic, P.J.D., and Myburgh, K.H., Antioxidant supplementation enhances neutrophil oxidative burst in trained runners following prolonged exercise, *Int. J. Sport Nutr. Exc. Metab.,* 13, 369, 2003.
39. Peters, E.M., Anderson, R., Nieman, D.C., Fickl, H. and Jogessar, V., Vitamin C supplementation attenuates the increases in circulating cortisol, adrenaline and anti-inflammatory polypeptides following ultramarathon running, *Int. J. Sports Med.,* 22, 537, 2001.
40. Zeman, F.J., *Clinical Nutrition and Dietetics,* 2nd ed., MacMillan Pub. Co., New York, 1991, 760.
41. Garry, P.J. and Appenzeller, O., Vitamins A and C and endurance races, *Ann. Sports Med.,* 1, 82, 1983.
42. Boddy, K., Hume, R., King, P.C., Weyers, E. and Rowan, T., Total body, plasma and erythrocyte potassium and leucocyte ascorbic acid in "ultra-fit" subjects, *Clin. Sci. Mol. Med.,* 46, 449, 1974.

43. Ferrandez, M., Maynar, M. and De la Fuente, M., Effects of a long-term training program of increasing intensity on the immune function on indoor Olympic cyclists, *Int. J. Sports Med.,* 17, 592, 1996.

44. Robertson, J., Maughan, R., Duthie, G. and Morrice, P., Increased blood antioxidant systems of runners in response to training load, *Clin. Sci.,* 80, 611, 1991.

45. Krause, R., Patruta, S., Daxbock, F., Fladerer, P, Biegelmayer, C. and Wenisch, C., Effect of vitamin C on neutrophil function after high-intensity exercise, *Eur. J. Clin. Invest.,* 31, 258, 2001.

46. Bacinskij, P.P., Effect of physical activity on the vitamin C and B1 supply of the body, *Vopr. Pitan.,* 18, 53, 1959.

47. Rokitzki, L., Hinkel, S., Klemp, C. Curl, D. and Keul, J., Dietary, serum and urine ascorbic acid status in male athletes, *Int. J. Sports Med.,* 15, 435, 1994.

48. Henschel, A., Taylor, H.L., Brozek, J., Mickelsen, O. and Keys, A., Vitamin C and the ability to work in hot environments, *Am. J. Trop. Med.,* 24, 259, 1944.

49. Visagie, M.E., du Plessis, J.P. and Laubscher, N.F., Effect of vitamin C supplementation on black mineworkers, *S. Afr. Med. J.,* 49, 889, 1975.

50. Karnaugh, N., Effect of physical work and heat microclimate on the excretion of 17-hydroxycorticosteroids and ascorbic acid, *Vrach. Delo,* 3, 134, 1976.

51. Strydom, N.B., Kotze, H.F., van der Walt, W.H. and Rogers, G.G., Effect of ascorbic acid on rate of heat acclimatization, *J. Appl. Physiol.,* 41, 202, 1976.

52. Kotze, H.F., van der Walt, W.H., Rogers, B.B. and Strydom, N.B., Effects of plasma ascorbic acid levels on heat acclimatization in man, *J. Appl. Physiol.,* 42, 771, 1977.

53. Staton, W.M., The influence of ascorbic acid in minimizing post-exercise muscle soreness in young men, *Res. Q. Am. Assoc. Health Phys. Educ. Recreat.,* 23, 356, 1952.

54. Thompson, D., Williams, C., Kingsley M., Nicholas, W.W., Lakomy, H.K., McArdle, F. and Jackson, M.J., Muscle soreness and damage parameters after prolonged intermittent shuttle-running following acute vitamin C supplementation, *Int. J. Sports Med.,* 22, 68, 2001.

55. Jakeman, P. and Maxwell, S., Effect of antioxidant vitamin supplementation on muscle function after eccentric exercise, *Eur. J. App. Physiol.,* 67, 426, 1993.

56. Thompson, D., Williams, C., McGregor, S.J., Nicholas, C.W., Mc Ardle, F., Jackson, M.J. and Powell, J.R., Prolonged vitamin C supplementation and recovery from demanding exercise, *Int. J. Sport Nutr. Exc. Metab.,* 11, 466, 2001.

57. Nieman, D.C., Henson, D.A., Butterworth, D.E., Warren, B.J., Davis, M.J., Fagoaga, O.R. and Nehlsen-Cannarella, S.L., Vitamin C supplementation does not alter the immune response to 2.5 hours of running, *Int. J Sports Nutr.,* 7, 173, 1997.

58. Peters, E.M., Goetzsche, J., Grobbelaar, B. and Noakes, T., Vitamin C supplementation reduces the incidence of post-race symptoms of upper respiratory tract infection in ultradistance runners, *Am. J. Clin. Nutr.,* 57, 170, 1993.

59. Peters, E.M., Goetzsche, J.M., Joseph, L.E. and Noakes, T.D., Vitamin C as effective as combinations of anti-oxidants nutrients in reducing symptoms of upper respiratory tract infection in ultramarathon runners, *S. Afr. J. Sports Med.,* 11, 23, 1996.

60. Hemila, H., Vitamin C and common cold incidence: a review of studies with subjects under heavy physical stress, *Int. J. Sports Med.,* 17, 379, 1996.

61. Himmelstein, S.A., Roberts, R.A., Koehler, K.M., Lewis, S.L. and Qualls, C.R., Vitamin C supplementation and upper respiratory tract infections in marathon runners, *J. Ex. Physiol.,* online, 1, 1998.

62. Guyton, A.C., *Textbook of Medical Physiology,* 6th ed., W.B. Saunders Co., Philadelphia, 1981, 948.

63. Nieman, D., Peters, E.M., Henson, D., Nevines, E. and Thompson, M., Influence of vitamin C supplementation on cytokine changes following an ultramarathon, *J. Interferon Cytokine Res.,* 20, 1029, 2000.

64. Peters, E.M., Anderson, R. and Theron, A.J., Attenuation of increase in circulating cortisol and enhancement of the acute phase protein response in vitamin C-supplemented ultramarathoners, *Int. J. Sports Med.,* 22, 120, 2001.

65. Basu, N.M. and Biswas, P., The influence of ascorbic acid on contractions and the incidence of fatigue of different types of muscles, *Indian J. Med. Res.,* 28, 405, 1940.

66. Bushnell, R.G. and Lehmann, A.G., Antagonistic effect of sodium ascorbate on ethanol-induced changes in swimming of mice, *Behav. Brain Res.,* 1, 351, 1980.

67. Richardson, J.H. and Allen, R.B., Dietary supplementation with vitamin C delays onset of fatigue in isolated striated muscle of rats, *Can. J. Appl. Sport Sci.,* 8, 140, 1983.

68. Lang, J., Gohil, K. and Packer, L., Effect of dietary vitamin C on exercise performance and tissue vitamin C, vitamin E and ubiquinone levels, *Fed. Proc.,* 45, 1747, 1986.

69. Sieburg, H., Redoxon as a tonic for sportsmen, *Deutsch. Med. Wochenschr.,* 63, Arzt. und Sport, 13, 11, 1937.

70. Wiebel, H., Studies of dosage with vitamin C in athletic female students, *Deutsch. Med. Wochenschr.,* 65, 60, 1939.

71. Basu, N.M. and Ray, G.K., The effect of vitamin C on the incidence of fatigue in human muscles, *Indian J. Med. Res.,* 28, 419, 1940.

72. Harper, A.A., MacKay, I.F.S., Raper, H.S. and Camm, G.L., Vitamins and physical fitness, *Br. Med. J.,* i, 243, 1943.

73. Hoitink, A.W., Vitamin C and work. Studies on the influence of work and of vitamin C intake on the human organism, *Verh. Nederlands Inst. Praevent. Geneesk,* 4, 176, 1946.

74. Hoogerwerf, A. and Hoitink, A.W., The influence of vitamin C administration on the mechanical efficiency of the human organism, *Int. Z. Angew. Physiol. Arbeitsphysiol.,* 20, 164, 1963.

75. Margolis, A.M., Vitamin C status of miners and some other population groups in the Don basin, *Vopr. Pitan.,* 23, 78,1964.

76. Spioch, F., Kobza, R. and Mazur, B., Influence of vitamin C upon certain functional changes and the coefficient of mechanical efficiency in humans during physical effort, *Acta Physiol. Pol.,* 17, 204, 1966.

77. Meyer,B.J., deBruin, E.J., Brown, J.M., Bieler, E.U., Meyer, A.C. and Grey, P.C., The effect of a predominately fruit diet on athletic performance, *Plant Foods Man,* 1, 223, 1975.

78. Howald, H., Segesser, B. and Korner, W.F., Ascorbic acid and athletic performance, *Ann. N.Y. Acad. Sci.,* 258, 458, 1975.

79. Samanta, S.C. and Biswas, K., Effect of supplementation of vitamin C on the cardiorespiratory endurance capacity of college women, *Snipes J.* 8, 55, 1985.

80. Jetzler, A. and Haffler, C., Vitamin C-bedarf bei einmaligar sportlicher dauerleistung, *Wein. Med. Wochenschr.,* 89, 332, 1939.

81. Fox, F.W., Dangerfield, L.F., Gottlich, S.F. and Jokl, E., Vitamin C requirements of native mine labourers. An experimental study, *Br. Med. J.,* ii, 143, 1940.

82. Jokl, E. and Suzman, H., A study of the effects of vitamin C upon physical efficiency, *Transvaal Mine Med. Off. Assoc. Proc.,* 19, 292, 1940.

83. Keys, A. and Henschel, A.F., Vitamin supplementation of U.S. Army rations in relation to fatigue and the ability to do muscular work, *J. Nutr.,* 23, 259, 1942.

84. Jenkins, G.N. and Yudkin, J., Vitamins and physiological function, *Br. Med. J.,* ii, 265, 1943.

85. Vinarickij, R., An attempt to improve the efficiency of medium distance runners by large doses of vitamin B_1, B_2 and C, *Scripta Med.,* 27, 1, 1954.

86. Rasch, P., Effects of vitamin C supplementation on cross country runners, *Sportzarztliche Praxis,* 5, 10, 1962.

87. Margaria, R., Agheno, P. and Rovelli, E., The effect of some drugs on the maximal capacity of athletic performance in man, *Int. Z. Angew. Physiol.,* 20, 281, 1964.

88. Snigur, O.I., Signs of fatigue in school children in different states of ascorbic acid supply, *Gig. Sanit.,* 7, 117, 1966.

89. Kirchhoff, H.W., Effect of vitamin C on energy expenditure and circulatory and ventilatory function in stress studies, *Nutr. Diet.,* 11, 184, 1969.

90. Gey, G.O., Cooper, K.H. and Bottenberg, R.A., Effect of ascorbic acid on endurance performance and athletic injury, *J. Am. Med. Assoc.,* 211, 105, 1970.

91. Bailey, D.A., Carron, A.V., Teece, R.G. and Wehner, H.J., Vitamin C supplementation related to physiological response to exercise in smoking and nonsmoking subjects, *Am. J. Clin. Nutr.,* 23, 905, 1970.

92. Bailey, D.A., Carron, A.V., Teece, R.G. and Wehner, H.J., Effect of vitamin C supplementation upon the physiological response to exercise in trained and untrained subjects, *Int. J. Vit. Res.,* 40, 435, 1970.

93. Bender, A.E. and Nash, A.H., Vitamin C and physical performance, *Plant Foods Man.,* 1, 217, 1975.

94. Horak, J. and Zenisek, A., Vitamin C blood level before and after laboratory load and its relation to cardiorespiratory performance parameters in top sportsmen, *Cas. Lek. Cesk.* 116, 679, 1977.

95. Keren, B. and Epstein, Y., Effect of high dosage vitamin C intake on aerobic and anaerobic capacity, *J. Sports Med. Phys. Fitness,* 20, 145, 1980.

96. Keith, R.E. and Merrill, E., The effects of vitamin C on maximum grip strength and muscular endurance, *J. Sports Med. Phys. Fitness,* 23, 253, 1983.

97. Keith, R.E. and Driskell, J.A., Lung function and treadmill performance of smoking and nonsmoking males receiving ascorbic acid supplements, *Am. J. Clin. Nutr.,* 36, 840, 1982.

98. Driskell, J.A. and Herbert, W.G., Pulmonary function and treadmill performance of males receiving ascorbic acid supplements, *Nutr. Rep. Int.,* 32, 443, 1985.

99. Peters, A.J., Dressendorfer, R.H., Rimar, J. and Keen, C.L., Diets of endurance runners competing in a 20-day road race, *Phys. Sportsmed.,* 14, 63, 1986.

100. Nieman, D.C., Butler, J.V., Pollett, L.M., Dietrich, S.J. and Lutz, R.D., Nutrient intake of marathon runners, *J. Am. Diet. Assoc.,* 89, 1273, 1989.

101. Hickson, J.F., Duke, M.A., Risser, W.L., Johnson, C.W., Palmer, R. and Stockton, J.E., Nutritional intake from food sources of high school football athletes, *J. Am. Diet. Assoc.,* 87, 1656, 1987.

102. Nowak, R.K., Knudsen, K.S. and Schulz, L.O., Body composition and nutrient intakes of college men and women basketball players, *J. Am. Diet. Assoc.,* 88, 575, 1988.

103. Burke, L.M. and Read, R.S.D., Diet patterns of elite Australian male triathletes, *Phys. Sportsmed.,* 15, 140, 1987.

104. Bazzarre, T.L., Kleiner, S.M., and Ainsworth, B.E., Vitamin C intake and lipid profiles of competitive male and female bodybuilders, *Int. J. Sport Nutr.,* 2, 260, 1992.

105. Niekamp, R.A. and Baer, J.T., In-season dietary adequacy of trained male cross-country runners, *Int. J. Sport Nutr.,* 5, 45, 1995.

106. Berning, J.R., Troup, J.P., van Handel, P.J., Daniels, J. and Daniels, N., The nutritional habits of young adolescent swimmers, *Int. J. Sport Nutr.,* 1, 240, 1991.

107. Rankinen, T., Fogelholm, M., Kujala, U., Rauramaa, R., and Uusitupa, M., Dietary intake and nutritional status of athletic and nonathletic children in early puberty, *Int. J.Sport Nutr.,* 5, 136, 1995.

108. Fogelholm, M., Rehenen, S., Gref, C-G., Laakso, J.T., Lehto, J., Ruokonen, I. and Himberg, J-J., Dietary intake and thiamin, iron, and zinc status in elite nordic skiers during different training periods, *Int. J. Sport Nutr.,* 2, 351, 1992.

109. Ellsworth, N.M., Hewitt, B.F. and Haskell, W.L., Nutrient intake of elite male and female nordic skiers, *Phys. Sportsmed.,* 13, 78, 1985.

110. Short, S.H. and Short, W.R., Four-year study of university athletes' dietary intake, *J. Am. Diet. Assoc.,* 82, 632, 1983.

111. Hickson, J.F., Schrader, J.W., Pivarnik, J.M. and Stockton, J.E., Nutritional intake from food sources of soccer athletes during two stages of training, *Nutr. Rep. Int.,* 34, 85, 1986.

112. DeBolt, J.E., Singh, A., Day, B.A. and Deuster, P.A., Nutritional survey of the US Navy SEAL trainees, *Am. J. Clin. Nutr.,* 48, 1316, 1988.

113. Evers, C.L., Dietary intake and symptoms of anorexia nervosa in female university dancers, *J. Am. Diet. Assoc.,* 87, 66, 1987.

114. Moffat, R.J., Dietary status of elite female high school gymnasts: Inadequacy of vitamin and mineral intake, *J. Am. Diet. Assoc.,* 84, 1361, 1984.

115. Hickson, J.F., Schrader, J. and Trischler, L.C., Dietary intakes of female basketball and gymnastics athletes, *J. Am. Diet. Assoc.,* 86, 251, 1986.

116. Keith, R.E., O'Keeffe, K.A. and Alt, L.A., Dietary status of trained female cyclists, *J. Am. Diet. Assoc.,* 89, 1620, 1989.

117. Benson, J., Gillien, D.M., Bourdet, K. and Loosli, A.R., Inadequate nutrition and chronic calorie restriction in adolescent ballerinas, *Phys. Sportsmed.,* 13, 79, 1985.

118. Steen, S.N. and McKinney, S., Nutrition assessment of college wrestlers, *Phys. Sportsmed.,* 14, 100, 1986.

119. Loosli, A.R., Benson,J., Gillien, D.M. and Bourdet, K., Nutrition habits and knowledge in competitive adolescent female gymnasts, *Phys. Sportsmed.,* 14, 118, 1986.

120. Reeves, S., and Collins, K., The nutritional and anthropometric status of Gaelic football players, *Int. J. Sport Nutr. Exc. Metab.,* 13, 539, 2003.

121. Rico-Sanz, J., Frontera, W.R., Mole, P.A., Rivera, M.A., Rivera-Brown, A. and Meredith, C.N., Dietary and performance assessment of elite soccer players during a period of intense training, *Int. J. Sport Nutr.,* 8, 230, 1998.

122. Subudhi, A.W., Davis, S.L., Kipp, R.W. and Askew, E.W., Antioxidant status and oxidative stress in elite alpine ski racers, *Int. J. Sport Nutr. Exc. Metab.,* 11, 32, 2001.

123. Papadopoulou, S.K., Papadopoulou, S.D. and Gallos, G.K., Macro- and micro-nutrient intake of adolescent Greek female volleyball players, *Int. J. Sport Nutr. Exc. Metab.,* 12, 73, 2002.
124. Jonnalagadda, S.S., Benardot, D. and Nelson, M., Energy and nutrient intake of the United States national women's artistic gymnastics team, *Int. J. Sport Nutr.,* 8, 331, 1998.
125. Mullins, V.A., Houtkooper, L.B., Howell, W.H., Going, S.B. and Brown, C.H., Nutritional status of U.S. elite female heptathletes during training, *Int. J. Sport Nutr. Exc. Metab.,* 11, 299, 2001.

3 Thiamin

Enas K. Al-Tamimi and Mark D. Haub

CONTENTS

I. INTRODUCTION

Thiamin, also known as vitamin B1, was the first chemically identified component of B-complex vitamins. Since thiamin is a water-soluble vitamin, it cannot be stored in the body and must be consumed regularly. Thiamin plays a significant role in carbohydrate and protein metabolism, particularly metabolism of branched-chain amino acids. It also serves as an enzyme cofactor in substrate metabolism, especially with pyruvate dehydrogenase, transketolase and 2-oxo-glucarate dehydrogenease to produce adenosine triphosphate.[1] In addition, thiamin is known to affect neural function, nerve conduction, and neurotransmitters.[2] Thus, thiamin is necessary for the normal functioning of the nervous system and skeletal and cardiac musculature.[3] Thiamin deficiency causes many complications, including beriberi, loss of appetite, weakness, insomnia, loss of weight, vague aches and pains, mental depression, constipation and heart problems. The importance of thiamin in sports nutrition pertains to its importance in energy metabolism. Furthermore, thiamin deficiency may lead to health problems in individuals with high carbohydrate and protein demands, including athletes. It has been reported that some athletes may be at least marginally thiamin deficient.[4,5] This marginal deficiency might result from exercise-induced increases in thiamin-dependent amino acid catabolism.[6,7] This chapter will review the chemical and functional properties of thiamin and then apply that information to athletic endeavors.

II. CHEMICAL PROPERTIES OF THIAMIN

A. CHEMICAL STRUCTURE

Thiamin contains pyrimidine and thiazol moieties attached by a methylene group with a molecular weight of about 300.8 Da as thiamin hydrochloride (Figure 3.1).[8] Those functional groups give thiamin the property of high water solubility. Thiamin is very sensitive to alkali, and the thiazol moiety easily opens at room temperature when pH is above 7.

Moisture greatly accelerates the destruction of thiamin, and thus makes it less stable to heat in fresh foods than in dry foods. In dry conditions, thiamin is stable at 100°C for several hours.[9]

Thiamin is found in several forms, including thiamin monophospahate (TMP), thiamin pyrophosphate (TPP), which is also known as thiamin diphosphate, and thiamin triphosphate (TTP). Each of these forms has a specific physiological function, but only the roles of TPP are well established. Thiamin pyrophosphate, which is the active and most abundant form of thiamin in body tissues (about 80% of total thiamin), is the product of thiamin phosphorylation by thiamin diphosphotransferasein in brain and liver cells.[10] Thiamin is necessary as a cofactor for the carbohydrate metabolic enzyme pyruvate dehydrogenase and α-ketoglutarate dehydrogenase in the citric acid cycle (CAC), which catalyzes reactions as well as the transketolase catalyzes reactions of the pentose phosphate pathway.[11]

On the other hand, anti-thiamin activity is common, and includes chemical structures that act as antagonists in a competitive inhibition pattern. Pyrithiamine is one thiamin antagonist that not only blocks the esterification with phosphoric acid to produce the phosphorylated forms, but also inhibits thiamin coenzyme cocarboxylase. Likewise, oxythiamine transfers cocarboxylase, whereas amprolium inhibits absorption of thiamin from the intestine and blocks thiamin phosphorylation.[2] Thiamin activity is also decreased by action of the thiamin hydrolysis enzyme, thiaminase, which attenuates thiamin activity by altering the structure of the vitamin, rendering it ineffective.[12,13]

B. SEPARATION, DETERMINATION AND PURIFICATION

Thiamin is isolated in pure form as thiamin hydrochloride. New techniques have been used for thiamin separation. Supercritical fluid chromatography is efficient at thiamin separation, particularly when the mobile phase has been modified.[14]

Many procedures have been used for thiamin determination, including biological, microbiological and chemical methods. The conventional chemical methods are time consuming, i.e., gravimetric and titration, whereas spectrophotometric and chromatographic techniques[15–17] are more rapid and have been used to assess thiamin deficiency.[18] The procedure of thiamin determination differs depending on the sample whether it is food,[15] pharmaceutical preparation[16] or a clinical specimen.[17] In general, the first step of thiamin determination is extraction, and this step requires

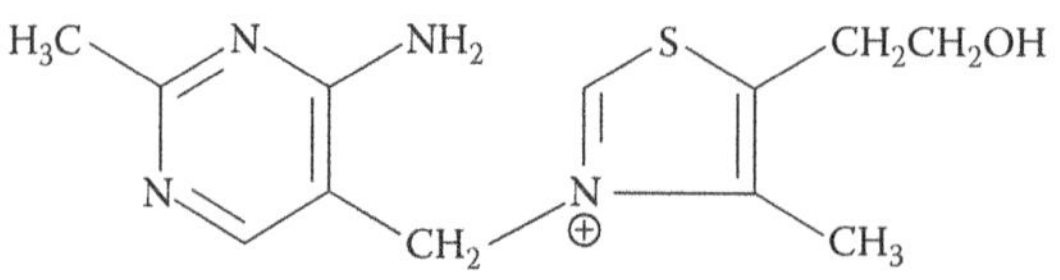

FIGURE 3.1 Structure of thiamin.

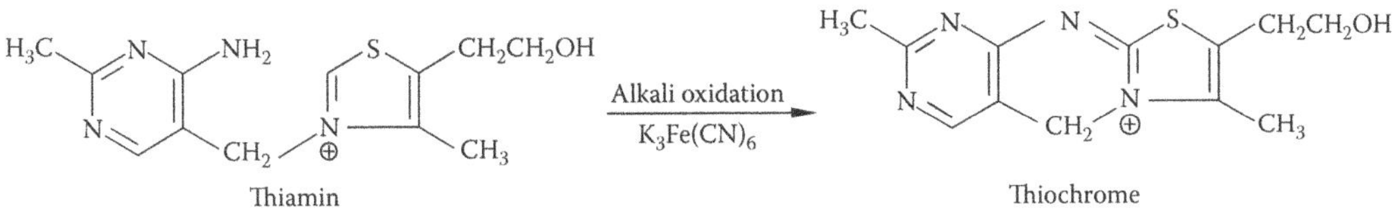

FIGURE 3.2 Thiochrome, the detectable form of thiamin, after alkali oxidation.

separating thiamin from other components, particularly proteins, which are removed by precipitation. Another step of thiamin determination is derivatization, and this can be accomplished by alkaline oxidation of thiamin into thiochrome, which is the detectable form of thiamin (Figure 3.2). Thiochrome emits light that can be captured by the detector,[15] or UV detector with Fourier-transform infrared detection.[19] Liu et al.[20] evaluated the spectrophotometric method for thiamin determination of pharmaceutical preparations using several dyes that react with thiamin at a wavelength between 420 and 450 nm. They reported that the spectrophotometric method is an effective and sensitive method for determining of thiamin in an aqueous solution.

C. SYNTHESIS

Industrially, thiamin, in its phosphorylated form, can be synthesized using chemical or enzymatic methods. Enzymatic methods achieve higher yields of phosphorylated thiamin than chemical methods, which require many steps including phosphorylation of thiamin, purification and crystallization.[21] However, chemical methods are more convenient than enzymatic methods, but the low yield is considered a problematic issue.[21,22] To address this problem, some researchers have overcome the negative aspects of the chemical methods by reducing the processing steps and using 5'-monophosphate as a precursor with plenty of phosphoric acid in the reactant. The result was a 70% increase in thiamin yield compared with the conventional chemical method.[22]

While humans cannot synthesize thiamin,[23] microorganisms provide a rich environment for thiamin enzymatic biosynthesis which is, to some extent, well established.[24–29] Melnick et al.[29] reported that 71% of TPP could be enzymatically synthesized in *Escherichia coli* via thiazol kinase, pyrimidine kinase, thiamin phosphate synthase, and thiamin phosphate kinase.

III. METABOLISM OF THIAMIN

Thiamin has a relatively short biological half-life (9–18 days), is stored in small quantities (25–30mg), and is readily excreted in urine, with small amounts also appearing in perspiration.[30] Therefore, thiamin must be consumed on a regular basis. Thus, the digestion and absorption of the thiamin are important processes in thiamin metabolism.

A. DIGESTION

Thiamin is readily digested from the food sources, either in its free or phosphorylated forms, but sufficient production of hydrochloric acid in the stomach is necessary for its digestion. In the stomach, acid hydrolysis occurs that yields free thiamin, and a phosphoric ester is obtained.

B. ABSORPTION

In the small intestine, particularly the proximal part, free thiamin is directly absorbed. Thiamin is transported by active absorption and passive diffusion from the brush border membrane and basolateral membrane in the small intestine.[8,31,32] Active sodium transport occurs at low concentrations of thiamin, and simple diffusion occurs at higher thiamin concentrations.[33] With transportation of free thiamin through the intestine, some phosphorylation of thiamin occurs in everted jejunal sacs and in isolated enterocytes.[8,34,35] Following absorption, the free and phosphorylated forms travel to the liver with a protein carrier via the portal vein, where further metabolism occurs.[36]

Excretion of absorbed thiamin occurs in both the urine and feces, and small amounts in sweat.[30] The excretion in sweat may increase thiamin requirements in athletes.

C. PHOSPHORYLATION

In the liver, and less so in the brain, heart and muscles, phosphorylation of thiamin occurs under the action of adenosine triphosphate (ATP) and thiamin diphosphokinase to form TPP, the meta-bolically active form of thiamin, and acts as a cofactor for the metabolic enzymes in the CAC and the pentose phosphate pathway.[36,37] On the other hand, enzymatic phosphorylation of thiamin into TTP in the brain and liver is required to activate the chloride ion channel in nerves and muscles.[36,38]

D. THIAMIN IN THE CITRIC ACID CYCLE

The CAC extracts energy nutrients throughout a chain of cyclic reactions. Thiamin pyrophosphate is the key coenzyme for α-ketoacid dehydrogenases, which catalyzes two reactions of CAC, the oxidative decarboxylation of pyruvate to acetyl CoA and the oxidative decarboxylation of α-ketoglutarate to succinyl CoA. These reactions lead to the reduction of nicotinamide adenine dinucleotide (NAD+) to NADH and production of a molecule of CO_2 for release.

Thiamin pyrophosphate is also the cofactor for the pyruvate dehydrogenase component of the complex. Pyruvate dehydrogenase catalyzes the oxidative decarboxylation of pyruvate. Other com-ponents of the enzyme complex complete the conversion of pyruvate to acetyl CoA. Other reactions that require TPP involve α–ketoglutarate and branched-chain α-keto acids. This reaction has a similar metabolic pathway to that of pyruvate.[37] Alpha-ketoglutarate is decarboxylated and the product is transferred to CoA to give succinyl CoA by action of TPP dependent α-ketoglutarate dehydrogenase. Also, in BCAA catabolism, TPP is required as a coenzyme for branched-chain keto-acid dehydrogenase for the oxidative decarboxylation of α-ketoglutarate and branched chains derived from certain amino acids (valine, luecine, isoluecine).[38]

E. THIAMIN IN THE PENTOSE PHOSPHATE PATHWAY

The pentose phosphate pathway transforms energy from carbohydrate molecules and stores it in the form of nicotinamide adenine dinucleotide phosphate (NADPH), which is important as an electron donor for several biosynthetic reactions in the cell such as reducing reactive oxygen species and lipids.[36,39] Moreover, the pentose phosphate pathway has a role in the production of 5-carbon sugars such as ribose, which is used in the synthesis of polysaccharides, coenzymes, DNA and RNA. Thiamin, in TPP form, is the coenzyme for the transketolase (TK),[37,39] which has the primary function of TK is to transfer a 2-carbon unit from an α-ketose to an aldose.

IV. PHYSIOLOGICAL FUNCTION OF THIAMIN

Thiamin, as TPP, serves as a coenzyme in carbohydrate and BCAA metabolism.[1,38,40] A magnesium ion along with TPP are essential for α-ketols formation. Thiamin is needed for the oxidation of α-keto acids pyruvate, α-ketoglutarate, and branched-chain α-keto acids by dehydrogenase complex enzymes in CAC.[36,39] However, when thiamin is deficient, there is a decline in carbohydrate metabolism, and consequently, this affects amino acid metabolism and neural function due to a decrease in the acetylcholine formation.[39]

Thiamin also has an independent non-cofactor role in electrical generative cells such as nerves, brain and muscles, particularly glial cells.[38,39,41,42] It is believed that TTP has a role in chloride channel regulation and trophic effects on neuronal cells.[42] This has been confirmed by a study on rat brain incubated with TPP.[43] The results showed that not only is TTP synthesized, but they also showed a direct correlation between TTP content and increased chloride uptake, which indicates the activation role of TTP on chloride channels.[43] Some researchers reported that TTP is necessary for the synthesis of acetylcholine, a neurotransmitter that affects several brain functions including memory, and acetylcholine maintains muscle tone of the stomach, intestines and heart.[44] Acetylcholine stimulation of nerves results in the release of TMP and free thiamin with a concomitant decrease of intracellular TPP and TTP.[42,45]

V. DEFICIENCY OF THIAMIN

Thiamin deficiency occurs among individuals who consume inadequate intakes of thiamin. It is more common in developing and undeveloped countries, and in the regions where rice is the staple food item.[1,44] Also, breastfed infants of low socio-economic families,[46] alcoholics,[36,47] and total parental nutrition patients may present with thiamin deficiency.[48,49]

Since thiamin acts as a coenzyme for several metabolic enzymes to generate energy, thiamin deficiency generally affects substrate metabolism, leading to weight loss, weakness, cardiac abnormalities and neuromuscular dysfunction.[1,50,51] Hence, two metabolic syndromes (beriberi and Wernicke-Korsakoff syndrome) are the typical consequence of thiamin deficiency.[1,44]

A. BERIBERI

Beriberi, the most common thiamin deficiency syndrome in humans, is characterized by peripheral neuropathy, exhaustion and anorexia that progress to edema, cardiovascular diseases and neurologic and muscular degeneration.[51–53] Beriberi strikes in three major types: dry beriberi, wet beriberi and infantile beriberi. Beriberi is considered an epidemic disease in some parts of Southeast Asia[54] and Cuba[55] where refined rice is a staple diet, and these regions have inadequate thiamin-enrichment programs.

B. WERNICKE-KORSAKOFF SYNDROME

Wernicke-Korsakoff syndrome, or Wernicke's encephalopathy, the acute thiamin-deficient disease that occurs most often in Western developed countries, is linked to alcoholism.[39,56] Patients with alcoholism, HIV-AIDS and malabsorption disorders are at a greater risk of acquiring Wernicke-Korsakoff syndrome. However, patients with alcoholism will likely develop Wernicke's encephalopathy more often than the others for several reasons, including insufficient diet intake of thiamin,[57] increased metabolic demands of thiamin due to increased alcohol consumption and the fact that alcoholism induces malabsorption of thiamin and consequently inhibits thiamin-dependent enzymes.[39,58] Wernicke-Korsakoff syndrome symptoms are similar to those of wet beriberi, being characterized by defects in motor, sensory and cognitive systems.[36,59] Moreover, with progression of Wernicke-Korsakoff syndrome, psychosis may develop, with coma occurring in severe cases.

VI. ASSESSMENT OF THIAMIN

The total thiamin concentration in the body is about 25–30 mg, where TPP is the primary form. In addition, about 80% of the thiamin in whole blood is present in erythrocytes.[60] Because the body cannot store thiamin for long periods, thiamin deficiency may develop without adequate regular ingestion of thiamin. Therefore, thiamin assessment provides a useful tool not only in identifying thiamin deficiency, but also to evaluate the nutritional status of different groups.

Many procedures are used to estimate thiamin status, requirements and deficiency. These include measurements of urinary thiamin excretion, erythrocyte transketolase (ETK) activity, erythrocyte TPP[30,61] and, to a lesser extent, blood pyruvate and lactate levels.[30,62] The urinary excretion rate of the thiamin is one of the oldest methods used to evaluate the thiamin status, and the presence of thiamin and its derivatives in urine tends to reflect thiamin intake.[60] However, this method does not necessary reflect the thiamin status as much as it reflects recent thiamin intake.[60] The ETK activity assay is an indirect method that reflects TPP levels in blood, which represents the most abundant form of thiamin.[63] This assay derives an activity coefficient based on basal TPP stimulation.[64] A higher activity coefficient (i.e., >1.25) indicates thiamin deficiency, whereas coefficient values of 1.00–1.15, and 1.20–1.25 are considered normal and marginally deficient, respectively.[65]

Baines and Davies[61] suggest that it is useful to determine erythrocyte TPP directly because TPP is less susceptible to factors that influence enzyme activity. There are methods for determining thiamin and its phosphate esters in whole blood using high-performance liquid chromatography (HPLC) instead of erythrocytes.[64] Talwar et al.[64] compared the direct HPLC method to assess TPP with the indirect assay to measure ETK activity. The results showed that HPLC can be used to separate and directly measure not only TPP in blood, but also thiamin and TMP status as accurately as the ETK activation test, with slightly better detection of thiamin deficiency detection obtained using the HPLC method over the ETK test.[64,65] Sgouros et al.[30] used the HPLC direct method to detect thiamin deficiency status in individuals with alcohol-dependence syndrome before and after administration of thiamin treatment. The results demonstrated the effectiveness of HPLC in identifying thiamin deficiency in erythrocytes with an inter-batch precision of 5.7%. For urinary excretion, administration of 5 mg loading dose of thiamin was suggested to evaluate thiamin status, and the cut point to be considered thiamin deficient was a value of <20µg of thiamin or its derivatives.[60]

VII. THIAMIN IN PHYSICAL ACTIVITY AND EXERCISE

Thiamin is important for physically active individuals, given its critical role in carbohydrate and amino acid metabolism. Manore[67] reported that thiamin, riboflavin, vitamin B-6, niacin, pantothenic acid and biotin are involved in energy production during exercise. Consequently, it has been suggested that thiamin deficiency may lead to decreased athletic performance.[68] To investigate whether physical activity and exercise increase the dietary requirements of thiamin, researchers have compared whether thiamin intake is different between athletes and less active individuals.[69–72] Others have also studied the effects of thiamin supplementation on physical performance.[73,74] The results of these studies demonstrate that athletes seem to consume different amounts of thiamin, yet supplementing with thiamin or thiamin derivatives over a short period of time does not seem to improve athletic performance.

Since thiamin is required for the production of adenosine triphosphate, its requirements have usually been expressed relative to energy intake, which tends to vary according to the level of physical activity. For instance, Niekamp and Baer[75] reported the average energy and CHO intakes for trained male cross-country runners were 3,248 ± 580 kcal and 497 ± 134 g/day, respectively, levels that were higher than the average recommended intakes of less active men in the same age group. Thiamin intake also tended to be higher (2.1 mg/day) than the recommended intake when energy and CHO intakes were higher.[75] Similar findings of thiamin intake have been reported by Fogelholm et al.[76] However, Elmafda et al.[77] observed that thiamin status decreased when relative carbohydrate intake increased during isoenergetic diets. That is, while maintaining a constant energy intake, increasing the relative intake of carbohydrates seems to decrease thiamin status, albeit the enzymatic activity of relevant metabolic pathways remains unchanged. Taken together, athletes who increase total energy intake seem to minimize the risk for thiamin deficiency, even with increased carbohydrate intake (in absolute terms).

Rokitzki et al.[71] estimated the nutritional needs of athletes from several sports (marathon, football or American soccer, handball, basketball and wrestling). They observed significant differences in dietary and energy intakes between well-trained athletes and controls, and the athletes' serum thiamin levels were twofold higher. Another study by Rokitzki et al.[78] reported that 35.4% of the athletes tested had lower thiamin intake than the German recommendation for thiamin intake (0.5 mg/1000 kcal), and about 87% of the athletes had less than satisfactory blood thiamin levels. Based on the correlations between thiamin intake and blood concentrations of thiamin, they suggested the two measurements could be an effective means of determining thiamin status in athletes. In a similar study, Rankinen et al.[79] compared the nutritional habits of Finnish ski jumpers with age-matched controls. They reported that body weight and energy intake were lower in the ski jumpers than control subjects, yet thiamin intakes were similar between groups.

While some studies have demonstrated differences between athletes and controls, others have shown no effect of training or exercise on thiamin status.[80,81] Nutter et al.[82] compared the seasonal changes of dietary intake between athletes and non-athletes and showed no differences between groups for energy or thiamin intake.[82] Also, following prolonged exercise (a 100-km race walk) no differences in thiamin status were observed relative to pre-exercise values.[83]

As for the efficacy of thiamin supplementation, several studies have investigated whether dietary supplementation of B-complex vitamins affects exercise performance in athletes and non-athletes. For example, Suzuki and Itokawa[84] studied the metabolic effect of a high dose of thiamin (100mg/d) on exercise recovery in cyclists. The result showed that a high dose of thiamin seems to enhance subjective attributes of recovery following exercise-induced fatigue.[84] In addition, thiamin (300mg/d and 90mg/d) has been shown to improve neurological and motor function in target-shooting sports compared with a control group that experienced a decline in physical and motor performance.[85] That study also observed that performance improved with the duration of supplementation, indicating that the potential neurological benefits of thiamin supplementation result from chronic supplementation instead of an acute response.

Doyle et al.[73] studied the effects of allithiamin on isokinetic exercise performance in healthy college students (n=15). A randomized, double-blind, counterbalanced crossover design was used. The supplementation scheme consisted of consuming allithiamin (1 g/day) or a placebo for 5 consecutive days. The exercise testing consisted of isokinetic knee extensions and flexions for six sets. They observed no differences in peak or average torque, average power output or total work performed between treatments. Using lactate accumulation in the blood as a surrogate of glycolytic activity, they observed no differences in lactate accumulation during or following the exercise.

In a similar study from the same group, Webster[86] investigated the effects of derivatives of thiamin (allithiamin) and pantothenic acid (pantethine) on 2,000m time trial performance in trained cyclists (VO_2max=61.8 ± 2.1 ml O2/kg/min; n=6). The subjects supplemented with the intervention compound (1 g of allithiamin and 1.8 g of a pantethine–pantothenic acid compound) or a placebo for 7 days. A randomized double-blind crossover design was used so that each subject served as his or her own control. On the testing days, the cyclists performed a steady-state 50 km ride at 60% of their VO_2max followed by the 2,000m time trial. Performance times were not different (p=0.58) between the treatment ride (170.7 ± 10.2 s) or the placebo ride (178 ± 8.4 s). However, even though the rides were not statistically different, the 8-second difference between groups might be of athletic importance. The results from these two studies seem to indicate that supplementation with thiamin derivatives does not enhance glycolytic-dependent exercise in trained or untrained men.

Using a longer supplementation period, Fogelholm et al.[70] observed that 5 weeks of supplementation with a B-complex vitamin in physically active college students (n=42) did not enhance exercise performance even though the activation coefficients were different (p < 0.001) between the supplement group and the placebo group. They stated that although there were differences in the activity coefficients, exercise-induced lactate accumulation was not different. This study also demonstrates that improvements in vitamin status (as the students had marginal vitamin status), do not always equate to alterations in exercise metabolism. This outcome is supported by another study[68] that reported thiamin restriction does not decrease short-duration high-intensity-exercise performance. Also, they did not report any correlations between thiamin status and exercise performance.[68]

Collectively, the available data seem to indicate that some athletes may be at risk for thiamin deficiency; however, that deficiency may not affect athletic performance in competitions relying heavily on glycolytic energy production. Likewise, supplementation with thiamin and thiamin derivatives does not seem to affect glycolytic energy production, but may be of value to athletes competing in sports that rely heavily on neurologic activity (e.g., hand-eye coordination). Table 3.1 summarizes the results of some studies that were performed to assess the thiamin status in physically active individuals.

TABLE 3.1
Results of Some Studies Performed to Assess the Thiamin Status in Physically Active Individuals

Reference	Subjects (n)	Intervention	Thiamin/Exercise Assessment	Thiamin Intake
Frank et al.[83]	Leisure athletes (42)	100-km race (walk)	Total blood thiamin Initial = 16.2 ± 8.8nmol/l After finish = 23.1 ± 9.4nmol/l ETK = 3.58 ± 0.66ukat/l	ND*
Ziegler et al.[80]	Elite figure skaters (41)	Descriptive	ND	1.6 ± 1.4 mg/day
Rokitzki et al.[78]	Trained athletes (various sports) (62)	Descriptive	Total blood thiamin = 151–308nmol/l ETK = 1.09–1.21 Urine = 0.99–1.42 umol/g Cr.	1.3–1.9 mg/day
Fogelholm[81]	Fitness exercised females (21) Controls (18)	Descriptive	ETK-AC Exercised = 1.16 Control = 1.14	Exercised = 1.3 mg Control = 1.3 mg
Berning et al.[72]	Swimmers(43)	Descriptive	ND	2.5 ± 0.09 mg
Rankinen et al.[79]	Elite ski jumpers (21) Controls (20)	Descriptive	No difference in hematological differences between groups	Ski jumpers = 1.6mg Control = 2.0mg $p = 0.07$
Fogelholm et al.[70]	Healthy college students Supplemented (n = 22) Placebo (n = 20)	Supplementation 15 mg/d	Supplementation Decreased EKT	ND
Doyle et al.[73]	Allithiamin (1 g/d) (15) Placebo (15)	Supplementation (5 days) 1g/d	No differences in isokinetic exercise performance	ND
Webster et al.[74]	Thiamin tetrahydrofurfuryl Disulfide (1 g/d) (14) Placebo (14)	Supplementation (4 days)	No difference in performance outcomes	ND
Webster[86]	Allithiamin + Pantethine (n = 6) (1 g allithiamine + 1.8 g pantethine/pantothenic acid) Placebo (n = 6)	Supplementation (7 days)	No difference in 2,000m time trial performance	ND

* Not determined

TABLE 3.2
Recommended Dietary Allowance of Thiamin

Life Stage	Age	Males (mg/day)	Females (mg/day)
Infants	0–6 months	0.2 (AI)*	0.2 (AI)
	7–12 months	0.3 (AI)	0.3 (AI)
Children	1–3 years	0.5	0.5
	4–8 years	0.6	0.6
	9–13 years	0.9	0.9
Adolescents	14–18 years	1.2	1.0
Adults	19 years and older	1.2	1.1
Pregnancy		—	1.4
Lactating		—	1.4

*AI = Adequate Intake

VIII.   THIAMIN RECOMMENDATION

The dietary requirement for thiamin is generally proportional to the caloric intake of the diet and ranges from 1.0–1.5 mg/day for normal adults. If the carbohydrate content of the diet is excessive, an increased thiamin intake is recommended.[77]

Dietary recommendations for thiamin are different according to the age, sex and physiological status of the individuals. The recommendations for thiamin are given in Table 3.2.

IX.   FOOD SOURCES OF THIAMIN

Thiamin is found in small quantities in many plant and animal foods. Good sources of thiamin include lean pork, beef, liver, yeast, whole grains, enriched grains and legumes. Table 3.3 shows some sources and content of thiamin.

TABLE 3.3
Some Food Sources of Thiamin

Food	Serving	Thiamin (mg)
Worthington Food, Morningstar Farm "Burger" crumbles	1 cup (240 ml)	9.92
Cereals ready-to-eat	3/4 cup (180 ml)	2.11
General Mills, whole Grain Total		
Fortified breakfast cereal (different types)	1 cup (240 ml)	0.5–2.0
Pork, lean (cooked)	3 ounces (90 g)	0.98
Oat bran (cooked)	1 cup (240 ml)	0.35
Peas (cooked)	1/2 cup (120 ml)	0.21
Long-grain white rice, enriched (cooked)	1 cup (240 ml)	0.44
Long-grain white rice (cooked)	1 cup (240 ml)	0.26
Pecans	1 ounce (30 g)	0.13
White bread, enriched	1 slice (30 g)	0.12
Orange	1 fruit	0.11
Whole wheat bread	1 slice (30 g)	0.10
Milk	1 cup (240 ml)	0.10
Spinach (cooked)	1/2 cup (120)	0.09
Egg (cooked)	1 large	0.03

X. BIOAVAILABILITY OF THIAMIN

In general, thiamin bioavailability is affected by many factors, including:

1. Interaction with compounds that are present in the same food sources, including polyphenolic and sulfite compounds; and thiamin analogues that directly affect thiamin bioavailability.[87]
2. Food processing and processing conditions (i.e., high temperature; added compounds such as alkaline solutions that are used in the food industry can degrade thiamin and reduce bioavailability.[62]
3. Drug–nutrient interaction: low blood levels of thiamin have been reported in patients taking anticonvulsant medication.[88] Additionally, 5-Fluorouracil, a drug used in cancer therapy, inhibits the phosphorylation of thiamin to thiamin pyrophosphate (TPP).[89]
4. As stated previously, high consumption of alcohol interferes with absorption of thiamin;[90] likewise, diuretics, especially furosemide, may increase the risk of thiamin deficiency in individuals with marginal thiamin intake due to increased urinary excretion of thiamin.[91,92]

XI. SUPPLEMENTATION OF THIAMIN

Thiamin is available in nutritional supplements and fortification in two forms — thiamin hydro-chloride and thiamin nitrate. Because alcohol inhibits thiamin absorption, high doses of thiamin are typically administered in the treatment of alcoholism. Thiamin supplementation may also be prescribed for those with sepsis, since infections increase cellular energy requirements and therefore thiamin requirements. To treat beriberi, thiamin administration ranges from 50–100 mg given intravenously or intramuscularly for 1 or 2 weeks. The dose can then be decreased to 10 mg until the patient recovers. A dose of 100mg/d has been suggested for athletes for recovering from exercise-induced fatigue.[84]

XII. TOXICITY OF THIAMIN

Toxicity is generally not a problem with thiamin because renal clearance is very rapid. Because there is no evidence of toxic effects of excess thiamin intake, no tolerable upper level has been set for its intake from food sources and through long-term supplementation up to 200mg/d.[65]

XIII. FUTURE RESEARCH

Thiamin has been studied for more than 50 years as an important cofactor for carbohydrate and protein metabolism and for its non-cofactor function as a neuro-protective nutrient. Thiamin intake has also been assessed in active and sedentary individuals. However, there is no supporting evidence to determine whether physical activity increases thiamin requirement. Therefore, future research should focus on the metabolism of thiamin status in sedentary and physically active groups to determine whether the physically active individuals do indeed require a greater intake of thiamin.

XIV. SUMMARY

Thiamin is an important micronutrient for energy metabolism and for neurological functions in humans, with requirements differing according to the physiological status and energy intake. Athletes may require more energy intake than other individuals, but further research is needed to better understand the role of thiamin in athletic performance.

REFERENCES

1. Thiamine. Monograph, *Altern Med Rev* 8 (1), 59–62, 2003.
2. Rindi, G., Patrini, C., Nauti, A., Bellazzi, R. and Magni, P., Three thiamine analogues differently alter thiamine transport and metabolism in nervous tissue: An *in vivo* kinetic study using rats, *Metab Brain Dis* 18 (4), 245–63, 2003.
3. Smidt, L.J., Cremin, F.M., Grivetti, L.E. and Clifford, A.J., Influence of thiamin supplementation on the health and general well-being of an elderly Irish population with marginal thiamin deficiency, *J Gerontol* 46 (1), M16–22, 1991.
4. Hickson, J.F., Jr., Schrader, J., Pivarnik, J.M. and Stockton, J.E., Nutritional intake from food sources of soccer athletes during two stages of training, *Nutr Rep Int* 34 (85), 1986.
5. Guilland, J.C., Penaranda, T., Gallet, C., Boggio, V., Fuchs, F. and Klepping, J., Vitamin status of young athletes including the effects of supplementation, *Med Sci Sports Exerc* 21 (4), 441–9, 1989.
6. Henderson, S.A., Black, A.L. and Brooks, G.A., Leucine turnover and oxidation in trained rats during exercise, *Am J Physiol* 249 (2 Pt 1), E137–44, 1985.
7. Layman, D.K., Paul, G., and Olken, M.H., Amino acid metabolism during exercise, in *Nutrition in Exercise and Sport*, 2nd ed., Wolinsky, I., Hickson, J.F. and Hickson, J.F., Jr. CRC Press, Boca Raton, FL, 1994.
8. Rindi, G. and Laforenza, U., Thiamine intestinal transport and related issues: Recent aspects, *Proc Soc Exp Biol Med* 224 (4), 246–55, 2000.
9. Wostheinrich, K. and Schmidt, P.C., Polymorphic changes of thiamine hydrochloride during granulation and tableting, *Drug Dev Ind Pharm* 27 (6), 481–9, 2001.
10. Molina, P.E., Myers, N., Smith, R.M., Lang, C.H., Yousef, K.A., Tepper, P.G. and Abumrad, N.N., Nutritional and metabolic characterization of a thiamine-deficient rat model, *J Parenter Enteral Nutr (JPEN)*, 18 (2), 104–11, 1994.
11. Egi, Y., Koyama, S., Shioda, T., Yamada, K. and Kawasaki, T., Identification, purification and reconstitution of thiamin metabolizing enzymes in human red blood cells, *Biochim Biophys Acta* 1160 (2), 171–8, 1992.
12. Bos, M. and Kozik, A., Some molecular and enzymatic properties of a homogeneous preparation of thiaminase I purified from carp liver, *J Protein Chem* 19 (2), 75–84, 2000.
13. Boros, L. G., Population thiamine status and varying cancer rates between western, Asian and African countries, *Anticancer Res* 20 (3B), 2245–8, 2000.
14. Pyo, D., Separation of vitamins by supercritical fluid chromatography with water-modified carbon dioxide as the mobile phase, *J Biochem Biophys Meth* 43 (1–3), 113–23, 2000.
15. Sanchez-Machado, D.I., Lopez-Cervantes, J., Lopez-Hernandez, J. and Paseiro-Losada, P., Simultaneous determination of thiamine and riboflavin in edible marine seaweeds by high-performance liquid chromatography, *J Chromatogr Sci* 42 (3), 117–20, 2004.
16. Markopoulou, C.K., Kagkadis, K.A. and Koundourellis, J.E., An optimized method for the simultaneous determination of vitamins B1, B6, B12 in multivitamin tablets by high performance liquid chromatography, *J Pharm Biomed Anal* 30 (4), 1403–10, 2002.
17. Mancinelli, R., Ceccanti, M., Guiducci, M.S., Sasso, G.F., Sebastiani, G., Attilia, M.L. and Allen, J.P., Simultaneous liquid chromatographic assessment of thiamine, thiamine monophosphate and thiamine diphosphate in human erythrocytes: A study on alcoholics, *J Chromatogr B Analyt Technol Biomed Life Sci* 789 (2), 355–63, 2003.
18. Tallaksen, C.M., Bell, H. and Bohmer, T., Thiamin and thiamin phosphate ester deficiency assessed by high performance liquid chromatography in four clinical cases of Wernicke encephalopathy, *Alcohol Clin Exp Res* 17 (3), 712–6, 1993.
19. Li, Y. and Brown, P.R., The optimization of HPLC-UV conditions for use with FTIR detection in the analysis of B vitamins, *J Chromatogr Sci* 41 (2), 96–9, 2003.
20. Liu, S., Zhang, Z., Liu, Q., Luo, H. and Zheng, W., Spectrophotometric determination of vitamin B1 in a pharmaceutical formulation using triphenylmethane acid dyes, *J Pharm Biomed Anal* 30 (3), 685–94, 2002.
21. Grandfils, C., Bettendorff, L., de Rycker, C. and Schoffeniels, E., Synthesis of [gamma-32P]thiamine triphosphate, *Anal Biochem* 169 (2), 274–8, 1988.

22. Bettendorff, L., Nghiem, H. O., Wins, P. and Lakaye, B., A general method for the chemical synthesis of gamma-32P-labeled or unlabeled nucleoside 5(')-triphosphates and thiamine triphosphate, *Anal Biochem* 322 (2), 190–7, 2003.

23. Boulware, M.J., Subramanian, V.S., Said, H.M. and Marchant, J.S., Polarized expression of members of the solute carrier SLC19A gene family of water-soluble multivitamin transporters: implications for physiological function, *Biochem J* 376 (Pt 1), 43–8, 2003.

24. Begley, T.P., The biosynthesis and degradation of thiamin (vitamin B1), *Nat Prod Rep* 13 (3), 177–85, 1996.

25. Settembre, E., Begley, T.P. and Ealick, S.E., Structural biology of enzymes of the thiamin biosynthesis pathway, *Curr Opin Struct Biol* 13 (6), 739–47, 2003.

26. Leonardi, R. and Roach, P.L., Thiamine biosynthesis in *Escherichia coli: In vitro* reconstitution of the thiazole synthase activity, *J Biol Chem* 279 (17), 17054–62, 2004.

27. Morett, E., Korbel, J.O., Rajan, E., Saab-Rincon, G., Olvera, L., Olvera, M., Schmidt, S., Snel, B. and Bork, P., Systematic discovery of analogous enzymes in thiamin biosynthesis, *Nat Biotechnol* 21 (7), 790–5, 2003.

28. Park, J.H., Dorrestein, P.C., Zhai, H., Kinsland, C., McLafferty, F.W. and Begley, T.P., Biosynthesis of the thiazole moiety of thiamin pyrophosphate (vitamin B1), *Biochemistry* 42 (42), 12430–8, 2003.

29. Melnick, J.S., Sprinz, K.I., Reddick, J.J., Kinsland, C. and Begley, T.P., An efficient enzymatic synthesis of thiamin pyrophosphate, *Bioorg Med Chem Lett* 13 (22), 4139–41, 2003.

30. Sgouros, X., Baines, M., Bloor, R.N., McAuley, R., Ogundipe, L.O. and Willmott, S., Evaluation of a clinical screening instrument to identify states of thiamine deficiency inpatients with severe alcohol dependence syndrome, *Alcohol Alcohol.* 39 (3), 227–32, 2004.

31. Rindi, G., Some aspects of thiamin transport in mammals, *J Nutr Sci Vitaminol* (Tokyo) Spec No, 379–82, 1992.

32. Dudeja, P.K., Tyagi, S., Kavilaveettil, R.J., Gill, R. and Said, H.M., Mechanism of thiamine uptake by human jejunal brush-border membrane vesicles, *Am J Physiol Cell Physiol* 281 (3), C786–92, 2001.

33. Rindi, G. and Ferrari, G., Thiamine transport by the small intestine *in vitro*, *Experientia* 33, 211–213, 1997.

34. Ricci, V. and Rindi, G., Thiamin uptake by rat isolated enterocytes: Relationship between transport and phosphorylation, *Arch Int Physiol Biochim Biophys* 100 (3), 275–9, 1992.

35. Rindi, G., Ricci, V., Gastaldi, G. and Patrini, C., Intestinal alkaline phosphatase can transphosphorylate thiamin to thiamin monophosphate during intestinal transport in the rat, *Arch Physiol Biochem* 103 (1), 33–8, 1995.

36. Singleton, C.K. and Martin, P.R., Molecular mechanisms of thiamine utilization, *Curr Mol Med* 1 (2), 197–207, 2001.

37. Butterworth, R.F., Kril, J.J. and Harper, C.G., Thiamine-dependent enzyme changes in the brains of alcoholics: relationship to the Wernicke-Korsakoff syndrome, *Alcohol Clin Exp Res* 17 (5), 1084–8, 1993.

38. Bender, D.A., Optimum nutrition: thiamin, biotin and pantothenate, *Proc Nutr Soc* 58 (2), 427–33, 1999.

39. Martin, P.R., Singleton, C.K. and Hiller-Sturmhofel, S., The role of thiamine deficiency in alcoholic brain disease, *Alcohol Res Health* 27 (2), 134–42, 2003.

40. La Selva, M., Beltramo, E., Pagnozzi, F., Bena, E., Molinatti, P.A., Molinatti, G.M. and Porta, M., Thiamine corrects delayed replication and decreases production of lactate and advanced glycation end-products in bovine retinal and human umbilical vein endothelial cells cultured under high glucose conditions, *Diabetologia* 39 (11), 1263–8, 1996.

41. Czerniecki, J., Chanas, G., Verlaet, M., Bettendorff, L., Makarchikov, A.F., Leprince, P., Wins, P., Grisar, T. and Lakaye, B., Neuronal localization of the 25-kDa specific thiamine triphosphatase in rodent brain, *Neuroscience* 125 (4), 833–40, 2004.

42. Bettendorff, L., A non-cofactor role of thiamine derivatives in excitable cells? *Arch Physiol Biochem* 104 (6), 745–51, 1996.

43. Bettendorff, L., Hennuy, B., De Clerck, A. and Wins, P., Chloride permeability of rat brain membrane vesicles correlates with thiamine triphosphate content, *Brain Res* 652 (1), 157–60, 1994.

44. Butterworth, R. F., Thiamin deficiency and brain disorders, *Nutr Res Revs* 16 (2), 277–283, 2003.

45. Bettendorff, L., Michel-Cahay, C., Grandfils, C., De Rycker, C. and Schoffeniels, E., Thiamine triphosphate and membrane-associated thiamine phosphatases in the electric organ of *Electrophorus electricus, J Neurochem* 49 (2), 495–502, 1987.
46. Soukaloun, D., Kounnavong, S., Pengdy, B., Boupha, B., Durondej, S., Olness, K., Newton, P.N. and White, N.J., Dietary and socio-economic factors associated with beriberi in breastfed Lao infants, *Ann Trop Paediatr* 23 (3), 181–6, 2003.
47. Harper, C., Dixon, G., Sheedy, D. and Garrick, T., Neuropathological alterations in alcoholic brains. Studies arising from the New South Wales Tissue Resource Centre, *Prog Neuropsychopharmacol Biol Psychiatry* 27 (6), 951–61, 2003.
48. Svahn, J., Schiaffino, M.C., Caruso, U., Calvillo, M., Minniti, G. and Dufour, C., Severe lactic acidosis due to thiamine deficiency in a patient with B-cell leukemia/lymphoma on total parenteral nutrition during high-dose methotrexate therapy, *J Pediatr Hematol Oncol* 25 (12), 965–8, 2003.
49. Hahn, J.S., Berquist, W., Alcorn, D.M., Chamberlain, L. and Bass, D., Wernicke encephalopathy and beriberi during total parenteral nutrition attributable to multivitamin infusion shortage, *Pediatrics* 101 (1), E10, 1998.
50. Pitkin, S.R. and Savage, L.M., Age-related vulnerability to diencephalic amnesia produced by thiamine deficiency: the role of time of insult, *Behav Brain Res* 148 (1–2), 93–105, 2004.
51. Morin, K., Thiamine (vitamin B1) revisited, MCN *Am J Matern Child Nurs* 29 (3), 200, 2004.
52. Tatibouet, L. and Tatibouet, M.H., [Congestive heart failure due to chronic alcoholism (author's transl in French,)], *Sem Hop* 58 (16), 991–6, 1982.
53. Betrosian, A.P., Thireos, E., Toutouzas, K., Zabaras, P., Papadimitriou, K. and Sevastos, N., Occidental beriberi and sudden death, *Am J Med Sci* 327 (5), 250–2, 2004.
54. Krishna, S., Taylor, A.M., Supanaranond, W., Pukrittayakamee, S., ter Kuile, F., Tawfiq, K.M., Holloway, P.A. and White, N.J., Thiamine deficiency and malaria in adults from southeast Asia, *Lancet* 353 (9152), 546–9, 1999.
55. Roman, G.C., An epidemic in Cuba of optic neuropathy, sensorineural deafness, peripheral sensory neuropathy and dorsolateral myeloneuropathy, *J Neurol Sci* 127 (1), 11–28, 1994.
56. Robinson, K., Wernicke's encephalopathy, *Emerg Nurse* 11 (5), 30–3, 2003.
57. Nicolas, J.M., Fernandez-Sola, J., Robert, J., Antunez, E., Cofan, M., Cardenal, C., Sacanella, E., Estruch, R. and Urbano-Marquez, A., High ethanol intake and malnutrition in alcoholic cerebellar shrinkage, *QJM* 93 (7), 449–56, 2000.
58. Stacey, P.S. and Sullivan, K.A., Preliminary investigation of thiamine and alcohol intake in clinical and healthy samples, *Psychol Rep* 94 (3 Pt 1), 845–8, 2004.
59. Homewood, J. and Bond, N.W., Thiamin deficiency and Korsakoff's syndrome: failure to find memory impairments following nonalcoholic Wernicke's encephalopathy, *Alcohol* 19 (1), 75–84, 1999.
60. Finglas, P.M., Thiamin, *Int J Vitam Nutr Res* 63 (4), 270–4, 1993.
61. Baines, M. and Davies, G., The evaluation of erythrocyte thiamin diphosphate as an indicator of thiamin status in man and its comparison with erythrocyte transketolase activity measurements, *Ann Clin Biochem* 25 (Pt 6), 698–705, 1988.
62. Gregory, J.F., III, Bioavailability of thiamin, *Eur J Clin Nutr* 51 Suppl 1, S34-7, 1997.
63. Mataix, J., Aranda, P., Sanchez, C., Montellano, M.A., Planells, E. and Llopis, J., Assessment of thiamin (vitamin B_1) and riboflavin (vitamin B_2) status in an adult Mediterranean population, *Br J Nutr* 90 (3), 661–6, 2003.
64. Talwar, D., Davidson, H., Cooney, J. and St. James O'Reilly, D., Vitamin B_1 status assessed by direct measurement of thiamin pyrophosphate in erythrocytes or whole blood by HPLC: comparison with erythrocyte transketolase activation assay, *Clin Chem* 46 (5), 704–10, 2000.
65. *Thiamin in Dietary Reference Intakes: Thiamin, Riboflavin, Niacin, Vitamin B-6, Vitamin B12, Pantothenic Acid, Biotin and Choline.* National Academy Press, Washington D.C., 1998, pp. 58–86.
66. Howard, J. M., Assessment of vitamin B(1) status, *Clin Chem* 46 (11), 1867–8, 2000.
67. Manore, M.M., Effect of physical activity on thiamine, riboflavin and vitamin B6 requirements, *Am J Clin Nutr* 72 (2 Suppl), 598S–606S, 2000.
68. van der Beek, E.J., van Dokkum, W., Wedel, M., Schrijver, J. and van den Berg, H., Thiamin, riboflavin and vitamin B6: Impact of restricted intake on physical performance in man, *J Am Coll Nutr* 13 (6), 629–40, 1994.

69. Fogelholm, M., Rehunen, S., Gref, C.G., Laakso, J.T., Lehto, J., Ruokonen, I. and Himberg, J.J., Dietary intake and thiamin, iron and zinc status in elite Nordic skiers during different training periods, *Int J Sport Nutr* 2 (4), 351–65, 1992.

70. Fogelholm, M., Ruokonen, I., Laakso, J. T., Vuorimaa, T. and Himberg, J. J., Lack of association between indices of vitamin B_1, B_2 and B_6 status and exercise-induced blood lactate in young adults, *Int J Sport Nutr* 3 (2), 165–76, 1993.

71. Rokitzki, L., Berg, A. and Keul, J., Blood and serum status of water- and fat-soluble vitamins in athletes and non-athletes, *Int J Vitam Nutr Res Suppl* 30, 192–7, 1989.

72. Berning, J.R., Troup, J.P., VanHandel, P.J., Daniels, J. and Daniels, N., The nutritional habits of young adolescent swimmers, *Int J Sport Nutr* 1 (3), 240–8, 1991.

73. Doyle, M.R., Webster, M.J. and Erdmann, L.D., Allithiamine ingestion does not enhance isokinetic parameters of muscle performance, *Int J Sport Nutr* 7 (1), 39–47, 1997.

74. Webster, M.J., Scheett, T.P., Doyle, M.R. and Branz, M., The effect of a thiamin derivative on exercise performance, *Eur J Appl Physiol Occup Physiol* 75 (6), 520–4, 1997.

75. Niekamp, R.A. and Baer, J.T., In-season dietary adequacy of trained male cross-country runners, *Int J Sport Nutr* 5 (1), 45–55, 1995.

76. Fogelholm, M., Tikkanen, H., Naveri, H. and Harkonen, M., High-carbohydrate diet for long distance runners: A practical viewpoint, *Br J Sports Med* 23 (2), 94–6, 1989.

77. Elmadfa, I., Majchrzak, D., Rust, P. and Genser, D., The thiamine status of adult humans depends on carbohydrate intake, *Int J Vitam Nutr Res* 71 (4), 217–21, 2001.

78. Rokitzki, L., Sagredos, A., Logemann, E., Sauer, B., Buchner, M. and Keul, J., Vitamin B_1 status in athletes of various types of sports, *Med Exerc Nutr Health* 3, 240–247, 1994.

79. Rankinen, T., Lyytikainen, S., Vanninen, E., Penttila, I., Rauramaa, R. and Uusitupa, M., Nutritional status of Finnish elite ski jumpers, *Med Sci Sports Exerc* 30 (11), 1592–7, 1998.

80. Ziegler, P.J., Nelson, J.A. and Jonnalagadda, S.S., Nutritional and physiological status of U.S. national figure skaters, *Int J Sport Nutr* 9 (4), 345–60, 1999.

81. Fogelholm, M., Micronutrient status in females during a 24-week fitness-type exercise program, *Ann Nutr Metab* 36 (4), 209–18, 1992.

82. Nutter, J., Seasonal changes in female athletes' diets, *Int J Sport Nutr* 1 (4), 395–407, 1991.

83. Frank, T., Kuhl, M., Makowski, B., Bitsch, R., Jahreis, G. and Hubscher, J., Does a 100-km walking affect indicators of vitamin status? *Int J Vitam Nutr Res* 70 (5), 238–50, 2000.

84. Suzuki, M. and Itokawa, Y., Effects of thiamine supplementation on exercise-induced fatigue, *Metab Brain Dis* 11 (1), 95–106, 1996.

85. Bonke, D. and Nickel, B., Improvement of fine motoric movement control by elevated dosages of vitamin B_1, B_6 and B_{12} in target shooting, *Int J Vitam Nutr Res Suppl* 30, 198–204, 1989.

86. Webster, M.J., Physiological and performance responses to supplementation with thiamin and pantothenic acid derivatives, *Eur J Appl Physiol Occup Physiol* 77 (6), 486–91, 1998.

87. Rains, T.M., Emmert, J.L., Baker, D.H. and Shay, N.F., Minimum thiamin requirement of weanling Sprague-Dawley outbred rats, *J Nutr* 127 (1), 167–70, 1997.

88. Botez, M.I. and Young, S.N., Effects of anticonvulsant treatment and low levels of folate and thiamine on amine metabolites in cerebrospinal fluid, *Brain* 114 (Pt 1A), 333–48, 1991.

89. Schumann, K., Interactions between drugs and vitamins at advanced age, *Int J Vitam Nutr Res* 69 (3), 173–8, 1999.

90. van den Berg, H., van der Gaag, M. and Hendriks, H., Influence of lifestyle on vitamin bioavailability, *Int J Vitam Nutr Res* 72 (1), 53–9, 2002.

91. Rieck, J., Halkin, H., Almog, S., Seligman, H., Lubetsky, A., Olchovsky, D. and Ezra, D., Urinary loss of thiamine is increased by low doses of furosemide in healthy volunteers, *J Lab Clin Med* 134 (3), 238–43, 1999.

92. da Cunha, S., Albanesi Filho, F.M., da Cunha Bastos, V.L., Antelo, D.S. and Souza, M.M., Thiamin, selenium and copper levels in patients with idiopathic dilated cardiomyopathy taking diuretics, *Arq Bras Cardiol* 79 (5), 454–65, 2002.

4 Riboflavin

Susan H. Mitmesser, Ph.D.

CONTENTS

I. INTRODUCTION

Riboflavin (7,8-dimethyl-10-ribityl-isoalloxazine) was first isolated from milk whey in 1879 and occurs naturally in a wide variety of foods. Its most important biologically active forms participate in many of the redox reactions that are absolutely crucial to the function of aerobic cells and are cofactors for many metabolic reactions that produce energy. There is particular interest in the role riboflavin may play as an ergogenic aid due to these metabolic properties. Is it reasonable to assume that, as a person becomes more physically active and energy and protein intakes increase, riboflavin needs increase? Micronutrient needs may not rise with increased energy and protein intake if adequate dietary choices are made. However, if energy and protein intake are restricted while physical activity is increased, the need for certain micronutrients may further increase. This chapter will address relevant research concerning the effects of physical activity on riboflavin status, as well as recent evidence for the use of riboflavin as a performance enhancer.

II. CHEMICAL STRUCTURE AND METABOLIC ROLES

Riboflavin, or vitamin B_2, is a water-soluble vitamin involved in many metabolic reactions. Consisting of an isoalloxazine ring, it is chemically referred to as 7,8-dimethyl-10-(1'-D-ribity).[1] Riboflavin is responsible for the synthesis of coenzymes, flavin mononucleotide (FMN) and flavin adenine dinucleotide (FAD), which are important in the metabolism of glucose, fatty acids, glycerol and amino acids for energy.[1,2] Specifically, FMN and FAD are critical coenzymes involved in glycolysis, tricarboxylic acid cycle (TCA) and β-oxidation. These coenzymes act as electron carriers and assist in redox reactions classified as dehydrogenases, oxidases and monooxygenases by serving as either one-electron (FMNH, FADH) or two-electron ($FMNH_2$, $FADH_2$) acceptors or donors.[1] Additionally, riboflavin is involved in the conversion of vitamin B_6 into its functional coenzyme.[3–6]

The majority of riboflavin found in food is in the form of FAD. Smaller amounts are present in the form of FMN and free riboflavin, which is an isoalloxazine ring bound to a ribitol side chain, with the absorption half-life of about 1.1 h.[7] Flavins that are covalently bound do not appear to be available for absorption. However, FAD and FMN are predominantly in a non-covalently-bound form attached to an enzyme. FAD and FMN must be hydrolyzed to riboflavin before absorption can occur. Nonspecific phosphatases in the brush border membranes of enterocytes are responsible for this catalysis.[8] Once in the enterocytes, free riboflavin undergoes ATP-dependent phosphorylation, which is catalyzed by cytosolic flavokinase to form FMN; it can now enter the plasma and small intestine. However, most of this is further converted to FAD by the FAD-dependent FAD synthetase.[9] In the rare instance when riboflavin may be in excess, it is excreted in the urine as riboflavin, 7-hydroxymethylriboflavin (7-α-hydroxyriboflavin), or luminflavin.[10]

III. DIETARY SOURCES

Riboflavin is a water-soluble B-complex vitamin found in animal and vegetable products. The primary food sources of riboflavin include: eggs, lean meats, milk, dairy products, broccoli and enriched breads and cereals.[1,3] In the western diet, milk and dairy products contribute the greatest amount of riboflavin. Naturally occurring grain products contain low amounts of riboflavin. However, fortification practices have allowed bread and cereal products to become very good sources of riboflavin. Although relatively heat-stable, riboflavin is readily degraded by light. The oxidative products of photolysis can damage milk lipids and are associated with flavor changes. This was an important consideration when milk was delivered in glass bottles.

There are no known toxicities associated with riboflavin. However, there is evidence of a possible dietary interaction; dietary fiber may reduce the absorptive ability of riboflavin. Roe et al. studied the effect of dietary fiber from wheat bran and psyllium gum on the absorption of riboflavin in healthy women. Determined by fluorometric techniques, psyllium gum and a combination of fiber supplements significantly reduced the 24-hour absorption of riboflavin by 31.8% and 26.1%, respectively. The wheat bran supplement had no effect on riboflavin aborption.[11]

IV. RECOMMENDED DIETARY ALLOWANCE

Riboflavin deficiency can lead to a variety of clinical abnormalities including degenerative changes in the nervous system, anemia, endocrine dysfunction and skin disorders, and can lead to an increase in the susceptibility to carcinogens.[12–14] Feeding studies, in which clinical signs and symptoms of riboflavin deficiency were observed, were used to determine the recommended dietary allowance (RDA).[15] The 1989 RDA for riboflavin was determined on the basis of energy and protein intake (0.6 mg/1000 kcal).[3] Specifically, men 23 to 50 years of age need 1.7 mg and women 23 to 50 years of age need 1.3 mg of riboflavin. Individuals 50+ years of age are recommended to consume less, based on lower energy requirements. The dietary reference intake (DRI) for riboflavin set in 1998 suggests an intake of 1.3 mg/d for men and 1.1 mg/d for women 19 to 70 years of age.[4]

V. ASSESSMENT OF STATUS

Assessment of riboflavin status should include direct and indirect biochemical measures, as well as dietary intake data (Table 4.1). While the degree of urinary riboflavin excretion is a direct reflection of tissue saturation, urinary excretion is not a sensitive marker of very low riboflavin intakes.[16] More appropriately, riboflavin status is determined by an oxidation-reduction reaction in which oxidized glutathione is reduced by GSSH in an FAD-dependent glutathione reductase reaction.[17,18] Specifically, riboflavin status is obtained by determining the erythrocyte riboflavin

TABLE 4.1
Biochemical Measures and Values Considered Inadequate of Riboflavin Status

Biochemical Measure	Inadequate Value
Plasma riboflavin	< 0.24 µmol/L
Erythrocyte riboflavin	< 270 nmol/L
Erythrocyte glutathione reductase activity coefficient	> 1.25
Urinary riboflavin	< 30 µg/g creatinine
Urinary riboflavin	< 40 µg/d

Source: Adapted from Fischbach[26] and Gibson.[27]

concentration measured by the urinary excretion of riboflavin. The erythrocyte glutathione reductase activity coefficient (EGRAC) can be calculated from the erythrocyte riboflavin concentration. EGRAC and the erythrocyte transketolase enzyme activity coefficient (ETKAC) are determined by dividing the stimulated enzyme activity (with added FAD) by the basal enzyme activity (without added FAD). Thus, a high EGRAC indicates impaired riboflavin status (low riboflavin excretion indicates deficiency). This technique of determining riboflavin status has been confirmed by human depletion studies.[2] Table 4.2 depicts frequently used cutoff values for EGRAC. The sensitivity of EGRAC, found to be useful in determining impaired riboflavin status, is the preferred method for assessing riboflavin status.[19] In women, it is important to note that the phase of the menstrual cycle should be considered when assessing riboflavin status, due to some blood and urinary assessment indexes influenced by recent nutrient intakes. Martini et al. found that riboflavin intakes were significantly higher in the midluteal phase than in the midfollicular phase of menstruating women.[20]

Few studies have actually determined riboflavin intake of athletes compared with their non-athletic counterparts. In a study conducted by Rokitzki et al., serum and blood concentrations of riboflavin were measured in athletes and non-athletes by high-pressure liquid chromatography (HPLC). Compared with non-athletes, the riboflavin status of body builders, cross-country cyclists, cross-country skiers and 3,000-m steeplechase athletes was greater.[21] According to Weight et al., the mean daily intake of riboflavin in athletes was above the RDA. Furthermore, blood riboflavin concentrations remained within the normal range throughout the study and no clinical evidence of toxicity was evident.[22] These studies reinforce the notion that athletes consuming a well balanced diet do not require vitamin and mineral supplements.[23–25]

TABLE 4.2
Frequently Used Cutoff Values for EGRAC Indicating Riboflavin Deficiency

Deficiency Status	Value
Adequate	<1.2
Low	1.2–1.4
Deficient	>1.4

Source: Adapted from McCormick, D.B. and Institute of Medicine.[1,4]

VI. EFFECTS OF PHYSICAL PERFORMANCE

Due to riboflavin's involvement in many metabolic functions critical to exercise performance, its use as a performance enhancer has emerged. Specifically, riboflavin is involved in muscle cell energy metabolism. Recall that FAD and FMN are important in the metabolism of glucose, fatty acids, glycerol and amino acids for energy. When physical activity is performed, stress is put upon the biochemical pathways involved in the metabolism of these substrates.[1,2,28]

Before we can examine riboflavin's role as an ergogenic aid, we need to evaluate the research available as to whether physical activity can actually influence the riboflavin requirement. To date, many studies have addressed this very issue.[2,28–32] However, it is important to note that several differences have emerged among the pool of research studies; such as exercise interventions in men versus women, the methodology in assessing riboflavin status and the length of the studies (i.e., 5 to 40 weeks). Several studies have examined the effect of vitamin deficiency on work performance.[2, 33–36] In particular, Suboticanec et al. found that 19% of 12–14 y boys enrolled in the study had poor riboflavin status.[33] After supplementation of 2 mg riboflavin was given for 6 days/week for 2 months, a linear relationship between EGRAC and maximal work capacity was observed. Thus, as EGRAC improved, work capacity improved. This suggests that subclincial deficiencies in riboflavin negatively affect aerobic capacity in young boys. Furthermore, work capacity has the potential to improve as the deficiency is corrected. Additionally, Haralambie examined the influence of riboflavin supplementation on neuromuscular irritability in athletes. After 10 mg riboflavin was administered, neuromuscular irritability was moderately lowered.[37]

A series of well documented studies conducted by Belko et al. examined exercise as an influence on riboflavin requirements.[28, 30, 38] To achieve EGRAC values under the 1.2 cutoff, researchers found that women needed to take in 0.96 µg/kcal and 1.16 µg/kcal riboflavin under sedentary and exercise conditions (6 weeks of running), respectively. The authors concluded that the RDA of 0.6 mg/1000 kcal was not sufficient to meet the needs of the study subjects, whether sedentary or exercising. Additionally, Belko and colleagues examined the relationship between riboflavin intake and aerobic performance. They concluded that riboflavin status was not related to aerobic capacity. When a riboflavin load (1.16 µg/kcal) was given, no improvement in aerobic capacity was observed.[38]

Winters et al.[32] repeated one of the first studies conducted by Belko et al.[30] Active women 50–67 y of age were fed a diet containing 1793–1983 kcal/day and either 0.14 mg/239 kcal or 0.22 mg/239 kcal riboflavin for 5 weeks. During the weeks the subjects were required to exercise (2.5 h/week), EGRAC significantly increased compared with the weeks when no exercise was performed. Furthermore, during the exercised weeks, 0.22 mg riboflavin was required to maintain mean EGRAC values within the normal range. This indicates that dieting alone or exercise alone may increase riboflavin requirements above the RDA. Additionally, dieting (1243 kcal/day) plus exercise (2.5–5 h/week) increased the requirement up to 0.38 mg/day.[28,32]

As the population ages, more and more people are becoming aware of the importance an exercise routine can play in overall health. The effect of supplementation on an aging population was addressed by Winters et al.[32] in a crossover-study design that implement an exercise intervention of 4 weeks to determine the effects of exercise on riboflavin requirements in older women. The researchers determined that exercise does, indeed, affect riboflavin status (assessed by measuring EGRAC and urinary riboflavin excretion) in women 50–67 y of age. However, upon receiving 0.6–0.9 mg/kcal riboflavin, improvements in exercise endurance were not enhanced.[32]

While nutrient requirements are similar for the non-athlete, physical activity does influence the amount of some nutrients needed by the athlete. However, the 1989 RDA recommendation does not take physical activity into account. For the most part, an athlete has higher energy, water, sodium, potassium, thiamin, riboflavin and niacin needs than the non-athlete. A few studies have indicated that riboflavin status of elite athletes is no different from that of nonathletic control subjects, indicating athletes consume more calories, which can counterbalance the extra demands placed upon the body by exercise.[39,40] Thus, riboflavin supplementation will most likely not improve athletic performance unless initial status is severely compromised prior to supplementation.[34]

Likewise, research has shown that riboflavin deficiency can impair physical performance. If the deficiency is corrected, performance will usually improve. Riboflavin supplementation for an athlete already consuming a well-balanced diet has not been shown to improve performance. Deficiencies in riboflavin due to poor dietary intakes may decrease the ability to do work, especially maximal work.[30,39,40]

VII. SUMMARY AND RECOMMENDATIONS FOR ATHLETES

Based on available research, riboflavin requirements appear to increase with exercise demands. Despite the anticipated effect of riboflavin deficiency on physical exercise, relatively few studies have shown a relationship. Many research studies have indicated that physical activity may deplete riboflavin status. However, there is no evidence that the riboflavin status in well nourished athletes is different from well nourished non-athletic controls. Furthermore, to date, limited data is available for riboflavin status in individuals who exercise strenuously. While the amount of additional riboflavin needed to cover losses or the increase in needs is small, it can be easily met through a well balanced diet. In addition, metabolic studies examining active women, exercise, dieting for weight loss and dieting plus exercise appeared to increase the need for riboflavin above the 1989 RDA and the 1998 DRI.[28,30–38]

The hypothesis that athletes may have compromised riboflavin status seems plausible because many studies have indicated that exercise alters biochemical indices of riboflavin status.[2,28,30–38] Researchers have begun to examined riboflavin status to evaluate if, indeed, trained athletes are at higher risk for riboflavin deficiency.[37,41–44] As long as a well balanced diet is consumed and calorie consumption rises as physical activity increases, athletes should be able to maintain adequate riboflavin status. It is important to note that several studies indicate the current RDA to be sub par in meeting riboflavin needs of normal healthy individuals, let alone athletes. There appears to be no clinical evidence of riboflavin toxicity and little likelihood that toxic side effects will develop. While it is difficult to prove whether a positive effect of vitamin supplementation on physical performance was due to a preexisting vitamin deficiency or on the basis of normal serum and blood vitamin status, future research needs to accurately determine riboflavin status and the metabolic processes responsible for absorption and utilization in energy production. In addition, further investigation is warranted to determine the long-term effects of exercise on riboflavin status and riboflavin supplementation on elite athletic performance.

REFERENCES

1. McCormick, D.B. Riboflavin. In: *Modern Nutrition in Health and Disease*, 9th ed. (Shiles, M.E., Olson, J.A., Shike, M. and Ross, A.C., Eds.). Williams & Wilkins, Baltimore, MD, 1999:391–399.
2. Soares, M.J., Satyanarayana, K., Bamji, M.S., Jacob, C.M., Ramana, Y.V. and Rao, S.S. The effect of exercise on the riboflavin status of adult men. *Br. J. Nutr.*, 69, 541–551, 1993.
3. National Research Council. Recommended Dietary Allowances. 10th ed. National Academy Press, Washington, D.C., 1989.
4. Institute of Medicine. Dietary reference intakes. Thiamin, riboflavin, niacin, vitamin B_6, folate, vitamin B_{12}, pantothenic acid, biotin and choline. National Academy Press, Washington, D.C., 1998.
5. Leklem, J.E., Miller, L.T., Hardin, K., and Ridlington, J. Effect of two levels of riboflavin on the metabolism of pyridoxine and pyridoxal. *FASEB J.*, 10, A465, 1996.
6. Leklem, J.E. Vitamin B_6: of reservoirs, receptors and requirements. *Nutr. Today*, Sept./Oct., 4–10, 1988.
7. McCormick, D.B. The fate of riboflavin in the mammal. *Nutr. Rev.*, 30, 75–79, 1972.

8. Jusko, W.J. and Levy, G. Absorption, metabolism and excretion of riboflavin 5'-phosphate in man. *J. Pharm. Sci.*, 56, 58–62, 1967.

9. Zempleni, J., Galloway, J.R., and McCormick, D.B. Pharmacokinetics of orally and intravenously administered riboflavin in healthy humans. *Am. J. Clin. Nutr.*, 63, 54–66, 1996.

10. Chastain, J.L. and McCormick, D.B. Flavin catabolites: identification and quantitationin human urine. *Am. J. Clin. Nutr.*, 46, 830–834, 1987.

11. Roe, E.A., Kalkwarf, H., and Stevens, J. Effect of fiber supplements on the apparent absorption of pharmacological does of riboflavin. *J. Am. Diet. Assoc.*, 88, 211–213, 1988.

12. Cooperman, J.M. and Lopez, R. Riboflavin. In: *Handbook of Vitamins: Nutritional Biochemical and Clinical Aspects* (Machlin, L.J., Ed.). Marcel Dekker, New York, 1984, p. 299–327.

13. Goldsmith, G.A. Riboflavin deficiency. In: *Riboflavin* (Rivlin, R.S., Ed.). Plenum, New York, 1975, p. 221–244.

14. Pangrekar, J., Krishnaswamy, K., and Jagadeesan, V. Effects of riboflavin deficiency and riboflavin administration on carcinogen-DNA binding. *Food Chem. Toxicol.*, 31, 745–750, 1993.

15. National Academy of Sciences, Water-soluble vitamins. In: Recommended Dietary Allowances. National Academy Press, Washington, D.C., 1989.

16. Biosvert, W.A., Mendoza, I., and Castenada, C. Riboflavin requirement of healthy elderly humans and its relationship to the macronutrient composition of the diet. *J. Nutr.*, 123, 915–925, 1993.

17. Glatzle, D., Korner, Christeller, S., and Wiss, O. Method for the detection of a biochemical riboflavin deficiency stimulation of $NADPH_2$-dependent glutathione reductase from human erythrocytes by FAD in vitro investigations on the vitamin B_2 status in healthy people and geriatric patients. *Int. J. Vitam. Res.*, 40, 166, 1970.

18. Sauberlich, H.E., Dowdy, R.P., and Skala, J.H. *Laboratory Tests for the Assessment of Nutritional Status*. CRC Press, Boca Raton, FL, 1974, 30.

19. Gibson, R.S. *Principles of Nutritional Assessment*. Oxford University Press, New York, NY, 1990.

20. Martini, M.C., Lampe, J.W., Slavin, J.L., and Kurzer, M.S. Effect of the menstrual cycle on energy and nutrient intake. *Am. J. Clin. Nutr.*, 60, 895–899, 1994.

21. Rokitzki, L., Berg, A., and Keul, J. Blood and serum status of water and fat soluble vitamins in athletes and nonathletes. *Int. J. Vit. Nutr. Res. Suppl.*, 30, 192, 1989.

22. Weight, L.M., Noakes, T.D., Labadarios, D., Graves, J., Jacobs, P., and Berman, P.A. Vitamin and mineral status of trained athletes including the effects of supplementation. *Am. J. Clin. Nutr.*, 47, 186, 1988.

23. Williams, M.L. *Nutritional Aspects of Human Physical and Athletic Performance*. Charles C. Thomas, Springfield, IL, 1976.

24. Barnett, D.W. and Conlee, R.K. The effects of commercial dietary supplementation on human performance. *Am. J. Clin. Nutr.*, 40, 586–90, 1984.

25. van der Beek, E.J. Vitamins and human training. Food for running or faddish claims? *Sports Med.*, 2, 175–97, 1985.

26. Fischbach, F.A. *A Manual of Laboratory and Diagnostic Tests.* 5th ed. Lippincott-Raven, Philadelphia, PA, 1996.

27. Gibson, R.S. *Principles of Nutritional Assessment*. Oxford University Press, New York, NY, 1990.

28. Belko, A.Z., Obarzanek, E., and Kalkwarf, H.J. Effects of exercise on riboflavin requirements of young women. *Am. J. Clin. Nutr.*, 37, 509–517, 1983.

29. Ohno, H., Yahata, T., Sato, Y., Yamamura, K., and Taniguchi, N. Physical training and fasting erythrocyte activities of free radical scavenging enzyme systems in sedentary men. *Eur. J. Appl. Physiol.*, 57, 173, 1988.

30. Belko, A.Z., Obarzanek, E., and Roach, R. Effects of aerobic exercise and weight loss on riboflavin requirements of moderately obese, marginally deficient young women. *Am. J. Clin. Nutr.*, 40, 553–561, 1984.

31. Evelo, C.T., Paimen, N.G., Artur, Y., and Janssen, G.M. Changes in blood glutathione concentrations and in erythrocyte glutathione reductase and glutathione S-transferase activity after running training and after participation in contests. *Eur. J. Appl. Physio.*, 64, 354, 1992.

32. Winters, L.R., Yoon, J.S., Kalkwarf, H.J., Davies, J.C., Berkowitz, M.G., Haas, J., and Roe, D.A. Riboflavin requirements and exercise adaptation in older women. *Am. J. Clin. Nutr.*, 56, 526–532, 1992.

33. Suboticanee, K., Stavljenic, A., Schalch, W., and Buzina, R. Effects of pyridoxine and riboflavin supplementation on physical fitness in young adolescents. *Int. J. Vit. Nutr. Res.*, 60, 81–88, 1990.

34. van der Beek, E.J., van Dokkum, W., and Schrijver, J. Thiamin, riboflavin, and vitamins B_6 and C: Impact of combined restricted intake on functional performance in man. *Am. J. Clin. Nutr.*, 48, 1451–1462, 1988.

35. van der Beek, E.J., van Dokkum, W., Wedel, M., Schrijver, J., and van den Berg, H. Thiamin, riboflavin and vitamin B_6: impact on restricted intake on physical performance in man. *J. Am. Coll. Nutr.*, 13, 629–640, 1994.

36. Powers, H.J., Bates, C.J., Lamb, W.H., Singh, J., Gelman, W., and Webb, E. Effects of a multivitamin and iron supplement on running performance in Gambian children. *Hum. Nutr. Clin. Nutr.*, 39C, 427–437, 1985.

37. Haralambie, G. Vitamin B2 status in athletes and the influence of riboflavin administration on neuromuscular irritability. *Nutr. Metab.*, 20, 1–8, 1976.

38. Belko, A.Z., Meredith, M.P., and Kalkwarf, H.J. Effects of exercise on riboflavin requirements: Biological validation in weight reducing women. *Am. J. Clin. Nutr.*, 41, 270–277, 1985.

39. Neikamp, R.A. In season dietary adequacy of trained male cross-country runners. *J. Sports Nutr.*, 5, 45–55, 1995.

40. Rankinen, T., Lyytikainen, S., Vanninen, E., Penttila, I., Rauramaa, R., and Uusitupa, M. Nutritional status of the Finnish elite ski jumpers. *Med. Sci. Sports Exerc.*, 30, 1592–1597, 1998.

41. Keith, R.E. and Alt, L.A. Riboflavin status of female athletes consuming normal diets. *Nutr. Res.*, 11, 727, 1991.

42. Guilland, J., Penaranda, T., Gallet, C., Bogglo, V., Fuchs, F., and Klepping, J. Vitamin status of young athletes including the effects of supplementation. *Med. Sci. Sport Exercise*, 21, 441, 1989.

43. Temblay, A., Boiland, F., Breton, M., Bessette, H., and Roberge, A.G. The effects of a riboflavin supplementation on the nutritional status and performance of elite swimmers. Nutr. Res., 4, 201, 1984.

44. Singh, A., Moses, F.M., and Deuster, P.A. Vitamin and mineral status in physically active men: effects of a high-potency supplement. *Am. J. Clin. Nutr.*, 55, 1, 1992.

5 Niacin

Edward M. Heath

CONTENTS

I. INTRODUCTION

Niacin has a rich and intriguing history. Its discovery dates to the identification by a Spanish physician named Casals in 1735 of pellagra, the disease now known to be caused by niacin deficiency. Pellagra was widespread for the next two centuries in populations with high consumption of corn. It was rampant throughout rural areas of the southern United States, where a physician named Joseph Goldberger was sent by the U.S. Public Health Service in the 1920s to investigate what they thought was an infectious disease. Goldberger, who recognized that changes in the diet to include milk, meat and fresh vegetables resulted in a substantial decrease in the symptoms of pellagra, was convinced that the disease could be cured by changes in diet. In 1937, Elvehjem demonstrated that nicotinic acid (the acid form of niacin synthesized roughly 50 years before) could treat lesions caused by pellagra in dogs, and within the year, it was reported to cure pellagra in humans.[1-3]

The role for supplying fuel for physical activity is filled predominantly by carbohydrates and fats, plus a small donation from proteins. The contribution from each of these macronutrients during an exercise bout is dependent upon the fitness level and the nutritional status of the individual, as well as the intensity and duration of the activity. Niacin, in its coenzyme form, is involved in numerous reactions, including glycolysis, tricarboxylic acid (TCA) cycle and electron transport, to produce ATP from carbohydrates, fats and proteins in the major metabolic pathways. Because of the extensive role of niacin as a coenzyme in the metabolic process, it is conceivable that the level of niacin should be increased for those involved in a vigorous training program.[1,4] This chapter will investigate the possibility of an increased requirement for niacin with a review of the structure, general properties (Recommended Dietary Allowance (RDA) and dietary sources) and the metabolic functions of niacin. In addition, this chapter will address the history and current status of the use

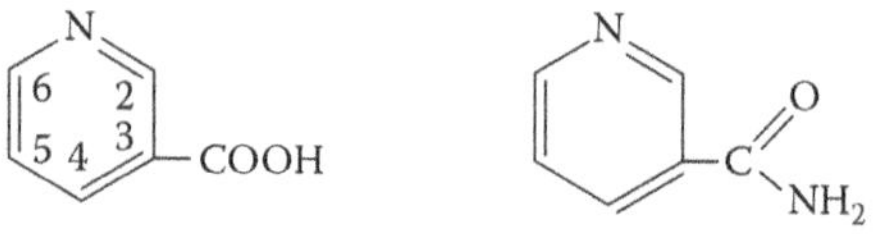

FIGURE 5.1 The acid (nicotinic acid) and the amide (nicotinamide) forms of niacin. (From Berdanier, C.D., *Advanced Nutrition: Micronutrients,* CRC Press, Boca Raton, FL, 1998.)

of pharmacologic doses of niacin to improve cholesterol profile, and the changes in fuel utilization on these mega doses of niacin and how these changes may affect performance. Finally, the chapter will review recommendations for exercise and sport performance and future research directions.

II. CHEMICAL STRUCTURE

Niacin is a generic term for the water-soluble vitamin in the B complex that occurs as an acid (nicotinic acid) or as an amide (nicotinamide) (Figure 5.1). Both nicotinic acid and nicotinamide are stable in the dry state and soluble in water, although nicotinamide has a much higher solubility. Nicotinamide is the main component of the coenzymes nicotinamide adenine dinucleotide (NAD) and nicotinamide adenine dinucleotide phosphate (NADP), which have a major role in the catabolic reactions of metabolism.[3,5]

III. GENERAL PROPERTIES—RECOMMENDED DIETARY ALLOWANCE AND DIETARY SOURCES

The RDA for niacin is based on early studies with the intention of preventing or treating pellagra. Niacin is found in a variety of common foods and can also be synthesized in the body from the essential amino acid tryptophan. Therefore, the RDA for niacin is expressed in niacin equivalents (NE). It takes 60 mg of tryptophan to produce 1 mg of niacin, thus 1 NE equals 1 mg of preformed niacin or 60 mg of tryptophan. Lean meats, poultry and fish are excellent sources of niacin because they are all rich in both niacin and tryptophan. Sources rich in niacin alone are brewer's yeast, peanuts and peanut butter. Milk and eggs contain large amounts of tryptophan. Smaller amounts can be found in beans, peas, other legumes, nuts and enriched whole-grain cereal products. Because of the extensive metabolic role of the coenzymes derived from nicotinamide, NAD and NADP, the RDA for niacin is determined by energy intake and expressed per 1,000 kcal. The RDA for niacin is 6.6 mg/1,000 kcal (16–19 NE for adult males and 13–14 NE for adult females).[5-7]

IV. METABOLIC FUNCTIONS

More than 200 enzymes are dependent on the coenzymes NAD and NADP in metabolic processes.[1] These coenzymes are pervasive in metabolism, serving as carriers of reducing equivalents in glycolysis, the TCA cycle and electron transport. They also serve similar functions in ß-oxidation and in fat and protein biosynthesis.

These coenzymes play a critical role in fast glycolysis, where NAD is reduced in the glyceraldehyde-3- phosphate to 1, 3 biphosphoglycerate step, and then the hydrogen ions are used in converting pyruvate to lactate (Figure 5.2). Under slow glycolysis these hydrogens are transported to the ETC. In the TCA cycle, NAD serves as an electron acceptor for a number of enzymes including pyruvate dehydrogenase, isocitrate dehydrogenase, α-ketogluterate dehydrogenase and malate dehydrogenase (Figure 5.3). The resulting NADH is then moved to the ETC to be reoxidized to NAD and generates ATP as a result (Figure 5.4).[1-4]

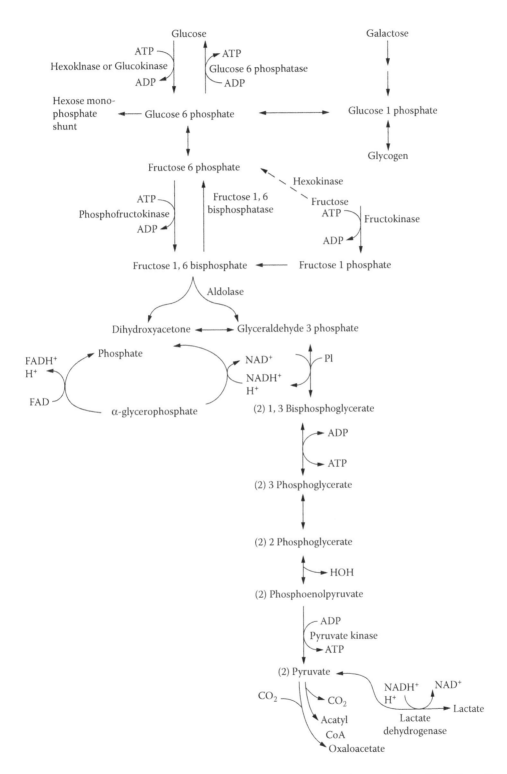

FIGURE 5.2 Glycolysis. (From Berdanier, C.D., *Advanced Nutrition: Macronutrients,* CRC Press, Boca Raton, FL, 1995.)

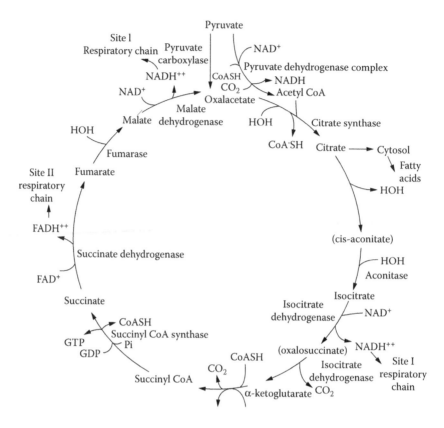

FIGURE 5.3 Tricarboxylic acid cycle. (From Berdanier, C.D., *Advanced Nutrition: Macronutrients,* CRC Press, Boca Raton, FL, 1995.)

V. NICOTINIC ACID DOSES

Large doses of nicotinic acid, with no reported toxicity, have been used for a wide variety of purposes including as a purported ergogenic aid,[8,9] to treat schizophrenia,[10] to treat pellagra,[5] to examine the effects on bouts of exercise,[11–21] to reduce plasma FFA levels,[22,23] and most commonly as an agent to improve cholesterol profile.[24–36] The amount of the nicotinic acid dose and the time for treatment varies considerably for the purposes mentioned above. As a possible ergogenic aid,

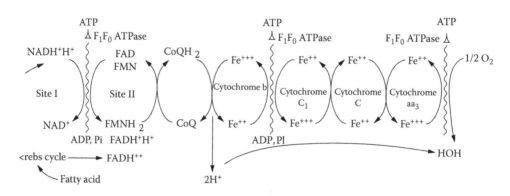

FIGURE 5.4 Electron Transport System. (From Berdanier, C.D., *Advanced Nutrition: Macronutrients,* CRC Press, Boca Raton, FL, 1995.)

Hilsendager and Karpovich[9] used two 75-mg nicotinic acid doses and Frankau[8] used 3 days of a 40–50-mg dose of nicotinamide. Osmond and Hoffer[10] reported use of up to 5 g/day for extended periods in the treatment of schizophrenia. Administration of 40–250 mg/day has been reported to be successful in the treatment cases of pellagra.[1]

Of particular interest for this chapter are the amounts of nicotinic acid used to affect substrate utilization during bouts of exercise, to affect plasma free fatty acid (FFA) levels and to affect cholesterol levels. Two investigations demonstrated significant changes in respiratory exchange ratio (RER) with infusion of 1.4 g of nicotinic acid over 4 h of rest and exercise[12] and 1.6 g (1 g intravenous and 600 mg orally) of nicotinic acid given in a 2 h period prior to exercise.[11] Two other studies reported significant decreases in plasma FFA levels with ingestion of 200 mg of nicotinic acid 10 min prior to testing[22] and 3.2 mg/kg (235 mg for a 70-kg person) 2 h prior to testing with 1.6 mg/kg administered every 30 min thereafter.[23] Other exercise studies to report on the amount of nicotinic acid administered were Jenkins[16] with 200 mg at the start and 100 mg after 1 h, and Lassers et al.[18] with a 200-mg IV bolus and continuous intravenous of 3.8 mg/min. Both Heath et al.[14,15] studies used 1 g 1 h prior to exercise, Norris et al.[19] used 2 g and Pernow and Saltin[21] administered 1.2 g — half of the dose intravenous and the rest ingested.

A variety of nicotinic acid doses, progressions of doses and durations of nicotinic acid treatment have been used to achieve similar changes in plasma cholesterol levels. The doses vary from 1.2 g/day[29] to 4 g/day,[29] with the most common dose being 3 g/day.[26,28,30,31] The investigators varied in how fast they increased the dose of nicotinic acid to the target dose. One group of researchers increased the dose from 0.5 g/day to 3 g/day in 3–6 days[30] and another group took 6 months to increase from 1 g/day to 3 g/day.[26] The doses of the new formulation, extended-release niacin, used in the more recent studies ranged from 1–3 g/d.[27,34]

A. TOLERANCE OF NICOTINIC ACID

Large doses of nicotinic acid have been used to bring about changes in cholesterol levels for more than 50 years,[32] despite annoying side effects. Flushing, a reddening of the skin with the sensation of heat or itching, is the most common side effect. This flushing response mainly affects the upper body and face, occurring 1 to 2 h after ingestion, and the symptoms usually disappear after repeated nicotinic acid administration. Reduced oral glucose tolerance has also been commonly reported in the past with ingestion of nicotinic acid, but recent evidence demonstrates that niacin can be used safely and effectively in diabetics who have good glucose control.[33,34] Although the use of pharmacologic doses of niacin have been associated with adverse side effects like flushing, liver dysfunction and gastrointestinal stress, newer formulations of niacin (extended-release) demonstrate minimal side effects with comparable effectiveness.[35]

VI. NICOTINIC ACID AND CHOLESTEROL LEVELS

Pharmocologic doses of niacin have been used to treat hyperlipidemia since the middle 1950s. The use of niacin for this purpose had declined considerably since its more widespread use early, but there has been a renewed interest in the last decade. The extended-release formulation of niacin has lessened the adverse side effects and may be in large part responsible for its resurgent use.[35]

Niacin is an over-the-counter medication that is arguably the best cholesterol-lowering agent available. In its new formulation, it is safe, inexpensive and effective. It has proved to significantly increase high-density lipoprotein cholesterol (HDL-C) with greater effectiveness than any other medication. In addition, it decreases total cholesterol, low-density lipoprotein cholesterol (LDL-C), lipoprotein (a) and triglycerides.[27,35] Niacin has also recently been used in combination with other medications such as lovastatin and, because of their different mechanisms of action, cholesterol profile has improved more than with one medication alone.[34,36]

VII. NICOTINIC ACID AND SUBSTRATE AVAILABILITY/PERFORMANCE

A. NICOTINIC ACID EFFECTS ON FUEL UTILIZATION AT REST

Numerous investigators have demonstrated changes in FFA mobilization as a result of ingesting or infusing nicotinic acid. The articles that were reviewed all indicated that plasma or serum FFA levels were lowered by the presence of nicotinic acid.

Havel, Carlson, Ekelund and Holmgren[37] investigated the effects of norepinephrine and nicotinic acid on energy metabolism in seven 21–26-year-olds. They ingested 1–3 g of nicotinic acid daily for 3 days before the testing to become accustomed to the flushing response caused by nicotinic acid, and then reported to the laboratory at 0800 h after a 12–15 h fast. During the entire procedure (just over 4 h) the participants were supine, with a catheter in an antecubital vein and a brachial artery, while expired air was collected intermittently. Norepinephrine was infused between minutes 45 and 60, and plasma concentrations of FFA, glycerol and glucose rose rapidly. At minute 120, nicotinic acid (100 or 200 mg) infusion started at 15 min intervals up to minute 225, when another infusion of norepinephrine started. The plasma concentration of FFA, glycerol and glucose decreased after the first infusion of nicotinic acid and stabilized in 30 min. The RER was increased after administration of nicotinic acid. The effect of norepinephrine on FFA and glycerol levels was almost completely blocked by nicotinic acid.

Two groups of investigators took advantage of the decreasing plasma levels of FFA caused by administration of nicotinic acid to investigate cold exposure in man. Hanson et al.[22] used four males (aged 21–25 years) to examine the effects of nicotinic acid ingestion on plasma FFA in acute cold exposure in a fasted state. A 200-mg dose of nicotinic acid was taken 10 min before the start of the cold exposure. The plasma FFA level was significantly lower in the conditions of the experiment that involved ingestion of nicotinic acid. More recently, Martineau and Jacobs[23] also investigated plasma FFA levels using nicotinic acid, although the cold exposure was in water. Eight males (aged 19–32 years) performed two cold-water immersions 1 week apart following a 14–16 h fast. Both immersions were preceded by ingestion of nicotinic acid or placebo (3.2 mg/kg 2 h prior to immersion and 1.6 mg/kg at 30 min intervals before immersion). Plasma FFA levels were significantly lower before and during immersion in the trials with previous ingestion of nicotinic acid. The plasma FFA values with nicotinic acid ingestion were still significantly less than without nicotinic acid ingestion after immersion, despite a 73% increase in FFA levels.

These findings demonstrate that nicotinic acid has a significant effect on fat utilization at rest. Butcher, Baird and Sutherland[38] revealed the manner by which nicotinic acid effectively suppresses fat metabolism. Adenosine 3', 5'-monophosphate (cyclic AMP) has been implicated as an intracellular second messenger. A decrease in cyclic AMP, caused by nicotinic acid, blocks the breakdown of white adipose tissue triglycerides to FFA and glycerol. Madsen and Malchow-Møller[39] stated that nicotinic acid inhibited the stimulation of adenylcyclase in adipocytes, causing decreased intracellular concentrations of cyclic AMP, which interfered with the activation of hormone-sensitive lipase. Nicotinic acid also has a direct inhibiting effect on the hormone-sensitive lipase.

B. NICOTINIC ACID EFFECTS ON FUEL UTILIZATION DURING BOUTS OF EXERCISE

A number of investigations have focused on the effects of nicotinic acid administration on exercise metabolism; more specifically on the contribution of fat and carbohydrate sources to fuel acute or prolonged exercise. Nicotinic acid has been used in these studies because of its marked effect on FFA availability during exercise by the same mechanism as in resting conditions explained earlier. The importance of mobilizing FFA from adipose tissue to fuel exercise is readily apparent because there is only a small amount of stored fat within the skeletal muscles, thus, circulating FFA is essential for continued fat metabolism in the muscle.[40] The common findings of these studies was that nicotinic acid decreased fat utilization in a variety of exercise conditions.[11–21]

Carlson and co-workers[12] investigated the effect of nicotinic acid on plasma glycerol and glucose as well as the appearance, oxidation and turnover of FFA at rest and during exercise in two college-aged males. They were infused with 200 mg of nicotinic acid in the middle of the first rest period, followed by 100 mg of nicotinic acid every 15 min throughout the 2 h of exercise and the following 1 h of rest. Expired air and blood samples were collected intermittently. Nicotinic acid decreased the concentration and turnover rate of FFA and profoundly inhibited the usual increase in concentration and turnover rate found in fasted subjects during exercise. The normal increase in concentration of glycerol in fasted exercise was not present in one of the nicotinic acid-infused subjects. In the other nicotinic acid-infused subject, there was an increase in glycerol concentration and turnover rate of FFA during exercise, although the absolute values were lower than the controls. The plasma glucose concentration did not change significantly in the controls. The subject that demonstrated the greatest decrease in turnover rate of FFA had a large drop in the plasma glucose concentration (105 to 68 mg/100 ml) at the end of exercise while the other nicotinic acid-infused subject had little change. Both nicotinic acid-infused subjects had higher plasma glucose concentrations than the controls. Until the last hour of rest, the nicotinic acid-infused subject, who had the lowest glucose level during exercise, had a higher RER than the control subjects. After administration of nicotinic acid, the other subject demonstrated a progressive rise in RER to a higher level than the control subjects at the end of exercise. The levels of lactate and pyruvate in the nicotinic acid-infused subjects changed little during exercise and were comparable to the values of the control subjects. Nicotinic acid did not affect the rate of removal of FFA from the blood, oxidation of FFA, heart rate or mechanical efficiency. The most noteworthy results of the study were that nicotinic acid markedly decreased the rate of FFA mobilization at rest and inhibited the normal increase in FFA mobilization that occurs when fasted subjects exercise.

Jenkins[16] followed the work of Carlson et al.[12] to determine the metabolic response after nicotinic acid ingestion on a treadmill at 3.5 mph and 10% grade for either 1.5 h (n = 2) or 2.5 h (n = 1). Compared with the control exercise session, the session with prior ingestion of 200 mg of nicotinic acid showed significantly lower plasma FFA levels and a significantly higher RER. Unlike the Carlson[12] study, Jenkins[16] reported an increase with blood glucose after the nicotinic acid ingestion, which he speculated was caused indirectly by the drop in FFA.

Bergström et al.[11] examined the effect of nicotinic acid on physical work capacity and muscle glycogen stores, with particular focus on the possibility of increased glycogen utilization when nicotinic acid blocked mobilization of FFA. In the first series, two males performed a two-leg cycle ergometer protocol that increased work load every 6 min up to a near maximal level. After a 2 h rest, during which 1.6 g of nicotinic acid (1 g intravenous and 0.6 g orally) was given, the same procedure was performed. In the second series, 13 males used one-leg cycle ergometry at a constant load for 60–90 min with a 1 h rest period in between conditions (with and without nicotinic acid). When the work was gradually increased to a near maximal level in the first series, the participants performed the same amount of exercise whether nicotinic acid was administered or not. After nicotinic acid administration, the RER was higher at rest and at lower work loads, although there was no difference in RER at higher work intensities. Arterial lactate and glucose concentrations were lower in the nicotinic acid exercise. In the second series, where the opposite leg was used for the nicotinic acid exercise, they performed the same amount of work, although the second bout of exercise was more fatiguing. The resting heart rate was similar before the two exercise sessions, however, the increase in heart rate during exercise before nicotinic acid administration was significantly higher with a mean difference of 20 beats/min at the end of the exercise. The VO_2 was slightly higher in the cycling with prior administration of nicotinic acid ($p < 0.10$). The RER was slightly higher at rest in the nicotinic acid condition, but was significantly ($p < 0.005$) higher at the end of exercise in the nicotinic acid trial (0.93 ± 0.03 to 0.77 ± 0.03). There was an increased rate of glycogen utilization after administration of nicotinic acid both at 45–60 min of exercise ($p < 0.025$) and after 90 min of exercise ($p < 0.005$). Arterial glucose had large individual variations and was less at rest after nicotinic acid administration and showed no differences during exercise.

The lactate concentration was significantly higher during exercise after nicotinic acid administration. The resting levels of FFA were lower after nicotinic acid in four of five subjects and the normal increase during exercise was almost completely blocked. One nicotinic acid-administered subject showed an increase in FFA concentration with exercise, although the values were lower than the control exercise. The glycerol concentration was lower after nicotinic acid administration both at rest and during exercise.

Pernow and Saltin[21] investigated work capacity and substrate utilization with and without 1.2 g of nicotinic acid using one-leg cycling to exhaustion under conditions of glycogen depletion. The glycogen depletion was caused by exhaustive one-leg cycling and a no-carbohydrate diet the previous 24 h, and verified by biopsy. The result of the trial with nicotinic acid showed a significant decrease in work load and time to exhaustion compared with both legs the previous day and with the other leg the same day. With the nicotinic acid blocking the release of FFA, exercise capacity was significantly reduced.

Unlike what many of the previous researchers might predict, Norris et al.[20] demonstrate no significant difference in the performance of a 10-mile run without (76 ± 3 min) and with nicotinic acid ingestion (78 ± 3 min). Ten habitual runners were randomized into ingesting 2 g of nicotinic acid or a placebo 2 h before a timed 10-mile run on a measured course. The runners who ingested nicotinic acid showed similarly depressed FFA levels as in previous studies, but did not demonstrate a decrease in performance as a result of the decreased fat oxidation. The authors suggested that the 10-mile run did not deplete glycogen levels enough to affect performance and that when carbohydrate stores are still plentiful, the decreased fat oxidation caused by nicotinic acid did not impair 10-mile run time.

Two other investigations demonstrated a decrease in performance when the exercise was presumably severe enough to deplete glycogen levels to the point where the lack of fat oxidation in the nicotinic acid trial impacted performance. In an abstract, Galbo et al.[13] reported a decrease in running time to exhaustion with prior ingestion of nicotinic acid. Seven participants ran at 60% of VO_2 max to exhaustion under normal conditions and with prior ingestion of nicotinic acid. The total time to exhaustion was significantly shorter in the nicotinic acid condition (122 ± 8 vs. 166 ± 10 min). In a similar study with cyclists, Heath and collaborators[15] published abstract showed significantly decreased time to exhaustion cycling at 68% of VO_2 peak but not at 86% of VO_2 peak with prior ingestion of nicotinic acid. Five highly trained male cyclists who fasted for 12 h participated in four time-to-exhaustion rides at 68% and 86% of their VO_2 peak. The work rates were equivalent at each of the two intensities with 1 g of nicotinic acid ingested before one of the trials at each intensity. The order of the four trials was randomized and conducted at least 1 week apart. The ingestion of nicotinic acid significantly decreased pre- and post-exercise FFA levels, and time to exhaustion was significantly reduced in the niacin trials at 68% VO_2 peak (101.6 ± 40.2 vs. 142.3 ± 51.0 min), while there was no effect for the 86% VO_2 peak trials (13.9 ± 6.5 vs. 20.3 ± 7.8 min). Most of the difference in the high-intensity time-to-exhaustion rides was from one participant who recorded 25 min 1 s without nicotinic acid and 5 min 55 s with nicotinic acid, showing considerable variation in his response to the metabolic effects of nicotinic acid. Because of the drastic decrease in the nicotinic acid trial at 86% of VO_2 peak with this participant, the trial with nicotinic acid was repeated and the results were similar. This confirmed the possibility of marked individual metabolic differences affecting the rides to exhaustion. The authors concluded that, as expected, the inhibition on FFA mobilization caused by nicotinic acid impaired performance at the moderate-intensity exercise. However, at the higher-intensity exercise, where fat utilization has a more minor role, the inhibiting effects of nicotinic acid on FFA availability did not result in differences in performance time.

Supplementation of carbohydrates during prolonged exercise, similar to nicotinic acid, causes a blunted release of FFA, but also has the effect of increasing performance because of its glycogen-sparing effect.[41] Murray and co-workers[19] predicted that carbohydrate supplementation in combination with nicotinic acid ingestion would enhance performance because of the proven effect of nicotinic acid's increasing carbohydrate reliance. Under four conditions, 10 participants cycled at 68% VO_2 peak for 120 min and then completed a 3.5-mile time trial. Every 15 min during the exercise, the participants ingested one of four beverages: (1) water placebo (WP), (2) WP + 280 mg nicotinic acid (NA) per liter (WP + NA), (3) 6% carbohydrate electrolyte drink (CE) and (4) CE + NA. In the two NA conditions (WP + NA & CE + NA) the NA attenuated FFA rise during exercise but the NA + CE condition, although it showed an increase in carbohydrate oxidation, did not demonstrate improved performance on the 3.5-mile cycling time trial. The performance times were 641.8 ± 17 s for CE, 685 ± 34 s for CE + NA, 730.6 ± 36 s for WP and 765.9 ± 59 s for WP + NA. The CE group was significantly better than both the WP and the WP + NA groups. Trends in the data are suggestive that NA ingestion may decrease performance (CE < CE + NA & WP < WP + NA). Comparison of performance times for CE + NA and WP + NA approached significance ($p = 0.0517$). Thus, Murray et al.'s hypothesis that combining nicotinic acid and carbohydrate electrolyte drink would improve performance compared with all other conditions except the CE trial did not come to fruition. The possibility exists that there was insufficient power to detect differences or that another performance test could have demonstrated the benefits of nicotinic acid and carbohydrate electrolyte ingestion combined.

There is little question that the administration of large doses of nicotinic acid has an adverse effect on fat utilization. This decrease in availability of lipid fuel sources could have a negative impact on lower-intensity exercise, where the contribution from fat sources is considerable. One of the intriguing aspects of this line of research is the relationship between beneficial effects of pharmacologic doses of niacin on cholesterol profiles and the physical activity recommendations to decrease the risk of coronary artery disease. Physical inactivity and the associated low exercise capacity is one of the most powerful changeable risk factors.[42] To investigate the possibility of an adaptation to the decreased fat utilization during single bouts of exercise, Heath et al.[14] assessed fuel utilization during 3 weeks of nicotinic acid administration. Eight trained male runners performed four 30-min submaximal treadmill runs at 60% of VO_2 max. The first treadmill run served as a control and the next three were at the onset, midpoint and end of 3 weeks of nicotinic acid administration. The nicotinic acid dose was built up to a typical regimen to impact cholesterol profile — 3 g/d ingested with meals three times per day. A 1-g nicotinic dose was ingested 1 h prior to the last three treadmill runs, which were conducted in the morning after a 12-h fast. Serum FFA and glycerol levels were significantly lower in the three treadmill runs with nicotinic acid compared with the control run, showing no adaptation over the 3 weeks of nicotinic acid administration. The RER showed a beginning of a possible adaptation starting at 0.871 ± 0.008 in the control condition and peaking with a significant increase at 0.919 ± 0.009 in the initial run with nicotinic acid. After, the RER showed a significant drop compared with the first nicotinic acid run — 0.898 ± 0.007 for the second nicotinic acid run and 0.896 ± 0.009 for the third nicotinic acid run. Although the values for the last two submaximal runs were significantly lower than the first run with nicotinic acid, they were significantly higher than the control run without the nicotinic acid. The possibility exists that a complete adaptation may take longer than 3 weeks. Interestingly, total cholesterol was significantly decreased (195 ± 9.2 to 174 ± 9.2 mg/dl) and HDL-C levels were significantly increased (56.2 ± 2.9 to 63.0 ± 3.9 mg/dl) in these habitual healthy runners with the 3 weeks of nicotinic acid administration.

In addition to the fuel utilization changes for skeletal muscle with nicotinic acid administration, Lassers et al.[18] demonstrated similar changes in the myocardial metabolism. They showed an estimated 42% decrease in lipid utilization during rest and a 56% decrease during exercise with nicotinic acid administration. There is scant evidence that niacin status impacts performance. Jetté et al.[17] investigated changes in VO_2 max following glycogen supercompensation accomplished by exhaustive exercise and followed by low- and high-carbohydrate diets. VO_2 max was slightly decreased following the high-carbohydrate diets where niacin intake and N1-methylnicotinamide excretion was lower compared with the high-protein, low-carbohydrate condition. The authors concluded that the decreased VO_2 max with the high-carbohydrate condition might have been associated with compromised oxidative metabolism from lower, although still adequate, niacin intake.

VIII. SUMMARY AND RECOMMENDATIONS FOR EXERCISE AND SPORTS PERFORMANCE

Although niacin has an important role in energy metabolism, few studies cite enhanced performance with administration of small amounts of niacin. Frankau[8] used 40–50-mg doses of nicotinamide and reported improved performance in an agility test. Hilsendager and Karpovich[9] showed no effect of 75 mg of niacin on a cycle or hand ergometer endurance test, and there certainly has been no research to show improved performance with doses of nicotinic acid large enough to impact cholesterol levels (3 g/d is the typical dose).

A number of new studies have touted the effectiveness of large doses of nicotinic acid to treat hyperlipidemia. With the new formulation of nicotinic acid that decreases the side effects, there appears to be greater interest for its use to positively affect cholesterol profiles. These large doses of nicotinic acid reduce the availability of FFA and make the individual more dependent on carbohydrate sources. There is the possibility that the ability to exercise could be affected, but to date, the only decrease in performance that has been demonstrated has been where carbohydrate availability becomes compromised.[15,21]

There is no question of the critical metabolic role of niacin, but there is no evidence that compromised niacin status in an athletic or general population causes decreased aerobic exercise performance. In addition, the substantial decrease in FFA availability with those on pharmacologic doses of nicotinic acid does not impact performance unless carbohydrate sources are limited.

IX. FUTURE RESEARCH DIRECTIONS

Because of the extensive involvement of niacin-derived coenzymes in metabolism, it would seem logical that there could be a possible ergogenic effect for niacin. Although no well controlled study has shown an ergogenic effect of niacin, it is predictable that studies like these would continue. Pharmacologic doses of niacin present some exceptional research possibilities because niacin causes decreased availability of FFA and its effect on lipid profiles. It would be interesting to investigate the effect on exercise of these large doses on individuals who have poor cholesterol profiles. More extensive and longer studies could ascertain the effect of the niacin on their ability to be physically active, and investigate a possible adaptation of increasing fat utilization back to normal. If there is an adaptation in fat utilization to chronic niacin administration, more involved studies could be designed to attempt to detect a mechanism for the adaptation.

REFERENCES

1. Swendseid, M.E. and Jacob, R.A., Niacin, in: *Modern Nutrition in Health and Disease.* Shils, M.E., Olson, J.A. and Shike, M., Eds., Lea & Feiger, Malvern, PA, 1994, pp. 376–382.
2. Wildman, R E.C. and Medeiros, D.M., *Advanced Human Nutrition.* CRC Press, Boca Raton, FL, 2000, pp. 195–200.
3. Berdanier, C.D., *Advanced Nutrition: Macronutrients,* CRC Press, Boca Raton, FL, 1998, pp. 94–99.
4. Lewis, R.D., Riboflavin and niacin, in: *Sports Nutrition: Vitamins and Trace Elements.* Wolinsky, I. and Driskell, J.A. CRC Press, Boca Raton, FL, 1997, 67–73.
5. Pike, R.L. and Brown, M.L., *Nutrition: An Integrated Approach* (3rd ed.). New York: Macmillan, 1986, 97–107.
6. National Academy of Science, Water-soluble vitamins, in *Recommended Dietary Allowances,* National Academy Press, Washington, D.C., 1989, pp. 115–118.
7. Williams, M.H., *Nutrition for Sport and Fitness* (4th ed.). Dubuque, IA: Wm. C. Brown, 1988, p. 194.
8. Frankau, I. M., Acceleration of coordinated muscular effort by nicotinamide, *Br. Med. J.,* 2, 601, 1943.
9. Hilsendager, D. and Karpovich, P.V., Ergogenic effect of glycine and niacin separately and in combination, *Res. Q.,* 35, 389, 1964.

10. Osmond, H. and Hoffer, A., Massive niacin treatment in schizophrenia: A review of a nine-year study, *Lancet,* 1, 316, 1962.

11. Bergström, J., Hultman, E., Jorfeldt, L., Pernow, B. and Wahren, J., Effect of nicotinic acid on working capacity and on metabolism of muscle glycogen in man, *J. Appl. Physiol.,* 26, 170, 1969.

12. Carlson, L.A., Havel, R.J., Ekelund, L.G. and Holmgren, A., Effect of nicotinic acid on the turnover rate and oxidation of plasma free fatty acid during exercise, *Metabolism,* 12, 837, 1963.

13. Galbo, H., Holst, J.J., Christnesen, N.J. and Hilsted, J., The effect of nicotinic acid and propanolol on glucagons and plasma catecholamine responses to prolonged exercise in man, *Diabetologia,* 11, 343, 1975.

14. Heath, E.M., Wilcox, A.R. and Quinn, C.M., Effects of nicotinic acid on respiratory exchange ratio and substrate levels during exercise, *Med. Sci. Sports Exercise,* 25, 1018, 1993.

15. Heath, E.M., Wilcox, A.R., Lickliter, K.L. and Kornatz, K.W., Effect of niacin on endurance performance in cyclists, *Med. Sci. Sports Exercise,* 28 (Suppl.), S2, 1996.

16. Jenkins, D.J.A., Effects of nicotinic acid on carbohydrate and fat metabolism during exercise, *Lancet,* 1, 1307, 1965.

17. Jetté, M., Pelletier, O., Parker, L. and Thoden, J., The nutritional and metabolic effects of a carbohydrate-rich diet in a glycogen supercompensation training regimen, *Am. J. Clin. Nutr.,* 31, 2140, 1978.

18. Lassers, B.W., Wahlqvist, M.L., Kaijser, J. and Carlson, L.A., Effect of nicotinic acid on myocardial metabolism in man at rest and exercise, *J. Appl. Physiol.,* 33, 72, 1972.

19. Murray, R., Bartoli, W.P., Eddy, D.E. and Horn, M.K., Physiological and performance responses to nicotinic-acid ingestion during exercise, *Med. Sci. Sports Exercise,* 27, 1057, 1995.

20. Norris, B., Schade, D.S. and Eaton, R.P., Effects of altered free fatty acid mobilization on the metabolic response to exercise, *J. Clin. Endocrinol. Metab.,* 46, 254, 1978.

21. Pernow, B. and Saltin, B., Availability of substrates and capacity for prolonged heavy exercise, *J. Appl. Physiol.,* 31, 416, 1971.

22. Hanson, P.G., Johnson, R.E. and Engel, G., Plasma free fatty acid changes in man during acute cold exposure and nicotinic acid ingestion, *Aerospace Med.,* November, 11, 1054, 1965.

23. Martineau, L. and Jacobs, I., Free fatty acid availability and regulation in cold water, *J. Appl. Physiol.,* 67, 2466, 1989.

24. Alderman, J.D., Pasternak, R.C., Sacks, F.M., Smith, H.S., Monard, E.S. and Grossman, W., Effect of a modified, well-tolerated niacin regimen on serum total cholesterol, high density lipoprotein cholesterol and the cholesterol to high density lipoprotein ratio, *Am. J. Cardiol.,* 64, 725, 1989.

25. Atmeh, R.F., Shepherd, J. and Packard, C.J., Subpopulations of apolipoprotein A-1 in human high-density lipoproteins their metabolic properties and response to drug therapy, *Biochem. Biophys. Acta.,* 751, 175, 1983.

26. The Coronary Drug Project Research Group, Clofibrate and niacin in coronary heart disease, *J. Am. Med. Assoc.,* 231, 360, 1975.

27. Goldberg, A.C., A meta-analysis of randomized controlled studies on the effects of extended-release niacin in women, *Am. J. Cardiol.,* 94, 121, 2004.

28. Gurakar, A., Hoeg, J.M., Kostner, G., Papadopoulos, N.M. and Brewer, H.B., Levels of lipoprotein Lp(a) decline with neomycin and niacin treatment, *Atherosclerosis,* 57, 293, 1985.

29. Hanefeld, M., Hora, C., Schulze, J., Rothe, G., Barthel, U. and Haller, H., Reduced incidence of cardiovascular complications and mortality in hyperlipoproteinemia (HPL) with effective lipid correction, *Atherosclerosis,* 57, 47–58, 1984.

30. Hoogwerf, B.J., Bantle, J.P., Kuba, K., Frantz, I.D. and Hunninghake, D.B., Treatment of type III hyperlipoproteinemia with four different treatment regimens, *Athersclerosis,* 15, 251, 1984.

31. Shepherd, J., Packard, C.J., Patsch, J.R., Gotto, A.M. and Taunton, O.D., Effects of nicotinic acid therapy on plasma high density lipoprotein subfraction distribution and composition and on apoprotein A metabolism, *J. Clin. Invest.,* 63, 858, 1979.

32. Atschul, R., Hoffer, A. and Stephen, J.D., Influences of nicotinic acid on serum cholesterol in man, *Arch. Biochem. Biophys.,* 54, 558, 1955.

33. Tavintharan, S. and Kashyap, M.L., The benefits of niacin in atherosclerosis, *Curr. Atheroscler. Rep.,* 3, 74, 2001.

34. Moon, Y.S. and Kashyap, M.L., Niacin extended-release/lovastatin: combination therapy for lipid disorders, *Expert Opin. Pharmacother.,* 3, 1763, 2002.

35. Ganji, S.H., Kamanna, V.S. and Kashyap, M.L., Niacin and cholesterol: role in cardiovascular disease (review), *J. Nutr. Biochem.,* 14, 298, 2003.

36. Hunninghake, D.B., McGovern, M.E., Koren, M., Brazg, R., Murdock, D., Weiss, S. and Pearson, T., A dose-ranging study of a new, once-daily, dual-component drug product containing niacin extended-release and lovastatin, *Clin. Cardiol.,* 26, 112, 2003.

37. Havel, R.J., Carlson, L.A., Ekelund, L.-G. and Holmgren, A., Studies on the relation between mobilization of free fatty acids and energy metabolism in man: Effects of norepinephrine and nicotinic acid, *Metabolism,* 13, 1402, 1964.

38. Butcher, R.W., Baird, C.E. and Sutherland E.W., Effects of lipolytic and antilipolytic substances on adenosine 3', 5'-monophosphate levels in isolated fat cells, *J. Biol. Chem.,* 243, 1705, 1968.

39. Madsen, J. and Malchow-Møller, A., Effects of glucose, insulin and nicotinic acid on adipose tissue blood flow in rats, *Acta. Physiol. Scand.,* 118, 175, 1983.

40. Gollnick, P.D. and Saltin, B. Fuel for muscular exercise: Role of fat, in *Exercise, Nutrition and Energy Metabolism,* Horton, E.S. and Terjung, R.L., Eds., Macmillan, New York, 1988, p. 72.

41. Coggan, A.R. and Coyle, E.F., Carbohydrate ingestion during prolonged exercise: Effects on metabolism and performance, in *Exercise and Sports Science Reviews,* Holloszy, J.O., Ed., Williams & Wilkins, Baltimore, MD, 1991, p. 1.

42. Meyers, J., Prakash, M., Froelicher, V., Do, D., Partington, S. and Atwood, J.E., Exercise capacity and mortality among men referred for exercise testing, *N. Engl. J. Med.,* 346, 793, 2002.

6 Vitamin B₆

Christine M. Hansen and Melinda M. Manore

CONTENTS

I. INTRODUCTION

The critical role vitamin B_6 plays in fuel utilization has directed attention to the vitamin from athletes and others interested in exercise performance. In this chapter, we will discuss the interactions between vitamin B_6 status and athletic performance. Because there are many excellent reviews available,[1-3] this chapter will provide only a brief discussion of vitamin B_6 metabolism, function, food sources and recommended intakes and status assessment.

II. VITAMIN B₆ CHEMISTRY AND METABOLISM

A. FORMS AND INTERCONVERSIONS

Vitamin B_6 is the commonly used term for all 3-hydroxy-5-hydroxymethyl-2-methyl pyridine derivatives. The three primary forms are the alcohol form (pyridoxine), the aldehyde (pyridoxal) and the amine (pyridoxamine); each of these may also be phosphorylated on the 5′ position. Metabolism of vitamin B_6 takes place primarily in the liver and the non-phosphorylated forms can be converted by pyridoxine kinase to their phosphorylated forms in an ATP- and zinc-requiring reaction. Pyridoxamine 5′-phosphate and pyridoxine 5′-phosphate can be converted by a flavin mononucleotide-dependent oxidase reaction to pyridoxal 5′-phosphate (PLP). The phosphorylated forms are dephosphorylated by alkaline phosphatase and pyridoxal (PL) can be irreversibly converted to 4-pyridoxic acid (4-PA), the major metabolic end product by an FAD-requiring aldehyde oxidase or an NAD-dependent dehydrogenase.[4]

B. FUNCTIONS

The primary biologically active form of vitamin B_6 is PLP, which functions as a coenzyme for more than 100 mammalian enzymes. Pyridoxal phosphate reacts with the ε-amino groups of lysine groups in enzymes, forming a Schiff base. Enzymes requiring PLP include aminotransferases, decarboxylases, racemases and enzymes involved in side-chain elimination and replacement reactions.[2] Cellular processes in which PLP-requiring reactions play a role include immune function, gluconeogenesis, niacin formation, red cell metabolism, nervous-system function and hormone modulation.[3] Of particular interest to athletes are the roles vitamin B_6 plays in the breakdown of amino acids for energy, the conversion of alanine to glucose in the liver and the utilization of muscle glycogen.

III.   DIETARY SOURCES AND RECOMMENDED INTAKES

Vitamin B_6 is found in a variety of fruits, vegetables, legumes, nuts and dairy products. The major form in animal products is pyridoxal phosphate, while pyridoxine and pyridoxamine and their phosphorylated forms are the major ones in plant foods. An additional form found in plants is pyridoxine glucoside, which has reduced bioavailability compared with pyridoxine.[3] In the United States, the food group that contributes the largest percentage of daily vitamin B_6 intake is fortified, ready-to-eat cereals.[5]

The current recommended dietary allowance (RDA) for vitamin B_6 is 1.3 mg/day for adults 50 years old and younger.[5] Because vitamin B_6 is required by many enzymes in protein metabolism, high dietary protein intakes may increase vitamin B_6 requirements.[6,7] This may be important for athletes who consume protein supplements. Although recommended protein intakes for athletes range from 1.2–1.8 g/kg body weight per day,[8] some athletes have reported protein intakes of as high as 4.3 g/kg body weight. The required ratio of dietary vitamin B_6 to protein has been estimated to be 0.015–0.020 mg/g.[9,10] For an individual consuming 136 g of protein (2.0 g/kg body weight for a 150 lb person), 2.7 mg of vitamin B_6 would be required to supply 0.020 mg/kg protein. Athletes and others consuming high-protein diets may need two or more times the current RDA to meet their metabolic need for vitamin B_6.

Although no adverse effects of high intakes of vitamin B_6 from food sources has been reported, peripheral neuropathy has been reported in individuals with chronic supplemental intakes between 1 and 4 g/d. Based on dose-response studies and the lack of reported adverse effects at doses less than 200 mg/d, the Tolerable Upper Intake Limit (UL) for vitamin B_6 has been set at 100 mg/d.[5]

IV.   VITAMIN B_6 STATUS ASSESSMENT

A variety of measures are used to assess vitamin B_6 status, but there is no consensus as to which measure is best or what levels indicate adequate status. Most investigators agree that more than one measure should be used. For a more detailed discussion of biochemical methods of status assessment, see the review by Reynolds.[11]

A. DIRECT METHODS

Direct methods are methods in which concentrations of the vitamers or 4-PA are measured in blood, urine or tissues. The most frequently used direct measure of vitamin B_6 status is plasma PLP concentration, which has been demonstrated to correlate with dietary intake.[12] Plasma PLP concentrations greater than 30 nmol/L have been suggested to indicate adequate vitamin B$_6$ status.[13] The Dietary Reference Intakes Committee based the current RDA on a plasma PLP concentration of 20 nmol/L, referring to a study in which the lowest reported plasma PLP concentration in apparently healthy men was 20 nmol/L.[5] They stated that "the more conservative cutoff of 20 nmol/L is not accompanied by observable health risks," but a study by Shultz et al. revealed increased lymphocyte DNA strand breaks in subjects whose mean plasma PLP concentration was 23.4 ± 8.5 nmol/L.[14]

Because plasma PLP concentrations can be influenced by plasma activity of alkaline phosphatase and conditions such as pregnancy, some researchers have proposed that measurement of plasma PLP plus PL gives a better assessment of nutritional status. However, not enough data are available to establish adequate values for plasma concentrations of PL or PLP plus PL. Plasma total vitamin B$_6$ concentration (sum of all vitamers) of 40 nmol/L has been suggested to indicate adequate status.[13]

Urinary excretion of 4-PA is also used regularly in vitamin B$_6$ status assessment. Urinary 4-PA responds rapidly to changes in vitamin B$_6$ intake and is considered a good short-term indicator of status. Excretion greater than 3.0 μmol/day has been suggested to indicate adequate vitamin B$_6$ status. Total urinary vitamin B$_6$ has also been used to assess status, but it is relatively insensitive to changes in intake.[11]

B. INDIRECT METHODS

Indirect measures of vitamin B$_6$ status involve measurement of metabolic products of vitamin B$_6$-dependent enzymatic reactions, or enzyme activity. The most commonly used indirect measures are activity coefficients (AC) of erythrocyte alanine or asparate aminotransferase (EALT or EAST). Activity coefficients are calculated by the ratio of enzyme activity with and without added PLP. When vitamin B$_6$ status is compromised, there is a greater increase in activity when exogenous PLP is added, resulting in a higher activity coefficient. Adequate status is indicated when EALT-AC is less than 1.25 or EAST-AC less than 1.80.[13]

Amino acid load tests have also been used as indirect measures of vitamin B$_6$ status. Urinary excretion of tryptophan or methionine metabolites after loading doses of these amino acids indicates availability of the coenzyme PLP for the metabolic enzymes. After a 2 g load of tryptophan, excretion of less than 65 μmol/day of xanthurenic acid indicates adequate vitamin B$_6$ status, or after a 3 g methionine load, excretion of less than 350 μmol/day of cystathionine.[13] Increase in plasma homocysteine concentration can also be measured after a methionine load, but adequate values have not been established.

All measures have both advantages and drawbacks and so a more complete assessment of vitamin B$_6$ status would include at least one direct measure, an indirect measure and evaluation of dietary vitamin B$_6$ and protein intakes.[15]

V. VITAMIN B$_6$ IN SPORTS AND EXERCISE

Vitamin B$_6$ is a cofactor for many metabolic reactions that produce energy, including the transamination of amino acids and the release of glucose from glycogen. Thus, it is not surprising that researchers would ask whether exercise and physical activity increases the need for vitamin B$_6$.

This section will review the current literature examining whether physical activity increases the need for vitamin B$_6$ due to training-induced changes in metabolism that require the vitamin. First, the exercise-related metabolic functions of vitamin B$_6$ will be reviewed. Then the impact of vitamin B$_6$ inadequacy or marginal vitamin status on exercise performance and work will be discussed. Next, we will review the vitamin B$_6$ intakes of active individuals and whether combining exercise with energy restriction for weight loss increase vitamin B-6 needs. Finally, the frequency and impact of vitamin B$_6$ supplementation in active individuals will be reviewed.

A. EXERCISE-RELATED METABOLIC FUNCTIONS

As mentioned above, vitamin B_6 (pyridoxine) has a number of functions related to energy metabolism and, thus, to exercise.[16–20] First, vitamin B_6 is required for the metabolism of proteins and amino acids. Pyridoxal 5′ phosphate, the most biologically active form of vitamin B_6, is a cofactor for transaminases, decarboxylases and other enzymes used in the metabolic transformations of amino acids and nitrogen-containing compounds.[21] In addition, during exercise, gluconeogenesis involves the breakdown of amino acids, with the carbon skeleton being used for energy. Thus, the link between protein intake and vitamin B_6 requirements is especially important for athletes, because active individuals typically have a higher protein requirement than sedentary individuals[8,22] and higher protein intakes, due in part to their higher energy intakes. Another primary function of vitamin B_6 related to physical activity is that PLP is required for glycogen phosphorylase, the key enzyme in the breakdown of muscle glycogen. Active individuals typically have higher glycogen stores and need adequate vitamin B_6 to assure that the energy stored in glycogen can be quickly released when it is needed for energy during exercise.

B. VITAMIN B_6 INADEQUACY AND EXERCISE

Do individuals who engage in physical activity have higher vitamin B_6 needs? Researchers have attempted to answer this question in a number of ways. First, researchers have identified individuals with poor vitamin B_6 status, or have fed diets low in vitamin B_6 and then determined the impact of low status on the ability to do exercise compared with periods of good status. Second, metabolic studies have fed trained and untrained individuals controlled levels of vitamin B_6 to determine whether trained individuals had higher B_6 needs to maintain status. Third, cross-sectional studies have examined the nutritional status of trained individuals to determine the frequency of poor status. At the moment, no longitudinal studies have controlled vitamin B_6 intake in active individuals and determined changes in nutritional status over time, or whether these changes impacted exercise performance or the ability to do work.

1. Exercise Performance and Poor Vitamin B_6 Status

Because of the role vitamin B_6 plays in energy production during exercise, it is generally assumed that individuals with poor vitamin B_6 status will have a reduced ability to perform physical activity. This hypothesis has been supported in studies examining the effect of vitamin B_6 deficiency on work performance.[23–25] For example, van der Beek et al.[25] depleted 24 healthy men of thiamin, riboflavin and vitamin B_6 over an 11-wk metabolic feeding period and then examined the effect of deficiency on physical performance. They found that B-vitamin depletion significantly decreased maximal work capacity (VO2max) by 12%, onset of blood lactate accumulation (OBLA) by 7%, oxygen consumption at OBLA by 12%, peak power by 9% and mean power by 7%. The research study was not designed to separate the impact of vitamin B_6 alone on exercise performance, but does support an earlier study by Suboticanec et al.,[23] who measured the vitamin B_6 status of 124 boys aged 12–14 y. They found that 24% had poor vitamin B_6 status (using erythrocyte aspartate aminotransferase activity coefficient [EAST-AC] >2.00). A subgroup ($n = 37$) of the original sample pool was given 2 mg of vitamin B_6 (pyridoxine) 6 d/wk for 2 months. At the beginning and end of the treatment period, physical work capacity was measured on a bicycle ergometer. The researchers reported a significant negative correlation ($p = 0.036$) between VO2max and E-ASTAC values. Thus, as vitamin B_6 status improved (i.e., EAST-AC values decreased), work capacity improved. These data suggest that subclinical deficiencies of vitamin B_6 can negatively affect the aerobic capacity of young boys and that correction of the vitamin deficiency improves work capacity. As expected, supplementation with vitamin B_6 significantly improved status ($p = 0.001$). In summary, these studies indicate that a deficiency of vitamin B_6 due to poor dietary intakes may decrease the ability to do work, especially maximal work and exercise.

2. Vitamin B$_6$ Metabolic Studies in Active Individuals

Metabolic studies done with active or sedentary individuals consuming known amounts of vitamin B$_6$ indicate that ~1.5–2.3 mg/d of vitamin B$_6$ are required to maintain plasma PLP concentrations above the cutoff value of 30 nmol/L.[7,13,26,27] As mentioned earlier, the 1989 RDA for vitamin B$_6$ was 1.6 mg/d for women and 2.0 mg/d for men,[28] while the 1998 RDA is 1.3 mg/d for both men and women (19–50 y of age).[5] Thus, studies report different adequacy levels for vitamin B$_6$ depending on when the study was done. A metabolic study by Dreon and Butterfield[29] examined vitamin B$_6$ status in men consuming 4.2 mg/d of vitamin B$_6$ and running either 5 or 10 miles/d for 29 d. Data from these active individuals were compared with those from sedentary male controls. In this study, as determined by a methionine load test, vitamin B$_6$ status did not change as individuals increased their running mileage from 5–10 miles/wk. However, subjects were consuming twice the 1989 RDA for vitamin B$_6$ (1.6–2.0 mg/d), which would be well above the current 1998 RDA (1.3 mg/d) and, thus, appeared to have adequate vitamin B$_6$ to cover all the metabolic costs of exercise. No daily measurements of 4-pyridoxic acid (4-PA) excretion were done to determine whether excretion increased on exercise days or was higher when more exercise was done.

In another metabolic study by Manore et al.,[30] three groups of women (recreationally active young, sedentary young, sedentary old) were fed known amounts of vitamin B$_6$ over a 7-wk period. Throughout the study, the active women continued to exercise (2–4 h/wk) and all subjects exercised on a cycle ergometer for 20 min at 80% VO2max four times during the study. Baseline mean plasma PLP concentrations for the active and sedentary young groups were within normal ranges (mean values: 35 and 42 nmol/L, respectively), while the baseline mean value of the sedentary older group was marginal (30 nmol/L). For all groups, mean plasma PLP concentrations improved when fed the metabolic diet providing 2.3 mg/d of vitamin B$_6$. For all groups, plasma PLP concentrations increased significantly during exercise and returned to baseline within 60 min. All individuals responded similarly. This phenomenon has been documented in a number of other studies,[31–33] with only Leonard and Leklem[34] documenting a decrease in PLP with exercise. This study was unique in that it was the first to assess change in vitamin B$_6$ status and PLP during an ultra-endurance run (50 km). The extreme physiological conditions experienced by the subjects during the race may have affected plasma PLP concentrations and may explain why they appeared to respond differently. The metabolic rationale for the increases in plasma PLP observed during exercise is not known, but a number of hypotheses have been proposed and focus on the movement of PLP from various body pools to the plasma during exercise.[16,30–34]

Plasma PLP concentrations typically increase within the first 5 min of exercise and stay elevated during exercise, which increases the probability that PLP will be metabolized to 4-PA and lost in the urine.[31] Thus, exercise can increase the turnover and loss of vitamin B$_6$. Indeed, researchers have documented higher 4-PA losses in active individuals compared with sedentary controls or during non-exercise periods,[30,35] and after a strenuous exercise bout.[31] In addition, Leonard and Leklem[34] found that 4-PA increased 21% in the plasma of individuals after participating in a 50-km run, but did not measure 4-PA urinary losses. Rokitzki et al.[36] recently calculated that marathon runners lost approximately 1 mg of vitamin B$_6$ during a race (26.2 miles), based on 4-PA excretion. However, no research has documented a decrease in plasma PLP concentrations due to exercise-induced 4-PA losses. In general, any loss of vitamin B$_6$ due to exercise is small and could easily be replaced by eating one to two servings of a high-vitamin-B$_6$ food.

3. Vitamin B$_6$ Status of Active Individuals

If exercise increases the need for vitamin B$_6$, then active individuals theoretically should have poor status while consuming the RDA for vitamin B$_6$. Much of the research examining whether exercise increases the need for vitamins has been done with athletes, with some being done in moderately active individuals (4–7 h/wk). Table 6.1 outlines studies that examined the nutritional status of active individuals consuming their free-living diets with no supplemental intakes of vitamin B$_6$.

TABLE 6.1
Incidence of Low or Marginal Vitamin B-6 Status in Studies of Nonsupplemented Active Individuals

Study	Assessment Indices	n	Type of Subjects	Low status (%)	Vitamin B-6 (mg/d)[a]
Fogelholm et al.[54]	EAST-AC[b] (>2.00)	42	Active subjects[c]	43	—
	EAST basal				
Guilland et al.[39]	EAST-AC	55	Male athletes	35	1.5 ± 0.1
	Plasma PLP[b]			17	
Leonard and Leklem[34]	Plasma PLP	11	50-km runners[c]	0	—
	Plasma 4-PA				
	Total B-6				
Manore et al.[30]	Plasma PLP	5	Active females	0	—
	Urine 4-PA				
Telford et al.[37]	EAST-AC	86		60	—
Rokitzki et al.[63]	EAST-AC (>1.50)	57	Athletes[c]	5	1.36–5.40[d]
	Urine 4-PA[b] (<2.73 umol/g creatinine)			18	
	Whole blood				
Weight et al.[64]	Plasma PLP	30	Female athletes	0	1.7 ± 0.6

[a] Mean ± Standard Deviation

[b] EAST-AC = Erythrocyte aspartic aminotransferase (EAST) activity coefficient (AC); 4-PA = 4-Pyridoxic acid; PLP = pyridoxal 5'-phosphate.

[c] Included both males and females.

[d] Researchers used 7-d weighed food records. Values reported are a range of intakes for various male and female athletes.

The number of assessment parameters measured for each study varies, but in most studies, poor status was based on more than one measurement as well as on dietary intake of vitamin B_6. The number of active individuals with poor B_6 status ranged from 0–60%, with the highest percentage reported by Telford et al.[37] They studied 86 male and female athletes before and after an 8-mo training period. During this time, half consumed a multivitamin/mineral supplement and a matched group took a placebo. They found that 60% of the athletes had poor vitamin B_6 status before any supplementation occurred. Fogelholm et al.[38] also examined vitamin B_6 status in 42 physically active college students (18–32 y) before and after 5 weeks of supplementation with vitamin B complex. At the beginning of the study, they found that 43% had poor vitamin B_6 status and, as expected, supplementation significantly increased ($p < 0.0001$) the erythrocyte aspartate aminotransferase activity coefficient (EAST-AC). These data suggest that some active individuals have poor or marginal vitamin B_6 status while consuming their free-living diet.

One reason for poor nutritional status in active individuals may be long-term marginal dietary intakes associated with either poor dietary choices or reduced energy intake.[25,39,40,41] This point was demonstrated by van der Beek et al.,[24,25] where they produced marginal vitamin B_6 deficiency in 8–11 weeks in active men by feeding a highly processed diet. Another reason for inconsistencies in these studies might be related to differences in the experimental design. For example, the studies could vary in the degree of dietary control, the type and intensity of exercise used, the type and number of status indices measured, the level of regular physical activity in which subjects are engaged, the type of subjects used or the lack of a control group. It is known that exercise can increase both energy and protein needs, and thus could increase the total daily needs of vitamin B_6 in active individuals. If active individuals consume adequate energy to maintain body weight and cover exercise energy expenditure, then dietary intakes of vitamin B$_6$ should be adequate unless dietary food choices are poor. For example, if athletes include low-fat animal (e.g., meat, fish and poultry) and plant foods (e.g., bananas, navy beans, walnuts) in their diet, then both protein and vitamin B$_6$ intakes will increase simultaneously. However, if active individuals restrict energy intake or eliminate food groups, then intake of vitamin B$_6$ will probably be low.

C. VITAMIN B$_6$ INTAKES OF ACTIVE INDIVIDUALS

Research examining the dietary vitamin B$_6$ intake of active adult individuals, excluding athletes, is limited. Thus, we reviewed current studies examining dietary intakes (collecting ≥ 3-d diet records) of athletes and active individuals published since 1995. In general, studies report adequate mean dietary intakes of vitamin B$_6$ in active men.[42–47] This can be attributed to the relatively high-energy intakes in these subjects, especially if the study examined intakes during a competitive training period where energy intake is especially high.[42] Only Paschoal et al.[46] reported one male swimmer consuming a mean intake of 0.89 mg B$_6$/d using a 4-d diet record. However, an earlier study by Guilland et al.[39] reported low mean intakes of vitamin B$_6$ in young male athletes (20 y of age), with 67% of their subjects consuming less than 100% of the 1989 RDA (2 mg/d) and having a vitamin B$_6$:protein ratio of 0.013. As expected, the dietary intakes of vitamin B$_6$ are generally lower in active females than males. Most studies report mean vitamin B-6 intakes greater than 66% of the 1989 RDA (1.6 mg/d) and 100% of the 1998 RDA (1.3 mg/d).[40,44,47–51] Those studies reporting lower dietary intakes of vitamin B$_6$ typically also report energy intakes less than 1900 kcal/d.[48,52,53] This point was demonstrated by Leydon and Wall,[53] who examined the intakes of male and female jockeys over a 7-d period in which the subjects alternated from energy-restricted to energy-adequate days depending on their "making weight" goals. Over this 7-d period, mean vitamin B$_6$ intake for all subjects was 0.95 ± 0.44 mg/d. Thus, it appears that unless an individual is restricting energy intake or consuming a diet high in refined foods, nutrient intakes of B$_6$ are near the 1998 RDA level.

D. EXERCISE AND DIETING FOR WEIGHT LOSS

The effect of dieting plus exercise has been examined to a limited extent for vitamin B$_6$. Fogelhom et al.[54] examined the effect of a 3-wk diet (7018 kJ/d or 1700 kcal/d) on male elite wrestlers and found a significant increase in EASTAC (p < 0.01). However, no dietary intake data for vitamin B$_6$ were given. Thus, the poor status might have been due to poor dietary intakes during the dieting period combined with high physical activity. In another study examining the effect of diet plus exercise, van Dale et al.[55] examined the effect of a 14-wk diet-only (3715 kJ/d or 900 kcal/d) or diet-plus-exercise period in 12 obese men (mean age = 40 y). They found that plasma PLP concentrations significantly decreased in the diet-plus-exercise group (54.5 to 40.0 nmol/L) compared with the diet only group (49.8 to 48.7 nmol/L). However, the dietary intake of vitamin B-6 was below the 1989 RDA (2 mg/d) for the last 9 wk of the study. Finally, Lovelady et al.* examined the effect of a 10-wk diet and exercise weight loss program on the B$_6$ status of overweight lactating women (Body Mass Index [BMI] Π25 and Σ30 kg/m^2). All women were consuming a 4-mg/d vitamin B$_6$ from diet and supplements. Results showed that this level of vitamin B$_6$ intake maintained vitamin B$_6$ status in the mothers, who lost ~4.4 kg in 10 wk. However, mean PLP concentrations of the weight loss group were consistently lower than the sedentary control group who was not dieting even though vitamin B$_6$ intakes were similar. In summary, there is limited research on changes in vitamin B$_6$ status in active individuals who diet for weight loss or who lose weight due to the high levels of physical activity they engage in while failing to increase energy intake.**

* Lovelady, C.A., Williams, J.P., Garner, K.E., Moreno, K.L., Taylor, M.L. and Leklem, J.E., Effect of energy restriction and exercise on vitamin B-6 status of women during lactation. *Med. Sci. Sports Exerc.*, 33(4), 512–518, 2001.
** Committee on Military Nutrition Research, Institute of Medicine, Food and Nutrition Board. *Nutrient Composition of Rations of Short-term, High-Intensity Combat Operations.* National Academy Press, 2005.

E. VITAMIN B$_6$ SUPPLEMENTATION IN ACTIVE INDIVIDUALS

Although marginal vitamin B$_6$ status appears to negatively impact exercise performance and the ability to do work, no data support that supplementation with vitamin B$_6$, above that necessary to produce good status, improves exercise performance.[58,59] Virk et al.[59] fed two different metabolic diets varying in vitamin B$_6$ content — either 2.3 mg/d or 22 mg/d — for 9 days to trained males who exercised to exhaustion on each diet. Vitamin B$_6$ intake had no effect on exercise times to exhaustion.

Based on recent surveys, ~36–47% of athletes report using a multivitamin or multivitamin-mineral supplement regularly ($\geq$ 5 times/week).[60–62] These types of supplements typically include vitamin B$_6$ at 100% or more of the daily value (2 mg/d). Participants typically reported they supplemented to improve overall health. Few athletes (1–4%) surveyed by Herbold et al.[61] and Froiland et al.[60] used single vitamin B$_6$ supplements, but Morrison et al.[62] found that 16% of individuals who exercised at a commercial gym used a B-complex supplement on a regular basis. Examination of supplement use in elite figure skates indicated that both male (61%) and female (83%) athletes were high users of multivitamin-mineral supplements.[47] Thus, active individuals, especially competitive athletes, appear to use supplements on a regular basis.

VI. SUMMARY AND CONCLUSIONS

Research examining the vitamin B$_6$ needs of active individuals is still limited, with most of the work being done in competitive athletes. Exercise appears to increase the loss of vitamin B$_6$ through urinary 4-PA excretion; however, the amount of additional vitamin B$_6$ needed to cover losses or increased need is small and could be easily met through good food choices. Little research is available on the effect of combining both diet and exercise for weight loss on vitamin B$_6$ status. If individuals are restricting energy intake for weight loss or making poor dietary choices, dietary intakes of vitamin B$_6$ will probably be low. Finally, no data are available on the effect of exercise or dieting plus exercise on vitamin B$_6$ status of individuals with chronic health problems that may increase the need for vitamin B$_6$, such as diabetes, cardiovascular disease, arthritis or hypertension.

REFERENCES

1. Dakshinamurti, K., Ed., Vitamin B$_6$, *Ann. N.Y. Acad. Sci.* 585, 1990.
2. Bender, D.A., Vitamin B$_6$, in *Nutritional Biochemistry of the Vitamins,* 2nd ed., Cambridge University Press, Cambridge, UK, 2003, pp. 232–269.
3. Leklem, J.E., Vitamin B$_6$, in *Handbook of Vitamins,* 3rd ed., Rucker, R.B., Suttie, J.W., McCormick, D.B. and Machlin, L.J., Eds., Marcel Dekker, Inc., New York, 2001, pp. 339–396.
4. Merrill, A.H. and Henderson, J.M., Vitamin B$_6$ metabolism by human liver, *Ann. N.Y. Acad. Sci.* 585, 110–117, 1990.
5. Institute of Medicine, *Dietary Reference Intakes for Thiamin, Riboflavin, Niacin, Vitamin B$_6$, Folate, Vitamin B$_{12}$, Pantothenic Acid, Biotin and Choline,* National Academy Press, Washington, D.C., 1998.
6. Miller, L.T., Leklem, J.E. and Shultz, T.D., The effect of dietary protein on the metabolism of vitamin B$_6$ in humans, *J. Nutr.,* 15, 1663–1672, 1985.
7. Hansen, C.M., Leklem, J.E. and Miller, L.T., Vitamin B-6 status of women with a constant intake of vitamin B-6 changes with three levels of dietary protein, *J. Nutr.* 126, 1891–1901, 1996.
8. Lemon, P.W.R., Beyond the zone: Protein needs of active individuals, *J. Am. Coll. Nutr.,* 19, 513S–521S, 2000.
9. Kretsch, M.J., Sauberlich, H.E., Skala, J.H. and Johnson, H.L., Vitamin B-6 requirement and status assessment: Young women fed a depletion diet followed by plant- or animal-protein diet with graded amounts of vitamin B-6, *Am. J. Clin. Nutr.,* 61, 1091–1101, 1995.
10. Hansen, C.M., Shultz, T.D., Kwak, HK, Memon, H.S. and Leklem, J.E. Assessment of vitamin B-6 status in young women consuming a controlled diet containing four levels of vitamin B-6 provides an estimated average requirement and recommended dietary allowance, *J. Nutr.,* 131, 1777–1786, 2001.

11. Reynolds, R.D., Biochemical methods for status assessment, in *Vitamin B-6 Metabolism in Pregnancy, Lactation and Infancy,* Raiten, D.J., Ed., CRC Press, Boca Raton, FL, 1995, pp. 41–59.

12. Shultz, T.D. and Leklem, J.E., Urinary 4-pyridoxic acid, urinary vitamin B$_6$ and plasma pyridoxal phosphate as measures of vitamin B$_6$ status and dietary intake of adults, in *Methods in Vitamin B$_6$ Nutrition,* Leklem, J.E. and Reynolds, R.D., Eds., Plenum Press, New York, 1981, pp. 297–320.

13. Leklem, J.E., Vitamin B-6: A status report. *J. Nutr.,* 120, 1503–1517, 1990.

14. Shultz, T.D., Hansen, C.M., Hunt, K.C., Hardin, K., Leklem, J.E., Huang, A. and Ames, B.N., Lymphocyte DNA strand breaks in smokers and nonsmokers are related to vitamin B-6 (B-6) intake and metabolite concentrations in plasma and urine, *FASEB J.* 17, A1156, 2003.

15. Leklem, J.E. and Reynolds, R.D., Recommendations for status assessment of vitamin B$_6$, in *Methods in Vitamin B$_6$ Nutrition,* Leklem, J.E. and Reynolds, R.D., Eds., Plenum Press, New York, 1981, pp. 389–392.

16. Manore, M.M., Vitamin B-6 and exercise. *Int. J. Sport Nutr.,* 4, 89–103, 1994.

17. Manore, M.M., The effect of physical activity on thiamin, riboflavin and vitamin B-6 requirements. *Am. J. Clin. Nutr.,* 72, 598S–606S, 2000.

18. Manore, M.M., Barr, S.I. and Butterfield, G.A., Position of the American Dietetic Association, Dietitians of Canada and the American College of Sports Medicine: Nutrition and athletic performance. *J. Am. Diet. Assoc.,* 100, 1543–1556, 2000.

19. Manore, M.M. and Thompson, J.L., *Sport Nutrition for Health and Performance.* Human Kinetics Publishers, Champaign, IL, 2000.

20. Maughan, R.J., Role of micronutrients in sport and physical activity. *Brit. Med. J.,* 55(3), 683–690, 1999.

21. Leklem, J.E., Vitamin B$_6$. in Shils, M.E., Olsen, J.A., Shike, M. and Ross, C.A. Eds. *Modern Nutrition in Health and Disease,* 9th ed. Philadelphia, PA: Lippincott, Willams and Wilkins, 1999, pp. 412–423.

22. Lemon, P.W.R., Effects of exercise on dietary protein requirements. *Int. J. Sport Nutr.,* 8, 426–447, 1998.

23. Suboticanec, K., Stavljenic, A., Schalch, W. and Buzina, R., Effects of pyridoxine and riboflavin supplementation on physical fitness in young adolescents. *Int. J. Vit. Nutr., Res.,* 60, 81–88, 1990.

24. van der Beek, E.J., van Dokkum, W. and Schrijver, J., et al., Thiamin, riboflavin and vitamins B$_6$ and C: Impact of combined restricted intake on functional performance in man. *Am. J. Clin. Nutr.,* 48, 1451–1462, 1988.

25. van der Beek, E.J., van Dokkum, W., Wedel, M., Schrijver, J. and van den Berg, H., Thiamin, riboflavin and vitamin B$_6$: Impact of restricted intake on physical performance in man. *J. Am. Coll. Nutr.,* 13, 629–640, 1994.

26. Hansen, C.M., Shultz, T.D., Kwak, H.K., Memon, S. and Leklem, J.E., Assessment of vitamin B-6 status in young women consuming a controlled diet containing four levels of vitamin B$_6$ provides an estimated average requirement and recommended dietary allowance. *J. Nutr.,* 131, 1777–1786, 2001.

27. Huang, Y., Chen, W., Evans, M.A., Mitchell, M.E. and Schultz, T.D., Vitamin B$_6$ requirement and status assessment of young women fed a high-protein diet with various levels of vitamin B-6. *Am. J. Clin. Nutr.,* 67, 208–220, 1998.

28. Food and Nutrition Board, National Research Council. *Recommended Dietary Allowances.* 10th ed., Washington, D.C.: National Academy Press, 1989.

29. Dreon, D.M. and Butterfield, G.E., Vitamin B$_6$ utilization in active and inactive young men. *Am. J. Clin. Nutr.,* 43, 816–824, 1986.

30. Manore, M.M., Leklem, J.E. and Walter, M.C., Vitamin B$_6$ metabolism as affected by exercise in trained and untrained women fed diets differing in carbohydrate and vitamin B$_6$ content. *Am. J. Clin. Nutr.,* 46, 995–1004, 1987.

31. Crozier, P.G., Cordain, L. and Sampson, D.A., Exercise-induced changes in plasma vitamin B$_6$ concentrations do not vary with exercise intensity. *Am. J. Clin. Nutr.,* 60, 552–58, 1994.

32. Leklem, J.E. and Shultz, T.D., Increased plasma pyridoxal 5′-phosphate and vitamin B$_6$ in male adolescents after a 4500-meter run. *Am. J. Clin. Nutr.,* 38, 541–548, 1983.

33. Hofmann, A., Reynolds, R.D., Smoak, B.L., Villanueva, V.G. and Deuster, P.A., Plasma pyridoxal and pyridoxal 5'-phosphate concentrations in response to ingestion of water or glucose polymer during a 2-h run. *Am. J. Clin. Nutr.,* 53, 84–89, 1991.

34. Leonard, S.W. and Leklem, J.E., Plasma B-6 vitamer changes following a 50-km ultramarathon. *Int. J. Sport Nutr. Exerc. Metab.,* 10, 302–314, 2000.

35. Dunton, N., Virk, R. and Leklem, J., The influence of vitamin B_6 supplementation and exercise to exhaustion on vitamin B_6 metabolism. *FASEB J.,* 6, A1374 (abstract), 1992.

36. Rokitzki, L., Sagredos, A.N., Reub, F., Buchner, M. and Keul, J., Acute changes in vitamin B_6 status in endurance athletes before and after a marathon. *Int. J. Sport Nutr.,* 4, 154–165, 1994.

37. Telford, R.D., Catchpole, E.A., Deakin, V., McLeay, A.C. and Plank, A.W., The effect of 7 to 8 months of vitamin/mineral supplementation on the vitamin and mineral status of athletes. *Int. J. Sport Nutr.,* 2, 123–134, 1992.

38. Fogelholm, G.M., Koskinen, R., Laakso, J., Rankinen, T. and Ruokonen, I., Gradual and rapid weight loss: Effects on nutrition and performance in male athletes. *Med. Sci. Sports Exerc.,* 25, 371–377, 1993.

39. Guilland, J.C., Penaranda, T., Gallet, C., Boggio, V., Fuchs, F. and Klepping, J., Vitamin status of young athletes including the effects of supplementation. *Med. Sci. Sports Exerc.,* 21, 441–449, 1989.

40. Beals, K.A. and Manore, M.M., Nutritional status of female athletes with subclinical eating disorders. *J. Am. Diet. Assoc.,* 98, 419–25, 1998.

41. Beals, K.A. and Manore, M.M., Subclinical eating disorders in physically active women. *Topics in Clin. Nutr.,* 14(3), 14–29, 1999.

42. Garcia-Roves, P.M., Terrados, N., Fernandez, S. and Patterson, A.M., Comparison of dietary intake and eating behavior of professional road cyclists during training and competition. *Int. J. Sport Nutr. Exerc. Metab.,* 10, 82–98, 2000.

43. Rico-Sanz, J., Frontera, W.R., Mole, P.A., Rivera, M.A., Rivera-Brown, A. and Meredith, C.N., Dietary and performance assessment of elite soccer players during a period of intense training. *Int. J. Sport Nutr.,* 8, 230–40, 1998.

44. Jonnalagadda, S.S., Ziegler, P.J. and Nelson, J.A., Food preferences, dieting behaviors and body image perceptions of elite figure skaters. *Int. J. Sport Nutr. Exerc. Metab.,* 14, 594–606, 2004.

45. Niekamp, R.A. and Baer, J.T., In-season dietary adequacy of trained male cross-country runners. *Int. J. Sport Nutr.,* 5, 45–55, 1995.

46. Paschoal, V.C.P. and Amancio, O.M.S., Nutritional status of Brazilian elite swimmers. *Int. J. Sport Nutr. Exerc. Metab.,* 14, 81–94, 2004.

47. Ziegler, P.J., Nelson, J.A. and Jonnalagadda, S.S., Use of dietary supplements by elite figure skaters. *Int. J. Sport Nutr. Exerc. Metab.,* 13, 266–276, 2003.

48. Clark, M., Reed, D.B., Crouse, S.F. and Armstrong, R.B., Pre- and post-season dietary intake, body composition and performance indices of NCAA Division I female soccer players. *Int. J. Sport Nutr. Exerc. Metab.,* 13, 303–319, 2003.

49. Beshgeteoor, D. and Nichols, J.F., Dietary intake and supplement use in female master cyclists and swimmers. *Int. J. Sport Nutr. Exerc. Metab.,* 13, 166–172, 2003.

50. Kopp-Woodroffe, S.A., Manore, M.M., Dueck, C.A., Skinner, J.S. and Matt, K.S., Energy and nutrient status of amenorrheic athletes participating in a diet and exercise training intervention program. *Int. J. Sport Nutr.,* 9, 70–88, 1999.

51. Mullins, V.A., Houtkooper, L.B., Howell, W.H., Going, S.B. and Brown, C.H., Nutritional status of U.S. elite female heptathletes during training. *Int. J. Sport Nutr. Exerc. Metab.,* 11, 299–314, 2001.

52. Papadopoulou, S.K., Papadopoulou, S.D. and Gallos, G.K., Macro- and micro-nutrient intake of adolescent Greek female volleyball players. *Int. J. Sport Nutr. Exerc. Metab.,* 12, 73–80, 2002.

53. Leydon, M.A. and Wall, C., New Zealand jockeys' dietary habits and their potential impact on health. *Int. J. Sport Nutr. Exerc. Metab.* 12, 220–237, 2002.

54. Fogelholm, M., Ruokonen, I., Laakso, J.T., Vuorimaa, T. and Himberg, J.J., Lack of association between indices of vitamin B_1, B_2 and B_6 status and exercise-induced blood lactate in young adults. *Int. J. Sport Nutr.,* 3, 165–176, 1993.

55. van Dale, D., Schrijver, J. and Saris, W.H.M., Changes in vitamin status in plasma during dieting and exercise. *Int. J. Vit. Nutr. Res.,* 60, 67–74, 1990.

56. Lovelady, C.A., Williams, J.P., Garner, K.E., Moreno, K.L., Taylor, M.L. and Leklem, J.E., Effect of energy restriction and exercise on vitamin B_6 status of women during lactation. *Med. Sci. Sports Exerc.,* 33(4), 512–518, 2001.

57. Committee on Military Nutrition Research, Institute of Medicine, Food and Nutrition Board. *Nutrient Composition of Rations of Short-term, High-Intensity Combat Operations.* National Academies Press, 2005.

58. van der Beek, E.J., Vitamin supplementation and physical exercise performance. *J. Sports Sci.,* 9: 77–89, 1991.

59. Virk, R.S., Dunton, N.J., Young, J.C. and Leklem, J.E., Effect of vitamin B$_6$ supplementation on fuels, catacholamines and amino acids during exercise in men. *Med. Sci. Sports Exerc.* 31(3), 400–408, 1999.

60. Froiland, K., Koszewski, W., Hingst, J. and Kopecky, L., Nutritional supplement use among college athletes and their sources of information. *Int. J. Sport Nutr. Exerc. Metab.,* 14, 104–120, 2004.

61. Herbold, N.H., Visconti, B.K., Frates, S. and Bandini, L., Traditional and nontraditional supplement use by college female varsity athletes. *Int. J. Sport Nutr. Exerc. Metab.,* 24, 586–593, 2004.

62. Morrison, L.J., Gizis, F. and Shorter, B., Prevalent use of dietary supplements among people who exercise at a commercial gym. *Int. J. Sport Nutr. Exerc. Metab.,* 14, 481–491, 2004.

63. Rokitzki, L., Sagredos, A.N., Reub, F., Cufi, D. and Keul, J., Assessment of vitamin B$_6$ status of strength and speedpower athletes. *J. Am. Coll. Nutr.,* 13, 87–94, 1994.

64. Weight, L.M., Noakes, T.D., Labadarios, D., Graves, J., Jacobs, P. and Berman, P.A., Vitamin and mineral status of trained athletes including the effects of supplementation. *Am. J. Clin. Nutr.,* 47, 186–191, 1988.

7 Folate

Wayne E. Billon

CONTENTS

I. INTRODUCTION

Folate is fast emerging as the vanguard of protection against many diseases. However, the specific role of folate in exercise performance has yet to be adequately defined. Because the functions of folate in the human body are necessary for optimal health, adequate folate is necessary for optimal athletic performance. This is particularly true of endurance athletes, as folate is necessary for the production of erythrocytes. Folate, a required constituent of certain enzymes involved in amino acid metabolism, has a critical role in cell reproduction, being required for the synthesis of DNA and RNA. This chapter discusses the requirement, status and function of folate in the general population with emphasis on the athlete and exercise performance.

A. BRIEF HISTORY

Over a period of several years, a number of compounds that had folate activity were independently discovered. In 1931, Lucy Wills, an English physician working in India, observed a macrocytic anemia in poor pregnant women. She found an extract in both liver and yeast that was effective in curing the anemia.[1] In 1935, Day, Langston and Shukers reported on an anemia that was produced in monkeys fed a refined diet.[2] In 1938, Langston et al. proposed that the substance missing in the refined diet was vitamin M.[3] In 1940, Snell and Peterson isolated a factor in liver and in yeast that enabled *Lactobacillus casei* to grow.[4] This substance became known as the *L. casei* growth factor. In 1940, Hogan and Parrott observed that chicks on a simplified diet failed to grow and developed anemia. A liver extract added to the diet cured the anemia. The researchers concluded that the substance was a B vitamin and named it vitamin B_c.[5] In 1941, Mitchell, Snell and Williams isolated a growth factor from spinach that promoted growth in *Streptococcus lactis R* similar to the *L. casei* growth factor and named it folic acid.[6] The name "folic acid" comes from *folium*, the Latin word for leaf. In 1943, Stokstad synthesized folic acid and Angier et al. published the results in 1945.[7] The synthesis of folate proved that the structure contained a pteridine ring, paraminobenozic acid and glutamic acid.[8] In time, it was realized that all of the above factors were in the same family and were called folates or folacin. Today, folacin, folates and folic acid are used interchangeably; however, it has been suggested that the term folacin no longer be used.[9]

B. CHEMICAL STRUCTURE

Folate is the generic term for a group of derivatives found in plants that have similar chemical structures and properties. All of the derivatives are reduced forms of the B vitamin, folic acid. Folate is the natural form found in plants, and folic acid is the synthetic form found in vitamin tablets and fortified food. Folates found naturally in plants usually have additional glutamate residues (up to nine[10]) bound together in peptide linkages to the gamma carboxyl group of the glutamate. The structure of folate consists of a double pteridine ring that is covalently bound to para-aminobenzoic acid (PABA) and glutamate, commonly called PGA.[11] The chemical formula is $C_{19}H_{19}N_7O_6$ (Figure 7.1).

C. GENERAL PROPERTIES

The biologically active form of folic acid in serum is tetrahydrofolic acid (THFA). It has two reactive sites in the pteridine ring, one each at the 5 and 10 nitrogens.[12] Either of these two sites can be methylated, with the most common methylation being N-5-methyltetrahydrofolic acid (MTHFA). Folate acts as a coenzyme and N-5-MTHFA is the primary active form.[13]

THFA is important in one-carbon transfer reactions, particularly those involved with amino acid metabolism and nucleotide bases for DNA and RNA biosynthesis.[12] Normal metabolism produces

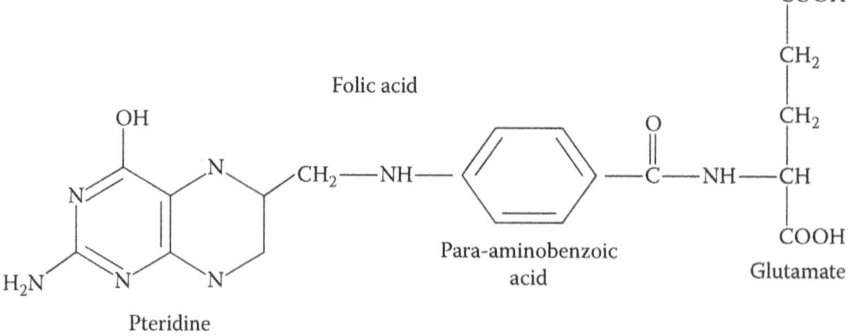

FIGURE 7.1 Structure of folic acid

several one-carbon fragments, such as methyl (–CH$_3$), methylene (–CH$_2$–), methenyl (=CH–), formyl (O=CH–),[14] or formimino (–CHNH).[15] The one-carbon group that is being transferred is bonded to the N^5 or to the N^{10} or to both. THFA can exist in three different oxidation states: the most reduced, the intermediate and the most oxidized form. The most reduced carries a methyl group, the intermediate a methylene and the most oxidized a methenyl, a formyl, or a formimino group.[15] Two basic methods are used to measure folate in blood: microbiological assays and radiometric techniques.[13]

D. METABOLIC FUNCTIONS

The role of folate in anemia is well established. Anemia was the first deficiency symptom associated with the vitamin.[1–3] Folate deficiency is characterized by the inability of erythrocytes to replicate normally,[16] resulting in a megaloblastic anemia.[17] This is important to athletes, particularly endurance athletes, because of the need to transport oxygen. The large oval cells of this anemia have less hemoglobin and a reduced capacity to carry oxygen through the blood.

Because folate is necessary for DNA synthesis, it is important in the reproduction of cells, particularly those that rapidly proliferate as erythrocytes, gastrointestinal epithelium and fetal cells. The relationship between folate deficiency and neural-tube defects is also well established. Folate supplementation around conception greatly decreases the risk of having an offspring with a neural-tube defect.[18–21]

The relationship between folic acid and homocysteine has been the focus of considerable research. Homocysteine is an intermediate sulfur-containing amino acid that is formed during normal metabolism and converted to the essential amino acid methionine. THFA, along with vitamins B$_6$ and B$_{12}$, is important in the conversion of homocysteine to methionine. Homocysteine is produced as a result of methylation reactions. The two most productive methyltransferases are guanidinoacetate methyltransferase and phosphatidylethanolamine N-methyltransferase. The first produces creatine and the latter produces phosphatidylcholine.[22] Both reactions increase plasma homocysteine. The methylation of guanidinoacetate to produce creatine requires more methyl groups than all other methylation reactions combined.[23] This is significant to athletes because creatine production is a vital factor in exercise. Because of the diseases associated with hyperhomocysteinemia, its production during exercise should be of concern to the athlete.

Hyperhomocysteinemia has been suspected as a risk factor for atherosclerosis,[24] particularly with diabetics.[25] Elevated homocysteine has now emerged as a major player in atherosclerosis[26–28] and Alzheimer's.[29–32] It may have a causative role in some cancers,[33–36] and possibly increases susceptibility to osteoporotic fractures.[37,38] It may cause chromosome damage,[42] and is elevated in stroke patients,[39] patients with depression,[40] dementia,[29] and those having Parkinson's disease who are taking L-DOPA.[22,41]

Simultaneous with homocysteine research, folic acid is emerging as the vanguard nutrient to possibly prevent all of the diseases mentioned, because it has been shown to lower plasma homocysteine.[43,44] Hyperhomocysteinemia has been correlated with decreased levels of either B$_{12}$ or folate.[25,45] Several studies have reported that folate treatments significantly reduced elevated homocysteine in chronic renal insufficiency and hemodialysis patients,[46] while others reported a beneficial effect from high daily doses of folate and B$_6$,[47] or with high daily dosing of folate, B$_6$ and B$_{12}$.[48] Research completed in the Netherlands found the combined supplementation of folate, B$_6$ and B$_{12}$ to reduce homocysteine by 30% compared with a placebo.[49]

Most of the research with homocysteine has to do with methylation. Feron and Vogelstein point out that the loss of DNA methylation has been shown to inhibit chromosome condensation and thus might lead to mitotic nondisjunction.[50] The U.S. Nurses' Health Study suggested that an increase in dietary folate and vitamin B$_6$ above the normal requirements may be a primary preventive measure against coronary heart disease[51] and the Kuopio Ischemic Heart Disease Risk Factor Study found a significant inverse relationship between folate intakes and acute coronary events in men.[52]

Clark and co-workers believe hyperhomocysteinemia to be a weak risk factor for asymptomatic extracranial carotid atherosclerosis.[53] Majors and co-workers suggested that homocysteine accumulation might promote an increase in both collagen production and total protein synthesis, which could increase the risk for vascular disease. Majors quotes others that indicate elevated homocysteine may promote the oxidation of LDL and have the potential to increase free radicals.[54] Moustapha et al. believe their research confirms that patients with elevated plasma homocysteine levels have a greater likelihood of developing thrombotic or atherosclerotic complications.[55] Stanger et al., investigating the management of homocysteine, folate and B vitamins in treatment of cardiovascular and thrombotic diseases, reported that a plasma homocysteine concentration of 10 μmol/l could produce a linear dose-response relationship for increased risk of cardiovascular disease. The researchers further stated that hyperhomocysteinemia, as an independent risk factor for cardiovascular disease, is thought to be responsible for 10% of the total risk.[56]

In a review of hyperhomocysteinemia, Virdis and co-workers conclude that experimental evidence exists to suggest hyperhomocysteinemia can be considered an independent risk factor for the recurrence of cardiovascular events and could be a predictor of new cardiovascular events.[26] Others also consider hyperhomocysteinemia to be an independent risk factor for coronary disease.[27,28] Despite all of the information relating homocysteine with cardiovascular disease, the American Heart Association has yet to declare hyperhomocysteinemia as a major risk factor for cardiovascular disease.[57]

Aside from folate's relationship with homocysteine, the latest-breaking news about folate is promising. Wilmink et al. completed a case-controlled study on the effect of folate and vitamin B_6 intake on peripheral arterial occlusive disease in men over the age of 50. Their model suggests that a daily increase of folate by one standard deviation decreased the risk of peripheral arterial occlusive disease by 46%. This was independent of serum levels of homocysteine.[58] Moat and others observed that folic acid supplementation could reverse endothelial dysfunction observed in patients with cardiovascular disease, also independent of homocysteine levels.[59] When adolescents and children with type 1 diabetes were given 5 mg of folic acid for 8 weeks, there was an improvement in endothelial function independent of homocysteine.[60]

The relationship between elevated homocysteine and athletes is important, because research suggests that endurance exercises may cause a significant increase in plasma homocysteine. Twenty-five percent of the recreational endurance athletes studied in one trial exhibited hyperhomocysteinemia in association with low intakes of folate and B_{12}.[61] Another study completed with rats indicated that exercise increased endothelial nitric oxide. If this is true in humans, it may have a protective effect against elevated homocysteine, which decreases nitric oxide.[62] A Dutch study did not find a significant effect on plasma homocysteine concentration due to exercise[63] while another study suggests that proper diet and exercise may lower homocysteine levels.[64]

Research at Tufts University indicated that the elderly are susceptible to metabolic and physiological changes that affect B_{12}, B_6 and folate status. Low gastric pH enhances the absorption of B_{12} and folate, and many of the elderly have decreased production of gastric acid.[65]

The serum homocysteine status is affected by many variables and, in most cases, elevated homocysteine is probably the result of a combination of factors, including gender, age, smoking, nutrition, coffee and alcohol.[66]

E. NUTRIENT STATUS ASSESSMENT

Clinical manifestations of folate deficiency occur only after severe depletion of the vitamin on the tissue level.[9] Folate deficiency could be prompted by several conditions:

A folate deficient diet for 2 to 4 months
Chronic alcoholism
Pregnancy or lactation without increased intake
Hypermetabolic states
Disorders of the intestines that cause a decrease in folate absorption
Medications such as oral contraceptives, phenytoin and other anticonvulsants
Folic acid antagonists used to treat cancer, such as methotrexate and aminopterin[13]

TABLE 7.1
Stages of Folate Deficiency

	1	2	3	4
Serum Folate ng/ml	<3*	<3	<3	<3
RBC Folate ng/ml	>200	<160	<120	<100
Serum Homocysteine μmol/L	Normal	Normal	High	High
Erythrocytes	Normal	Normal	Normal	Macrocytic
MCV	Normal	Normal	Normal	Elevated
Hgb g/dl	>12	>12	>12	<12
Clinical or Subclinical Evidence	Early negative balance	Folate depletion	Folate deficiency	Folate deficiency and anemia evident
Effects on exercise performance	Folate requiring enzymes inhibition may be occurring, but probably no measurable effect seen.	Folate requiring enzymes inhibition may be occurring, but probably not much of a measurable effect seen.	RBC production inhibited and O_2 availability to cells is reduced; performance inhibited, particularly high intensity.	RBCs enlarged; O_2 availability is reduced; endurance is decreased.

* Normal serum folate is >5. This is the first indication of an abnormality.

Adapted from Herbert, Chapter 26 Folic Acid *In Modern Nutrition in Health and Disease,* 9th ed. Sils, M.E., Olson, J.A., Shine, M. and Ross, A.C. (Eds.) 1995. Williams & Wilkins, Baltimore, Maryland and from Manore, M. and Thompson, *J. Sport Nutrition for Health and Performance.* 2000. Human Kinetics, United States.

The stages of folate deficiency have been characterized by Herbert (Table 7.1). In the first stage, folate drops below 3 ng/ml. This is serum only and does not reflect tissue levels. In stage II, folate drops in serum and erythrocytes. In the third stage, erythrocyte folate continues to decrease and homocysteine begins to rise. DNA synthesis is affected and erythropoiesis is inhibited.[67] Hemoglobin is still in the normal range, but could be decreased enough to affect oxygen availability to cells, particularly with intense exercise.[68] In the final stage, frank folate deficiency is manifested by megaloblastic anemia and decreased hemoglobin.[67]

Clinical symptoms of folate deficiency include glossitis, diarrhea, weight loss, nervous instability,[9] and dementia.[9,29,69] To determine subclinical deficiency and the true status of folate, biochemical measurements are necessary. The primary reason for looking at serum folate is suspected megaloblastic anemia.[13] Serum folic acid reflects recent folate intake and not total body stores. If serum folate levels are normal, it does not mean that the subject is not folate deficient. Erythrocyte folate is a better reflection of total body stores and shows the level of folate over the last 120 days.[70]

A deficiency of either folic acid or B_{12} can cause a megaloblastic anemia. If a deficiency of B_{12} is not corrected, nerve damage can occur because B_{12} deficiency can cause demyelination of nerves. Folic acid does not correct demyelination, but it can correct a megaloblastic anemia from B_{12} deficiency.[11] Therefore, it has been suggested that folic acid supplementation should not exceed 1,000 μg per day so as not to mask a B_{12} deficiency.[71] Other researchers emphasize that the masking of B_{12} is more likely in the elderly. When recommending greater than the tolerable upper limits of folic acid (not food folate), a multivitamin that includes B_{12} should also be recommended.[72]

There is no direct evidence that indicates an increased requirement of folate as a result of exercise. However, as the intensity of exercise increases, there is a need for increased creatine and methylation will increase.[23] Logically, the need for folate will increase, but logic does not always prove to be correct in such instances. Also, an increase in appetite and food consumption usually accompanies an increase in the duration and intensity of exercise. If the increase in consumption is balanced and contains an increase in natural folate or food fortified with folic acid, the athlete may not need additional folate. If the increased consumption is not balanced with an increase in folate, or if the athlete erroneously believes the increased intake should be primarily meat and protein, then the athlete may need additional folate. The bottom line dictates a need for additional research and the need for individual evaluation of each case by a qualified nutritional professional, such as a registered dietitian.

F. NATURAL FOLATE CONTENT OF FOOD

Mammals do not have the ability to synthesize folic acid so it is an essential nutrient and must be ingested by humans. The best sources are liver and organ meats. Beans, peas and green leafy vegetables are also good sources. A sample of common foods containing folic acid can be found in Table 7.2.

G. FOLATE ENRICHMENT OF FOOD

After many years of research, the Food and Drug Administration, in March of 1996, mandated enriched cereal-grain products to be fortified with 140 μg of folic acid per 100 g of flour. The mandate was implemented January 1, 1998.[74]

Providing vitamin and mineral supplementation periconceptionally results in significant prevention of neural-tube defects as well as urinary tract and cardiovascular defects, a decrease in limb deficiencies and congenital hypertropic pyloric stenosis.[75]

Food supplementation of less than 300 μg per day of folic acid lowered plasma homocysteine in one study, but the authors suggest that it may take more than 300 μg per day to substantially lower plasma homocysteine.[76] In a study completed on 41 Caucasian men ($\geq$ 58 years of age) who were taking in more than 400 μg of folate, supplementary intake of folic acid from fortified cereals did not have an additional lowering effect on homocysteine.[77] Jacques et al. used the Framingham Offspring Study cohort to see the effects of folic acid fortification of enriched grains on plasma folate and total homocysteine concentrations. They found the mean plasma folate concentrations increased significantly ($p < 0.001$) and the level of plasma homocysteine decreased significantly ($p < 0.001$).[78]

TABLE 7.2
Sources of dietary folate[1,2]

Serving size	Item	μg of Folate	Serving size	Item	μg of folate
3.5 oz (99g)	Cooked chicken liver	770	½ c (99g)	Lentils	179
3.5 oz (99g)	Cooked beef liver	220	½ c (86g)	Pinto beans, boiled	148
3.5 oz (99g)	Cooked salmon	34	1 c (248g)	Fresh orange juice	75
3.0 oz (85g)	Yellow fin tuna	1.7	1 oz (28g)	Peanuts, dry roasted	40.6
3.0 oz (85g)	Beef, ground	6.0	½ c (90g)	Spinach, boiled	131.4
4.0 oz (113g)	Chicken, light meat, raw	4.5	2 oz (57g)	Plain pasta	100.3
4.0 oz (113g)	Chicken, dark meat, raw	7.9	½ c (93g)	White rice, enriched, cooked	54.9
3.0 oz (85g)	Pork, center chop/raw	2.9	1 c (244g)	Milk, whole	12
1 whole (50g)	Cooked egg	22	1 slice (21g)	Swiss cheese	1.2
1 cup (28g)	Corn flakes[+]	98.8	1 slice (30g)	White bread	28.5
1 cup (47g)	Bran flakes[++]	165.9	1 whole (102g)	Generic cheeseburger	54.1

[1] Includes supplemented folate in processed grains
[2] Taken from Nutrients in Food by E.S. Hands[73]
[+] Range among three fortified brands = 98.8 to 133.3, weight varies
[++] Range among eight brands = 46.9 to 273.0, weight varies

H. TOXICITY

Whittaker et al. analyzed 29 breakfast cereals for iron and folic acid. They found the values for folate ranged from 98% to 320% of the label values. The values for iron ranged from 80% to 190%. They expressed concern that consumption of breakfast cereals may contribute to excessive intakes of iron and folate.[79] Sisk and co-workers studied 3-day diet records of 320 subjects to determine the total folate intake from food and supplements before and after the fortification of grains. They found only five subjects took over 1,000 µg (tolerable upper limits) of supplemental folate per day. They concluded that the fortification of grains with folic acid did not appear to be a risk of folate toxicity in the population studied.[80] Folate toxicity is not an outstanding problem, but there are concerns about excessive folic acid consumption that can be divided into three areas: (1) masking pernicious anemia of B_{12} deficiency and allowing for neurological damage; (2) possible interference with zinc function and (3) interference with certain medications.[81] Large doses of folic acid have been known to interfere with anticonvulsant drugs, particularly Dilantin.[82]

I. ABSORPTION, DISTRIBUTION AND ELIMINATION

Folate is absorbed primarily in the proximal third of the jejunum but can be absorbed anywhere in the small bowel. Most folates found naturally in plants are in a polyglutamate form and need to be hydrolyzed. This is accomplished by the conjugase, pteroylpolyglutamate hydrolase, found in the brush border of the small intestines.[67] In a review article, Hathcock summarizes an important relationship between folate and zinc. The conjugase responsible for hydrolyzing the polyglutamates is zinc dependent. Thus, folate absorption can theoretically be affected by zinc deficiency. Do high levels of folate affect zinc bioavailability or function in the small intestines? Considerable variation is found in the literature, indicating that as little as 350 µg can affect zinc function, while no harmful effects were noted with 4 mg per day.[81] Large, well-controlled clinical trials are necessary to determine the interactions of folate and zinc.

Active transport of folate is enhanced by glucose and galactose. A small amount of folate is absorbed by passive diffusion. Absorption is inhibited by unknown factors found in yeast and beans, acidic pH, alcohol, some medications (including Dilantin) and some diseases.[67] Once absorbed, the pteroylmonoglutamate is transported to the liver and is either stored as a polyglutamate or circulated. Some of the folate in plasma is bound to a low-affinity protein, primarily albumin.[12] Total-body folate stores usually range from 5 to 10 mg. About half of this is in the liver. Folate excretion is in the urine and bile of both the biologically active and inactive forms. The primary excretion product of folate in the urine is acetamindobenzoylglutamate.[67] Ninety-percent of the folate in the serum is either not bound or is loosely bound to albumin. The remaining 10% is bound to a specific protein called folic acid-binding protein (FABP).[13] Normal folate values for serum is 3.0–17.0 ng/ml. RBC folate is 280–903 ng/ml.[70]

II. INTAKE

A. GENERAL POPULATION

International approaches to food fortification with folate vary. The United States mandates folate fortification while the United Kingdom, some European countries, Australia and New Zealand have voluntary fortification policies. The voluntary fortification of food with folate at the level of 50% of the recommended daily dose resulted in a beneficial effect on the folate status of young South Australians, but not at the level required for maximal prevention of neural tube defects.[83]

In a report from the National Center for Health Statistics on the intake of selected vitamins in the United States for 1999 to 2000, it was found that males consumed from 267 to 435 µg per day. Those consuming 267 µg were in a group less than 6 years of age and excluded nursing infants and children. Those who consumed 435 µg were in the group for 20–39 years of age. The intake for females was lower for every category, with the range being 243–335 µg per day. Those consuming 243 µg were in a group less than 6 years of age and excluded nursing infants and children. Those that consumed 335 µg were in the group for 40–59 years of age. Requirements were met for all of the age groups for males except the 60-year-olds and older. Only the 6–11-year-old females met their requirements.[84]

B. ATHLETES

Generally speaking, a regular increase in exercise intensity will cause an increase in the need for additional nutrients, including vitamins and minerals.[85] Also, generally speaking, those who are more active are usually more health conscious and consume the recommended amount of vitamins and minerals.[16] Beitz et al., when using the German reference values, found moderately active adults to consume more nutrients than sedentary adults in Germany.[86] Athletic performance can be directly influenced by a deficiency of folate because of the anemia that would result, but Lukaski found that the use of vitamin and mineral supplements did not improve measures of performance when adequate diets were consumed.[16] The question has to be asked, was homocysteine reduced in these same subjects as a result of the supplements, thus improving overall health without showing a performance difference?

Niekamp and Baer studied 12 male cross-country runners to determine the adequacy of their dietary intake. Their diets were assessed using two 4-day self-recorded diet records. Their analysis showed the diet to be more than adequate for folate.[87]

The elderly athlete might be another concern. Sacheck and Roubenoff have suggested four considerations when making recommendations to the exercising elderly:

1. What change in needs occurs with age?
2. What change in needs occurs with exercise?
3. Are there any chronic illnesses or diseases?
4. Is the subject exercising for fitness, recreation, or competition?[88]

A decrease in stomach acid can cause a decrease in folate absorption.[65] High doses of folate may interfere with zinc metabolism.[89] Research has documented that, even with adequate energy intake, some older athletes have an insufficient micronutrient intake.[90] Campbell, Rachel and Geik list the vitamin and mineral intakes suggested for the elderly athlete, but they suggest that research to make specific suggestions is lacking. They suggest increasing folate because of a decrease in stomach acid that occurs with the elderly.[91]

The nutritional status of elite Finnish ski jumpers was evaluated concerning macro and micronutrient intake. Twenty-one male ski jumpers were compared with 20 non-athletic male controls. Several micronutrients were looked at besides folate. There were no differences in the absolute intake of folate between skiers and controls, but when the comparison was based on densities, the skiers consumed more folate ($p < 0.02$).[92]

III. BIOCHEMICAL STATUS IN ATHLETES

A. RESEARCH ON CURRENT STATUS

Several research reports are concerned with the biochemical status of folate in athletes. Telford et al. divided 86 Australian athletes into a treatment group ($n = 42$) and a placebo group ($n = 44$). Dietary recalls revealed that both groups were receiving adequate folate in their diet. The treatment group received an additional 200 µg of folate daily for 7 to 8 months of hard exercise.

The athletes were basketball players, gymnasts, swimmers, or rowers. The supplemented athletes were found to have a significant increase in serum folate (10.9 vs. 24.4 nmol/l, $p < 0.001$).[93]

Ziegler et al. studied the nutritional status of 18 competitive female figure skaters and found folate to be significantly higher in the preseason than in the competitive and off seasons. At least 20% of the skaters exhibited less than normal serum folate for all of the seasons.[94]

Forty male middle- and long-distance runners with 12 non-athletic controls were evaluated for several parameters, some of which were hemoglobin concentration, mean cell volume, erythrocyte count, serum and erythrocyte folate. The treatment groups were given iron, iron plus folate, or folate alone. There were essentially no differences between the athletes and non-athletes for any of the measured parameters except that the blood volume and hemoglobin of the athletes was 20% more than the controls.[95] It should be noted that there were not large numbers per treatment group in this study.

In 1991 a review article by Haymes reported that more than 50% of elite women distance runners, non-elite women marathon runners and triathletes, and iron man triathletes of both sexes regularly consume vitamin and mineral supplements. A large percentage of high school and college athletes also consumed vitamin and mineral supplements. Haymes concluded that vitamin deficiencies are not likely to be common among most athletes but, based on work published in the 1980s, the dietary intake of many girls were deficient in folate. The folate requirement has increased since then.[96] Haymes lists three primary reasons that it would be beneficial to supplement the diet of athletes with specific vitamins or minerals:

1. The diet of the athlete is deficient in one or more vitamin or mineral.
2. The athletes have a greater need than the general population.
3. The addition of certain vitamin or minerals improves performance.[96]

B. CONDITIONS THAT MAY CHANGE THE STATUS

The research relating folate to hyperhomocysteinemia in athletes is controversial. Following are several reports of elevated homocysteine levels as a result of exercise.

- Herrmann et al. studied the effects of 3 weeks of strenuous swimming on blood homocysteine, B_{12}, B_6, folate and methylmalonic acid of young healthy swimmers. They found a prolonged homocysteine increase during the 3 weeks (about 15%) that was significant at the 10% level. This did not reverse after 5 days of recovery training. Folate increased substantially during the training period but dropped by the end of the recovery training. The researchers proposed that the stimulation of the methionine cycle secondary to the increased demand for methyl groups during exercise might help explain the increase in homocysteine.[97]

- Konig et al. studied the effects of training volume and acute physical exercise on plasma levels of homocysteine and its interactions with plasma folate and B_{12}. The subjects were 42 well-trained male tri-athletes. Blood samples were obtained before and after a 30-day endurance-training period and before competitive exercise, at 1 hour and at 24 hours after competitive exercise. The athletes were divided into subgroups of low training and high training, depending on the number of hours of training per week. After the training period was over, no significant differences in homocysteine could be found in the group as a whole. When the subgroups were analyzed, the athletes in the highest training quartile exhibited a significant decrease in homocysteine ($p < 0.05$). At the same time, the plasma folate levels were significantly higher in this group ($p < 0.05$). When plasma was analyzed at 1 hour and 24 hours after training, homocysteine levels were elevated in all athletes regardless of the training volume ($p < 0.001$). After 1 hour of training, folate increased in all athletes ($p < 0.05$). Multivariate analysis indicated the increase in homocysteine levels was dependent on baseline levels of folate and training volume but not on B_{12} levels.[98]

- Bailey, Davis and Baker studied 34 physically active subjects who were randomly assigned to either a normoxia or a hypoxia-training group. The training involved 4 weeks of cycling. Each group inspired either a normobaric normoxic or a normobaric hypoxic gas under double-blind conditions. Plasma concentrations of resting total homocysteine decreased by 11% following hypoxic training ($p < 0.05$) but increased by 10% ($p < 0.05$) following normoxic training. Serum B_{12} and erythrocyte folate were determined to remain stable in both treatments.[99]

- Tapola and co-workers investigated the effects of mineral water fortified with folic acid and other vitamins and minerals that included B_6 and B_{12}. Serum and erythrocyte folate were measured along with plasma homocysteine. Sixty normohomocysteinemic subjects with normal folate levels completed the study that consisted of a 2-week running period followed by an 8-week intervention period. During the intervention period, the subjects consumed the fortified mineral water that contained 563 µg/day along with other vitamins and minerals or placebo water. Serum and erythrocyte folate increased ($p < 0.001$) and plasma homocysteine decreased ($p < 0.001$).[100]

- Herrmann et al. investigated 100 recreational endurance athletes (87 males and 13 females) who participated in a marathon race (n = 46), a 100-km run (n = 12), or a long-distance mountain bike race (n = 42). Blood was drawn before, 15 minutes and 3 hours after the race. Fourteen of the athletes (nine marathon runners and five cyclists) had additional blood drawn 24 hours after the race. The authors reported that mild to moderate hyperhomocysteinemia can frequently be found among recreational endurance athletes and these athletes frequently have folate and B_{12} deficiencies. Twenty-three percent of the athletes had elevated homocysteine levels before the race started. Since no strenuous training was performed 48 hours prior to the event, a possible explanation for the elevation was the fact that both folate and B_{12} were in the lower levels of the reference range. The post-exercise levels of homocysteine (overall) were significantly increased at 15 minutes (23%, $p < 0.0001$), at 3 hours (19%, $p < 0.0001$) and at 24 hours (33%, $p < 0.002$). Only 14 subjects had blood analyzed at 24 hours, with significant results; there was considerable variation. When the results of the individual races were observed, the marathon runners' homocysteine level was 64% higher after the event when compared with levels prior to the race. There were only 12 subjects in the 100-km race with considerable variation among them. Six had a considerable increase in homocysteine, three were unchanged and three had a decrease.[61]

- In the Intermountain Heart Collaborative Study, 2481 subjects were investigated to determine the effects of folic acid fortification of food on homocysteine plasma levels and mortality. Median homocysteine levels dropped modestly in the post-fortification group but there was an insignificant drop in mortality.[101]

IV. STUDIES RELATED TO EXERCISE PERFORMANCE

A. ANIMAL

At least one animal study is of significance to athletes. One of the concerns with hyperhomocysteinemia is the effect on endothelial function. Hyperhomocysteinemia results in decreased availability of nitric oxide and impairs vascular function, two early events in atherosclerosis. The effect of exercise on nitric oxide synthase, the enzyme necessary for nitric oxide production, was investigated using rats that were subjected to treadmill running. The exercise increased the activity of nitric oxide synthase and vasorelaxation in the exercise rats following homocysteine exposure but not in the sedentary control group.[62]

B. Human

Previously mentioned research completed by Telford et al. was concerned with the biochemical status of folate in athletes. In a similar parallel study completed by the same authors to determine the effects of vitamin and mineral supplementation on the performance of athletes already receiving the DRIs, little evidence of improved performance was obtained.[102] Considering research that states exercise raises homocysteine levels, the question has to be asked, did the supplementation decrease homocysteine as in other research efforts, thus improving the health of the athlete?

Matter et al. studied the effects of folate deficiency on 85 female marathon runners. The subjects were treated for 1 week with 5 mg/day of folic acid. When tested on a treadmill, maximum oxygen uptake, maximum treadmill running time, peak blood lactate levels and the running speed at the blood lactate turn point were not changed from the previous week before supplementation. The tests were repeated 10 weeks after treatment and were still unchanged.[103]

Weight et al. studied the effects of 3 months of vitamin and mineral supplementation that was 25 times the RDAs on the running performance of 30 well-trained male runners. Folic acid was one of the vitamins supplemented. None of the athletes had a vitamin deficiency during the trial and there was no measurable difference in performance as a result of vitamin supplementation.[104]

V. REQUIREMENTS

A. Recommended Dietary Allowances

The recommended dietary allowances (RDAs) are a means of describing the amount of a nutrient necessary to meet the needs of approximately 97 to 98% of all individuals in a certain age and gender group. The RDAs are a part of a larger classification, the dietary reference intakes (DRIs). Included in the DRIs are adequate intakes (AIs) and tolerable upper intake levels (ULs). The AIs are recommendations for the intake of those nutrients for which there is not enough research available to make a recommendation as definite as the RDAs. The UL is the maximum daily intake of a nutrient that can be taken without the likelihood of causing adverse health effects in almost all of the population in certain age and gender groups.[71] The ULs have not been determined for all nutrients. Table 7.3 lists the latest recommendations for folate.

In 1998, the National Academy of Sciences completed an exhaustive review of the evidence available on folate intake, status and health for all age groups. As a result of the review, they developed calculations to determine the estimated average requirement (EAR) of folate. They further determined recommended dietary allowances (RDAs) to be the EAR plus two standard deviations. This estimation agrees with the definition of the FAO/WHO recommended nutrient intake (RNI). The members of the FAO/WHO expert group agreed that the values published by the National Academy of Sciences were the best estimates of folate requirements based on current literature.[106] The National Academy of Sciences reports that folic acid taken with food is 85% bio-available and food folate is only 50% bioavailable. The bioavailability ratio of folic acid taken with food to folate found naturally in food is 85/50 or 1.7 times more available. When a mixture of synthetic folic acid and food folate is fed, dietary equivalents (DEFs) are calculated as follows to determine the estimated average requirements: μg of DEF provided = [μg of food folate + (1.7 × μg of synthetic folic acid)].

Only half as much folic acid is needed if taken on an empty stomach, so to be comparable to food folate, the American Academy of Sciences gives this explanation:

* 1 μg of DEF = 1 μg of food folate
* 1 μg of food folate = 0.5 μg of folic acid taken on an empty stomach
* 0.5 μg of folic acid on an empty stomach = 0.6 μg of folic acid with meals[107]

TABLE 7.3

Life Stage Group	RDA/AI* of Folate in μg/d	ULa in μg/d
Infants		
0–6 months	65*	ND^b
7–12 months	80*	ND
Children		
1–3 years	150	300
4–8 years	200	400
Males and Females		
9 > 13 years	300	600
14–18 years	400	800
19 > 70 years	400	1000
Pregnancy		
≤ 18 years	600	800
19–50 years	600	1000
Lactation		
≤ 18 years	500	800
19–50 years	500	1000

* Represents Recommended Dietary Allowances (RDAs) in bold type and Adequate Intakes (AIs) in ordinary type followed by an asterisk (*). RDAs and AIs may both be used as goals for individual intake. RDAs are set to meet the needs of almost all individuals in a group (97 to 98 percent). For healthy breastfed infants, the AI is the mean intake. The AI for other life stage groups is believed to cover the needs of all individuals in the group, but lack of data prevent being able to specify with confidence the percentage of individuals covered by this intake.

a Tolerable upper limits. The maximum level of daily nutrient intake that is likely to pose no risk of adverse effects. Unless otherwise specified, the UL represents total intake from food, water and supplements.

b ND = Not determinable due to lack of data of adverse effects in his age group and concern with regard to lack of ability to handle excess amounts. Source of intake should be from food only to prevent high levels of intake.

Source: Dietary Reference Intakes for Thiamin, Riboflavin, Niacin, Vitamin B[6], Folate, Vitamin B[12], Pantothenic Acid, Biotin and Choline. 1998. The Food and Nutrition and Board, the National Academy of Sciences.[71]

The FAO/WHO expert group agrees with the findings of the Food and Nutrition Board of the National Academy of Sciences.[106] The reduced folates found in food are less stable than folic acid. Large amounts of folate can be lost during cooking and folate can leach out of food during preparation.[12] The retention of folate in cooked food is variable and highly dependent on the type of food and the method of preparation.[108] Vitamin C may help prevent folate degradation during cooking.[109]

B. Specific Recommendations for Athletes

There is no official recommendation for folate by athletes that is different from the recommendation for the general public. To make such a specific recommendation, more research is necessary. Because there are young athletes, middle-aged athletes, "older" and elderly athletes, and because there are casual athletes and elite athletes, the word "athlete" must be adequately defined. The research reviewed in this chapter indicates that most serious athletes have an adequate to better-than-adequate intake of folic acid[87] and that an additional intake of folic acid beyond the requirement did not increase performance.[16,103,105] The effects of exercise on homocysteine is a new area of concern.[61] Because folate can have a positive effect on lowering homocysteine,[43,44] future recommendations may be different from those of today, not for the sake of increasing athletic performance, but for the sake of preventing disease processes caused by elevated homocysteine.

VI. FUTURE RESEARCH

There is a paucity of research expressly aimed at determining the need for additional folate for the athlete to support maximum performance and control the rises in serum homocysteine that occur as a result of exercise. The relationship between exercise and hyperhomocysteinemia needs to be explored further and there is a conspicuous need for additional research to determine whether an increase in the consumption of folate beyond the recommendation for the general population will benefit the athlete's performance or health by reducing elevated serum homocysteine levels.

VII. CONCLUSIONS

Folate is necessary for the synthesis of DNA and RNA. A deficiency of folate will affect many systems but is primarily manifested by a megaloblastic anemia. Any type of anemia could affect the performance of athletes, particularly endurance athletes. Supplementation with folate will correct the anemia and thus possibly improve the athletes' performance, but there is no strong evidence that an increase in folate beyond the amount recommended for the general population will produce a measurable increase in athletic performance. Additional research will determine whether an increase in folate consumption is needed by the athlete to prevent disease due to a possible increase in homocysteine levels secondary to exercise.

REFERENCES

1. Wills, L. Treatment of "pernicious anemia of pregnancy" and "tropical anemia." *Brit. Med. J.* 1:1059–1064, 1931.
2. Day, P.L., Langston, W.C. and Shukers, C.F. Leukopenia and anemia in the monkey resulting from vitamin deficiency. *J. Nutr.* 9:637–644, 1935.
3. Langston, W.C., Darby, W.J., Shukers, C.F. and Day, P.L. Nutritional cytopenia (vitamin M deficiency) in the monkey. *J. Exp. Med.* 68:923–940, 1938.
4. Snell, E.E. and Peterson, W.H. Growth factors for bacteria. Additional factors required by certain lactic acid bacteria. *J. Bact.* 39:273–285, 1940.
5. Hogan, A.G. and Parrott, E.M. Anemia in chicks caused by a vitamin deficiency. *J. Biol. Chem.* 132:507–517, 1940.
6. Mitchell, H.K., Snell, E.E. and Williams, R.J. The concentration of folic acid. *J. Am. Chem. Soc.* 63:2284, 1941.
7. Angier, R.B., Boothe, J.H., Hutchings, B.L., Mowat, J.H., Semb, J., Stokstand, E.L.R., Subarow, Y., Waller, C.W., Cosulich, D.B., Fahrenbach, M.J., Hultquist, M.E., Kuh, E., Northey, E.H., Seeger, D.R., Sickels, J.P. and Smith, Jr., J.M. Synthesis of a compound identical with the *L. casei* factor isolated from liver. *Sci.* 102:227–228, 1945.
8. Hoffbrand, A.V. and Weir, D.G. The history of folic acid. *Br. J. Haematol.* 13:579–589, 2001.
9. Boosalis, M.G. in Matarese, L.E. and Gottschlich, M.M. (Eds.) *Contemporary Nutrition Support Practice: A Clinical Guide.* Philadelphia: Saunders. 153, 1998.
10. Grooper, S.S., Smith, J.L. and Groff, J.L. *Advanced Nutrition and Human Metabolism.* 4th ed. Belmont, CA, Thomson Wadsworth. 301–309, 2005.
11. Stipanuk, M.H. *Biochemical and Physiological Aspects of Human Nutrition.* Philadelphia: W.B. Saunders. 484–485, 2000.
12. Gropper, S.S. *The Biochemistry of Human Nutrition.* 2nd ed. Belmount, CA: Wadsworth/Thompson. 91, 2000.

13. McNeely, M.D.D. Folic Acid. (CDRom) in Kaplan, L.A., Pesce, A.J. and Kazmierczak (Eds). *Clinical Chemistry: Theory, Analysis, Correlation*. 4th ed. St. Louis: C.V. Mosby Company. 2003.

14. Orten, J.M. and Neuhaus, O.W. *Human Biochemistry*. 10th ed. St. Louis: C.V. Mosby Company. 338, 1982.

15. Stryer, L. *Biochemistry*. 4th ed. New York: W.H. Freeman. pp. 719–721, 1995.

16. Lukaski, H.C. Vitamin and mineral status: effects on physical performance. *Nutrition* 20:632–644, 2004.

17. Chandra, J., Jain, V., Narayan, S., Sharma, S., Singh, V., Kapoor, A.K. and Batra, S. Folate and cobalamin deficiency in megaloblastic anemia in children. *Indian Pediatr.*, 39:453–457, 2002.

18. MRC Vitamin Study Research Group. Prevention of neural tube defects: results of the Medical Research Council Vitamin Study. *Lancet*. 338:131–137, 1991.

19. Czeizel, A.E. and Dudas, I. Prevention of the first occurrence of neural-tube defects by periconceptional vitamin supplementation. *N. Engl. J. Med.* 327:1832–1835, 1992.

20. Shaw, G.M., Schaffer, D., Velie, E.M., Morland, K. and Harris, J.A. Periconceptual vitamin use, dietary folate and the occurrence of neural tube defects. *Epidemiology*. 6:205–207, 1995.

21. Berry, R.J., Li, Z., Erickson, J.D., Li, S., Moore, C.A., Wang, H., Mulinare, J., Zhao, P., Wong, L.Y., Gindler, J., Hong, S.X. and Correa, A. Prevention of neural- tube defects with folic acid in China. China–U.S. Collaborative Project for Neural Tube Defect Prevention. *N. Engl. J. Med.* 11;341:1485–1490, 1999.

22. Brosnan, J.T., Jacobs, R.L., Stead, L.M. and Brosnan, M.E. Methylation demand: a key determinant of homocysteine metabolism. *Acta. Biochim. Pol.* 51:405–413, 2004.

23. Stead, L.M., Au, K.P., Jacobs, R.L., Brosnan, M.E. and Brosnan, J.T. Methylation demand and homocysteine metabolism: effects of dietary provision of creatine and guanidinoacetate. *Am. J. Physiol. Endocrinol. Metab.* 281: E1095–E1100, 2001.

24. Guo, H., Lee, J.D., Ueda, T., Shan, J. and Wang, J. Plasma homocysteine levels in patients with early coronary artery stenosis and high risk factors. *Jpn. Heart J.* 44:865–871, 2003.

25. Skibinska, E., Sawicki, R., Lewczuk, A., Prokop, J., Musial, W., Kowalska, I. and Mroczko, B. Homocysteine and progression of coronary artery disease. *Pol. Heart J.* 60, 2004.

26. Virdis, A., Ghiadoni, L., Salvetti, G., Versari, D., Taddei, S. and Salvetti, A. Hyperhomocysteinemia: Is this a novel risk factor in hypertension? *J. Nephrol.* 15:414–421, 2002.

27. Clarke, R., Daly, L., Robinson, K., Naughten, E., Cahalane, S., Fowler, B. and Graham, I. Hyperhomocysteinemia: an independent risk factor for vascular disease. *N. Engl. J. Med.* 26;325:966–967, 1991.

28. Barghash, N.A., Elewa, S.M., Hamdi, E.A., Barghash, A.A. and El Dine, R. Role of plasma homocysteine and lipoprotein (a) in coronary artery disease. *Br. J. Biomed. Sci.* 61:78–83, 2004.

29. Seshadri, S., Beiser, A., Selhub, J., Jacques, P.F., Rosenberg, I.H., D'Agostino, R.B., Wilson, P.W. and Wolf P.A. Plasma homocysteine as a risk factor for dementia and Alzheimer's disease. *N. Engl. J. Med.* 14;346:476–483, 2002.

30. Kruman, I.I., Kumaravel, T.S., Lohani, A., Pedersen, W. A., Cutler, R. G., Kruman, Y., Haughey, N., Lee, J. and Mattson, M.P. Folic acid deficiency and homocysteine impair DNA repair in hippocampal neurons and sensitize them to amyloid toxicity in experimenmtal models of Alzheimer's disease. *J. Neurosci.* 22:1752–1762, 2002.

31. Snowdon, D.A., Tully, C.L., Smith, C.D., Riley, K.P. and Markesbery, W.R. Serum Folate and the severity of atrophy of the neocortex in Alzheimer disease: Findings from the Nun Study 1–3. *Am. J. Clin. Nutr.* 71:993–998, 2000.

32. Clarke, R., Smith, A.D., Jobst, K.A., Refsum, H., Sutton, L. and Ueland, P.M. Folate, vitamin B_{12} and serum total homocysteine levels in confirmed Alzheimer disease. *Arch. Neurol.* 55:1449–1455, 1998.

33. Goelz, S.E., Vogelstein, B/, Hamilton, S.R. and Feinberg A.P. Hypomethylation of DNA from benign and malignant human colon neoplasms. *Sci.* 12;228:187–190, 1985.

34. Giovannucci, E., Stampfer, M.J., Colditz, G.A., Rimm, E.B., Trichopoulos, D., Rosner, B.A., Speizer, F.E. and Willet, W.C. Folate, methionine and alcohol intake and risk of colorectal adenoma. *J. Natl. Cancer Inst.* 2;85:875–884, 1993.

35. Ifergan, I., Shafran, A., Jansen, G., Hooijber, J.H., Scheffer, G.L. and Assaraf, Y.G. Folate deprivation results in the loss of breast cancer resistance protein (BCRP/ABCG2) expression. A role for BCRP in cellular folate homeostasis. *J. Biol. Chem.* 11;279:25527–25534, 2004.

36. Giovannucci, E., Stamper, M.J., Colditz, G.A., Hunter, D.J., Fuchs, C., Rosne, B.A., Speizer, F.E. and Willett, W.C. Multivitamin use, folate and colon cancer in women in the Nurses' Health Study. *Ann. Intern. Med.* 129;7:517–524, 1998.

37. van Meurs, J.B., Dhonukshe-Rutten, R.A., Pluijm, S.M., van der Klift, M., de Jonge, R., Lindemans, J., de Groot, L.C., Hofman, A., Witteman, J.C., van Leeuwen J.P., Breteler, M.M., Lips P., Pols H.A. and Uitterlinden, A.G. Homocysteine levels and the risk of osteoporotic fracture. *N. Engl. J. Med.* 350:2089–2090, 2004.

38. McLean, R.R., Jacques, P.F., Selhub, J., Tucker, K.L., Samelson, E.J., Broe, K.E., Hannan, M.T., Cupples, L.A. and Kiel, D.P. Homocysteine as a predictive factor for hip fracture in older persons. *N. Engl. J. Med.* 350:2042–2049, 2004.

39. Matsui, T., Arai. H., Yuzuriha, T., Yao, H., Miura, M., Hashimoto, S., Higuchi, S., Matsushita, S., Morikawa, M., Kato, A. and Sasaki, H. Elevated plasma homocysteine levels and risk of silent brain infarction in elderly people. *Stroke.* 32:1116–1119, 2001

40. Bottiglieri, T., Laundy, M., Crellin, R., Toone, B.K., Carney, M.W. and Reynolds, E.H. Homocysteine, folate, methylation and monoamine metabolism in depression. *J. Neurol. Neurosurg. Psychiatry.* 69:228–232, 2000.

41. Allain, P., LeBouil, A., Cordillet, E., Le Quay, L., Bagheri, H. and Montastrue, J.L. Sulfate and cysteine levels in the plasma of patients with Parkinson's disease. *Neurotoxicology.* 16:527–529, 1995.

42. Fenech, M., Aitken, C. and Rinaldi, J. Folate, vitamin B$_{12}$, homocysteine status and DNA damage in young Australian adults. 19:1163–1171. *Carcinogenesis,* 1998.

43. Refsum, H., Ueland, P.M., Nygard, O. and Vollset, S.E. Homocysteine and cardiovascular disease. *Annu. Rev. Med.* 49:31–62, 1998.

44. Hughes, K. and Ong, C.N. Homocysteine, folate, vitamin B12 and cardiovascular risk in Indians, Malays and Chinese in Singapore. *J. Epidemiol. Community Health.* 54:31–34, 2000.

45. Clarke, .R, Refsum, H., Birks, J., Evans, J.G., Johnston, C., Sherliker, P., Ueland, P.M., Schneede, J., Mcpartlin, J., Nexo, E and, Scott, J.M. Screening for vitamin B-12 and folate deficiency in older persons. *Am. J. Clin. Nutr.* 77:1241–1247, 2003.

46. Wilken, D.E., Dudman, N.P., Tyrrell, P.A. and Robertson, M.R. Folic acid lowers elevated plasma homocysteine in chronic renal insufficiency: possible implications for prevention of vascular disease. *Metabolism.* 37:697–701, 1998.

47. Arnadottir, M., Brattstrom, L., Simonsen, O., Thysell, H., Hultberg, B., Andersson, A. and Nilsson-Ehle, P. The effect of high-dose pyridoxine and folic acid supplementation on serum lipid and plasma homocysteine concentrations in dialysis patients. *Clin Nephrol.* 40:236–240, 1993.

48. Boston, A.G., Shemin, D., Lapane, K.L., Hume, A., Yoburn, D., Nadeau, M.P., Bendich, A., Selhub, J. and Rosenberg, I.H. High dose-B-vitamin treatment of hyperhomocysteinemia in dialysis patients. *Kidney Int.* 49:147–152, 1996.

49. Heijer, M.D., Brouwer, I.A., Bos, G., Blom, H.J., van der Put, N., Spaans, A.P., Rosendaal, F.R., Thomas, C., Haak, H.L., Wijermans, P.W. and Gerrits, W. Vitamin supplementation reduces blood homocysteine levels: A controlled trial in patients with venous thrombosis and healthy volunteers. *Arterioscler. Thromb. Vasc. Biol.* 18:356–361, 1998.

50. Fearon, E.R. and Vogelstein, B. A Genetic model for colorectal tumorigenesis. *Cell.* 61:759–767, 1990.

51. Rimm, E.B., Willet, W.C., Hu, F.B., Sampson, L., Colditz, G.A., Manson, J.E., Hennekens, C. and Stampfer, M.J. Folate and vitamin B$_6$ from diet and supplements in relation risk of coronary heart disease among women. *JAMA.* 4;279:359–364, 1998.

52. Voutilainen, S., Rissanen, T.H., Virtanen, J., Lakka, T.A. and Salonen, J.T. Low dietary folate intake is associated with an excess incidence of acute coronary events: The Kuopio Ischemic Heart Disease Risk Factor Study. *J. Am. Heart Assoc.* 103:2674–2680, 2001.

53. Clarke, R., Fitzgerald, D., O'Brien, C., O'Farrel,l C., Roche, G., Parker, R.A. and Graham, I. Hyperhomocysteinaemia: a risk factor for extracranial care artery artherosclerosis. *Ir. J. Med. Sci.* 161:61–65, 1992.

54. Majors, A., Ehrhart, L.A. and Pezacka, E.H. Homocysteine as a risk factor for vascular disease. *Arterioscler. Thromb. Vasc. Biol.* 17:2074–2081, 1997.

55. Moustapha, A., Naso, A., Nahlawi, M., Gupta, A., Arheart, K.L., Jacobsen, D.W., Robinson, K. and Dennis, V.W. Prospective study of hyperhomocysteinemia as an adverse cardiovascular risk factor in end-stage renal disease. *J. Am. Heart Assoc.* 97:711, 1998.

56. Stanger, O., Herrman, W., Pietrzik, K., Fowler, B., Geisel, J., Dierkes, J. and Weger, M. Clinical use and rational management of homocysteine, folic acid and B vitamins in cardiovascular and thrombotic diseases. *Z. Kardiol.* 93:439–453, 2004.

57. American Heart Association, Homocysteine, Folic Acid and Cardiovascular Disease. September 27, 2004. [Online] Available http://www.americanheart.org/presenter.jhtml?identifier=4677 (accessed 10/04).

58. Wilmink, A.B., Welch, A.A., Quick, C.R., Burns, P.J., Hubbard, C.S., Bradbury, A.W. and Day, N.E. Dietary folate and vitamin B6 are independent predictors of peripheral arterial occlusive disease. *J. Vasc Surg.* 39:513–516, 2004.

59. Moat, S.J., Lang, D., McDowell, I.F., Clarke, Z.L., Madhavan, A.K., Lewis, M.J. and Goodfellow, J. Folate, homocysteine, endothelial function and cardiovascular disease. *J. Nutr. Biochem.* 15:64–79, 2004.

60. Pena, A.S., Wiltshire, E., Gent, R., Hirte, C. and Couper, J. Folic acid improves endothelial function in children and adolescents with type 1 diabetes. *J. Pediatr.* 144:500–504, 2004.

61. Herrman, M., Schorr, H., Obeid, R., Scharhag, J., Urhausen, A., Kindermann, W. and Herrman, W. Homocysteine increases during endurance exersice. *Clin. Chem. Lab. Med.* 41:1518–1524, 2003.

62. Hayward, R., Ruangthai, R., Karnilaw, P., Chicco, A., Strange, R., McCarty, H. and Westerlind, K.C. Attenuation of homocysteine-induced endothelial dysfunction by exercise training. *Pathophysiology.* 9:207–214, 2003.

63. de Bree, A., Verschuren, W.M., Blom, H.J. and Kromhout, D. Lifestyle factors and plasma homocysteine concentrations in a general population sample. *Am. J. Epidemiol.* 15;154:150–154, 2001.

64. Koutoubi, S. and Huffman, F.G. Serum total homocysteine levels, folate and B-vitamins intake and coronary heart disease risk factors among tri-ethnic college students. *Ethn. Dis.* 14:160, 2004.

65. Rosenberg, I.H. and Miller, J. Nutritional factors in physical and cognitive functions of elderly people. *Am. J. Clin. Nutr.* 55:1237S–143S, 1992.

66. Schneede, J., Refsum, H. and Ueland, P.M. Biological and environmental determinants of plasma homocysteine. *Semin. Thromb. Hemost.* 26: 263–79, 2000.

67. Herbert, V. Folate. In Shills, M.E., Olson, J.A., Shike, M. and Ross, A.C. (Eds.) *Modern Nutrition in Health and Disease.* 9th ed. Baltimore, Maryland: Williams & Wilkins, pp. 335–336, 348–340, 1999.

68. Manore, M. and Thompson, J. *Sport Nutrition for Health and Performance.* Human Kinetics, p. 348, 2000.

69. Quadri, P., Fragiacomo, C., Pezzati, R., Zanda, E., Forloni, G., Tettamanti, M. and Lucca, U. Homocysteine, folate and vitamin B-12 in mild cognitive impairment, Alzheimer disease and vascular dementia. *Am. J. Clin. Nutr.* 80:114–122, 2004.

70. Lichtenstein, G.R .and Hopkins, B. In *Medical Nutrition & Disease*. Hark, L. and Morrison, G. (Eds.) 3rd ed. Malden, Massachusetts. Blackwell Science. 251–258, 2003.

71. Institute of Medicine. Food and Nutrition Board. Dietary Reference Intakes: Thiamin, riboflavin, niacin, vitamin B_6, folate, vitamin B_{12}, pantothenic acid, biotin and choline. National Academy Press. Washington, DC. 1998.

72. Rampersaud, G.C., Kauwell, G.P. and Bailey, L.B. Folate: a key to optimizing and reducing disease risk in elderly. *J. Am. Coll. Nutr.* 22:1–8, 2003.

73. Hands, E.S. *Nutrients in Food.* Baltimore: Lippincott Williams & Wilkins,. 2000.

74. U.S. Department of Health and Human Services, Food and Drug Administration Food standards: amendment of the standards of identity for enriched grain products to require addition of folic acid. *Federal Register.* 61:8781–8807, 1996.

75. Czeizel, A.E. Periconceptional folic acid containing multivitamin supplementation. *Eur. J. Obstet. Gynecol. Reprod. Biol.* 78: 151–161, 1998.

76. Alfthan, G., Laurinen, M.S., Valsta, L.M., Pastinen, T. and Aro, A. Folate intake, plasma folate and homocysteine status in random Finnish population. *Eur. J. Clin. Nutr.* 57; 81–88, 2003.

77. Holmes, T. and Gates, G. The effect of fortified breakfast cereal on plasma homocysteine concentrations in healthy older men already consuming a folate fortified diet. *Nutr. Res.* 23; 435–449, 2003.

78. Jacques, P.F., Selhub, J., Bostom , A.G., Wilson, P.W. and Rosenberg, I.H. The effect of folic acid fortification on plasma folate and total homocysteine concentrations. *N. Engl. J. Med.* 13;340:1449–54, 1999.

79. Whittaker, P., Tufaro, P.R and Rader, J.L. Iron and folate in fortified cereals. *J. Am. Coll. Nutr.* 20: 247–254, 2001.

80. Sisk, E.R., Lockner, D.W., Wold, R., Waters, D.L. and Baumgartner, R.N. The impact of folic acid fortification of enriched grains on an elderly population: the New Mexico Aging Process Study. *J. Nutr. Health Aging.* 8:140–143, 2004.

81. Hathcock, J.N. Vitamins and minerals: Efficacy and safety. *Am. J. Clin. Nutr.* 66:427–437, 1997.

82 Food and Drug Administration. Food labeling: Health claims and label statements; folate and neural tube defects; proposed rules. *Federal Register.* 58:53254–53288, 1993.

83. Wiltshire, E.J. and Couper, J.J. Improved folate status in children and adolescents during voluntary fortification of food with folate. *J. Paediatr. Child Health.* 40:44–47, 2004.

84. Ervin,R.B., Wright, J.D., Wang, C., Kennedy-Stephenson, J.U.S. Department of Health and Human Services, Centers for Disease Control and Prevention, National Center for Health Statistics, Division of Health and Nutrition Examination Surveys. No. 399, March 12, 2004.

85. Chen, J. Vitamins: effects of exercise on requirements. In: Maughan, RJ. (Ed.) *Nutrition in Sport. The Encyclopedia of Sports Medicine,* Vol VII. London: Blackwell Science. 281, 2000.

86. Beitz, R., Mensink, G., Henschel, Y., Fischer, B. and Erbersdobler, H.F. Dietary behavior of German adults differing in levels of sport activity. *Public Health Nutr.* 7:45–52, 2004.

87. Niekamp, R.A. and Baer, J.T. In-season dietary adequacy of trained male cross-country runners. *Int. J. Sport Nutr.* 5:45–55, 1995.

88. Sacheck, J.M. and Roubenoff, R. Nutrition in the exercising elderly. *Clin. Sports Med.* 18:565–584, 1999.

89. Fogelhom, M. Nutrition and the ageing athlete. In Burke L. and Deakin, V. (Eds.) *Clinical Sports Nutrition.* Melbourne: McGraw-Hill. 329, 2000.

90. Reaburn, P. Nutrition and the ageing athlete. In Burke L. and Deakin V. (Eds.) *Clinical Sports Nutrition.* Melbourne: McGraw-Hill. 611, 2000.

91. Campbell, W.W. and Geik, R.A. Nutritional considerations for the older athletes. *Nutr.* 20:603–604, 2004.

92. Rankinen, T., Lyytikainen, S., Vanninen, E., Penttila, I., Rauramaa, R. and Uusitupa, M. Nutritional status of the Finnish elite ski jumpers. *Med. Sci. Sports Exerc.* 30:11;1592–1597, 1998.

93. Telford, R.D., Catchpole, E.A., Deakin, V., McLeay, A.C. and Plank, A.W. The effect of 7 to 8 months of vitamin/mineral supplementation on the vitamin and mineral status of athletes. *Inter. J. Sport Nutr.* 2:123–134, 1992.

94. Ziegler, P., Sharp, R., Hughes, V., Evans, W. and Khoo, C. Nutritional status of teenage female competitive figure skaters. *J. Am. Diet. Assoc.* 101:374–379, 2001.

95. Brotherhood, J., Brozovic, B. and Pugh, L.G.C. Haematological status of middle- and long-distance runners. *Clin. Sci. Mol. Med.* 48:139–145, 1975.

96. Haymes, E.M. Vitamin and Mineral Supplementation to Athletes. *Inter. J. Sport Nutr.* 1:146–169, 1991.

97. Herrmann, M., Wilkinson, J., Schorr, H., Obeid, R., Georg, T., Scharhag, J., Urhausen, A., Kindermann, W. and Herrmann, W. Comparison of the influence of volume-oriented training and high-intensity interval training on serum homocysteine and its cofactors in young, healthy swimmers. *Clin. Chem. Lab. Med.* 41:1525–1, 2003.

98. Konig, D., Bisse, E., Deibert, P., Muller, H.M., Wieland, H. and Berg, A. Influence of training volume and acute physical exercise on the homocysteine levels in endurance-trained men: interactions with plasma folate and vitamin B_{12}. *Ann. Nutr. Metab.* 47: 114–118, 2003.

99. Bailey, D.M., Davies, B. and Baker, J. Training in hypoxia: modulation of metabolic and cardiovascular risk factors in men. *Med. Sci. Sports Exerc.* 32:1058–1066, 2000.

100. Tapola, N.S., Karvonen, H.M., Niskanen, L.K. and Sarkkinen, E.S. Mineral water fortified with folic acid, vitamins B_6, B_{12}, D and calcium improves folate status and decreases plasma homocysteine concentration in men and women. *Eur. J. Clin. Nutr.* 58: 376–385, 2004.

101. Anderson, KR Jensen, J.L., Carlquist, J.F. Blair, T.L. Horne, B.D. Muhlestein, J.B. Effect of folic acid fortification of food on homocysteine-related mortality. *Am. J. Med.* 116:158–164, 2004.

102. Telford, R.D., Catchpole, E.A., Deakin, V., Hahn, A.G. and Plank, A.W. The effect of 7 to 8 months of vitamin/mineral supplementation on athletic performance. *Inter. J. Sport Nutr.* 2:135–153, 1992.

103. Matter, M., Stittfall, T., Graves, J., Myburgh, K., Adams, B., Jacobs, P. and Noakes, T. The effect of iron and folate therapy on maximal exercise performance in female marathon runners with iron and folate deficiency. *Clin. Sci.* 72:415–422, 1987.

104. Weight, L.M., Noakes, T.D., Labadarios, D., Graves, J., Jacobs, P. and Berman, P.A. Vitamin and mineral status of trained athletes including the effects of supplementation. *Am. J. Clin. Nutr.* 47:186–191, 1988.

105. Wardlaw, G.M., Hampl, J.S. and DiSilvestro, R.A. *Perspectives in Nutrition.* 6th ed. McGraw-Hill. 46–49, 2004.

106. Human Vitamin and Mineral Requirements, report of a joint FAO/WHO expert consultation, Bangkok, Thailand. 2002.

107. Dietary Reference Intakes for Thiamin, Riboflavin, Niacin, Vitamin B_6, Folate, Vitamin B_{12}, Pantothenic Acid, Biotin and Choline The National Academy of Science, Institute of Medicine (IOM). [Online] Available http: http://www.nap.edu/books/0309065542/html/index.html. 210, 1998 (accessed 10/04).

108. McKillop, D.J., Pentieva, K., Daly, D., McPartlin, J.M., Hughes, J., Strain, J.J., Scott, J. M. and McNulty, H. The effect of different cooking methods on folate retention in various foods that are amongst the major contributors to folate intake in the U.K. diet. *Br. J. Nutr.* 88: 681–8, 2002.

109. Indrawati, C.A., Messagie, I., Nguyen, M.T., Van Loey, A. and Hendrickx, M. Comparative study on pressure and temperature stability of 5-methylterahydrofolic acid in model systems and in food products. *J. Ag. Food Chem.* 52:485–492, 2004.

8 Vitamin B$_{12}$

Kenneth E. McMartin

CONTENTS

I. INTRODUCTION

The role of vitamin B$_{12}$ (cobalamin) in sport and exercise is poorly defined today. Vitamin B$_{12}$ is crucial for DNA synthesis, hence is involved in cell division and growth. It is required for proper erythrocyte production, so could theoretically be important for endurance athletes, who need sufficient red blood cells to carry oxygen to benefit their aerobic performance. Cobalamin is also involved in other enzymatic steps that regulate amino acid and other cellular metabolic pathways. Thus, to maximize physiologic function during performance, many athletes take nutritional supplements, including those containing vitamin B$_{12}$. This chapter presents information on the intake and status of this vitamin in the general population as well as in athletic populations. In addition, evidence for its role in affecting exercise performance is discussed.

A. CHEMISTRY

Vitamin B$_{12}$ in the commercial form is generally cyanocobalamin. The chemical structure of cyano-cobalamin consists of a planar coordination complex of four conjoined pyrrole rings surrounding a central cobalt atom. This structure is similar to the iron porphyrins as in heme. The cyano (CN) group is attached to one of the available Cobalt (Co) sites, while attached to the other site is a ribonucleotide, which is additionally attached to the pyrrole ring structure by an aminopropanol linkage. There are three main physiologic cobalamins, in which the CN group is replaced with an OH group (hydroxoco-balamin, which is sometimes available commercially), a methyl group (methylcobalamin), or a 5′-deoxyadenosyl group (adenosylcobalamin). The latter two are the coenzyme forms of the vitamin in humans. Cyanocobalamin is used commercially and in most research studies because of its greater stability.[1] In addition to the cobalamins, human plasma often contains cobalamin analogues, which are generally inactive as coenzymes.[1]

B. METABOLIC FUNCTIONS

Cobalamins are critical for cell growth and division, by acting as coenzymes in two reactions, methylcobalamin in methionine synthase and adenosylcobalamin in methyl malonyl CoA mutase. The former reaction involves the remethylation of homocysteine using 5-methyltetrahydrofolate as methyl donor. Through this reaction, vitamin B_{12} is linked with the folate system.[2] In the absence of B_{12}, the methyl group cannot be transferred from the folate, leading to increased levels of 5-methyltetrahydrofolate. The latter cannot be converted to tetrahydrofolate by reversal of its formation, so the folate pool becomes "trapped" in the methyl form. Then tetrahydrofolate is not available to transfer one-carbon groups, especially in the thymidylate synthetase reaction, which leads to diminished DNA synthesis. Rapidly proliferating tissues such as the hematopoietic system, the gastrointestinal epithelium and the developing fetus have the greatest requirement for DNA synthesis and are therefore the major tissues affected in clinical cobalamin deficiency. Recently, vitamin B_{12} deficiency has been linked with an elevation in plasma homocysteine concentration, which has been recognized as an important risk factor for the development of atherosclerosis.[3] The second reaction, i.e., methyl malonyl mutase, converts methyl malonyl CoA to succinyl CoA and is involved in metabolism of propionate groups generated in fatty acid oxidation.

Because of the link with the folate system, vitamin B_{12}'s importance for athletes lies in proper erythropoiesis to maintain oxygen transport in the blood. In addition, cobalamin deficiency is associated with development of nervous-system damage leading to neurologic and mental symptoms, through as yet undetermined mechanisms. Hence, vitamin B_{12} may be needed for proper functioning of the nervous system. Athletes, who depend on central coordination of movement, timing, strength, etc., would probably be dependent on sufficient cobalamin to maintain proper CNS function.

Vitamin B_{12}, as a necessary cofactor for methionine synthetase, acts to help control the total plasma level of homocysteine. Recent epidemiologic studies have suggested that plasma homocysteine is inversely related to levels of physical fitness[4] or of physical exertion.[5] Because high levels of homocysteine are linked with an increased risk of cardiovascular disease,[3] the association of cardiovascular disease and lack of exercise could be related to increased homocysteine levels in such subjects. In turn, increased levels of homocysteine could result from a decrease in vitamin B_{12} levels or a dysfunction in B_{12} metabolism. In recent years, a number of studies have tried to determine whether there is a causal relationship between exercise and altered homocysteine levels. The theory behind such studies is that strenuous exercise could increase the usage of methylated substrates, which could affect homocysteine status because it is involved in recycling methyl groups.[6]

C. ABSORPTION, DISTRIBUTION AND ELIMINATION

The absorption of B_{12} is a highly regulated process and defects in it are the primary cause of deficiency.[7] Dietary B_{12} is cleaved from dietary and salivary proteins by acid in the stomach and by pancreatic proteases. B_{12} is then bound to intrinsic factor, a glycoprotein secreted by the gastric parietal cells.[7] Binding to intrinsic factor protects B_{12} from enzymatic digestion in the gastrointestinal tract. The cobalamin-intrinsic factor complex traverses the intestinal tract to the ileum, where it binds to specific receptors on ileal mucosal cells.[1] Following receptor-mediated uptake into mucosal cells, cobalamin is cleaved from intrinsic factor and transported into the portal circulation by binding to a specific protein, transcobalamin II. Absorption defects that contribute to B_{12}

deficiency include a decreased release of acid or decreased secretion of intrinsic factor by gastric parietal cells (secondary to gastric surgery), autoimmune diseases (antibodies to intrinsic factor) or various intestinal diseases leading to ileal damage. Some absorption of pharmacologic levels of B$_{12}$ can be mediated by a separate diffusion-type mechanism.[1]

Vitamin B$_{12}$ is carried in the circulation as a bound complex with transcobalamin II (hence, holo-TC) or with haptocorrins. Functional uptake into tissues, primarily the liver, occurs by binding of transcobalamin II to specific receptors, followed by receptor-mediated endocytosis.[1] Haptocorrin-bound B$_{12}$, comprising the majority of B$_{12}$ in the plasma, is not directly taken up by tissues. About 90% of the total body stores of cobalamin is found in the liver. Excretion via the urine and the feces is minor, accounting for the minimal daily requirement of 2–3 μg. Biliary secretion of cobalamin occurs, but most of the vitamin is reabsorbed in the ileum after binding to the intrinsic factor. Efficient conservation of vitamin B$_{12}$ can explain why deficiency takes years to develop even in cases of strict vegetarians, who consume almost no B$_{12}$.[8]

D. INDICATORS OF STATUS

Vitamin B$_{12}$ status can be assessed by biochemical measurements and by clinical indications, such as the presence of macrocytic anemia (increased mean cell volume (MCV) and decreased hemoglobin levels. However, the latter generally appear in severe deficiency so are of little use in diagnosing the initial development of deficiency.[9] The diagnosis of subclinical deficiency depends on demonstration of lower than normal tissue vitamin levels by biochemical measurements.

Many of the hematologic changes in B$_{12}$ deficiency are identical to those in folate deficiency, so are not true indicators of status of the individual vitamins. Megaloblastic changes in the bone marrow plus macroovalocytes and neutrophilic hypersegmentation in the peripheral blood are indicators of megaloblastic anemia, resulting from either folate or B$_{12}$ deficiency. Hence, laboratory methods are needed to distinguish the two types of deficiency — measurements of serum and red cell folate and of serum vitamin B$_{12}$ are needed to ascertain the cause of the macrocytic anemias. A wide range of neurologic signs and symptoms can indicate diminished cobalamin status. These include paresthesias of the extremities, loss of sensation, confusion, loss of memory and even, in severe cases, delusional psychosis. It is critically important to identify the cause of the hematologic abnormality because folate therapy for a cobalamin deficiency can reverse the megaloblastic symptomatology, but exacerbate the neurologic damage.[10]

The most common biochemical indicator of B$_{12}$ status is the demonstration of low serum or plasma cobalamin concentrations, which are usually associated with decreased tissue content of the vitamin. The lower levels of the normal range are about 200–250 pg/mL.[8] Serum B$_{12}$ levels can be determined by microbiological or radioisotope dilution assay. Although the latter procedures are used most often and are generally quite accurate, the presence of haptocorrins (transcobalamin analogues) in the plasma can sometimes obfuscate the binding of cobalamin,[7] leading to erroneous interpretations. For example, B$_{12}$ that is bound to haptocorrin is not available for cellular uptake, so subjects can have "normal" serum B$_{12}$ levels and still be deficient in available B$_{12}$ when there is an abnormally high level of B$_{12}$ bound to haptocorrin.

A specific indicator of diminished vitamin B$_{12}$ status is an increased plasma or urinary level of methylmalonate (because of the block in methylmalonate conversion to succinate). Recent studies have shown the value of urinary or plasma methylmalonate determinations for diagnosis of cobalamin deficiency.[11] Although these tests are not yet widely available, methylmalonate determinations are currently accepted as a prime indicator of functional B$_{12}$ deficiency. Another potential indication of cobalamin deficiency is an increase in plasma homocysteine, because of the block in conversion of homocysteine to methionine by cobalamin-dependent methionine synthetase. However, homocysteine is also elevated in folate deficiency, so it is not a specific indicator of B$_{12}$ deficiency.[12]

Holo-TC is the complex of vitamin B$_{12}$ and transcobalamin II in the plasma. Since holo-TC is the active form of B$_{12}$ (the only form that can be taken up by tissues), measurement of serum holo-TC levels is theoretically a measurement of active B_{12} levels.[13] Holo-TC is a minor component of circulating B_{12} because of the binding of the majority to haptocorrins in the plasma. An assay for holo-TC is in research development and may become useful in diagnosing functional B_{12} deficiency with greater specificity than the total plasma B_{12} determination.

There is no evidence that exercise has any direct effects on the biochemical or clinical indicators of vitamin B_{12} status per se. Nevertheless, exercise could change the optimal vitamin status by a decrease in availability or an increase in requirement. Availability of B_{12} is decreased when there is reduced dietary supply or reduced absorption of ingested vitamin. Dietary supply would primarily be determined by socioeconomic factors; if anything, exercise should increase dietary intake by stimulating the overall intake of food and the general concern of the exercising individual for health. Malabsorption of food B_{12} occurs in disorders of the intestinal tract such as in tropical sprue. Lack of intrinsic factor secretion (see Section I.C) is the most common cause of diminished vitamin B_{12} status. Gastric mucosal atrophy, such as in pernicious anemia, and loss of gastric function through surgical resection, are the major causes of loss of intrinsic factor secretion.

Vitamin B_{12} requirements are increased in persons who experience rapid growth (infants, pregnant and lactating women), suffer the presence of disease (malignancy, inflammation) and possibly use drugs that might alter cobalamin metabolism. Functional B_{12} deficiency can be produced by chronic exposure (24 hours) to high levels of the anesthetic gas nitrous oxide.[14] Nitrous oxide combines with the Co atom in cobalamin, hence specifically and irreversibly inhibiting the enzyme methionine synthase. Except for persons affected by such categories, there is no reason to expect exercise or sporting activities to increase the requirements for B_{12}. However, malabsorption of vitamin B_{12} increases in frequency with age, so that master athletes are more likely to have an increased requirement for B_{12}.

E. CONTENTS OF FOODS

Vitamin B_{12} is not biosynthesized by mammals, so must be ingested in order to achieve functional levels in the body. The ultimate sources of vitamin B_{12} are cobalamin-synthesizing microorganisms that are found in soil, water or the intestinal lumen of animals. Vegetable products do not contain cobalamins unless they are contaminated with such microorganisms. Hence, the primary source of vitamin B_{12} is the consumption of animal products such as meat, eggs and milk containing B_{12}. Small amounts of B_{12} are available from legumes, due to contamination with soil bacteria. Hence, because the daily requirement is only 2–3 µg, strict vegetarians often have marginal B_{12} status (see below). Also, infants breast-fed by strictly vegetarian mothers are susceptible to B_{12} deficiency because of the very low concentration of cobalamin in milk of mothers with diminished B_{12} intake.[15]

II. INTAKE

A. GENERAL POPULATION

Vitamin B_{12} deficiency is most often associated with absorption defects, so reduced intake per se may not be as relevant as for other water-soluble vitamins. Even so, population studies indicate that most humans in western societies consume more than adequate amounts of B_{12}. People at most risk for B_{12} deficiency would be the elderly, especially post 60 years, when increasing gastric atrophy contributes to malabsorption. Population studies of intake in the U.S. and U.K. reported 20–30 years ago (cited by Herbert[8]) suggest that vitamin B_{12} intakes range from 3–15 µg/d. A recent study of the Framingham Heart Study cohort of elderly subjects (>67 yr old) showed B_{12} intakes averaging 5–6 µg/d.[16] A study of the vitamin B_{12} status of a group of 132 Thai vegetarians (ingesting no animal products except milk) and a control group reported B_{12} intakes of 0.4 µg/d in the vegetarians, confirming the reduced levels of B_{12} in vegetarian diets.[17] As expected, the vegetarian group was relatively B_{12} deficient (mean serum levels of 117 and 152 pg/ml in males and females, compared with about 500 pg/ml in controls). Bissoli et al.[18] studied the long-term effects of diet on total serum B$_{12}$ levels in 31 strict vegans (no animal products), 14 lacto-ovo-vegetarians (LOVs) and 29 age- and sex-matched control subjects. The vegetarian groups had followed their respective diets for at least 5 years. Serum B$_{12}$ levels were decreased to 155 and 164 pmol/L in the vegans and LOVs, respectively, compared with the controls at 265 pmol/L, with the normal range defined as >220 pmol/L. The vegetarian groups also had a high prevalence (~40%) of subjects with very low vitamin B$_{12}$ levels (<127 pmol/L).

B. ATHLETES

Total B$_{12}$ intake by athletes does not seem to be much different from that of other groups that are active consumers of balanced diets and vitamin supplements, although such intake would be above those of the general population. Barry et al.[19] surveyed the reported intakes of 108 international- (I) class athletes and of 35 club- (C) class athletes (involving both endurance and strength sports) using weighed inventories over 3 alternative days. I- and C-class males consumed 19 and 13 µg of B$_{12}$/d (much higher than the existing RDA of 3 µg, probably due to a high meat consumption), while I-and C-class females consumed 3 and 6 µg/d, respectively. About 50% of both groups of athletes were active consumers of some type of vitamin supplement. Singh et al.[20] recorded the 4-d dietary records of ultramarathoners, who averaged 67 miles/wk in training. The estimated vitamin intake from food alone was 4.5–6 µg of B$_{12}$/d (compared with the existing RDA of 2 µg). Because 70% of this population used vitamin supplements, the total daily intakes were estimated at 50–55 µg B$_{12}$, well above the RDA. In a separate study of the effects of vitamin supplements on physically active men, Singh et al.[21] using baseline 4-d diet records (no subjects on supplements for 3 wk prior to baseline data), reported B$_{12}$ intakes were about 5.5 µg/d. Worme et al.[22] surveyed male and female participants in a forthcoming triathlon (about a 17% response). Subjects completed a 3-d dietary record during normal training periods within 6 wk after the event, including no competition during the 3 days. From food alone, daily B$_{12}$ intakes for both genders were about 5 µg/d. About 40% of the population consumed vitamin supplements on a regular basis, and the total B$_{12}$ intakes for males increased to 10 µg/d, but that for females remained the same as for food alone. The RDA cited at the time of this study was 3 µg/d for B$_{12}$. Hence, it would appear that total intake of cobalamin from this population was greater than the RDA. However, when the data were shown for individuals, it was noted that about 45% of the females and about 30% of the males consumed less than the RDA, including both food and supplements. The population means cited above were apparently inflated by the presence of a few excess consumers of food and supplements such that these populations included a significant number of active athletes with less than recommended vitamin consumptions.

A special concern should be noted because there are subsets of athletes who follow vegetarian diets for reasons of health or otherwise. As discussed above, the vitamin B$_{12}$ intake of strict vegetarians can be very low (0.4 µg/d,[17] compared with the current RDA of 2.4 µg/d) and long-term consumption of vegetarian diets may lead to reduced serum B$_{12}$ levels.[18] However, other studies suggest that vitamin B$_{12}$ intake by vegetarian athletes may be sufficient to maintain normal B$_{12}$ status. Eisenger et al.[23] combined a study of the effects of exercise on B$_{12}$ intake with a study of the effects of a vegetarian diet on exercise performance. For an "ultra" run involving a 1000-km run over a 20-d period, two groups of athletes were studied, 30 who consumed a regular western diet and 25 who consumed an LOV diet. Both diets were strictly controlled by study personnel and contained the same energy content and the same carbohydrate–fat–protein distribution. Partic-ipants consumed the diets *ad libitum*, although study personnel recorded the amount of consumption. Over the 20-d period, there was no difference in energy intake nor in the amount of weight loss between the two groups. The LOVs consumed a significantly lower amount of vitamin B$_{12}$, although this intake was still about twice the RDA. Analysis of serum B$_{12}$ levels in both groups showed no significant changes over the duration of the study. Thus, short-term consumption of a vegetarian diet, even in rigorously exercising endurance athletes, produces a reduced intake of vitamin B$_{12}$, but apparently the intake is sufficient to maintain normal serum B$_{12}$ levels.

An additional concern would be the athletic elderly. Because the high frequency of atrophic gastritis in elderly populations can diminish B_{12} absorption, high amounts of B_{12} may need to be ingested by the exercising elderly to maintain functional B_{12} status. Recommendations are to increase intake of B_{12} to 2.8 μg/d[24].

III.   BIOCHEMICAL STATUS IN ATHLETES

Several studies have examined the vitamin B_{12} status of humans and animals during training as well as the effects of vitamin supplements on such status. As noted above, recent evidence suggests a link between exercise and plasma levels of homocysteine, and by inference, a relationship with that of vitamin B_{12} or folate. While several studies have examined the effects of exercise on plasma homocysteine, only those that have also assessed the effects on vitamin B_{12} will be discussed here.

Studies that have simply screened B_{12} status show little difference between athletes and non-athletes. Brotherhood et al.[25] compared the status of numerous hematologic parameters in 40 male long-distance runners with 12 matched controls. They reported no differences between these groups in serum B_{12} levels. Matter et al.,[26] in a study of 85 female marathoners, reported normal vitamin B_{12} levels. The biochemical status of 17 of the I-class athletes, characterized by Barry et al.,[19] included serum B_{12} and folate levels in the normal range for all athletes. None of these athletes was an active consumer of vitamin supplements. Hermann et al.,[27] in a study of the effects of intense endurance exercise (running or bicycling) on homocysteine levels, measured the pre-race serum levels of vitamin B_{12} in those subjects who also had an elevated plasma homocysteine level. All 23 athletes with high homocysteine levels, out of the total of 100 athletes, had a low serum B_{12} level, suggesting that a substantial number of highly trained athletes are susceptible to a functional B_{12} deficiency. Vitamin B_{12} levels were not measured after the training period in these 100 athletes.

Several studies have examined the interaction between exercise and consumption of supplements. Singh et al.[20] reported on a group of ultramarathoners whose total B_{12} intake from foods and supplements was found to be significantly above the RDA. Their B_{12} levels averaged 226 pmol/L, in the middle of the reference range. Singh et al.[21] also reported on the status of physically active men before and during daily ingestion of a commercially available high-potency multivitamin and mineral supplement (200 μg B_{12}) for 12 wk. Blood B_{12} levels averaged about 200 pmol/L before supplementation, in the middle of the reference range, and significantly increased to 300 pmol/L by 6 wk of supplementation, with no further increase at 12 wk. The rise in B_{12} levels can readily be explained by the fact that the B_{12} content in the supplements was orders of magnitude greater than the RDA. Weight et al.[28] conducted a similar double-blind, placebo-controlled trial of multivitamin and mineral supplementation (60 μg B_{12}) in a group of male runners who averaged more than 40 miles per wk. Background (pre-supplementation) B_{12} status was normal in these endurance athletes — serum B_{12} was 340 pmol/L, in the middle of the normal range. Supplementation for up to 3 mo did not affect B_{12} status significantly; similarly, administration of a placebo did not affect this vitamin, suggesting that the control subjects maintained a well balanced diet throughout the study.

Vitamin B_{12} status has also been measured in controlled studies of exercise in endurance athletes. As noted above, Eisenger et al.[23] studied the effects of a 1000-km run over 20 d on serum B_{12} levels in 55 athletes consuming controlled diets, either regular western diets or LOV diets. In both groups, intake of B_{12} was well above the RDA, and there was no change in serum B_{12} levels in either group at the end of the 20 d. Konig et al.[29] studied 39 well-trained triathletes, both over the course of a 4-wk training and during a subsequent triathlon event (400-m swim, 25-km bicycle ride and 4-km run). Serum B_{12} levels were not affected by the 4 wk of strenuous endurance training (compared with the pre-training determination), nor by the intense exercise during the event. Hermann et al.[6] studied two groups of swimmers who underwent different levels of training, either high-intensity or volume training, for 3 wk. All 19 such athletes had normal serum B_{12} and methylmalonate levels before the training, and neither measure was changed by either type of training. It is interesting that, in this group of swimming athletes, this group found no pre-existing B$_{12}$ deficiency, while in an earlier study of runners and bicyclists, nearly one in four had a low serum B$_{12}$ level prior to training.

These studies of populations of heavy-endurance exercisers show that B$_{12}$ status is not related to exercise but may be related to the diets consumed, i.e., those who consume a well-balanced diet or supplements have normal or elevated status, while those who consume a marginal diet, such as a strict vegetarian diet without supplements, tend to have marginal B$_{12}$ status. Supplements, if they contain an elevated B$_{12}$ content, may actually raise B$_{12}$ levels to above normal status. In general, highly trained endurance athletes do not appear to be deficient in vitamin B$_{12}$. Short-term, but rigorous exercise has no effect of plasma B$_{12}$ levels in previously well-trained athletes.

Even in marginally healthy people, exercise does not appear to greatly alter B$_{12}$ status. De Jong et al.[30] conducted an intervention trial in 217 elderly (>70 yr) subjects over a 17-wk period including enriched foods or light exercise (45 min, 2 × wk). They found no changes in plasma vitamin B$_{12}$, total plasma homocysteine or serum methylmalonate levels between the exercise and control groups, suggesting that light exercise has no effect on B$_{12}$ status in the elderly. Bailey et al.[31] examined 32 young healthy male subjects who underwent a moderate cycling exercise program (30 min, 3 × wk) for 4 wk, during which they consumed their normal diets. Vitamin B$_{12}$ levels were unchanged after 4 wk. Randeva et al.[32] studied 12 overweight young women with polycystic ovary syndrome who followed a light exercise program (brisk walking for 20–60 min, 3 × wk for 6 wk, then 5 × wk up to 6 mo). The plasma B$_{12}$ levels at 6 mo in the exercising women did not differ from those in a control group of nine similarly afflicted women who did not exercise.

IV. STUDIES RELATED TO EXERCISE PERFORMANCE

A. ANIMAL

Apparently no studies that relate B$_{12}$ status or consumption of excess B$_{12}$ with changes in exercise performance have been conducted in animals.

B. HUMAN

Numerous studies have examined the effects of vitamin B$_{12}$ on exercise performance. Most of these have been conducted in conjunction with intake of other vitamins, especially other B vitamins (reviewed by Van der Beek[33]). Such studies are complicated in their interpretation as to the effects of B$_{12}$ per se. None of the studies of these vitamins individually have shown significant effects of B$_{12}$ on exercise performance, with the exception of a study[34] in which the subjects were already anemic, i.e., they were already suffering from deficiency symptoms.

Tin-May-Tan et al.[35] studied the effects of parenteral vitamin B$_{12}$ supplementation (1 mg, 3/wk for 6 wk) on physical performance in a double-blind placebo-controlled study in male students. B$_{12}$ supplementation had no effect on resting heart rate, on recovery heart rate after maximal exercise, on oxygen uptake (VO$_2$max) nor on measures of strength and coordination. Rodger et al.[36] reported on a mass screening study of a university population in which serum folate and B$_{12}$ levels in 300 subjects were compared with an assessment of exercise habits by questionnaire. The authors observed no significant relation between B$_{12}$ levels and levels of exercise in hr/wk in either men or women. Read and McGuffin[37] reported a double-blind placebo-controlled study of B vitamin supplementation in age-matched male college students. Subjects received 0.5 µg B$_{12}$ per day for 6 wk in a multivitamin complex containing near or above RDA levels of B$_1$, B$_2$, B$_6$, niacin and pantothenic acid. No significant effects of supplementation were noted in three tests of endurance capacity (treadmill) during the 6-wk period.

Although most sports require physical athletic exercise, others require mental conditioning and proper sensory-motor control such as marksmanship. Bonke and Nickel[38] studied the effects of megadoses of B_{12} in combination with B_1 (thiamine) and B_6 (pyridoxine) on performance by experienced marksman. In two studies, one of open design with 120 µg B_{12}/d for 8 wk and one as double blind design with 600 µg/d for 8 wk. In the latter study, the vitamin-treated group showed an increase in performance during the treatment period, with no such effect in placebos suggesting minimal effects of training per se on the increased performance. These results are intriguing, although a crossover study in the same subjects might have eliminated some bias. Also, the doses of all the B vitamins were 60–300 times the respective RDAs.

V. REQUIREMENTS

A. NRC Estimated Safe and Adequate Daily Dietary Intakes

The recommended dietary allowance (RDA) is the term used to describe the amount of intake of a necessary nutrient considered to be sufficient to meet the needs of most healthy persons, i.e., what is needed to prevent a deficiency. These allowances utilize certain margins of safety (mean requirement plus two standard deviations) to cover the degree of variability in requirements among people and in bioavailability from most food sources. The RDAs undergo changes, depending on the presence of new scientific data. For instance, the RDAs promulgated in 1998 (Table 8.1) represent a significant increase over those established in 1989.[39,40]

B. Specific Recommendations for Athletes

The popular or lay recommendation for intake of vitamin B_{12} by athletes appears to be to "take as much as you can," as it is often sterotyped as an ergonomic aid or as a tonic for tiredness and poor mental status. The reasons behind this hype are probably derived from the known rapid improvement

---

TABLE 8.1
Current Dietary Vitamin B_{12} Recommendations (µg/d)

Age/Gender	B_{12}
0–0.5 yr	0.4*
0.5–1 yr	0.5*
1–3 yr	0.9
4–8 yr	1.2
Males	
9–13 yr	1.8
14+ yr	2.4**
Females	
9–13 yr	1.8
14+ yr	2.4**
Pregnant	2.6
Lactating	2.8

Source: Recommended Dietary Allowance (RDA) determined by the Food and Nutrition Board of the National Academy of Sciences, 1998.[40]
*Adequate intake (not RDA) represents the mean intake for healthy infants; RDA represents the needs of almost all (97%) individuals in a group.
**Because of the higher degree of B_{12} absorption problems in those older than 50 yr, it is advised that these individuals reach their RDA by consuming foods fortified with B_{12} or supplements containing B_{12}.

---

in mental status that occurs when a person with the neurologic symptoms of B$_{12}$ deficiency is injected with B$_{12}$. Hence, it is "logically" derived that if B$_{12}$ works in such a situation, then B$_{12}$ should be good for other situations where a person feels the need to be stimulated by something healthy. Another potential misperception that promotes use of vitamin supplements to improve athletic performance is that exercise increases breakdown or excretion of vitamins, thus increasing the need for replacement. There is no indication that such changes in B$_{12}$ homeostasis happen because of exercise.

The intake studies that have been conducted in athletes show that a substantial portion of lay and highly trained athletes consume high-potency vitamin supplements on a regular basis.[19–21] Such consumption brings the B$_{12}$ status of these populations up to or above the recommended normal. In particular, B$_{12}$ levels are often elevated, since supplements are often super-fortified in B$_{12}$. Despite the fact that supplements have decreased the frequency of marginal or deficient status in exercising populations, the studies of performance have indicated that the added amounts of B$_{12}$ offer little if any improvement in endurance or athletic ability. Hence, there appears to be no need to recommend a different requirement of B$_{12}$ intake for athletes as compared with the general population. However, because of the increasing frequency of vitamin B$_{12}$ malabsorption with age and of the low level of B$_{12}$ in vegetarian diets, elderly athletes and athletes who are strict vegetarians should increase their B$_{12}$ intake above the current RDA, to 2.8 μg/d, or should consider supplementation.[24]

VI. SUMMARY

Vitamin B$_{12}$ is primarily needed to maintain proper growth and development of cells through DNA synthesis. Deficiency of vitamin B$_{12}$ leads to hematopoietic defects, and possibly to anemia or neurological damage in severe cases. In persons who have reached such morbidity, the administration of B$_{12}$ in diets or supplements will have marked effects, including increasing endurance and athletic performance. In the athlete with normal or marginal B$_{12}$ status, with no accompanying signs of deficiency, there is no scientific evidence that increased amounts of B$_{12}$ will provide any benefits in terms of athletic performance or exercise physiology. Hence, athletes and physically active persons should consume a well-balanced diet to obtain sufficient B$_{12}$. Supplements should be added to a vegetarian diet to ensure that the person does not suffer some of the subtle effects of marginal B$_{12}$ status, but there is no reason to recommend consumption of added amounts of B$_{12}$ to increase one's ability to exercise or perform athletically. Although vitamin B$_{12}$ is often given to patients complaining of tiredness, there is no evidence from controlled studies that B$_{12}$ improves alertness or wellbeing in non-deficient subjects.

REFERENCES

1. Ellenbogen, L. and Cooper, B.A., Vitamin B$_{12}$, *Handbook of Vitamins,* 2nd ed., Machlin, L.J., Ed., Marcel Dekker, New York, 1991, 491.
2. Shane, B. and Stokstad, E.L.R., Vitamin B$_{12}$-folate relationships, *Ann. Rev. Nutr.,* 5, 115, 1985.
3. Ueland, P.M. and Refsum, H., Plasma homocysteine, a risk factor for vascular disease: Plasma levels in health, disease, and drug therapy, *J. Lab. Clin. Med.,* 114, 473, 1989.
4. Nygard, O., Vollset, S.E., Refsum, H., Stensvold, I., Tverdal, A., Nordrehaug, J.E., Ueland, M. and Kvale G. Total plasma homocysteine and cardiovscular risk profile. The Hordaland Homocysteine Study. *JAMA,* 274, 1526–33, 1995.
5. Mennen, L.I., de Courcy, G.P., Guilland, J-C., Ducros, V., Bertarais, S., Nicolas, J-P., Maurel, M., Zarebska, M., Favier, J., Franchisseur, C., Hercberg, S. and Galan, P. Homocysteine, cardiovascular disease risk factors, and habitual diet in the French Supplementation with Antioxidant Vitamins and Minerals Study. *Am. J. Clin. Nutr.,* 76, 1279–89, 2002.
6. Hermann, M. Wilkinson, J., Schorr, H., Obeid, R., Georg, T., Urhausen, A., Scharhag, J., Kindermann, W. and Herrmann, W. Comparison of the influence of volume-oriented training and high-intensity interval training on serum homocysteine and its cofactors in young, healthy swimmers. *Clin. Chem. Lab. Med.* 41, 1525–31, 2003.

7. Nexø, E., Hansen, M., Rasmussen, K., Lindgren, A. and Gräsbeck, R., How to diagnose cobalamin deficiency, *Scand. J. Clin. Lab. Invest.*, 54, 61, 1994.

8. Herbert, V., Recommended dietary intakes (RDI) of vitamin B_{12} in humans, *Am. J. Clin. Nutr.*, 45, 671, 1987.

9. Herbert, V., Development of human folate deficiency, in *Folic Acid Metabolism in Health and Disease*, Picciano, M.F., Stokstad, E.L.R. and Gregory, J.F., Eds., Wiley-Liss, New York, 1990, 195.

10. Savage, D.G. and Lindenbaum, J., Folate-cobalamin interactions, in *Folate in Health and Disease*, Bailey, L.B., Ed., Marcel Dekker, New York, 1995, 237.

11. Marcell, P.D., Stabler, S.P., Podell, E.R. and Allen, R.H., Quantitation of methylmalonic acid and other dicarboxylic acids in normal serum and urine using capillary gas chromatography-mass spectrometry, *Anal. Biochem.*, 150, 55, 1985.

12. Snow, C.F. Laboratory diagnosis of vitamin B_{12} and folate deficiency. *Arch. Intern. Med.* 159, 1289–98, 1999.

13. Herzlich, B. and Herbert, V. Depletion of serum holotranscobalamin II. An early sign of negative vitamin B_{12} balance. *Lab. Invest.* 58, 332–7, 1998.

14. Amess, J.A.L., Burman, J.F., Rees, G.M., Nancekievill, D.G. and Mollin, D.L., Megaloblastic haemopoiesis in patients receiving nitrous oxide, *Lancet,* 2, 339, 1978.

15. Schneede, J., Dagnelie, P.C., Van Staveren, W.A., Vollset, S.E., Refsum, H. and Ueland, P.M., Methylmalonic acid and homocysteine in plasma as indicators of functional cobalamin deficiency in infants on macrobiotic diets, *Ped. Res.*, 36, 194, 1994.

16. Selhub, J., Jacques, P.F., Wilson, P.W.F., Rush, D. and Rosenberg, I.H., Vitamin status and intake as primary determinants of homocysteinemia in an elderly population, *JAMA,* 270, 2693, 1993.

17. Tungtrongchitr, R., Pongpaew, P., Prayurahong, B., Changbumrung, S., Vudhivai, N., Migasena, P. and Schelp F.P., Vitamin B_{12}, folic acid and haematological status of 132 Thai vegetarians, *Int. J. Vit. Nutr. Res.* 63, 201, 1993.

18. Bissoli, L., Di Francesco, V., Ballarin, A., Mandragons, R., Trespedi, R., Brocco, G., Caruso, B., Bosello, O. and Zamboni, M. Effect of vegetarian diet on homocysteine levels. *Ann. Nutr. Metab.* 46, 73–9, 2002.

19. Barry, A., Cantwell, T., Doherty, F., Folan, J.C., Ingoldsby, M., Kevany, J.P., O'Broin, J.D., O'Connor, H., O'Shea, B., Ryan, B.A. and Vaughan, J., A nutritional study of Irish athletes, *Brit. J. Sports Med.*, 15, 99, 1981.

20. Singh, A., Evans, P., Gallagher, K.L. and Deuster, P.A., Dietary intakes and biochemical profiles of nutritional status of ultramarathoners, *Med. Sci. Sports Exerc.*, 25, 328, 1993.

21. Singh, A., Moses, F.M. and Deuster, P.A., Vitamin and mineral status in physically active men: Effects of a high-potency supplement, *Am. J. Clin. Nutr.*, 55, 1, 1992.

22. Worme, J.D., Doubt, T.J., Singh, A., Ryan, C.J., Moses, F.M. and Deuster, P.A., Dietary patterns, gastrointestinal complaints, and nutrition knowledge of recreational triathletes, *Am. J. Clin. Nutr.*, 51, 690, 1990.

23. Eisenger, M., Plath, M., Jung, K. and Leitzmann, C. Nutrient intake of endurance runers with ovo-lacto-vegetarian diet and regular western diet. *Z. Ernahrungswiss.* 33, 217–29, 1994.

24. Sacheck, J.M. and Roubenoff, R. Nutrition in the exercising elderly. *Clin. Sports Med.* 18, 565–84, 1999.

25. Brotherhood, J., Brozović, B. and Pugh, L. G. C., Haematological status of middle- and long-distance runners, *Clin. Sci. Mol. Med.*, 48, 139, 1975.

26. Matter, M., Stittfall, T., Graves, J., Myburgh, K., Adams, B., Jacobs, P. and Noakes, T.D., The effect of iron and folate therapy on maximal exercise performance in female marathon runners with iron and folate deficiency, *Clin. Sci.*, 72, 415, 1987.

27. Hermann, M., Schorr, H., Obeid, R., Scharhag, J., Urhausen, A., Kindermann, W. and Hermann, H. Homocysteine increases during endurance exercise. *Clin. Chem. Lab. Med.* 41, 1518–24, 2003.

28. Weight, L.M., Noakes, T.D., Labadarios, D., Graves, J., Jacobs, P. and Berman, P.A., Vitamin and mineral status of trained athletes including the effects of supplementation, *Am. J. Clin. Nutr.*, 47, 186, 1988.

29. Konig, D., Bisse, E., Deibert, P., Muller, H-M., Wieland, H. and Berg, A. Influence of training volume and acute physical exercise on homocysteine levels in endurance-trained men: Interactions with plasma folate and vitamin B_{12}. *Ann. Nutr. Med.* 47, 114–8, 2003.

30. De Jong, N., Chin A Paw, M., de Groot, L., Rutten, R., Swinkels, D., Kok, F. and van Staveren, W. Nutrient-dense foods and exercise in frail elderly: Effects on B vitamins, homocysteine, methylmalonic acid, and neuropsychological functioning. *Am. J. Clin. Nutr.* 73, 338–46, 2001.

31. Bailey, D.M., Davies, B. and Baker, J. Training in hypoxia: Modulation of metabolic and cardiovascular risk factors in men. *Med. Sci. Sports Exerc.* 32, 1058–66, 2000.

32. Randeva, H.S., Lewandowski, K.C., Drzewoski, J., Brooke-Wavell, K., O'Callaghan, C., Czupryniak, L., Hillhouse, E.W. and Prelelevic, G.M. Exercise decreases plasma total homocysteine in overweight young women with polycystic ovary syndrome. *J. Clin. Endocrinol. Metab.* 87, 4496–501, 2002.

33. Van der Beek, E.J., Vitamins and endurance training, Food for running or faddish claims? *Sports Med.,* 2, 175, 1985.

34. Seshadri, S. and Malhotra, S., The effect of hematinics on the physical work capacity in anemics, *Indian Ped.,* 21, 529, 1984.

35. Tin-May-Tan, Ma-Win-May, Khin-Sann-Aung and Mya-Tu, M., The effect of vitamin B$_{12}$ on physical performance capacity, *Br. J. Nutr.,* 40, 269, 1978.

36. Rodger, R.S.C., Fletcher, K., Fail, B.J., Rahman, H., Sviland, L. and Hamilton, P.J., Factors influencing haematological measurements in healthy adults, *J. Chron. Dis.,* 40, 943, 1987.

37. Read, M.H. and McGuffin L., The effect of B-complex supplementation on endurance performance, *J. Sports Med.,* 23, 178, 1983.

38. Bonke, D. and Nickel, B., Improvement of fine motoric movement control by elevated dosages of vitamin B$_1$, B$_6$, and B$_{12}$ in target shooting, *Int. J. Vit. Nutr. Res. Suppl,* 30, 198, 1989.

39. Food and Nutrition Board, *Recommended Dietary Allowances,* 10th ed., National Academy of Sciences, Washington, D.C., 1989.

40. Food and Nutrition Board, Dietary reference intakes for thiamin, riboflavin, niacin, vitamins B$_6$, folate, vitamin B$_{12}$, pantothenic acid, biotin and choline. National Academy of Sciences, Washington, D.C., 1998.

9 Pantothenic Acid and Biotin

*Gabriela Camporeale, Rocío Rodríguez-Meléndez
and Janos Zempleni*

CONTENTS

I. INTRODUCTION

Pantothenic acid and biotin are water-soluble vitamins; chemical structures are depicted in Figure 9.1. In cells, pantothenic acid is converted to 4′-phosphopantetheine, which serves as a covalently linked coenzyme for acyl carrier protein; 4′-phosphopantetheine is further converted to coenzyme A (CoA), which is a ubiquitous cofactor in intermediary metabolism. Biotin serves as a coenzyme for carboxylases, but also plays roles in chromatin structure and cell signaling.

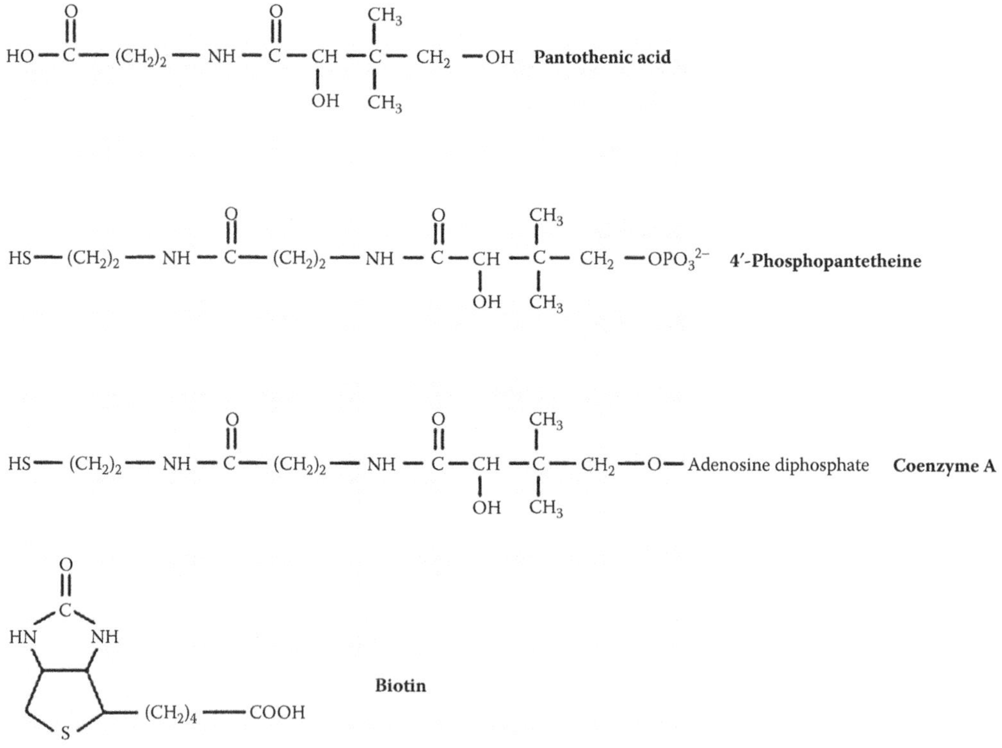

FIGURE 9.1 Chemical structures of pantothenic acid, 4′-phosphopantetheine, coenzyme A and biotin.

Pantothenic acid and biotin in vitamin supplements are obtained by chemical synthesis rather than by purification from natural sources. Isobutyraldehyde, formaldehyde and cyanide are used as starting materials in the chemical synthesis of pantothenic acid; the intermediate D-pantolactone is condensed with β-alanine to produce pantothenic acid.[1] Calcium salts of pantothenic acid are the most common commercial form of the vitamin. The chemical synthesis of biotin is based on using fumaric acid as a starting material.[2]

II. METABOLISM

A. PANTOTHENIC ACID

1. Digestion

The majority of pantothenic acid in foodstuffs is present as CoA or 4′-phosphopantetheine; both these compounds are hydrolyzed by pyrophosphatase and phosphatase in the intestinal lumen to release pantetheine.[3] Pantetheine is further hydrolyzed by luminal pantetheinase to release pantothenic acid. Some pantetheine is transported into mucosa cells, followed by intracellular hydrolysis by pantetheinase.

2. Intestinal Transport and Bioavailability

Uptake of pantothenic acid into intestinal cells is mediated by the sodium-dependent multivitamin transporter (SMVT).[4] This transporter has similar affinity for pantothenic acid, biotin and lipoic acid.[4–6] At high intestinal concentrations of pantothenic acid, absorption by passive diffusion is quantitatively more important than active transport.[7] It remains unknown whether bacterial synthesis in the intestine contributes substantially to pantothenic acid supply. Note that SMVT is also expressed in the colon, where the bulk of intestinal microorganisms reside. If microbial synthesis of pantothenic acid is substantial, balance studies in humans may have underestimated pantothenic acid turnover and requirements. The bioavailability of pantothenic acid from dietary sources is about 50% compared with synthetic pantothenate from vitamin supplements.[8] If supraphysiological doses of synthetic pantothenic acid (10–100 mg/day) are ingested orally, about 60% are excreted into urine.[9]

3. Coenzyme Forms of Pantothenic Acid

The two coenzyme forms of pantothenic acid that have been identified in humans are CoA and 4′-phosphopantetheine. The pathway of CoA synthesis is depicted in Figure 9.2; 4′-phosphopantetheine is an intermediate in CoA synthesis. Synthesis of CoA depends on ATP and CTP and involves phosphorylation and decarboxylation steps and a condensation with cysteine.[10] The sulfhydryl group in 4′-phosphopantetheine forms thioesters with acyl compounds groups to produce acyl-CoA derivatives, including acetyl-CoA.

Acetyl-CoA plays a central role in intermediary metabolism. Acetyl-CoA is generated in processes such as β-oxidation of fatty acids, oxidation of glucose and catabolism of amino acids. Acetyl-CoA is utilized in the generation of metabolic energy (ATP) in the tricarboxylic acid cycle and the respiratory chain.[11] Acetyl-CoA also participates in a number of acetylation reactions, including the formation of acetylcholine, melatonin, N-acetylglucosamine, N-acetylgalactosamine and N-acetylneuraminic acid.[12] Finally, acetyl-CoA is a substrate in the acetylation of histones (DNA-binding proteins), regulating transcriptional activity of chromatin.[13] Various acyl-CoA esters play roles in the synthesis of isoprenoid-derived compounds such as cholesterol, steroid hormones, dolichol, vitamin D and heme A. Acyl-carrier protein depends on 4′-phosphopantetheine as a prosthetic group in fatty acids synthesis.[12]

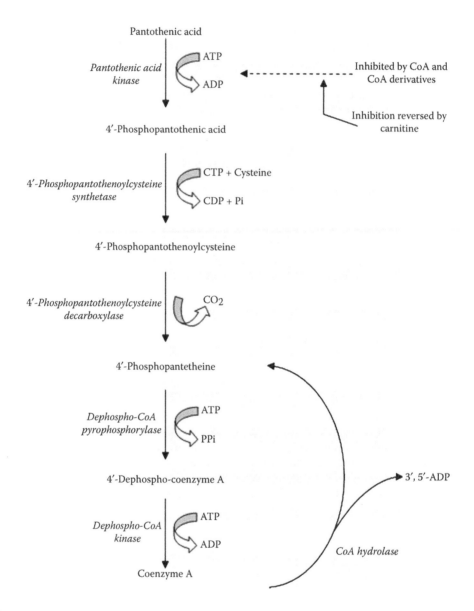

FIGURE 9.2 Conversion of pantothenic acid to 4-phosphopantetheine and coenzyme A.

4. Cellular Uptake of Pantothenic Acid

The cellular uptake of pantothenic acid is mediated by SMVT.[14] Activation of protein kinase C is associated with decreased SMVT activity.[15] Conversion of pantothenic acid to CoA prevents efflux of pantothenic acid from cells ("metabolic trapping"). Pantothenic acid kinase (Figure 9.2) plays an essential role in this process.[16] This kinase depends on magnesium and ATP and is inhibited by CoA and acyl-CoA esters, providing a negative feedback control. L-carnitine prevents the inhibition of pantothenic acid kinase by CoA. Insulin activates pantothenic acid kinase.[16]

5. Pantothenic Acid Excretion

The vitamin is excreted in urine primarily as intact pantothenic acid; CoA is hydrolyzed to release pantothenic acid before excretion.[17] The urinary excretion of pantothenic acid correlates with its dietary intake.[17]

B. BIOTIN

1. Digestion

Biotin in foods is largely protein bound; binding is mediated by an amide linkage between the valeric acid side chain in biotin and ε-amino groups in lysines.[18] Several gastrointestinal enzymes hydrolyze biotin-containing proteins to generate biotinyl peptides.[19] The amide bond between biotin and lysine in biotinyl peptides is hydrolyzed by intestinal biotinidase (E.C. 3.5.1.12) to release biotin. Biotinidase is found in pancreatic juice, secretions of the intestinal glands and brush-border membranes.[19] Biotinidase activities are similar in mucosa from duodenum, jejunum and ileum.[19]

2. Intestinal Transport and Bioavailability

Studies using jejunal segments from rats provided evidence that intestinal biotin uptake is mediated by both saturable and nonsaturable components.[20] At biotin concentrations less than 5 μM, biotin absorption proceeds largely by the saturable process, whereas at concentrations above 25 μM, non-saturable uptake predominates.[20] Transport of biotin is faster in the jejunum than in the ileum and is minimal in the colon. The intestinal transport of biotin is mediated by SMVT, i.e., the same transporter that also mediates pantothenic acid uptake (see above).[4,5] Biotin is absorbed nearly completely in humans, even if pharmacological doses are ingested.[21]

3. Biotin-Binding Proteins in Plasma

Biotinidase has one high-affinity and one low-affinity binding site for biotin and serves as a biotin-carrier protein in human plasma.[22] In addition, albumin, α-globulin and β-globulin have affinity for biotin and may play a role in biotin transport in plasma.[23] Evidence has been provided that 81% of the biotin in human plasma is free, 12% is covalently bound and 7% is reversibly bound.[24] A biotin-binding glycoprotein (mol. wt. 66,000) is present in serum from pregnant female rats [25] but not in serum from male rats.[23]

4. Cellular Biotin Uptake

Biotin uptake into mammalian cells is mediated by SMVT.[5,6,26] In addition, monocarboxylate transporter 1 mediates biotin uptake into human lymphoid cells and, perhaps, other tissues.[27] An inborn error of biotin transport has been described in humans.[28]

5. Biotin-Dependent Carboxylases

In mammals, biotin serves as a covalently bound coenzyme for four carboxylases (Figure 9.3): acetyl-CoA carboxylase (E.C. 6.4.1.2), pyruvate carboxylase (E.C. 6.4.1.1), propionyl-CoA carboxylase (E.C. 6.4.1.3) and β-methylcrotonyl-CoA carboxylase (E.C. 6.4.1.4).[29,30] The attachment of biotin to specific ε-amino groups of lysines in carboxylases is catalyzed by holocarboxylase synthetase (E.C. 6.3.4.10).[23]

For acetyl-CoA carboxylase, a cytosolic (denoted acetyl-CoA carboxylase "α") and a mitochondrial (denoted acetyl-CoA carboxylase "β") form have been identified.[31] Both acetyl-CoA carboxylase α and β catalyze the binding of bicarbonate to acetyl-CoA to form malonyl-CoA; the latter is a substrate of fatty acid synthesis. Acetyl-CoA carboxylase α and β have distinct roles in intermediary metabolism due to their subcellular localization. Acetyl-CoA carboxylase α controls fatty acid synthesis in the cytoplasm by generating malonyl-CoA. In contrast, acetyl-CoA carboxylase β controls fatty acid oxidation in mitochondria. This effect of acetyl-CoA carboxylase β is

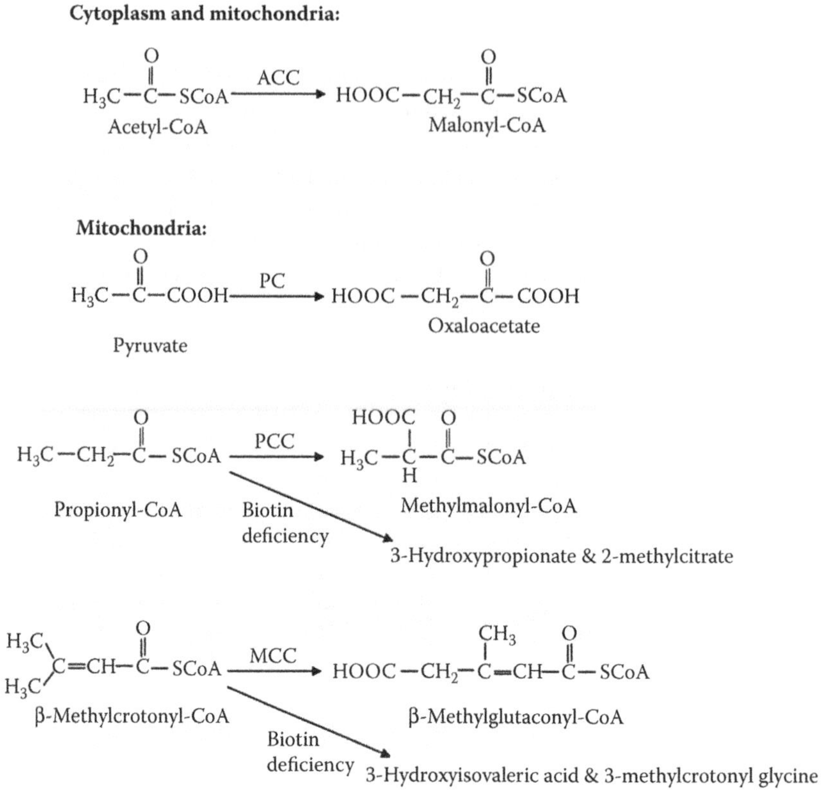

Cytoplasm and mitochondria:

$$H_3C-\overset{\overset{O}{\|}}{C}-SCoA \xrightarrow{\text{ACC}} HOOC-CH_2-\overset{\overset{O}{\|}}{C}-SCoA$$

Acetyl-CoA   Malonyl-CoA

Mitochondria:

$$H_3C-\overset{\overset{O}{\|}}{C}-COOH \xrightarrow{\text{PC}} HOOC-CH_2-\overset{\overset{O}{\|}}{C}-COOH$$

Pyruvate   Oxaloacetate

$$H_3C-CH_2-\overset{\overset{O}{\|}}{C}-SCoA \xrightarrow{\text{PCC}} H_3C-\overset{\overset{HOOC}{|}}{\underset{H}{C}}-\overset{\overset{O}{\|}}{C}-SCoA$$

Propionyl-CoA   Biotin   Methylmalonyl-CoA
                 deficiency
                          ⟶ 3-Hydroxypropionate & 2-methylcitrate

$$\underset{H_3C}{\overset{H_3C}{>}}C=CH-\overset{\overset{O}{\|}}{C}-SCoA \xrightarrow{\text{MCC}} HOOC-CH_2-\overset{\overset{CH_3}{|}}{C}=CH-\overset{\overset{O}{\|}}{C}-SCoA$$

β-Methylcrotonyl-CoA   β-Methylglutaconyl-CoA
                  Biotin
                  deficiency ⟶ 3-Hydroxyisovaleric acid & 3-methylcrotonyl glycine

FIGURE 9.3 Biotin-dependent steps in intermediary metabolism. ACC, acetyl-CoA carboxylase; PC, pyruvate carboxylase; PCC propionyl-CoA carboxylase; MCC, β-methylcrotonyl-CoA carboxylase.

also mediated through malonyl-CoA, which is an inhibitor of fatty acid transport into mitochondria. Acetyl-CoA carboxylase β may also play a role in biotin storage.[32]

Pyruvate carboxylase, propionyl-CoA carboxylase and β-methylcrotonyl-CoA carboxylase are located in mitochondria. Pyruvate carboxylase is a key enzyme in gluconeogenesis. Propionyl-CoA carboxylase catalyzes an essential step in the metabolism of isoleucine, valine, methionine, threonine, the cholesterol side chain and odd-chain fatty acids. β-Methylcrotonyl-CoA carboxylase catalyzes an essential step in leucine metabolism.

6. Storage

Mitochondrial acetyl-CoA carboxylase (isoform β) may serve as a reservoir for biotin; neither cytosolic acetyl-CoA carboxylase (isoform α) nor the mitochondrial pyruvate carboxylase, propionyl-CoA carboxylase, or β-methylcrotonyl-CoA carboxylase are quantitatively important biotin reservoirs.[32] A significant percentage of ingested biotin accumulates in the liver.[33]

7. Recycling of Biotin

Proteolytic degradation of holocarboxylases leads to the formation of biotinyl peptides. These peptides are further degraded by biotinidase to release biotin, which can then be used for the synthesis of new holocarboxylases.[19]

8. Biotinylation of Histones

Chromatin comprises (1) DNA; (2) a group of proteins named histones; and (3) various non-histone proteins. The folding of DNA into chromatin is mediated primarily by histones.[34] Five major classes of histones have been identified in mammals: H1, H2A, H2B, H3 and H4. Histones consist of a globular domain and a more flexible and charged amino terminus (histone "tail"). Lysines, arginines, serines and glutamates in the amino terminus are targets for acetylation, methylation, phosphorylation, ubiquitination, poly (ADP-ribosylation) and sumoylation.[13,34–37] These modifications of histones regulate processes such as gene expression, replication and DNA repair.[34] All five classes of histones are also modified by covalent attachment of biotin.[38–40] Biotinylation of histones is mediated by biotinidase [38] and holocarboxylase synthetase.[41] Evidence has been provided that biotinylation of histones might play a role in gene silencing and in the cellular response to DNA damage.[40–43]

9. Biotin and Gene Expression

The following three mechanisms are likely to mediate effects of biotin on gene expression; these mechanisms are not mutually exclusive but might coexist in human cells. The reader is referred to a recent review for an in-depth presentation of biotin-dependent gene expression.[44]

1. Activation of soluble guanylate cyclase by biotinyl-AMP. Biotinyl-AMP activates soluble guanylate cyclase, increasing the generation of cyclic guanosine monophosphate.[45] Subsequently, cyclic guanosine monophosphate-dependent protein kinase phosphorylates and activates proteins that enhance transcriptional activity of genes.
2. Nuclear abundance of transcription factors NF-κB and Sp1/Sp3. Biotin deficiency is associated with increased nuclear translocation of nuclear factor κB (NF-κB), mediating activation of NF-κB-dependent genes.[46] Biotin supplementation is associated with increased nuclear abundance of Sp1 and Sp3;[47] these ubiquitous proteins may act as transcriptional activators or repressors, depending on the context.[48,49]
3. Remodeling of chromatin by biotinylation of histones (see above).

10. Catabolism

Two pathways of biotin catabolism have been identified in mammals and microorganisms in a series of classical studies by McCormick and co-workers (Figure 9.4): (1) β-oxidation of the valeric acid side chain,[50–54] leading to the formation of bisnorbiotin, tetranorbiotin and related metabolites that are known to result from β-oxidation of fatty acids. (2) Sulfur oxidation in the heterocyclic ring, leading to the formation of biotin-l-sulfoxide, biotin-d-sulfoxide and biotin sulfone.[50,51] Combinations of both pathways also occur. Biotin catabolites are quantitatively important in mammalian tissues and body fluids; biotin catabolites account for approximately 50 to 70 mole% of the total biotinyl compounds.[52,53,55] Recent studies have provided evidence that biotin catabolites have biotin-like activities with regard to gene expression.

11. Biotin Excretion

Healthy adults excrete approximately 100 nmoles of biotin plus catabolites per day into urine.[55] Biotin accounts for approximately half of the total urinary biotin; the catabolites bisnorbiotin, biotin-d,l-sulfoxides, bisnorbiotin methyl ketone, biotin sulfone and tetranorbiotin-l-sulfoxide account for most of the balance.[53,55] Biotin in the glomerulum filtrate is reabsorbed by a saturable sodium-dependent transport mechanism, as evidenced by studies using brush-border membrane vesicles from human kidney cortex.[56] Apparent K_m and V_{max} values of this biotin transporter are 31 μM and 82 nmol biotin μg protein^{-1} • 30 • sec^{-1}, respectively.

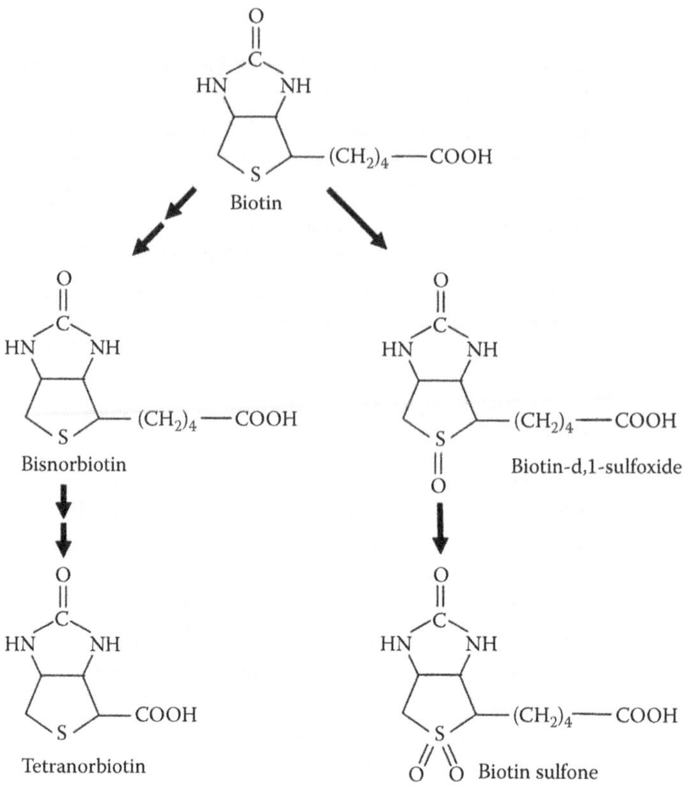

FIGURE 9.4 Biotin catabolism.

The biliary excretion of biotin and catabolites is quantitatively minor. Less than 2% of an intravenous dose of [^{14}C]biotin was recovered in rat bile but more than 60% of the dose was excreted in urine.[57]

III. DIETARY INTAKE AND STATUS ASSESSMENT

A. DIETARY AND SUPPLEMENTAL SOURCES

1. Pantothenic Acid

a. Adequate Intakes

Human requirements for pantothenic acid have not yet been quantified. Hence, recommendations for adequate intake (AI) are based on the average daily intake in healthy individuals.[58] The AI is 5 mg/day of pantothenic acid for adults of both genders. The AI of pantothenic acid in pregnant and lactating women is 6 mg/day and 7 mg/day, respectively.[17,58]

b. Intake and Food Sources

Pantothenic acid is widely distributed in plant, animal and microbial cells. In foodstuffs, the majority of pantothenic acid is present as CoA and 4′-phosphopantetheine. Rich dietary sources of pantothenic acid include chicken, beef, liver, egg yolk, potatoes, whole cereals, broccoli and cauliflower (containing more than 50 mg/g of pantothenic acid). Cow's milk and human milk contain approximately 3.5 mg/l and 2 mg/l pantothenic acid, respectively.[12,59]

Pantothenic acid degrades rapidly when exposed to heat. Hence, a significant fraction of pantothenic acid in foodstuffs may be destroyed during food preparation; cooking may destroy up to 78% of the vitamin, depending on the food source and preparation techniques.[60]

c. Supplemental Sources

Calcium salts of D-pantothenate are the typical sources of pantothenic acid in oral vitamin supplements. Dexpanthenol (pantothenyl alcohol) is a synthetic analog of pantothenic acid that is commonly used for topical applications. Dexpanthenol can be converted to pantothenic acid by mammalian cells.[58]

2. Biotin

a. Adequate Intakes

The Food and Nutrition Board of the National Research Council has released recommendations for AI of biotin.[58] The AI is 30 μg/day of biotin for adults of both genders; the AI of biotin in lactating women is 35 μg/day. These recommendations are based on estimated biotin intakes (not to be confused with requirements) in a group of healthy people. Some drugs may cause increased biotin requirements (see below).

b. Intake and Food Sources

The content of free and protein-bound biotin varies among foods. The majority of biotin in meats and cereals appears to be protein bound.[18] Most measurements of biotin content in food have used microbial bioassays. Despite potential analytical limitations due to interfering endogenous substances, protein binding and lack of chemical specificity for biotin versus catabolites, there is reasonably good agreement among the published reports and some worthwhile generalizations can be made.[18] Biotin is widely distributed in natural foodstuffs. Foods relatively rich in biotin include egg yolk, liver and some vegetables. The dietary biotin intake in western populations has been estimated to be 35 to 70 μg/d.[18] Infants who ingest 800 ml of mature breast milk per day receive approximately 6 μg of biotin.[61]

B. BIOMARKERS

1. Pantothenic Acid

a. Direct Measures

Typically, pantothenic acid status is assessed by quantifying concentrations of the vitamin in whole blood and urinary excretion. The urinary excretion of pantothenic acid correlates with recent dietary intake.[62,63] Concentrations of pantothenic acid are much lower in plasma compared with whole blood because plasma does not contain coenzyme forms of pantothenic acid.

b. Indirect Measures

Variables such as enzyme activities do not play an important role in the assessment of pantothenic acid status.

2. Biotin

a. Direct Measures

The most commonly used direct measures to determine biotin status are the serum concentration and the urinary excretion of biotin and catabolites. The urinary excretion of biotin and biotin catabolites decreases rapidly and substantially in biotin-deficient individuals,[64] suggesting that the urinary excretion is an early and sensitive indicator of biotin deficiency. In contrast, serum concentrations of biotin, bisnorbiotin and biotin-*d,l*-sulfoxide do not decrease in biotin-deficient individuals[64] and in patients on biotin-free total parenteral nutrition [65] during reasonable periods of observation. Thus, serum concentrations are not good indicators of marginal biotin deficiency.

b.   Indirect Measures

Activities of biotin-dependent carboxylases may be useful as indicators of biotin status in humans. Lymphocytes, which are easily accessible in human blood, contain detectable quantities of propionyl-CoA carboxylase and β-methylcrotonyl-CoA carboxylase. The use of an activation index of carboxylases in lymphocytes has been proposed to assess biotin status.[65] The carboxylase activation index is the ratio of carboxylase in cells after *in-vitro* incubation with biotin to the activity in cells that are incubated without biotin. High values for the activation index suggest that a substantial fraction of the carboxylase is in the apo form, consistent with biotin deficiency.

Reduced activity of β-methylcrotonyl-CoA carboxylase causes a metabolic block in leucine catabolism (Figure 9.3). As a consequence, β-methylcrotonyl-CoA is shunted to alternative pathways, leading to an increased formation of 3-hydroxyisovaleric acid and 3-methylcrotonyl glycine. Biotin deficiency studies in humans suggest that the urinary excretion of 3-hydroxyisovaleric acid is an early and sensitive indicator of biotin status.[64] In contrast, pathways that depend on propionyl-CoA carboxylase are not sensitive indicators of biotin status,[66,67] and pathways depending on acetyl-CoA carboxylase and pyruvate carboxylase have not been extensively tested in this regard.

C.   Toxicity

1.   Pantothenic Acid

Doses of pantothenic acid that exceed the normal dietary intake are considered safe. Excess pantothenic acid is rapidly excreted into urine. Diarrhea and gastrointestinal disturbances have been reported after oral administration of single doses exceeding the AI of pantothenic acid by 1,000 times.[17]

2.   Biotin

Classically, ingestion of pharmacologic doses of biotin has been considered safe. For example, no overt signs of toxicity have been observed in patients with inborn errors of biotin metabolism (e.g., biotinidase deficiency) who are empirically treated with biotin doses that exceed the normal dietary intake by 300 times;[68] and test subjects treated with acute oral and intravenous doses of biotin that exceeded the dietary biotin intake by up to 600-fold.[21]

The arrival of advanced techniques in molecular biology has raised some concerns regarding the safety of biotin supplements. Evidence has been provided that supplementation with pharmacological doses of biotin is associated with substantial changes in gene expression patterns.[69,70] Some of these changes may not be desirable. For example, evidence has been provided that biotin supplementation is associated with increased expression of the gene encoding cytochrome P450 1B1,[71] which mediates metabolic activation (hydroxylation) of pro-carcinogens. Moreover, biotin supplementation decreases expression of the sarco-/endoplasmic reticulum calcium ATPase 3 (unpublished observation); this is associated with decreased transport of calcium into the endoplasmic reticulum and, perhaps, impaired folding of secretory proteins.

IV.   INTERACTIONS WITH NUTRIENTS AND DRUGS

A.   Pantothenic Acid

Biotin, lipoic acid and pantothenic acid share the same transport system for cellular uptake.[26,72,73] Hence, interference of biotin and lipoic acid with the cellular transport of pantothenic acid needs to be considered when evaluating the safety of biotin and lipoate supplements. Pharmacological doses of biotin (~ 10 mg), as used to treat holocarboxylase synthetase deficiency and biotinidase deficiency, might cause pantothenic acid deficiency. Likewise, pharmacological doses of lipoic acid are administered to treat heavy-metal intoxications, to reduce signs of diabetes and to enhance glucose disposal in patients with noninsulin-dependent diabetes mellitus;[74] theoretically, these treatments might jeopardize pantothenic acid status.

B. BIOTIN

1. Anticonvulsants

Biotin requirements may be increased during anticonvulsant therapy. The anticonvulsants primidone and carbamazepine inhibit biotin uptake into brush-border membrane vesicles from human intestine.[75,76] Long-term therapy with anticonvulsants increases the urinary excretion of biotin catabolites and 3-hydroxyisovaleric acid.[77,78] Phenobarbital, phenytoin and carbamazepine displace biotin from biotinidase, conceivably affecting plasma transport, renal handling or cellular uptake of biotin.[22] During anticonvulsant therapy, the plasma concentration of biotin may be decreased.[79,80] Administration of carbamazepine is associated with decreased abundance and activity of pyruvate carboxylase in rats.[81,82]

2. Pantothenic Acid and Lipoic Acid

Pantothenic acid and lipoic acid may compete with biotin for the transporter SMVT (see above); hence, supplements containing large doses of pantothenic and lipoic acid may decrease cellular uptake of biotin. Indeed, chronic administration of pharmacologic doses of lipoic acid decreases the activities of pyruvate carboxylase and β-methylcrotonyl-CoA carboxylase in rat liver to 64% to 72% of controls.[74]

3. Egg White

Raw egg white contains the protein avidin, which has great affinity for biotin.[83] Binding of biotin to avidin renders biotin unavailable for absorption,[67,83] potentially triggering biotin deficiency. Hence, dietary supplements containing raw (spray-dried) egg white might impair biotin status. This may be of importance to athletes ingesting large amounts of protein supplements based on egg white.

V. EFFECTS ON PHYSICAL PERFORMANCE

A. PANTOTHENIC ACID

There is no conclusive evidence that pharmacological doses of pantothenic acid enhance physical performance. Note, however, that acetyl-CoA plays a key role in the regulation of glycogen synthesis. Glycogen is an important source of metabolic energy during exercise. Hence, theoretically, pantothenic acid might affect glycogen homeostasis and physical performance. Indeed, previous studies suggested that pantothenic acid-deficient mice have reduced exercise tolerance and low glycogen stores compared with controls.[63] The dietary and supplemental intake of pantothenic acid by athletes is unknown.

B. BIOTIN

No studies that address effects of biotin on physical performance have been published. Performance-enhancing effects of biotin are conceivable, based on the following lines of reasoning: (1) biotin is a coenzyme in pathways of gluconeogenesis (pyruvate carboxylase) and fatty acid metabolism (acetyl-CoA carboxylase; propionyl-CoA carboxylase); and (2) biotin plays a role in enhancing the expression of the gene encoding glucokinase,[84–87] a key enzyme in glycolysis. The dietary and supplemental intake of biotin by athletes is unknown.

VI.   RECOMMENDATIONS AND FUTURE RESEARCH DIRECTIONS

Clearly, there is a lack of well-designed studies to address performance-enhancing effects of pantothenic acid and biotin. There is a possibility that supplementation of athletes with these two vitamins might enhance physical performance, given their essential roles in intermediary metabolism. However, both pantothenic acid and biotin are ubiquitous in human diets and we believe that athletes can maintain vitamin sufficiency simply by selecting a well-balanced diet. Note that pantothenic acid and biotin deficiency are not commonly observed in healthy humans. Finally, there are a few uncertainties associated with the safety of pharmacological doses of pantothenic acid and biotin in cell signaling and gene expression. Those athletes who insist on using supplements are advised to use physiological doses rather than pharmacological doses. Future research should include both tests of adverse side effects of pantothenic acid and biotin and double-blinded studies to determine whether pantothenic acid and biotin enhance physical performance.

VII.   SUMMARY

Both pantothenic acid and biotin serve as essential coenzymes in the metabolism of amino acids, glucose, fatty acids and other intermediates. In addition, biotin plays a role in cell signaling and chromatin structure. Both pantothenic acid and biotin are ubiquitous in human diets, and signs of frank deficiency are rare. Some compounds have been identified that interfere with the normal metabolism of pantothenic acid and biotin. For example, use of anticonvulsants interferes with biotin metabolism. Individuals treated with these drugs may want to consider using vitamin supplements.

ACKNOWLEDGMENT

This work was supported by NIH grants DK 60447 and DK 063945.

REFERENCES

1. Miller, S.L. and Schlesinger, G., Prebiotic syntheses of vitamin coenzymes: II. Pantoic acid, pantothenic acid and the composition of coenzyme A. *J. Mol. Evol.* 36, 308, 1993.
2. Choi, C.Y., Tian, S.-K. and Deng, L., A formal catalytic asymmetric synthesis of (+)-biotin with modified cinchona alkaloids. *Synthesis* 11, 1737, 2001.
3. Shibata, K., Gross, C.J. and Henderson, L.M., Hydrolysis and absorption of pantothenate and its coenzymes in the rat small intestine. *J. Nutr.* 113, 2207, 1983.
4. Prasad, P., Wang, H., Huang, W., Fei, Y.-J., Leibach, F.H., Devoe, L.D. and Ganapathy, V., Molecular and functional characterization of the intestinal Na+-dependent multivitamin transporter. *Arch. Biochem. Biophys.* 366, 95, 1999.
5. Prasad, P.D., Wang, H., Kekuda, R., Fujita, T., Fei, Y.-J., Devoe, L.D., Leibach, F.H. and Ganapathy, V., Cloning and functional expression of a cDNA encoding a mammalian sodium-dependent vitamin transporter mediating the uptake of pantothenate, biotin and lipoate. *J. Biol. Chem.* 273, 7501, 1998.
6. Wang, H., Huang, W., Fei, Y.-J., Xia, H., Fang-Yeng, T.L., Leibach, F.H., Devoe, L.D., Ganapathy, V. and Prasad, P.D., Human placental Na+-dependent multivitamin transporter. *J. Biol. Chem.* 274, 14875, 1999.
7. Fenstermacher, D.K. and Rose, R.C., Absorption of pantothenic acid in rat and chick intestine. *Am. J. Physiol.* 250, 155, 1986.

8. Tarr, J.B., Tamura, T. and Stokstad, E.L., Availability of vitamin B_6 and pantothenate in an average American diet in man. *Am. J. Clin. Nutr.* 34, 1328, 1981.
9. Fry, P.C., Fox, H.M. and Tao, H.G., Metabolic response to a pantothenic acid deficient diet in humans. *J. Nutr. Sci. Vitaminol.* 22, 339, 1976.
10. Bucovaz, E.T., MacLeod, R.M., Morrison, J.C. and Whybrew, W.D., The coenzyme A-synthesizing protein complex and its proposed role in CoA biosynthesis in baker's yeast. *Biochem.* 79, 787, 1998.
11. Garrett, R.H. and Grisham, C.M., *Biochemistry* 1995, Fort Worth, TX: Saunders College Publishing.
12. Plesofsky-Vig, N., Pantothenic acid, in *Modern Nutrition in Health and Disease,* Shils, M.E., Olson, J.A., Shike, M. and Ross, A.C., Eds. Baltimore, MD: Willams & Wilkins 1999, p. 423.
13. Fischle, W., Wang, Y. and Allis, C.D., Histone and chromatin cross-talk. *Curr. Opin. Cell Biol.* 15, 172, 2003.
14. Said, H.M., Cellular uptake of biotin: mechanisms and regulation. *J. Nutr.* 129, 490, 1999.
15. Lopaschuk, G.D., Michalak, M. and Tsang, H., Regulation of pantothenic acid transport in the heart. Involvement of a Na+-cotransport system. *J. Biol. Chem.* 262, 3615, 1987.
16. Fisher, M.N., Robishaw, J.D. and Neely, J.R., The properties of and regulation of pantothenate kinase from rat heart. *J. Biol. Chem.* 256, 15745, 1992.
17. Miller, J.W., Rogers, L.M. and Rucker, R.B., Pantothenic Acid, in *Present Knowledge in Nutrition,* Bowman, B.A. and Russell, R.M., Eds. Washington, D.C.: ILSI Press, 2001, p. 253.
18. Zempleni, J. and Mock, D.M., Biotin biochemistry and human requirements. *J. Nutr. Biochem.* 10, 128, 1999.
19. Wolf, B., Heard, G.S., McVoy, J.R.S. and Grier, R.E., Biotinidase deficiency. *Ann. NY Acad. Sci.* 447, 252, 1985.
20. Bowman, B.B., Selhub, J. and Rosenberg, I.H., Intestinal absorption of biotin in the rat. *J. Nutr.* 116, 1266, 1986.
21. Zempleni, J. and Mock, D.M., Bioavailability of biotin given orally to humans in pharmacologic doses. *Am. J. Clin. Nutr.* 69, 504, 1999.
22. Chauhan, J. and Dakshinamurti, K., Role of human serum biotinidase as biotin-binding protein. *Biochem. J.* 256, 265, 1988.
23. Dakshinamurti, K. and Chauhan, J., Biotin-binding proteins, in *Vitamin Receptors: Vitamins as Ligands in Cell Communication,* Dakshinamurti, K., Ed. Cambridge University Press: Cambridge, 1994, p. 200.
24. Mock, D.M. and Malik, M.I., Distribution of biotin in human plasma: Most of the biotin is not bound to protein. *Am. J. Clin. Nutr.* 56, 427, 1992.
25. Seshagiri, P.B. and Adiga, P.R., Isolation and characterization of a biotin-binding protein from the pregnant-rat serum and comparison with that from the chicken egg-yolk. *Biochem. Biophys.* Acta 916, 474, 1987.
26. Prasad, P.D., Ramamoorthy, S., Leibach, F.H. and Ganapathy, V., Characterization of a sodium-dependent vitamin transporter mediating the uptake of pantothenate, biotin and lipoate in human placental choriocarcinoma cells. *Placenta* 18, 527, 1997.
27. Daberkow, R.L., White, B.R., Cederberg, R.A., Griffin, J.B. and Zempleni, J., Monocarboxylate transporter 1 mediates biotin uptake in human peripheral blood mononuclear cells. *J. Nutr.* 133, 2703, 2003.
28. Mardach, R., Zempleni, J., Wolf, B., Cannon, M.J., Jennings, M.L., Cress, S., Boylan, J., Roth, S., Cederbaum, S. and Mock, D.M., Biotin dependency due to a defect in biotin transport. *J. Clin. Invest.* 109, 1617, 2002.
29. Wood, H.G. and Barden, R.E., Biotin enzymes. *Ann. Rev. Biochem.* 46, 385, 1977.
30. Knowles, J.R., The mechanism of biotin-dependent enzymes. *Ann. Rev. Biochem.* 58, 195, 1989.
31. Kim, K.-H., McCormick, D.B., Bier, D.M. and Goodridge, A.G., Regulation of mammalian acetyl-coenzyme A carboxylase. *Ann. Rev. Nutr.* 17, 77, 1997.
32. Shriver, B.J., Roman-Shriver, C. and Allred, J.B., Depletion and repletion of biotinyl enzymes in liver of biotin-deficient rats: Evidence of a biotin storage system. *J. Nutr.* 123, 1140, 1993.
33. Petrelli, F., Coderoni, S., Moretti, P. and Paparelli, M., Effect of biotin on phosphorylation, acetylation, methylation of rat liver histones. *Molec. Biol. Rep.* 4, 87, 1978.
34. Wolffe, A., *Chromatin* 3rd ed. 1998, San Diego, CA: Academic Press.
35. Jenuwein, T. and Allis, C.D., Translating the histone code. *Science* 293, 1074, 2001.

36. Boulikas, T., Bastin, B., Boulikas, P. and Dupuis, G., Increase in histone poly(ADP-ribosylation) in mitogen-activated lymphoid cells. *Exp. Cell Res.* 187, 77, 1990.

37. Shiio, Y. and Eisenman, R.N., Histone sumoylation is associated with transcriptional repression. *Proc. Natl. Acad. Sci. USA* 100, 13225, 2003.

38. Hymes, J., Fleischhauer, K. and Wolf, B., Biotinylation of histones by human serum biotinidase: assessment of biotinyl-transferase activity in sera from normal individuals and children with biotinidase deficiency. *Biochem. Mol. Med.* 56, 76, 1995.

39. Stanley, J.S., Griffin, J.B. and Zempleni, J., Biotinylation of histones in human cells: effects of cell proliferation. *Eur. J. Biochem.* 268, 5424, 2001.

40. Camporeale, G., Shubert, E.E., Sarath, G., Cerny, R. and Zempleni, J., K8 and K12 are biotinylated in human histone H4. *Eur. J. Biochem.* 271, 2257, 2004.

41. Narang, M.A., Dumas, R., Ayer, L.M. and Gravel, R.A., Reduced histone biotinylation in multiple carboxylase deficiency patients: a nuclear role for holocarboxylase synthetase. *Hum. Mol. Genet.* 13, 15, 2004.

42. Peters, D.M., Griffin, J.B., Stanley, J.S., Beck, M.M. and Zempleni, J., Exposure to UV light causes increased biotinylation of histones in Jurkat cells. *Am. J. Physiol. Cell Physiol.* 283, 878, 2002.

43. Kothapalli, N. and Zempleni, J., Double strand breaks of DNA decrease biotinylation of lysine-12 in histone H4 in JAr cells. *FASEB J.* 18, 103, 2004.

44. Rodriguez-Melendez, R. and Zempleni, J., Regulation of gene expression by biotin. *J. Nutr. Biochem.* 14, 680, 2003.

45. Solorzano-Vargas, R.S., Pacheco-Alvarez, D. and Leon-Del-Rio, A., Holocarboxylase synthetase is an obligate participant in biotin-mediated regulation of its own expression and of biotin-dependent carboxylases mRNA levels in human cells. *Proc. Natl. Acad. Sci. USA* 99, 5325, 2002.

46. Rodriguez-Melendez, R., Schwab, L.D. and Zempleni, J., Jurkat cells respond to biotin deficiency with increased nuclear translocation of NF-κB, mediating cell survival. *Int. J. Vitam. Nutr. Res.* 74, 209, 2004.

47. Griffin, J.B., Rodriguez-Melendez, R. and Zempleni, J., The nuclear abundance of transcription factors Sp1 and Sp3 depends on biotin in Jurkat cells. *J. Nutr.* 133, 3409, 2003.

48. Birnbaum, M.J., van Wijnen, A.J., Odgren, P.R., Last, T.J., Suske, G., Stein, G.S. and Stein, J.L., Sp1 trans-activation of cell cycle regulated promoters is selectively repressed by Sp3. *Biochemistry* 34, 16503, 1995.

49. Black, A., Black, J.D. and Azizkhan-Clifford, J., Sp1 and Krüppel-like factor family of transcription factors in cell growth regulation and cancer. *J. Cell. Physiol.* 188, 143, 2001.

50. McCormick, D.B. and Wright, L.D., The metabolism of biotin and analogues, in *Metabolism of Vitamins and Trace Elements,* Florkin, M. and Stotz, E.H., Eds. Amsterdam, The Netherlands: Elsevier Publishing Company 1971, p. 81.

51. Kazarinoff, M.N., Im, W.-B., Roth, J.A., McCormick, D.B. and Wright, L.D., Bacterial degradation of biotin VI. Isolation and identification of β-hydroxy and β–keto compounds. *J. Biol. Chem.* 247, 75, 1972.

52. Lee, H.M., Wright, L.D. and McCormick, D.B., Metabolism of carbonyl-labeled [14C] biotin in the rat. *J. Nutr.* 102, 1453, 1972.

53. Zempleni, J., McCormick, D.B. and Mock, D.M., Identification of biotin sulfone, bisnorbiotin methyl ketone and tetranorbiotin-*l*- sulfoxide in human urine. *Am. J. Clin. Nutr.* 65, 508, 1997.

54. Zempleni, J., Biotin, in *Present Knowledge in Nutrition,* Bowman, B.A. and Russell, R.M., Eds. Washington, D.C.:ILSI Press 2001, p. 241.

55. Mock, D.M., Lankford, G.L. and Cazin, J., Jr., Biotin and biotin analogs in human urine: Biotin accounts for only half of the total. *J. Nutr.* 123, 1844, 1993.

56. Baur, B. and Baumgartner, E.R., Na(+)-dependent biotin transport into brush-border membrane vesicles from human kidney cortex. *Pflugers Archiv — Eur. J. Physiol.* 422, 499, 1993.

57. Zempleni, J., Green, G.M., Spannagel, A.U. and Mock, D.M., Biliary excretion of biotin and biotin metabolites is quantitatively minor in rats and pigs. *J. Nutr.* 127, 1496, 1997.

58. National Research Council, Dietary reference intakes for thiamin, riboflavin, niacin, vitamin B_6, folate, vitamin B_{12}, pantothenic acid, biotin and choline. Food and Nutrition Board, Institute of Medicine, National Academy Press, Washington, DC, 1998.

59. Walsh, J., Wyse, B. and Hansen, R., Pantothenic acid content of 75 processed and cooked foods. *J. Am. Diet. Assoc.* 78, 140, 1981.

60. Tahiliani, A. and Beinlich, C., Pantothenic acid in health and disease. *Vitamins and Hormones* 46, 165, 1991.

61. Mock, D.M., Stratton, S.L. and Mock, N.I., Concentrations of biotin metabolites in human milk. *J. Pediatr.* 131, 456, 1997.

62. Eissenstat, B., Wyse, B. and Hansen, R., Pantothenic acid status of adolescents. *Am. J. Clin. Nutr.* 44, 931, 1986.

63. Plesofsky-Vig, N., Pantothenic acid, in *Present Knowledge in Nutrition,* Ziegler, E.E. and L.J. Filer, J., Eds. Washington, D.C.: ILSI Press 1996, p. 236.

64. Mock, N., Malik, M., Stumbo, P., Bishop, W. and Mock, D., Increased urinary excretion of 3-hydroxyisovaleric acid and decreased urinary excretion of biotin are sensitive early indicators of decreased status in experimental biotin deficiency. *Am. J. Clin. Nutr.* 65, 951, 1997.

65. Velazquez, A., Zamudio, S., Baez, A., Murguia-Corral, R., Rangel-Peniche, B. and Carrasco, A., Indicators of biotin status: A study of patients on prolonged total parenteral nutrition. *Eur. J. Clin. Nutr.* 44, 11, 1990.

66. Mock, N.I., Evans, T. and Mock, D.M., Urinary 3-hydroxypropionic acid is not an early indicator of biotin deficiency. *FASEB J.* 12, 247, 1998.

67. Mock, D.M., Henrich-Shell, C.L., Carnell, N., Stumbo, P. and Mock, N. I., 3-Hydroxypropionic acid and methylcitric acid are not reliable indicators of marginal biotin deficiency in humans. *J. Nutr.* 134, 317, 2004.

68. Wolf, B. and Heard, G.S., Biotinidase deficiency, in *Advances in Pediatrics*, Barness, L. and Oski, F., Eds. Chicago: Book Medical Publishers 1991, p.1.

69. Wiedmann, S., Eudy, J.D. and Zempleni, J., Biotin supplementation causes increased expression of genes encoding interferon-γ, interleukin-1β and 3-methylcrotonyl-CoA carboxylase and causes decreased expression of the gene encoding interleukin-4 in human peripheral blood mononuclear cells. *J. Nutr.* 133, 716, 2003.

70. Wiedmann, S., Rodriguez-Melendez, R., Ortega-Cuellar, D. and Zempleni, J., Clusters of biotin-responsive genes in human peripheral blood mononuclear cells. *J. Nutr. Biochem.* 15, 433, 2004.

71. Rodriguez-Melendez, R., Griffin, J.B. and Zempleni, J., Biotin supplementation increases expression of the cytochrome P450 1B1 gene in Jurkat cells, increasing the occurrence of single-stranded DNA breaks. *J. Nutr.* 134, 2222, 2004.

72. Said, H.M., Ortiz, A., McCloud, E., Dyer, D., Moyer, M.P. and Rubin, S., Biotin uptake by human colonic epithelial NCM460 cells: A carrier-mediated process shared with pantothenic acid. *Am. J. Physiol. Cell Physiol.* 275, 1365, 1998.

73. Chatterjee, N.S., Kumar, C.K., Ortiz, A., Rubin, S.A. and Said, H.M., Molecular mechanism of the intestinal biotin transport process. *Am. J. Physiol.* 277, 605, 1999.

74. Zempleni, J., Trusty, T.A. and Mock, D.M., Lipoic acid reduces the activities of biotin-dependent carboxylases in rat liver. *J. Nutr.* 127, 1776, 1997.

75. Said, H.M., Redha, R. and Nylander, W., Biotin transport and anticonvulsant drugs. *Am. J. Clin. Nutr.* 49, 127, 1989.

76. Said, H.M., Redha, R. and Nylander, W., Biotin transport in the human intestine: inhibition by anticonvulsant drugs. *Am. J. Clin. Nutr.* 49, 127, 1989.

77. Krause, K.-H., Kochen, W., Berlit, P. and Bonjour, J.-P., Excretion of organic acids associated with biotin deficiency in chronic anticonvulsant therapy. *Int. J. Vitam. Nutr. Res.* 54, 217, 1984.

78. Mock, D.M. and Dyken, M.E., Biotin catabolism is accelerated in adults receiving long-term therapy with anticonvulsants. *Neurology* 49, 1444, 1997.

79. Krause, K.-H., Berlit, P. and Bonjour, J.-P., Vitamin status in patients on chronic anticonvulsant therapy. *Int. J. Vitam. Nutr. Res.* 52, 375, 1982.

80. Krause, K.-H., Berlit, P. and Bonjour, J.-P., Impaired biotin status in anticonvulsant therapy. *Ann. Neurol.,* 12, 485, 1982.

81. Rathman, S.C., Blanchard, R.K., Badinga, L., J.F. Gregory, R., Eisenschenk, S. and McMahon, R.J., Dietary carbamazepine administration decreases liver pyruvate carboxylase activity and biotinylation by decreasing protein and mRNA expression in rats. *J. Nutr.,* 133, 2119, 2003.

82. Rathman, S.C., Gregory, J.F., III and McMahon, R.J., Pharmacological biotin supplementation maintains biotin status and function in rats administered dietary carbamazepine. *J. Nutr.* 133, 2857, 2003.

83. Green, N.M., Avidin. *Adv. Protein Chem.* 29, 85, 1975.

84. Dakshinamurti, K. and Cheah-Tan, C., Liver glucokinase of the biotin deficient rat. *Can. J. Biochem.* 46, 75, 1968.
85. Spence, J.T. and Koudelka, A.P., Effects of biotin upon the intracellular level of cGMP and the activity of glucokinase in cultured rat hepatocytes. *J. Biol. Chem.* 259, 6393, 1984.
86. Chauhan, J. and Dakshinamurti, K., Transcriptional regulation of the glucokinase gene by biotin in starved rats. *J. Biol. Chem.* 266, 10035, 1991.
87. Borboni, P., Magnaterra, R., Rabini, R.A., Staffolani, R., Porzio, O., Sesti, G., Fusco, A., Mazzanti, L., Lauro, R. and Marlier, L.N.J.L., Effect of biotin on glucokinase activity, mRNA expression and insulin release in cultured beta-cells. *Acta Diabetol.* 33, 154, 1996.

10 Choline*

Patricia A. Deuster and Jamie A. Cooper

CONTENTS

I. INTRODUCTION

Choline, a quaternary amine and natural component of most plants and meats, is found in cell membranes, particularly nervous tissue, with brain tissue having the highest concentration.[1-3] Choline, which was named after the Greek word for anger "chole," was first characterized in bile as a nitrogen-containing substance by the German chemist, AFL Strecker in 1862.[4] Despite its identification, it was not until the 1930s that choline became recognized as an important dietary constituent.[5] The term "lipotropic" was used in association with choline based on the finding that it prevented the accumulation of lipids in the liver.[6] In 1977 Wurtman et al.[7] reported that choline administration

---

* The opinions and assertions expressed herein are those of the authors and should not be construed as reflecting those of the U.S. Army, the Uniformed Services University of the Health Sciences (USUHS), or the Department of Defense.

was associated with an increase in the neurotransmitter acetylcholine (ACh) and this finding stimulated much interest in choline. However, it was not until 1998 that choline was classified as an essential nutrient by the National Academy of Sciences. This resulted in the establishment of an adequate intake level (AI) for humans by the Food and Nutrition Board of the Institute of Medicine.[8]

The establishment of choline as an essential nutrient was based on the growing body of literature indicating the significant role served by choline in growth and development and overall human health.[1-3,8] For example, choline has been found to be important in fetal brain development, in memory function and in the prevention of heart disease, fatty liver and neural tube defects.[1-3] The present review will focus on a general overview of choline metabolism, supplemental dietary choline and the role of choline in physical performance.

II. CHOLINE METABOLISM

A. CHOLINE STRUCTURES

The chemical structure of choline and other compounds derived from choline are presented in Table 10.1; the synthetic pathways are presented in Figure 10.1. The scientific name(s) for choline are 2-Hydroxy-N, N, N-trimethylethanaminum, trimethylethanolamine and/or (beta-hydroxyethyl)

TABLE 10.1
Chemical Structures of Choline and Its Derivatives

BETAINE
$$^-O-\underset{\underset{O}{\|}}{C}-CH_2N^+(CH_3)_3$$

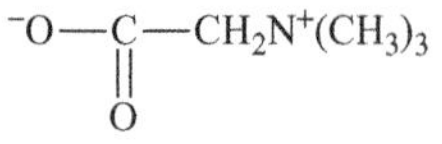

CHOLINE
$$HOCH_2CH_2N^+(CH_3)_3$$

ACETYLCHOLINE
$$CH_3-\underset{\underset{}{\overset{\overset{O}{\|}}{C}}}{}-O-CH_2CH_2N^+(CH_3)_3$$

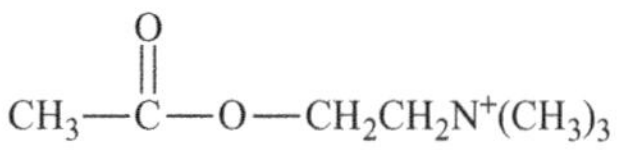

SPHINGOMYELIN
$$\overset{Ceramide \qquad\qquad Phosphorylcholine}{RCHOH-\underset{\underset{NHOCR^i}{|}}{CHCH_2}-OPO_3CH_2CH_2N^+(CH_3)_3}$$

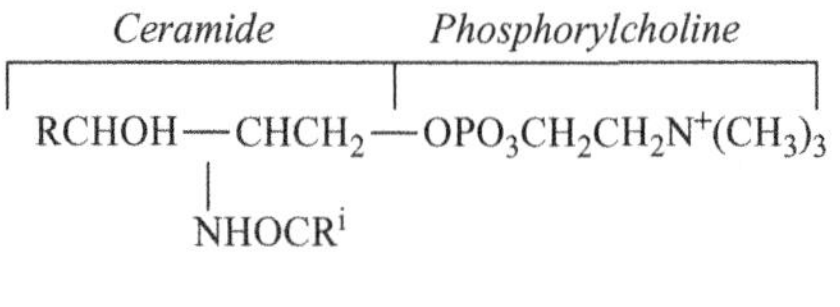

LYSOPHOSPHATIDYLCHOLINE
$$\begin{array}{l} CH_2-OOCR^l \\ | \\ HO-CH \\ | \\ CH_2-OPO_3-CH_2CH_2N^+(CH_3)_3 \end{array}$$

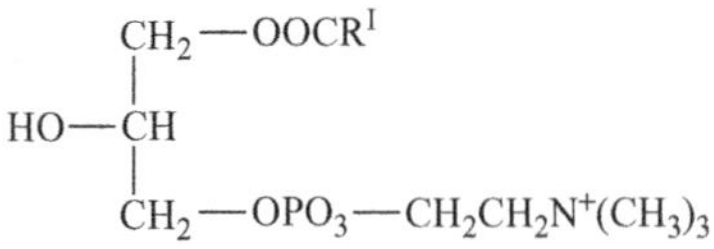

α-GLYCEROPHOS PHORYLCHOLINE
$$\begin{array}{l} CH_2-OH \\ | \\ HO-CH \\ | \\ CH_2-OPO_3-CH_2CH_2N^+(CH_3)_3 \end{array}$$

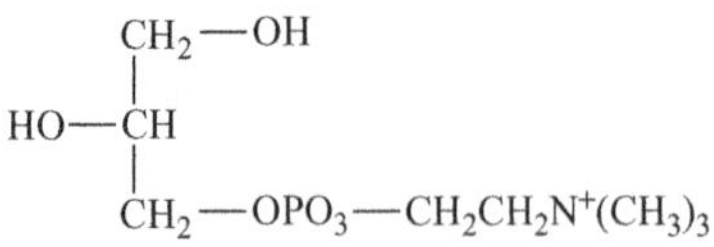

PHOSPHATIDYLCHOLINE
$$\begin{array}{l} \qquad\qquad CH_2-O-C-R_1 \\ \quad\overset{O}{\|}\qquad | \\ R_2-C-O-CH \\ \qquad\qquad | \\ \qquad\qquad CH_2-OPO_3-CH_2CH_2N^+(CH_3)_3 \end{array}$$

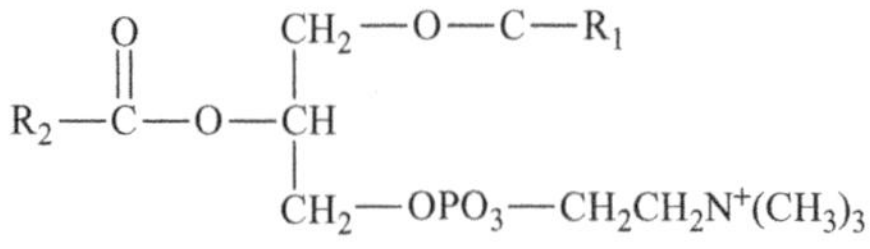

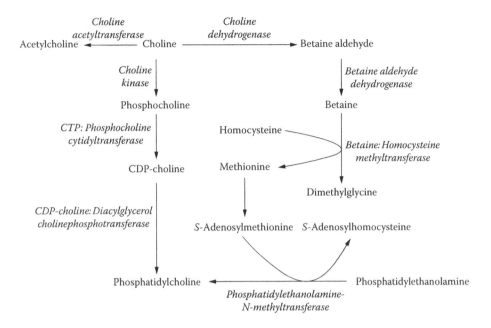

FIGURE 10.1 Synthetic Pathways of Choline. Adapted from Canty and Zeisel.[94]

trimethylammonium hydroxide, but choline as a simple compound has several common names, depending on the particular form.[1–3] Some of these names/forms include choline chloride, choline citrate, choline bitartrate, Intrachol™, Lipotropic Factor and methylated phosphatidylcholine.[9] Other forms of choline include cytidine 5-diphosphocholine (also known as CDP-choline or citocoline), phosphatidylcholine (commonly called lecithin) and L-alphaglycerylphosphorylcholine (Alpha GPC).

B. CHOLINE IN THE HUMAN BODY

1. Tissue Distribution

Choline is abundant in the human body, existing in all cell membranes as a constituent of phosphatidylcholine, sphingomyelin and choline plasmalogens, with phosphatidylcholine and sphingomyelin being the more common forms.[2,10,11] All tissues accumulate choline where it participates in various metabolic reactions. In the liver and kidney, choline is oxidized to form the methyl donor betaine. Nerve tissue, in particular the brain, contains the greatest concentration of choline. The choline content of human brain varies by regions, with average values ranging from 3.7 ± 0.6 mM in the parietal section to 7.7 ± 1.0 mM in the pons.[12] Within the brain, choline is transported across the blood-brain barrier by a specific carrier mechanism where the majority is converted to ACh.[13,14] Acetylcholine is commonly found in epithelial, mesothelial, endothelial, muscle, immune and neuronal cells. The choline phospholipids in brain and nerve tissue constitute a large precursor pool of choline for ACh synthesis, which could be important in neurons when the demand to sustain ACh release is high.[3,14] Choline acetyltransferase (ChAT), the enzyme that catalyzes the synthesis of ACh,[15,16] is also found in brain, skeletal muscle, spleen and placental tissue.[1–3]

Choline in blood exists as free choline, phospholipid-bound choline and erythrocyte choline. Free plasma choline levels in the adult male are quite low, averaging 7.4 μM, with a range from about 5.0 to 20 μM.[17] Approximately 98 to 99% of circulating choline exists in the form of phosphatidylcholine, where it is an integral component of lipoprotein particles, especially high-density lipoprotein (HDL).[18] The phospholipid composition of plasma HDL is approximately 81% phosphatidylcholine and 13% sphingomyelin, with an average phosphatidylcholine concentration of 1.3 mM. Plasma very low-density lipoprotein (VLDL) phospholipids are approximately 71% phosphatidylcholine and 23% sphingomyelin, with average phosphatidylcholine concentrations of 0.43 mM.[19] If plasma HDL or VLDL levels were to increase or decrease, total plasma choline levels would follow the same direction.

Erythrocytes also contain choline as part of the cell membrane where it participates in enzymatic reactions to synthesize ACh. The typical choline content of erythrocytes in normal controls averages 17 µM, but has been shown to range from 10 to more than 200 µM.[20,21] Finally, human breast milk also contains choline, which is very important for brain development in infants.[22] Total choline concentrations in breast milk between 7 and 22 days after birth average 1.28 mM.[22]

2. Absorption of Choline

Choline is absorbed throughout the small intestine by means of transporter proteins in the intestinal cells; after absorption it is delivered to the liver via the portal circulation. [23–25] Some choline is metabolized to and absorbed as trimethylglycine (betaine) and trimethylamine in the intestine before being transported to the liver. Phosphatidylcholine, the primary delivery form of choline from foods, can be absorbed in several ways, but most is absorbed through the intestine.[23,26]

It is of interest that 60% of choline ingested orally as choline chloride or other choline salts is transformed by intestinal bacteria into trimethylamine, which is metabolized and excreted as trimethylamine-N-oxide.[25] In contrast, only 26% of choline, when ingested as lecithin, is transformed into trimethylamine.[25] The transformation to trimethylamine is a function of intestinal bacteria, and as such, the proportion of choline transformed can be modified by altering the intestinal flora.[25] Overall, it appears these studies indicate that choline from lecithin is more effectively absorbed than choline alone and would be a preferred delivery form.[7,25]

3. Biosynthesis of Choline

Although choline is ingested in various foods, it is also synthesized *de novo* within the body, primarily in liver and kidneys, in two ways.[18] The first pathway begins with the decarboxylation of the amino acid serine to ethanolamine, followed by methylation of ethanolamine to form choline.[1,2,11,27] Methionine appears to be the primary methyl donor for choline, although S-adenosyl methionine (SAM), which is synthesized from the amino acid methionine as a methyl group donor, can also provide the methyl group for choline.[5,28] Because amino acids can contribute to the biosynthesis of choline, the amount of protein in the diet may affect dietary choline requirements.[1–3] Figure 10.1 presents a summary of the synthetic pathways of choline.

The second pathway for choline synthesis involves the conversion of phosphatidylethanolamine to phosphatidylcholine.[3] Three methylation reactions are required, with each using SAM as a methyl group donor. S-adenosyl methionine becomes S-adenosyl homocysteine after donating its methyl group and is metabolized to homocysteine, which can be converted to methionine in a reaction that requires methyl tetrahydrofolate (THF) and a vitamin B12-dependent enzyme. Thus, a close relationship exists between the synthesis of choline, methionine and folate.[1]

C. Metabolism and Mechanisms of Action

Choline is needed for both structural and functional roles in the body, as shown in Figure 10.2. First, choline is an integral component of several lipids that maintain cell membrane integrity.[29] These include phosphatidylcholine (lecithin) in the phospholipid bilayer of cell membranes; sphingomyelin, a critical component of the myelin sheath that surrounds nerve fibers;[17] choline plasmalogens, which make up 35 to 41% of the phospholipids in human cardiac tissue;[10] and lysophosphatidylcholine.[30]

Second, choline serves as a methyl donor.[31] Although its role as a methyl donor is primarily for the generation of betaine, choline can also serve as a methyl donor for creatine synthesis.[5,28] Once betaine is formed, it in turn donates methyl groups to homocysteine to form or regenerate methionine

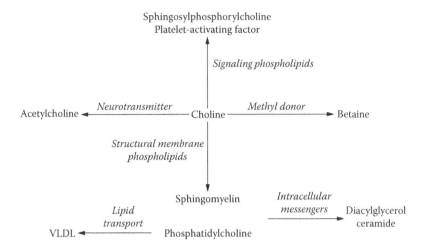

FIGURE 10.2 Metabolic Pathways of Choline. Adapted from Blusztajn.[27]

in the liver. The betaine pathway also provides methionine for protein synthesis.[32] Third, choline is a precursor for compounds that serve critical cell signaling functions, including phosphorylcholine;[33] platelet-activating factor, (PAF), a choline plasmalogens; and sphingophosphorylcholine.[34] In addition, the choline-containing phospholipids, phosphatidylcholine and sphingomyelin, are precursors for two other molecules that serve as intracellular messengers: diacylglycerol and ceramide.[2,11,33,34]

Choline also serves a role in lipid transport and metabolism. This role became apparent when a choline deficiency was found to result in the accumulation of lipids in the liver of rats and humans.[35] Subsequent investigations demonstrated that the accumulation of lipids reflected impaired secretion of VLDL particles from the liver and that phosphatidylcholine was a required component of VLDL particles.[35,36] Yao et al.[35] showed a reduction in plasma VLDL levels, but not HDL levels, as a consequence of choline deficiency in rats. Moreover, recent evidence demonstrated that a choline deficiency compromised assembly of nascent VLDLs and that blockage of phosphatidylcholine synthesis in the liver by the phosphatidylethanolamine N-methyltransferase (PEMT) pathway inhibited VLDL secretion in PEMT-deficient mice.[36]

The choline structure Alpha-GPC is a precursor for phospholipid biosynthesis and serves an important role in the recycling of phospholipids and in renal osmotic balance.[37-39] In the kidneys, Alpha-GPC is considered an organic osmolyte that can accumulate to high levels in response to elevated salt and urea concentrations. As a counteracting solute, Alpha-GPC allows cells to adapt osmotically and protects them from denaturation during extracellular hypertonic stress.[38,40]

The choline structure lysophosphatidylcholine may have adverse actions, as it has been implicated in the pathogenesis of cardiovascular disease through modulation of endothelial cell function.[41] The association with adverse actions is derived from the findings that levels of lysophosphatidylcholine are elevated in hyperlipidemia, atherosclerotic tissue, oxidized lipoproteins and ischemic hearts.[41] For example, the concentration of lysophosphatidylcholine in plasma from healthy adults is approximately 130–150 μM as compared with 1.7 mM in patients with hyperlipidemia.[30,41] Although the mechanism is uncertain, Murugesan et al.[30] demonstrated that lysophosphatidylcholine induces the release of chemokines in endothelial cells to recruit distinct leukocyte subsets to sites of inflammation. Further, it has been suggested that lysophosphatidylcholine serves as a positive modulator for self-generation *in vivo*.[41] Prolonged activation of this positive feedback system would adversely affect endothelial cells and cell function by allowing lysophosphatidylcholine to accumulate. Thus, the preferred pathway for lysophosphatidylcholine is either deacetylation or reacetylation so it does not accumulate.[41]

Finally, choline is a precursor for ACh, which is released from nerve terminals to activate nicotinic or muscarinic ACh receptors in presynaptic or postsynaptic membranes.[1,3,29] After ACh is released, it is hydrolyzed into choline and acetate by acetylcholinesterase. [1,3,29] Although ACh appears to regulate its own synthesis by feedback inhibition of ChAT and might be the rate-limiting step for ACh synthesis,[16] choline is requisite. Because cholinergic nerve cells cannot synthesize choline, they must transport it into the cells. To date, at least two choline transport systems have been identified to accomplish this function.[16,42]

D. CHOLINE TRANSPORT SYSTEMS

Choline can be transported into cells by at least two membrane uptake systems. The first is a high-affinity choline uptake (HACU) system that is temperature-, energy- and sodium-dependent.[11,36] This transport system, which is located in cholinergic nerve terminals, appears to be the primary mechanism by which choline is transported into neurons for ACh synthesis. Thus, the HACU system may be a rate-limiting step in the production of the ACh.[42] As extracellular choline levels increase, choline will be taken up via a low-affinity choline uptake (LACU) system, which is located in neurons as well as other cell types.[16] The LACU system is less energy- and sodium-dependent than the HACU system and appears to be activated when the metabolic demands for ACh are exceptionally high.[16] Instead of being stored within the cells as choline, the choline is immediately converted to and released as ACh.[16]

III. CHOLINE REQUIREMENTS AND CHOLINE STATUS

The recognition that humans have a dietary requirement for choline was long in coming.[8] As early as 1941, Du Vigneaud[43] had shown that biologically labile methyl donors, such as methionine and choline, must be supplied in the diet. However, it was only in 1998 that the Food and Nutrition Board (FNB) of the Institute of Medicine established a dietary reference intake (DRI) for choline.[8] The FNB estimated an AI level based on age and gender because insufficient data were available to establish a "recommended dietary allowance" or RDA for choline. An RDA could not be established because the evidence suggested that the dietary requirement for choline might depend on the availability of other methyl group donors, such as folate and SAM. Table 10.2 provides the AI values put forward by the FNB. As indicated in Table 10.2, the AIs for choline are greatest during pregnancy and lactation. During pregnancy, the availability of choline over during the first 3 months of gestation may be critical for normal development[11,22,44–47] and an adequate dietary intake of choline

---

TABLE 10.2
Adequate Intake Values for Choline by Age and Gender

Life Stage	Age	Males (mg/day)	Females (mg/day)
Infants	0–6 months	125	125
Infants	7–12 months	150	150
Children	1–3 years	200	200
Children	4–8 years	250	250
Children	9–13 years	375	375
Adolescents	14–18 years	550	400
Adults	≥19 years	550	425
Pregnancy	All ages		450
Breastfeeding	All ages		550

Source: Adapted from the Institute of Medicine Dietary Reference Intakes.[8]

---

would be required so that maternal stores would not be depleted. This is based on recent work suggesting that low dietary intakes of choline are associated with increased risk of neural-tube defects and that periconceptional dietary intake of choline is below the AI for pregnancy.[48] With respect to lactation, Holmes et al.[22] have shown that human breast milk contains large amounts of choline, an indication that lactating mothers need to obtain the requisite dietary choline during this period to support infant growth.

Sensitive and valid biologic markers of choline status are needed because a choline deficiency can lead to liver damage, compromise renal function and inhibit growth and development.[2,31] Based on human choline deficiency studies, it appears that plasma choline and phosphatidylcholine are good markers of choline status.[1–3,49] Fasting plasma choline concentrations typically range from 5 to 20 μM, with 10 μM being the more common value[17] and do not appear to change as a function of circadian rhythm.[18] In addition, concentrations appear to remain stable between 8 am and 4 pm, unless foods containing choline are consumed.[18] Jope et al.[21] have clearly demonstrated that ingestion of choline increases plasma and erythrocyte choline concentrations, with the greatest increases noted for plasma choline 3 to 4 hours after ingestion. Despite its stability, one concern is that plasma choline levels do not usually drop below 50% of normal unless the deficiency is severe.[17,49] As such, its sensitivity may be limited in terms of assessing choline status.

One issue with respect to choline status relates to the use of plasma or serum. Holm et al.[50] examined serum and plasma concentrations of choline, betaine and dimethylglycine under fed and fasted conditions and concluded that dietary intake affected choline and betaine, but not dimethylglycine. Furthermore, plasma choline concentrations were significantly higher in serum as compared with plasma under fasting (9.8 μM vs. 8.0 μM) and fed (11.9 μM vs 10.5 μM) conditions. Thus, the particular tissue used must be carefully considered and specified when assessing choline status.

Other tissues for assessing choline status include urinary and erythrocyte choline.[20,21] Although erythrocyte choline may indicate choline status, it appears to be markedly elevated in patients with manic-depressive illness and to be increased by lithium.[20,21] Thus, it may not be a viable biologic marker. Other possibilities are plasma and urinary betaine, but the validity of these measures has not been determined. More recently, da Costa et al.[51] suggested that serum levels of the MM isoform of creatine phosphokinase (CK), derived from skeletal muscle, not brain or heart, might prove to be a marker for choline status. Serum CK levels increased markedly in three of four men fed a choline-deficient diet, but levels returned to normal following repletion with choline.[51] The increase in serum CK would suggest a disruption in the muscle cell membrane, but this will require further investigation. It is clearly of interest with respect to the role of choline in muscle metabolism.

IV. DIETARY AND SUPPLEMENTAL SOURCES

Only recently have the concentrations and content of choline and choline-containing compounds in foods become readily available. In 2003 Zeisel et al.[32] published the concentrations of choline and betaine in common foods so that choline intake could be assessed with a higher degree of accuracy than before and to establish a choline database. Such a database will be important for determining the dietary requirement for choline, developing nutrient recommendations and designing research studies relating choline intake to human performance and disease risk. It is anticipated that the choline database will be posted on the United States Department of Agriculture Nutrient Data Laboratory web site.[52]

Based on the available data, the major dietary sources of choline are eggs, meats, vegetables, soy and dairy products.[52] Eggs, liver and soybeans contain choline in the form of lecithin, whereas vegetables such as cauliflower and lettuce provide free choline.[37] Because choline data are now available for foods and choline has been deemed an essential nutrient, the Food and Drug Administration (FDA) has allowed a nutrient content claim to be placed on labels of choline-containing foods. The claim can include "good" or "excellent" source of choline; to be rated "excellent," the food must contain at least 110 mg of choline per serving, whereas for a "good" claim, the food

TABLE 10.3
Choline and Betaine Concentrations in Common Foods

Food Product	Choline*	Betaine*
Dairy and Eggs		
Cream cheese	27.3	0.7
Egg, raw	251.0	0.6
Meat, Poultry and Fish		
Bacon, cured, cooked	124.7	3.5
Beef liver, pan fried	418.3	6.3
Chicken liver, pan fried	308.5	12.9
Chicken roasted	78.7	5.7
Cod, cooked	83.7	9.7
Ground beef, 95% lean, broiled	85.4	7.4
Pork Sausage	66.8	3.6
Fruits and Vegetables		
Avocados	14.1	0.7
Broccoli, cooked	40.1	0.1
Brussel sprouts, cooked	40.7	0.2
Cauliflower, cooked	39.1	0.1
Grains and Nuts		
Peanut butter, smooth, salted	65.6	0.8
Pistachio nuts, dry roasted, salted	71.5	0.8
Soybeans, raw	115.9	2.1
Wheat bran	74.5	1505.6
Beverages and Sweets		
Decaf. Coffee powder	101.9	0.7
Milk chocolate	46.1	2.6
Muffins, blueberry	51.8	35.8

*Numbers listed as mg choline moiety/100 grams of food.

Source: Adapted from USDA Database for the Choline Content of Common Foods (Supported by the United States Department of Agriculture, the National Institutes of Health and the National Cattlemen's Beef Association).

must contain at least 55 mg of choline per serving. Table 10.3 presents the total choline and betaine content of selected foods with the highest choline concentrations.[32]

Although food sources appear to be the best way to obtain choline, supplements are available. Choline as a nutrient is a generally recognized as safe (GRAS) substance, according to the Code of Federal Regulations, Title 21 — Food and Drugs, Part 182.[53] Specifically, choline bitartrate and choline chloride have been designated GRAS items when used in accordance with good manufacturing practices.[53] Thus, choline can be sold over the counter as a supplement in various forms without approval by the FDA.

Choline supplements are available in many forms, including the choline salts (choline bitartrate, choline citrate and choline chloride), phosphatidylcholine, lecithin, Alpha-GPC and cytidine 5-diphosphocholine (CDP-choline). Table 10.4 presents a list of some commercially available choline supplements and the more common doses. Lecithin, which also has GRAS status,[53] is a better choice than choline salts, because choline from lecithin appears to be more bioavailable.[7] Wurtman et al.[7] showed that plasma choline levels increased by 265% after ingestion of lecithin as compared

---

TABLE 10.4
Commercially Available Choline Supplements

Common Supplements

Choline Bitartrate (650 mg)
Choline Bitartrate (500 mg)
Choline Citrate (1,300 mg)
Choline Bitartrate (250 mg) and Inositol (250 mg)
Choline Bitartrate (103 mg) and Inositol (250 mg) in tablet form
Phosphatidylcholine (900 mg)
Phosphatidylcholine: Lecithin (1,200 mg) and Phosphatidyl Choline (420 mg)
Lecithin Choline: Soy Lecithin (1200 mg)
Phosphatidyl Choline Complex: Soy Lecithin (2400 mg); Phosphatidyl Choline (840 mg)
Leci-Choline
CDP Choline (250 mg)
Cognizin™ (Citicoline)
Alpha-GPC (300 mg)
Alpha-GPC (600 mg)
GPC Choline (450 mg)
Sport Supplement Beverages (100 mg choline bitartrate)
Choline Supreme™: GPC (200 mg) and Uridine (75 mg)
Lipotropic Fat Burner Capsules (Choline: 150 mg)

Source: Adapted from the www.naturaldatabase.com and many other Internet sources

---

with 86% after taking choline chloride (2–3 grams). Moreover, plasma levels were maintained above normal for 12 hours after lecithin as compared with only 4 hours following choline chloride.

The supplements CDP-choline and Alpha-GPC are both natural, water-soluble compounds. CDP-choline, also called citicoline, CDPC and citocholine, is an essential intermediate in the biosynthesis of phosphatidylcholine, and Alpha-GPC is a product of phosphatidylcholine degradation. Other names for Alpha-GPC include choline alfoscerate, choline alphoscerate, choline-glycerophosphate, glycerophosphorylcholine, glycerophosphorylcholine and GPC.

CDP-choline has been used in Europe for a number of years at doses up to 1.0 gram/day, but only became available over the counter in the U.S. in 1998.[54] A parenteral form of CDP-choline (citicoline) is marketed in Europe as a drug, and an oral form is being developed as a drug in the United States for treatment of ischemic stroke.[54] Citicoline is hydrolyzed in the small intestine and absorbed as choline and uridine[55] because most of the cytidine is deaminated by cytidine deaminase in the gastrointestinal tract and liver.[56] The uridine must be phosphorylated to uridine triphosphate, which must then be converted to cytidine triphosphate before resynthesis to citicoline. Oral ingestion of citicoline may preserve systemic choline stores and inhibit breakdown of membrane phospholipids.[55]

Alpha-GPC, when ingested as a supplement, is hydrolyzed, for the most part, to choline and glycerol-3-phosphate by phosphodiesterases in the intestinal mucosa and then absorbed.[57] It has been suggested, based on the work of Kim et al.,[40] that taking Alpha-GPC with caffeine, a phosphodiesterase inhibitor, would prevent hydrolysis and allow Alpha-GPC to be absorbed directly. Kim et al.[40] demonstrated in a canine kidney epithelial cell line that caffeine stimulated Alpha-GPC synthesis and accumulation by increasing the activity of phospholipase A2, a rate-limiting enzyme for Alpha-GPC synthesis. Such issues have not been researched but will be important for determining the most effective choline supplements.

Overall, lecithin, phosphatidylcholine, Alpha-GPC and CDP-choline are the major delivery forms of supplemental choline. Each supplement provides a different amount of choline, depending on the product and formulation. Typical commercial lecithin supplements contain 20 to 30%

phosphatidylcholine, which, assuming that approximately 15% of the weight of phosphatidylcholine is choline, would translate into 3 to 4.5% of lecithin as choline. In contrast, 40% of Alpha-GPC and 21% of CDP-choline are choline.[58] Differences in absorption, dose, formulation and other factors raise a number of questions regarding supplementation. The various effects of choline supplementation, which are of interest to both health professionals and the lay community, will be discussed later.

V. CHOLINE AND EXERCISE INTERACTIONS

A role for choline in physical activity evolved based on the importance of ACh in neuromuscular function.[7,11,16,17] It was reasonable to postulate that, as a neurotransmitter released at the neuro-muscular junction in response to nerve stimulation, ACh may be rate limiting for exercise performance. In particular, if release of ACh by cholinergic neurons were related to the level of physical activity,[16] then as the duration or intensity of the physical activity increased, comparable increases in ACh for neurotransmission would be needed. A constant supply of choline should be able to maintain ACh synthesis and release, whereas a reduction in choline availability could slow excitation-contraction coupling across the muscle membrane.[59] Failure of neuromuscular transmission might be one explanation for exercise-induced fatigue, and a depletion of ACh could account for such a failure.[16]

Athough it is rare for physiologic or pharmacologic manipulations to produce large changes in steady-state levels of ACh,[16] Conlay et al.[18] provided the first evidence in 1986 that choline availability might be compromised during prolonged exercise; marathon running decreased plasma choline concentrations by approximately 40%. Their initial results were confirmed in a subsequent study.[59] Other investigators have demonstrated similar declines in plasma choline with exercise.[31,60,61] Buchman et al.[61] showed that both plasma-free and phospholipid-bound choline concentrations decreased significantly after a marathon. In addition, Sandage et al.[60] noted significant decreases in plasma choline after only 20 miles. Von Allwörden et al.[31] studied triathletes between 23 and 28 years of age and found a significant decline in plasma choline concentrations (−16.9%) after 2 hours of cycling as compared with pre-exercise levels. Their range of reductions in plasma choline was wide, with a low of 3.6% and a high of 54.7%, which indicated that individuals have strikingly different plasma choline responses to strenuous exercise. Table 10.5 provides plasma choline concentrations before and after exercise in the studies published to date.

The exact mechanism(s) that might account for a decrease in plasma choline during prolonged exercise is unknown. However, several possibilities have been proposed. Choline may be needed during exercise for the increased demands for ACh synthesis or as an intramuscular methyl donor.[37] Alternatively, as plasma choline is synthesized in the liver for incorporation into phospholipids and lipoproteins or ACh synthesis, a decrease in hepatic choline release or secretion of VLDL particles could explain the exercise-induced reduction in plasma choline.[18] Another explanation may simply be a transient move in the choline pool as a result of fluid compartment redistribution during exercise.[37]

It is important to note that not all investigators have observed reductions in plasma choline with long-term exercise.[31,62,63] For example, Deuster et al.[62] showed slight, but nonsignificant reductions in plasma choline (−10.1%) when men underwent 2 hours of load carriage with a pack weighted at 40% of their body weight. Although not a marathon, the load carriage was very stressful and fatiguing, as indicated by marked increases in plasma levels of cortisol and lactate. As previously noted by Von Allwörden et al.,[31] Deuster et al.[62] found a striking range of change in plasma choline — one participant had a 41% decline and another a 14% increase, which suggested that some individuals might be more susceptible to choline depletion by exercise than others. In another study, Spector et al.[63] exercised cyclists to exhaustion and, although the decline in plasma choline was negatively correlated with time to exhaustion, the average decline in plasma choline was not significant. In other words, participants riding the longest had the greatest reductions in plasma choline. Finally, in contrast to the triathletes, Von Allwörden et al.[31] found no reduction in plasma choline

TABLE 10.5
Plasma Concentrations (Mean ± SD) of Choline (μM) before and after Exercise and Percent Change with and without Choline Supplementation

Lead Author	Supplementation	Pre–Exercise	Post–Exercise	%Change
Conlay [59]	None	10.1 ± 0.4 μM	6.2 ± 1.2 μM	−39%
Conlay [18]	None	14.1 ± 1.2 μM	8.4 ± 0.6 μM	−40%
Buchman [61]	Placebo	9.6 ± 3.6 μM	7.0 ± 3.6 μM	−27%
Deuster [62]	Placebo	7.9 ± 2.6 μM	7.1 ± 1.7 μM	−10.4%
von Allwörden [31]	Placebo: Triathletes	12.1 ± 1.5 μM	10.0 ± 2.1 μM	−17%
von Allwörden [31]	Placebo: Runners	14.5 ± 2.8 μM	14.9 ± 1.7 μM	+3%
Spector [63]	Placebo	~8.8 μM	~10.0 μM	~ +12%
Warber [73]	Placebo	8.1 ± 1.8 μM	7.9 ± 1.0 μM	−2%
Buchman [61]	2.2 g of choline from lecithin	8.0 ± 1.2 μM	11.7 ± 3.6 μM	+45.8%
Deuster [62]	0.050 g/kg as choline citrate	8.8 ± 3.9 μM	12.2 ± 4.4 μM	+41.9%
von Allwörden [31]	Triathletes: 0.2 g/kg of lecithin	10.8 ± 0.6 μM	11.1 ± 0.6 μM	+10%
von Allwörden [31]	Runners: 0.2 g/kg of lecithin	13.9 ± 2.1 μM	16.3 ± 2.8 μM	+18%
Spector [63]	2.43 g as choline bitartrate	~9.3 μM	~16.5 μM	+44%
Warber [73]	6.0 g as choline citrate	7.7 ± 1.3 μM	17.5 ± 3.9 μM	+128%

concentrations of adolescent runners aged 14 to 20 years who ran cross-country races lasting between 30 and 60 minutes. In fact, there was a slight rise in plasma choline, which could reflect hemoconcentration from the high-intensity exercise bout. However, this possibility was not addressed.

We are uncertain as to why Von Allwörden et al.[31] found differences in his two study populations. It can be postulated that the lack of a reduction in plasma choline for the adolescents might be explained by the shorter exercise time period (≤ 2 hours) or the age of the participants. Alternative explanations include dietary intake of choline, as the studies reporting significant exercise-induced decreases in plasma choline did not adequately control for or mention pre-race dietary intakes of choline-rich foods. Dietary control and standardizing the time before the last meal would be very important because plasma choline concentrations are known to peak about 3 to 5 hours after choline ingestion and remain elevated a number of hours afterward.[13,21] Moreover, none of the investigators corrected post-exercise plasma choline for changes in plasma volume, which would be expected to occur during long-duration exercise without fluid replacement. In the study by Deuster et al.,[62] no changes in plasma volume were observed, which indicated that post-exercise choline concentrations required no adjustments. Finally, changes in plasma VLDL and HDL levels before and after exercise should be considered, as phosphatidylcholine is a primary component of each. It is well known that HDL levels increase markedly with exercise,[64] and this would be expected to yield higher total plasma choline values.[65] Such issues should be addressed in all future studies of interactions between choline and exercise.

Another potential, but unexplored, choline and exercise interaction relates to the role of choline in creatine synthesis. The commercial marketing communities have promoted the ability of choline to enhance creatine synthesis and most athletes are well aware of the role of creatine in exercise performance. Thus, a creatine-boosting mechanism might be one additional way wherein choline might delay fatigue during marathon-type efforts. However, Stekol et al.[5] showed in 1953 that creatine synthesis was not enhanced in the presence of choline and that the primary methyl donor for creatine was SAM, not choline.[28] Moreover, methylation of tissue creatine in rats was relatively independent of dietary choline.[5] Although these early data would discount any choline, creatine and exercise interactions, no human studies have been conducted to address the interactions. Recent evidence that a choline deficiency in humans is associated with increased levels of serum CK suggests that choline may be important in maintaining the functional capacities and integrity of muscle cell membranes.[51] However, this is an unexplored area.

Finally, another area where choline and exercise may interact relates to lipid metabolism.[66,67] Choline is a well established lipotropic agent[17] and is known to interact with carnitine, a nutrient essential for the translocation of fatty acids into the mitochondria of skeletal muscle cells.[17,68] However, all work in this area has focused on choline supplementation and, as such, will be discussed under the section on choline supplementation.

VI. CHOLINE SUPPLEMENTATION

Dietary supplementation with vitamins, minerals, amino acids, cofactors and other such nutrients or food constituents is prevalent among the general population. Despite supplementation by many, the evidence to support beneficial actions is often lacking. Such is the case with choline. A number of studies have been conducted to evaluate the effects of choline supplementation on its various functional and structural roles. These studies include *in vitro* and *in vivo* as well as animal and human studies.

In some of the first studies, Bierkamper and Goldberg[16] examined how exogenous choline affected the synthesis and release of ACh in a rat phrenic nerve-hemidiaphragm preparation. They reported that increasing the availability of choline increased stimulated, but not spontaneous, release of ACh at the neuromuscular junction.[69] Wurtman et al.[55] demonstrated that choline administered increased both ACh synthesis and release in peripheral neurons. Further work by Ulus et al.,[70] who used perfused brain slices from rats, provided additional evidence that an increase in extracellular choline was associated with greater evoked, but not basal, release of ACh. They concluded that increases in tissue choline enhanced ACh synthesis.[70] However, they also found that ACh synthesis continued with repeated stimulation in the absence of choline, which led to a decrease in the phospholipid content of cell membranes.[70] This was interpreted as evidence that choline from membrane lipids could be liberated when the need for choline was high.[70]

Although this supported a justification for providing choline exogenously, the studies were carried out in animal preparations rather than whole animals or humans. Further work was required to demonstrate comparable responses *in vivo*. Zeisel et al.[71] demonstrated a greater decay in muscle conduction velocity when humans were fed a choline-deficient diet as compared with a control diet. These investigations helped form the basis for research on choline supplementation in humans under a variety of physiologic and pathologic conditions. Of particular interest was the role of choline in long-duration exercise where fatigue could limit performance.

A. Physical Performance and Metabolic Effects

It had been hypothesized that long-duration exercise might deplete ACh if choline availability were limited — without adequate ACh, the ability to perform physical work could be significantly diminished.[16,71,72] Accordingly, investigations on choline supplementation and physical performance have used long-duration, fatiguing aerobic exercise as a model for examining choline and exercise interactions. Variations in exercise methodologies, such as mode, intensity and duration, have affected the results of published studies, as have the dose, timing, form and characteristics of the choline supplements. For example, the specific form of choline (citrate, bitartrate and lecithin) and doses, in terms of absolute amounts and timing, have differed. Furthermore, dietary intake and choline status have not usually been evaluated and variations in these factors are known to affect plasma choline. In fact, no dietary intake data for choline are available. Given that plasma choline can increase for up to 5 hours after ingestion of a choline-containing food or supplement, plasma choline levels measured during and after exercise could be greatly affected if dietary intake were not comparable among participants. Each and all of these specific experimental issues would affect the results and could account for discrepancies across studies of choline supplementation for aerobic performance.

One of the first exercise and choline supplementation studies was conducted by Von Allwörden et al.,[31] who examined the effects of lecithin supplementation in two different populations: triathletes and adolescent runners. The lecithin was provided in orange juice 1 hour prior to the exercise, such that the amount of actual choline ingested was unknown but could have ranged from 7.5 to approximately 27 mg/kg, depending on the amount of phosphatidylcholine in the lecithin. In their study, choline supplementation did result in higher post-exercise plasma choline concentrations relative to baseline levels for both groups, but the percent increase was less in the triathletes (+10%) who cycled for 2 hours than the adolescents, who ran for 30 to 60 minutes (+18%). Providing the lecithin supplement in the absence of exercise increased plasma choline concentrations by 27% and 54% for the triathletes and runners, respectively.[31] They concluded that changes in plasma choline levels with exercise were dependent upon exercise duration and intensity.[31]

Although Von Allwörden et al.[31] demonstrated that choline supplementation prevented exercise-induced declines in plasma choline, they did not examine performance. However, four other studies on choline supplementation and exercise performance have shown negative results. In 1994 Spector et al.[63] sought to determine whether choline supplementation would improve the performance of cyclists engaged in brief, high-intensity (150% of maximal capacity) or sustained (70% of maximal capacity) cycle exercise. Approximately 45 minutes before the exercise, participants, who were asked to avoid choline-rich foods, were provided 2.45 g of choline bitartrate in a fruit drink that also contained potassium and B vitamins. Fatigue times and total work performed were similar in the placebo and supplemented groups for both exercise sessions, and plasma choline concentrations were significantly higher in both exercise groups as a function of supplementation.[63]

In a study by Deuster et al.,[62] participants underwent two load carriage treadmill tests while carrying 40% of body weight for 2 hours on separate days under conditions of placebo and choline. The load carriage task was followed by a strenuous physical battery that included a handgrip strength and endurance test, maximal number of steps completed in 1 minute while wearing a 20-kg pack and as many pull-ups as possible. In addition, they underwent a cognitive test battery after the exercise was completed. No improvement in any aspect of physical performance was seen with ingestion of choline as compared with placebo, despite marked increases in plasma choline.[62] Load carriage times, number of pull-ups, number of stairs stepped and handgrip strength and endurance were unaffected by choline. Interestingly, the dose of choline in this study was higher than most others (50mg/kg) and the increase in plasma choline under conditions of supplementation was also larger, with an average increase of 41.9%. The choline, which was in a liquid form as choline citrate with glycerine, was given 30 minutes before and 60 minutes after starting the exercise. As indicated by plasma choline values in Figure 10.3, the choline was clearly bioavailable. Of note is the finding that plasma choline decreased 41% after exercise under placebo conditions in one participant who had a very low plasma choline value (5.4 µM) prior to starting the exercise, and plasma choline increased 74% after exercise when choline was provided. This finding points to the importance of ensuring adequate choline status prior to enrollment, as well as the need to assess individual differences and not just group averages. Although strict dietary control was not maintained, the participants were given a list of choline-rich foods and instructed to avoid them prior to exercise. In addition, the participants ingested the same meal the evening prior to both tests. Thus, the influence of dietary choline should have been minimal.

Warber et al.[73] conducted a double-blind crossover study on plasma choline and performance by having participants undergo 4 hours of load carriage with a 34.1-kg pack, followed by a time-to-exhaustion treadmill run and squat tests. A placebo or choline-containing beverage (8.425 g choline citrate) was provided prior to and midway through the load carriage exercise. Despite marked increases in plasma choline (+ 128%) with the choline beverage, no significant improvements on any performance measures were noted. They concluded, as did Deuster et al.,[62] that

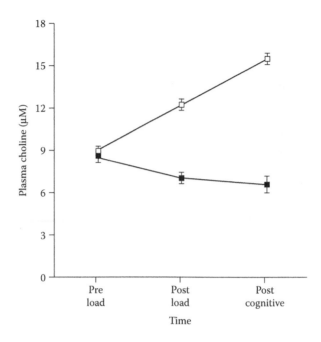

FIGURE 10.3 Mean plasma choline concentrations for choline (open squares) and placebo (closed squares) load carriage test sessions. Plasma choline concentrations were measured before (Pre Load) and after (Post Load) load carriage treadmill exercise and again 60 minutes later after completing a cognitive battery (Post Cognitive). (From Deuster et al.[62])

plasma choline was not depleted as a result of prolonged exhaustive exercise and that choline supplementation had no performance-enhancing benefit.

Finally, Buchman et al.[61] provided 2.2 g of choline as lecithin to runners on each of 2 days — the day prior to and the day of a marathon competition; plasma free and phospholipid bound choline, as well as urinary choline were measured. Unlike the other supplementation studies, this was not a crossover design, so that participants were assigned to either a placebo or choline group. However, consistent with other studies, performance in the choline-supplemented group was not superior to that of the placebo group, despite significantly higher plasma choline levels in the supplemented (+45.8%) as compared with the placebo (−26.2%) group. Urinary choline was reported to have been less after exercise in both groups, which suggested conservation of choline after strenuous exercise. This issue remains to be explored.

Only one study has demonstrated a performance improvement with choline. Sandage et al.[60] provided choline citrate (2.4 grams) or placebo to 10 runners 1 hour prior to and at 10 miles into a 20-mile run. Mean time to complete the 20 miles was significantly shorter (about 5 minutes) when they ingested choline as compared with placebo. Moreover, plasma choline levels, which declined under placebo conditions, were significantly increased with choline supplementation. As this research effort was published in abstract form and not yet published in a peer-reviewed journal, the results must be viewed with some caution.

It appears that a significant decrease or loss of choline during exercise occurs during long-duration exercise. However, the intensity of exercise may also be important. Warber et al.[73] found no improvement in physical performance with choline supplementation after 4 hours of treadmill walking. Running for more than 20 miles and swimming for more than 2 hours has led to significant decreases in plasma choline levels, while short-duration running or cycling showed no change in plasma choline levels.[60] This suggests that duration, intensity and possibly mode of exercise may determine changes in plasma choline levels with exercise. When plasma choline concentrations are normal, supplementing with choline appears to have no beneficial effect on performance. In contrast, although more evidence is needed, providing supplemental choline in a choline-deficient state might improve physical performance.

Another area of choline supplementation and exercise relates to interactions between choline and carnitine. Although a choline:carnitine interaction has been clearly established, an understanding of the implications has not been fully resolved. Early on it was determined that rats fed a choline-deficient diet had significant reductions in the levels of carnitine in skeletal muscle, liver and heart as compared with choline-sufficient animals.[2,74] Moreover, provision of choline reversed the reduction.[2] Subsequent to those studies, several investigators demonstrated that choline supplementation brought about a noticeable conservation of urinary carnitine in animals and humans [67,68,75] as well as carnitine accretion in the skeletal muscle of guinea pigs.[67] Rein et al.[68] also showed that chronic choline administration to rats decreased plasma and kidney carnitine, but increased liver concentrations. These efforts led to the suggestion that choline supplementation may facilitate redistribution of carnitine across specific body compartments.

Subsequent work has provided additional evidence that choline-supplemented guinea pigs had significantly lower total body fat and higher body proteins, but not different body weights, as compared with the nonsupplemented animals.[67,69] Because the respiratory exchange ratios of the groups were comparable, they speculated that acyl groups generated by the oxidation of fatty acids were not oxidized to carbon dioxide, but rather transferred by carnitine from one body pool to another.[67] As a consequence of these findings, they conducted a very complicated study wherein choline and carnitine supplements were provided to healthy women in combination with exercise.[66] In the first phase, one supplementation group took choline and another took carnitine, and in the second phase this was reversed, such that the group taking choline alone took carnitine and vice versa. After phase two, the two supplements were given in combination and exercise was imposed. The investigators concluded that the two supplements in combination reversed urinary conservation of carnitine and shifted fatty acid metabolism toward incomplete oxidation[66] as compared with the no supplementation group. Unfortunately, the outcome variables did not include anthropometric or exercise data with a single supplement so the study did not provide a clear picture of how each supplement alone and in combination with exercise altered lipid metabolism. Further studies may clarify the issues.

In addition to their efforts with choline and carnitine, caffeine, which has been discussed above with respect to choline absorption and metabolism, was added to animal studies of choline and carnitine supplementation.[69,76] The combination of choline, caffeine and carnitine was chosen based on the key roles of each compound — choline to promote entry of carnitine into the skeletal muscle cells, caffeine to enhance the release of fatty acids from adipose tissue and carnitine to facilitate translocation of fatty acids into muscle mitochondria.[76] The results of the studies have interesting implications that will need to be fully addressed in humans. Overall, providing choline in combination with carnitine and caffeine to rats for a 3-week period resulted in significantly lower epididymal, inguinal and perirenal fat pad weights and serum leptin levels as compared with nonsupplemented rats. These effects were enhanced when exercise was imposed 5 days a week.[69] Furthermore, the supplement combination resulted in significant decreases in serum and increases in skeletal muscle triglycerides. However, unlike exercise alone, the supplementation paradigm did not decrease body weight or weight gain over the study period. The authors concluded that choline, caffeine and carnitine in combination promote fat loss to the same extent as exercise alone and that the effects are not interactive.[69]

Sachan et al.[76] explored the possibility that this combination might improve exercise performance. At the end of a 3-week period, animals in the supplemented group had significantly higher maximal aerobic capacities and lower lactate levels, as well as a trend indicating increased endurance capacity.[76] In addition, biochemical markers supported enhancement of fatty acid oxidation by the supplement combination.[76] The results reported for rats must both be replicated and followed up by human studies to ascertain whether comparable outcomes will emerge. It is important to note that the amount of carnitine used by these investigators was extraordinarily high—150-fold higher than the non-supplemented group and 5- to 10-fold greater than what has been used in humans.[76] Nonetheless, the results are intriguing. Clearly the role of choline supplementation in association with physical activity and exercise performance has not been fully established.

B. COGNITIVE EFFECTS

Choline's involvement in brain development and function has been the basis for many choline supplementation studies, particularly in the area of memory and cognition, under both usual and altered physiological conditions.[14,24,77] A series of studies looked at the effects of choline supplementation on brain development during gestation and postnatally.[24,27,37,44–47,77,78] Overall, supplementing choline during fetal development improved spatial memory, timing and temporal memory, problem solving and attention in rats.[27,37,44–47,78] Conversely, a lack of choline led to impairments in attention and certain memory tasks.[27] A molecular basis for these findings was provided by Li et al.[45] who demonstrated that when choline was given prenatally, it altered the structure and function of hippocampal pyramidal cells. Although such studies have not been conducted in humans, these choline studies were the basis for recommending a higher choline intake during pregnancy.

Supplemental choline has been given to adult animals and humans to alter brain functioning.[7,13,14,41,62,78,79] Such studies were initiated based on the discovery that administration of choline would increase brain, as well as plasma, choline concentrations.[7,13] Since that discovery, a number of studies have been conducted, but to date, only one study of healthy adults has demonstrated benefits of choline in the absence of some underlying problem. Deuster et al.[62] saw no effect of 50 mg/kg of choline supplementation on reaction time, logical reasoning, vigilance, spatial memory or working memory in healthy adults as compared with placebo. Likewise, Harris et al.[78] were unable to demonstrate any significant change in memory performance or psychomotor speed after providing a single 20-gram dose of lecithin 5 hours before testing. Furthermore, they found no relationship between plasma choline levels and performance on a memory test.[78]

In contrast to the negative results, Ladd et al.[79] examined the effects of providing 10 or 25 grams of lecithin on explicit memory. Participants ingested 1.5 or 3.75 grams of choline as lecithin in a milk-based beverage either 60 or 90 minutes prior to a serial learning task. A significant reduction in the number of trials required to achieve criterion was found for the 25-gram lecithin dose at both 60 and 90 minutes, but not for the 10-gram dose.[79] Further examination of the data suggested the possibility of slow and fast learners and additional analyses revealed that choline supplementation appeared to benefit the slow, more than the fast, learners.[79] These results provide the first indication that supplemental choline may be beneficial only in those who have some pathology.

Several investigators have examined choline supplementation in the aged and those with compromised cognitive capacities. Overall, the value of choline as a supplement in aging has been inconclusive. Cohen et al.[13] showed that oral administration of choline bitartrate resulted in decreased brain uptake of choline by older (mean age 73 years) as compared with younger (mean age 32 years) adults. They postulated that the decreased uptake might contribute to dementia and other neurodegenerative changes of aging. However, Tan et al.[80] attempted to replicate the Cohen study and were unable to demonstrate increases in the choline content of brain in response to choline ingestion. They encouraged additional trials before promoting choline for neurodegenerative changes of aging.[80]

Despite the conflicting human data, animal models provide convincing evidence for choline supplementation. Old mice (28 months old) have significantly lower ACh levels in the hippocampus, frontal cortex and posterior cortex as compared with young mice (5 months old) and old mice show impairments in both working memory and reference memory.[81] Strong correlations between learning performance and ACh levels in the hippocampus and cerebral cortex may explain the behavioral impairment in spatial learning and habituation in old mice.[81] Providing exogenous choline in supplemental forms improved the observed deficits. Crespo et al.[82] reported that providing old mice with CDP-choline for 45 days positively affected memory and modified hippocampal formation, such that the neuronal characteristics and mitochondrial morphology of old animals treated with CDP-choline resembled that of younger animals. Additionally, Lee et al.[83] presented evidence that providing soy isoflavones to old rats influenced the brain cholinergic system by reducing age-related neuron loss and conferring benefit on cognitive functioning in old male rats.

A number of clinical studies with choline supplementation have also been conducted because the breakdown of cellular membranes is characteristic of neuronal degeneration and choline is rate-limiting for phospholipid biosynthesis.[24,77,84] The more recent human studies, which provide interesting results in the aged and diseased states, have used CDP-choline (citicoline) and Alpha-GPC as the delivery form of choline. Interestingly, citicoline has been approved in Europe and Japan for use in stroke, head trauma and other neurological disorders, and is being evaluated as a treatment for stroke in the United States.[54] As would be expected, some, but not all, results are positive.[29,54,84] In addition to its effect in stroke and ischemic brain injury, citicoline is being examined as a safe treatment for Alzheimer's disease (AD), cognitive decline in the elderly, memory enhancement and glaucoma.[29,54,84,85] Recent reviews[29,54,84,85] present the multiple research efforts with citicoline. Although the results are mixed, the compound is of great interest because of the apparent limited toxicity and high bioavailability of citicoline.[29,54] Clearly, more research is needed.

Alpha-GPC is also of great interest and may have multiple uses. Parnetti et al.[39] reviewed the literature on the clinical efficacy of Alpha-GPC in dementia disorders and acute cerebrovascular disease and concluded that most published studies of dementia had positive outcomes. Thus, unlike choline and lecithin, Alpha-GPC appeared to be effective in improving cognitive function in the dementia of stroke, degenerative disease and vascular disorders.[39] In addition, Moreno[86] published results from a multicenter trial designed to evaluate the effectiveness of Alpha-GPC (1,200 mg) in treating cognitive impairment due to mild to moderate AD. Overall, GPC was both useful and well tolerated over a period of 180 days and significant improvements in all outcome measures were noted at 90 and 180 days in the treated as compared with the placebo group.[86] Fewer studies have been published regarding stroke, but the results suggest that Alpha-GPC may assist in the functional recovery of patients.[39] Further work will be required to determine the efficacy.[39]

Overall, the potential for these choline derivatives that serve as delivery vehicles for choline is exciting from the perspective of physical performance, cognition, aging and neurodegenerative disorders. Previous studies of cognitive performance in healthy men and women should be reconsidered in light of the potential effectiveness of CDP-choline and Alpha-GPC. Thus, further work is clearly needed to confirm and further explore their boundaries.

C. EFFECTIVENESS

Choline is very important for a variety of functions, which is why many people are interested in taking supplemental choline for medical purposes and performance enhancement. Although a clear demonstration of effectiveness is lacking for most situations, choline supplementation has been and still is used orally for liver disease (including chronic hepatitis and cirrhosis), hypercholesterolemia, depression, memory loss, schizophrenia, AD, dementia and athletic performance. It is also added to infant formulas. Despite these many uses, there are only two areas where support for effectiveness has been consistent.[9]

First, choline supplementation appears to be effective for treating TPN-associated hepatic steatosis.[49,87] In fact, the hepatic steatosis associated with long-term TPN may be prevented with the addition of choline. Second, choline appears to be effective in decreasing symptom severity and frequency, as well as the need for bronchodilators, in asthmatics.[88,89] However, the preferred dosage for this application has not been determined.[88,89]

Finally, the first trials using choline and lecithin to test the cholinergic hypothesis for stroke and in the cognitive dysfunction of aging and AD were discouraging. Results with citicoline and

Alpha-GPC choline are more promising and demonstrate that the delivery form of choline may be critical for effectiveness.

D. SAFETY AND TOXICITY

Overall, the use of choline appears to be safe. However, as of 2004, insufficient data were available to establish a "no observed adverse effect level" (NOAEL). In contrast, a "lowest observed adverse effect level"(LOAEL) has been proposed. The term NOAEL reflects levels considered safe that require no application of a safety factor to determine a safe intake, whereas LOAEL refers to levels that should NOT be considered safe for everyone and may require the application of a safety factor to calculate a safe intake. Based on two clinical studies in humans, a LOAEL of 7.5 grams daily has been proposed. At 7.5 grams of choline daily, nausea, diarrhea and a small decrease in blood pressure were reported in some patients.[58] The upper limit (UL) for adults is 3.5 grams daily. Future research may change these limits, but at this point, less than 3.5 grams of choline daily should be considered safe and non-toxic.

E. DOSAGE AND ADMINISTRATION

Typical doses of choline range from 0.3 to 1.2 grams daily, with the major forms being choline chloride, choline bitartrate, phosphatidylcholine, lecithin, Alpha-GPC and CDP-choline. Choline is also added to some infant and TPN formulations. People who ingest less than 0.5 grams each day through their diet may need to consider supplementation to ensure adequate intakes. The most commonly recommended dose of choline (as a salt) for adults is 3 to 3.5 grams per day, which, as discussed, is well below the LOAEL of 7.5 grams. In contrast, an upper limit of 20 to 30 grams per day has been proposed for phosphatidylcholine. A common dose for Alpha-GPC is 0.5 to 1.0 grams daily and a typical dose of CDP-choline is 0.5 to 2.0 grams daily.

For pregnant or lactating women, doses of up to 3.5 grams each day appear acceptable, whereas for children up to 8 years old, 1 gram has been recommended. For children 9–13 years of age, 2 grams daily is adequate, and for adolescents between 14–18 years, 3 grams a day is recommended.[9] A liquid form of choline may be preferred because of the high bioavailability and rapid absorption.

F. NUTRIENT AND DRUG INTERACTIONS

Choline, as a methyl donor and precursor for betaine, works in concert and interacts with other nutrients. In particular, as part of the SAM cycle, choline status is linked to the intake or availability of vitamins B_6 and B_{12}, methionine and folate.[1-3] The compounds that actively exchange and provide methyl groups for the SAM cycle depend on folic acid, which accepts methyl groups from other molecules.[1-3] As noted earlier, Jacob et al.[90] fed diets that varied in folate and choline content to 21 men and women and concluded that choline is used as a methyl group donor when folate intake is low, and that synthesis of phosphatidylcholine is compromised when dietary folate and choline intakes are minimal. Thus, diets limited in folate increase the dietary requirement for choline, such that folate status is closely linked to choline status.[90]

Another choline–nutrient interaction that needs further investigation is choline and carnitine. Several studies have reported conservation of carnitine in guinea pigs and humans,[67,68,75,91] and carnitine accretion in skeletal muscle of guinea pigs[91] supplemented with choline. Future work will unravel the implications and concerns, if any, with regard to choline and carnitine interactions.

Although very few drug interactions have been identified, such interactions must always be considered. Two known drug and choline interactions are with methotrexate and phenobarbital. Methotrexate, a drug used for treating forms of cancer, rheumatoid arthritis and psoriasis, and anticonvulsant drugs have both been shown to increase risk of choline deficiency by compromising absorption.[58] Interestingly, choline supplementation seems to reverse the fatty liver caused by methotrexate administration in rats.[92]

G. Adverse Reactions

Minimal adverse reactions have been associated with ingestion of choline at doses of 3.5 grams per day, but it is possible to ingest toxic levels. Large dosages of choline (10 to 16 grams/day) may be associated with hypotension, sweating, salivation, vomiting or diarrhea and a fishlike body odor.[9] In addition, high doses of choline bitartrate have been associated with depression or symptoms of depression in some instances.[58]

The fishy body odor associated with high intakes of choline reflects excessive production and excretion of trimethylamine, a metabolite of choline.[1–3] Trimethylamine is eliminated from the body through urination, sweating, respiration and other bodily secretions. In contrast to choline, ingestion of phosphatidylcholine does not typically cause a fishlike odor, because its conversion to trimethylamine is limited. Some individuals (0.1 to 11.0% of the population) have a metabolic disorder, trimethylaminuria, where large amounts of trimethylamines are formed and excreted in the urine.[93] Trimethylaminuria may be inherited as an autosomal dominant genetic trait or acquired as a result of treatment with large doses of L-carnitine.[93] The disorder arises from a lack or impairment in the ability of the liver enzyme, trimethylamine-N-oxide synthetase, to convert the odorous compound trimethylamine to the non-odorous trimethylamine-N-oxide. Persons with this metabolic disorder should restrict their intake of choline.[93] In addition, persons with various types of liver and renal disease, depression and Parkinson's disease may be at increased risk when taking supplemental choline.

H. Recommendations

Choline supplementation has not been shown to be effective for improving exercise performance in long-duration events. However, a number of areas with regard to choline supplementation and exercise remain unexplored. If a person is unable to get the recommended amount of choline through dietary intake, choline supplementation is one way to ensure adequate amounts. Based on the literature, Alpha-GPC, CDP-choline or citicoline and lecithin would be the supplements of choice. However, no exercise studies with humans have used either Alpha-GPC or CDP-choline. Moreover, Alpha-GPC at this time is very expensive. It is important to note that lecithin supplements usually contain about 35% phosphatidylcholine, of which only 15% is choline. Therefore, people consuming lecithin in hopes of increasing plasma choline concentrations may not see the results that they might when using another choline supplement. Finally, persons who choose to take supplemental choline should keep in mind that ingested choline reaches its maximum level 3 to 4 hours after ingestion.[21]

VII. CONCLUSIONS AND FUTURE ISSUES

A. Summary

Choline is an essential nutrient that is only beginning to be fully appreciated and understood. There is little doubt that choline serves a multitude of important roles, both functional and structural, that can influence overall health and physical and cognitive performance. Whether supplementation with choline will overcome existing deficits, enhance selected physical activity and performance or provide a safe and effective approach for treating various illness and disorders remains to be critically evaluated. Most past studies used forms of choline that may not be optimal for the intended function. It is an exciting area, given that it achieved "essential" status only in 1998.[8] This review has attempted to provide and highlight some of the old and new information relating to this important nutrient.

B. Future Research Directions

A long list of interesting research projects could be proposed based on the current state of choline and choline supplementation with regard to physical activity and exercise. First and foremost, the particular forms of supplemental choline need to be examined to determine the most bioavailable and bioactive form for using before and during exercise. Also, dietary intake data are needed to determine ranges of choline intake. In addition, more appropriate outcome variables need to be established in future testing of choline during long-duration exercise. For example, given the reported role of choline in skeletal muscle membrane integrity,[51] outcome measures such as plasma levels of CK, recovery from exercise, muscle fatigue, muscle damage and energy stores should be considered. In addition, the role of choline on markers of lipid metabolism in the absence of carnitine should be considered. Furthermore, choline has never been studied in association with short-term anaerobic or eccentric exercise. Given the rapid turnover of ACh during anaerobic exercise and the muscle damage from eccentric activities, these paradigms are potential avenues for choline actions.

In all future research efforts regarding choline supplementation and exercise, care must be taken to control, account or adjust for differences in initial choline status, choline intake, caffeine intake, carnitine status, lipoprotein profiles and changes in plasma volume. Alone and together, these factors will influence results. Finally, appropriate markers of choline status and tissue redistribution need to be carefully evaluated so that the results can be adequately interpreted.

REFERENCES

1. Zeisel SH, Da Costa KA, Franklin PD, Alexander EA, Lamont JT, Sheard NF, Beiser A. Choline, an essential nutrient for humans. *FASEB J.* 1991;5:2093–98.
2. Zeisel SH, Blusztajn JK. Choline and human nutrition. *Ann Rev Nutr* 1994;14:269–96.
3. Zeisel SH. Choline and phosphatidylcholine, in Shils ME, Olson JA, Shike M, Ross AC (Eds.), *Nutrition in Health and Disease,* 9th ed. Baltimore: Williams and Wilkins, 1999; p. 513–523.
4. Strecker A. Uber einige neue bestandtheile der schweingalle. *Ann Chem Pharmacie* 1862;123:353–60.
5. Stekol JA, Weiss S, Smith P, Weiss K. The synthesis of choline and creatine in rats under various dietary conditions. *J Biol Chem.* 1953;201:299–316.
6. Best CH, Huntsman ME. The effects of the components of lecithine upon deposition of fat in the liver. *J Physiol* 1932;75:405–12.
7. Wurtman RJ, Hirsch MJ, Growdon JH. Lecithin consumption raises serum-free-choline levels. *Lancet* 1977;2:68–69.
8. Institute of Medicine, Food and Nutrition Board. Dietary Reference Intakes: Thiamin, Riboflavin, Niacin, Vitamin B-6, Vitamin B-12, Pantothenic Acid, Biotin and Choline. Washington, D.C.: National Academy Press; 1998. p. 390–422.
9. Jellin JM, Gregory PJ, Batz F, Hitchens Kea. Pharmacist's Letter/Prescriber's Letter Natural Medicines Comprehensive Database, 6th ed. Stockton, CA: Therapeutic Research Faculty; 2004.
10. Nagan N, Zoeller RA. Plasmalogens: Biosynthesis and functions. *Prog Lipid Res.* 2001;40:199–229.
11. Blusztajn JK, Wurtman RJ. Choline and cholinergic neurons. *Science* 1983;221:614–20.
12. Tong Z, Yamaki T, Harada K, Houkin K. *In vivo* quantification of the metabolites in normal brain and brain tumors by proton MR spectroscopy using water as an internal standard. *Magn Reson Imaging* 2004;22:735–42.
13. Cohen BM, Renshaw PF, Stoll AL, Wurtman RJ, Yurgelun-Todd D, Babb SM. Decreased brain choline uptake in older adults. An *in vivo* proton magnetic resonance spectroscopy study. *JAMA* 1995; 274: 902–07.
14. Hirsch MJ, Growdon JH, Wurtman RJ. Increase in hippocampal acetylcholine after choline administration. *Brain Res* 1977;125:383–85.
15. Dobransky T, Rylett RJ. Functional regulation of choline acetyltransferase by phosphorylation. *Neurochem Res* 2003;28:537–42.
16. Bierkamper GG, Goldberg AM. Release of acetylcholine from the vascular perfused rat phrenic nerve-hemidiaphragm. *Brain Res* 1980;202:234–37.
17. Zeisel SH. Choline: Needed for normal development of memory. *J Am Coll Nutr* 2000;19:528S–531.
18. Conlay LA, Wurtman RJ, Blusztajn K, Coviella IL, Maher TJ, Evoniuk GE. Decreased plasma choline concentrations in marathon runners. *N Engl J Med.* 1986;315:892.

19. Phillips GB. The phospholipid composition of human serum lipoprotein fractions separated by ultra-centrifugation. *J Clin Invest* 1959;38:489–93.

20. Jope RS, Jenden DJ, Ehrlich BE, Diamond JM, Gosenfeld LF. Erythrocyte choline concentrations are elevated in manic patients. *Proc Natl Acad Sci USA* 1980;77:6144–46.

21. Jope RS, Domino EF, Mathews BN, Sitaram N, Jenden DJ, Ortez A. Free and bound choline blood levels after phosphatidylcholine. *Clin Pharmacol Ther.* 1982;31:483–87.

22. Holmes HC, Snodgrass GJ, Iles RA. Changes in the choline content of human breast milk in the first 3 weeks after birth. *Eur J Pediatr.* 2000;159:198–204.

23. Zierenberg O, Grundy SM. Intestinal absorption of polyenephosphatidylcholine in man. *J Lipid Res.* 1982;23:1136–42.

24. Klein J. Membrane breakdown in acute and chronic neurodegeneration: focus on choline-containing phospholipids. *J Neural Transm.* 2000;107:1027–63.

25. De La Huer, Popper H. Factors influencing choline absorption in the intestinal tract. *J Clin.Invest* 1952;31:598–603.

26. Le Kim D, Betzing H. Intestinal absorption of polyunsaturated phosphatidylcholine in the rat. *Hoppe Seylers Z Physiol Chem.* 1976;357:1321–31.

27. Blusztajn JK. Choline, A vital amine. *Science* 1998;281:704–05.

28. Stekol JA anderson EI, Weiss S. S-Adenosyl-L-methionine in the synthesis of choline, creatine and cysteine *in vivo* and *in vitro*. *J Biol Chem.* 1958;233:425–29.

29. Conant R, Schauss AG. Therapeutic applications of citicoline for stroke and cognitive dysfunction in the elderly: A review of the literature. *Altern Med Rev.* 2004;9:17–31.

30. Murugesan G, Sandhya Rani MR, Gerber CE, Mukhopadhyay C, Ransohoff RM, Chisolm GM, Kottke-Marchant,K. Lysophosphatidylcholine regulates human microvascular endothelial cell expression of chemokines. *J Mol Cell Cardiol.* 2003;35:1375–84.

31. von Allwörden HN, Horn S, Kahl J, Feldheim W. The influence of lecithin on plasma choline concentrations in triathletes and adolescent runners during exercise. *Eur J Appl Physiol Occup Physiol* 1993;67:87–91.

32. Zeisel SH, Mar MH, Howe JC, Holden JM. Concentrations of choline-containing compounds and betaine in common foods. *J Nutr.* 2003;133:1302–07.

33. Cuadrado A, Carnero A, Dolfi F, Jimenez B, Lacal JC. Phosphorylcholine: a novel second messenger essential for mitogenic activity of growth factors. *Oncogene* 1993;8:2959–68.

34. Latorre E, Aragones MD, Fernandez I, Catalan RE. Platelet-activating factor modulates brain sphingomyelin metabolism. *Eur J Biochem.* 1999;262:308–14.

35. Yao ZM, Vance DE. Reduction in VLDL, but not HDL, in plasma of rats deficient in choline. *Biochem Cell Biol.* 1990;68:552–58.

36. Noga AA, Vance DE. Insights into the requirement of phosphatidylcholine synthesis for liver function in mice. *J Lipid Res.* 2003;44:1998–2005.

37. Kanter MM, Williams MH. Antioxidants, carnitine and choline as putative ergogenic aids. *Int J Sport Nutr.* 1995;5 Suppl:S120–S131.

38. Kwon ED, Zablocki K, Peters EM, Jung KY, Garcia-Perez A, Burg MB. Betaine and inositol reduce MDCK cell glycerophosphocholine by stimulating its degradation. *Am J Physiol* 1996;270:C200– C207.

39. Parnetti L, Amenta F, Gallai V. Choline alphoscerate in cognitive decline and in acute cerebrovascular disease: an analysis of published clinical data. *Mech Ageing Dev.* 2001;122:2041–55.

40. Kim DK, Jung KY. Caffeine causes glycerophosphorylcholine accumulation through ryanodine-inhibitable increase of cellular calcium and activation of phospholipase A2 in cultured MDCK cells. *Exp Mol Med.* 1998;30:151–58.

41. Wong JT, Tran K, Pierce GN, Chan AC, O K, Choy PC. Lysophosphatidylcholine stimulates the release of arachidonic acid in human endothelial cells. *J Biol Chem* 1998;273:6830–36.

42. Okuda T, Haga T. High-affinity choline transporter. *Neurochem Res* 2003;28:483–88.

43. Du Vigneaud V, Cohn M, Chandler JP, Schenck JR, Simmonds S. The utilization of the methyl group of methionine in the biological synthesis of choline and creatine. *J Biol Chem* 1941;140:625–41.

44. Cermak JM, Holler T, Jackson DA, Blusztajn JK. Prenatal availability of choline modifies development of the hippocampal cholinergic system. *FASEB J.* 1998;12:349–57.

45. Li Q, Guo-Ross S, Lewis DV, Turner D, White AM, Wilson WA, Swartzwelder, HS. Dietary Prenatal Choline Supplementation Alters Postnatal Hippocampal Structure and Function. *J Neurophysiol* 2004; 91:1545–55.

46. Meck WH, Williams CL. Perinatal choline supplementation increases the threshold for chunking in spatial memory. *Neuroreport* 1997;8:3053–59.

47. Mellott TJ, Williams CL, Meck WH, Blusztajn JK. Prenatal choline supplementation advances hippocampal development and enhances MAPK and CREB activation. *FASEB J* 2004;18:545–47.

48. Shaw GM, Carmichael SL, Yang W, Selvin S, Schaffer DM. Periconceptional dietary intake of choline and betaine and neural tube defects in offspring. *Am J Epidemiol.* 2004;160:102–09.

49. Buchman AL, Dubin MD, Moukarzel AA, Jenden DJ, Roch M, Rice KM, Gornbein J, Ament ME. Choline deficiency: a cause of hepatic steatosis during parenteral nutrition that can be reversed with intravenous choline supplementation. *Hepatology* 1995;22:1399–403.

50. Holm PI, Ueland PM, Kvalheim G, Lien EA. Determination of choline, betaine and dimethylglycine in plasma by a high-throughput method based on normal-phase chromatography-tandem mass spectrometry. *Clin.Chem.* 2003;49:286–94.

51. Da Costa KA, Badea M, Fischer LM, Zeisel SH. Elevated serum creatine phosphokinase in choline-deficient humans: mechanistic studies in C2C12 mouse myoblasts. *Am J Clin Nutr.* 2004;80:163–70.

52. United States Department of Agriculture. 2004. http://www.nal.usda.gov/fnic/foodcomp

53. Food and Drug Administration Department of HHS. Code of Federal Regulations; Title 21 — Food and Drugs; Part 182 — Substances Generally Recognized as Safe. U.S. Government Printing Office; 2003.

54. D'Orlando KJ, Sandage BW, Jr. Citicoline (CDP-choline): Mechanisms of action and effects in ischemic brain injury. *Neurol Res.* 1995;17:281–84.

55. Wurtman RJ, Regan M, Ulus I, Yu L. Effect of oral CDP–choline on plasma choline and uridine levels in humans. *Biochem Pharmacol.* 2000;60:989–92.

56. Weiss GB. Metabolism and actions of CDP-choline as an endogenous compound and administered exogenously as citicoline. *Life Sci.* 1995;56:637–60.

57. Abbiati G, Fossati T, Lachmann G, Bergamaschi M, Castiglioni C. Absorption, tissue distribution and excretion of radiolabelled compounds in rats after administration of [14C]-L-alpha-glycerylphosphorylcholine. *Eur J Drug Metab Pharmacokinet.* 1993;18:173–80.

58. Physicians' Desk Reference for Nonprescription Drugs and Dietary Supplements. Montvale, NJ: Medical Economics Co.; 2003.

59. Conlay LA, Sabounjian LA, Wurtman RJ. Exercise and neuromodulators: choline and acetylcholine in marathon runners. *Int J Sports Med.* 1992;13 Suppl 1:S141–S142.

60. Sandage, B. W., Jr., Sabounjian, L. A., White, R. and Wurtman, R. J. Choline citrate may enhance athletic performance. *Physiologist* 35, 236. 1992.

61. Buchman AL, Awal M, Jenden D, Roch M, Kang SH. The effect of lecithin supplementation on plasma choline concentrations during a marathon. *J Am Coll Nutr.* 2000;19:768–70.

62. Deuster PA, Singh A, Coll R, Hyde DE, Becker WJ. Choline ingestion does not modify physical or cognitive performance. *Mil Med.* 2002;167:1020–25.

63. Spector SA, Jackman MR, Sabounjian LA, Sakkas C, Landers DM, Willis WT. Effect of choline supplementation on fatigue in trained cyclists. *Med Sci Sports Exerc.* 1995;27:668–73.

64. Park DH, Ransone JW. Effects of submaximal exercise on high-density lipoprotein-cholesterol subfractions. *Int J Sports Med.* 2003;24:245–51.

65. Thompson PD, Crouse SF, Goodpaster B, Kelley D, Moyna N, Pescatello L. The acute versus the chronic response to exercise. *Med Sci Sports Exerc.* 2001;33:S438–S445.

66. Hongu N, Sachan DS. Carnitine and choline supplementation with exercise alter carnitine profiles, biochemical markers of fat metabolism and serum leptin concentration in healthy women. *J Nutr.* 2003;133:84–89.

67. Daily JW, III Hongu N, Mynatt RL, Sachan DS. Choline supplementation increases tissue concentrations of carnitine and lowers body fat in guinea pigs. *J Nutr Biochem* 1998;9:464–70.

68. Rein D Krasin B, Sheard NF. Dietary choline supplementation in rats increases carnitine concentration in liver, but decreases plasma and kidney carnitine concentrations. *J Nutr Biochem* 1997; 8:68–73.

69. Hongu N, Sachan DS. Caffeine, carnitine and choline supplementation of rats decreases body fat and serum leptin concentration as does exercise. *J Nutr.* 2000;130:152–57.

70. Ulus IH, Wurtman RJ, Mauron C, Blusztajn JK. Choline increases acetylcholine release and protects against the stimulation-induced decrease in phosphatide levels within membranes of rat corpus striatum. *Brain Res.* 1989;484:217–27.

71. Zeisel SH. Choline: Human requirements and effects on human performance, in Marriott BM (Ed.) *Food Components to Enhance Performance,* Food and Nutrition Board, Institute of Medicine; Washington, D.C.: National Academy Press; 1994; p. 381–406.

72. Wurtman RJ, Hefti F, Melamed E. Precursor control of neurotransmitter synthesis. *Pharmacol Rev.* 1980;32:315–35.

73. Warber JP, Patton JF, Tharion WJ, Zeisel SH, Mello RP, Kemnitz CP, Lieberman HR. The effects of choline supplementation on physical performance. *Int J Sport Nutr Exerc Metab* 2000;10: 170–81.

74. Carter AL, Frenkel R. The relationship of choline and carnitine in the choline deficient rat. *J Nutr.* 1978;108:1748–54.

75. Dodson WL, Sachan DS. Choline supplementation reduces urinary carnitine excretion in humans. *Am J Clin Nutr.* 1996;63:904–10.

76. Sachan DS, Hongu N. Increases in VO(2)max and metabolic markers of fat oxidation by caffeine, carnitine and choline supplementation in rats. *J Nutr Biochem.* 2000;11:521–26.

77. Klein J, Koppen A, Loffelholz K. Uptake and storage of choline by rat brain: influence of dietary choline supplementation. *J Neurochem.* 1991;57:370–75.

78. Harris CM, Dysken MW, Fovall P, Davis JM. Effect of lecithin on memory in normal adults. *Am J Psychiat* 1983;140:1010–12.

79. Ladd SL, Sommer SA, LaBerge S, Toscano W. Effect of phosphatidylcholine on explicit memory. *Clin Neuropharmacol.* 1993;16:540–49.

80. Tan J, Bluml S, Hoang T, Dubowitz D, Mevenkamp G, Ross B. Lack of effect of oral choline supplement on the concentrations of choline metabolites in human brain. *Magn Reson Med.* 1998; 39:1005–10.

81. Ikegami S. Behavioral impairment in radial-arm maze learning and acetylcholine content of the hippocampus and cerebral cortex in aged mice. *Behav Brain Res.* 1994;65:103–11.

82. Crespo D, Megias M, Fernandez-Viadero C, Verduga R. Chronic treatment with a precursor of cellular phosphatidylcholine ameliorates morphological and behavioral effects of aging in the mouse [correction of rat] hippocampus. *Ann NY Acad Sci.* 2004;1019:41–43.

83. Lee YB, Lee HJ, Won MH, Hwang IK, Kang TC, Lee JY, Nam SY, Kim KS, Kim E, Cheon SH, Sohn HS. Soy isoflavones improve spatial delayed matching-to-place performance and reduce cholinergic neuron loss in elderly male rats. *J Nutr.* 2004;134:1827–31.

84. Adibhatla RM, Hatcher JF. Citicoline mechanisms and clinical efficacy in cerebral ischemia. *J Neurosci Res.* 2002;70:133–39.

85. McDaniel MA, Maier SF, Einstein GO. "Brain-specific" nutrients: a memory cure? *Nutrition* 2003;19:957–75.

86. Moreno M. Cognitive improvement in mild to moderate Alzheimer's dementia after treatment with the acetylcholine precursor choline alfoscerate: A multicenter, double-blind, randomized, placebo-controlled trial. *Clin Therap;* 2003;25:178–93.

87. Shronts EP. Essential nature of choline with implications for total parenteral nutrition. *J Am Diet Assoc.* 1997;97:639–46, 649.

88. Gaur SN, Agarwal G, Gupta SK. Use of LPC antagonist, choline, in the management of bronchial asthma. *Indian J Chest Dis Allied Sci.* 1997;39:107–13.

89. Gupta SK, Gaur SN. A placebo controlled trial of two dosages of LPC antagonist—choline in the management of bronchial asthma. *Indian J Chest Dis Allied Sci.* 1997;39:149–56.

90. Jacob RA, Jenden DJ, Allman-Farinelli MA, Swendseid ME. Folate nutriture alters choline status of women and men fed low choline diets. *J Nutr.* 1999;129:712–17.

91. Daily JW, III, Sachan DS. Choline supplementation alters carnitine homeostasis in humans and guinea pigs. *J Nutr.* 1995;125:1938–44.

92. Freeman-Narrod M. Choline antagonism of methotrexate liver toxicity in the rat. *Med Pediatr Oncol.* 1977;3:9–14.

93. Rehman HU. Fish odor syndrome. *Postgrad Med J* 1999;75:451–52.

94. Canty DJ, Zeisel SH. Lecithin and choline in human health and disease. *Nutr Rev.* 1994;52:327–39.

11 Vitamin A

Maria Stacewicz-Sapuntzakis and Gayatri Borthakur

CONTENTS

I. INTRODUCTION

Fat-soluble vitamin A is an essential factor for vision, growth and reproduction of all vertebrate animals, including humans. It is derived from certain carotenoid pigments synthesized by plants, long-chained hydrocarbon compounds, constructed of eight 5-carbon isoprene units (C_{40}). To possess provitamin A activity, the carotenoids must have at least one cyclical structure of the β-ionone ring on either end. β-Carotene, the orange-red pigment of carrots, theoretically may yield two molecules of vitamin A aldehyde (retinal)[1] by central cleavage (Figure 11.1). The resulting 20-carbon structure contains one β-ionone ring and a tetraene side chain. The aldehyde group can be irreversibly oxidized to retinoic acid, or reversibly reduced to a hydroxyl group (retinol), which in turn is esterified by long-chain fatty acids to form retinyl esters. The most common form of vitamin A is all-*trans*, but 11-*cis*-retinol is formed in the photoreceptors of retina as a necessary component of our visual system.[2]

II. SOURCES OF VITAMIN A

The major sources of vitamin A in our diet include the easily absorbed retinyl esters found in foods of animal origin, and the provitamin A carotenoids from fruits and vegetables, which usually have low bioavailability. Among 600 known carotenoids[3] about 50 are consumed by humans in their diet, but only a few serve as precursors for vitamin A. The most abundant provitamin A carotenoids are β-carotene, α-carotene and β-cryptoxanthin.[4] β-Carotene is the predominant carotenoid in orange-colored fruits and vegetables (carrots, pumpkin, squash, sweet potato, apricots, mango), as well as dark-green vegetables (spinach, collards, broccoli). Carrots, pumpkin and squash are also rich in α-carotene, while β-cryptoxanthin is found mainly in tangerines, orange juice, red peppers and persimmons.[5] The nutritional value of provitamin A carotenoids in the human body is based on their conversion rate to vitamin A, which depends on food matrix, presence of dietary fat, efficiency of absorption and health of the subjects.[6]

The conversion factors for provitamin A activity of carotenoids reflect the changing views on carotenoid bioavailability. In 1967 the World Health Organization (WHO) derived those factors from the studies of young vitamin A-deficient rats, and assumed that one-sixth of the

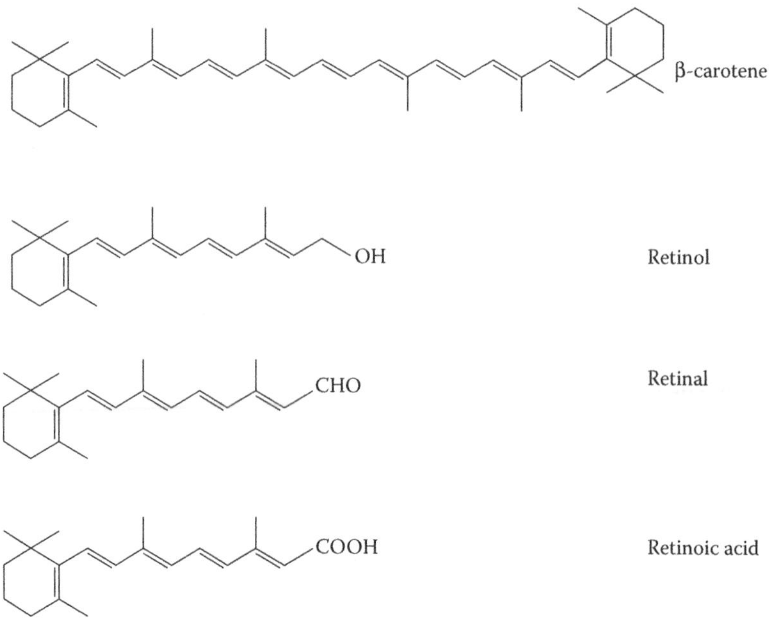

FIGURE 11.1 Structures of β–carotene and vitamin A compounds.

dietary provitamin A carotenoids are converted to retinol in humans.[7] Therefore, retinol equivalent (1 μg RE = 1 μg retinol) was defined as 6 μg β-carotene or 12 μg of other provitamin A carotenoids. However, more recent studies of stable isotope labeled vegetables ingested by well nourished human volunteers indicated much lower absorption and conversion rate.[8] Pureed carrots yielded only 1 μg of retinol from 15 μg of β-carotene, and spinach was even less productive (1 μg of retinol from 21 μg of β-carotene). In underdeveloped countries of Southeast Asia, plant-derived food was found to have very low vitamin A activity in combating vitamin A deficiency despite high carotenoid content.[9] In 2001, a new term, retinol activity equivalent (1 μg RAE = 1 μg retinol), was introduced by the U.S. Institute of Medicine.[4] It reduced the vitamin A activity of provitamin A carotenoids in plant-derived foods to half of their former value (1 RAE = 12 μg β-carotene or 24 μg of other provitamin A carotenoids), decreasing their share in total vitamin A intake, and also lowering the estimate of total vitamin A for any mixed food. However, the food and supplement labels still list total vitamin A content in International Units (1 IU = 0.3 μg retinol or 0.6 μg β-carotene), which were also used in many older reports of vitamin A nutrition among athletes and the general population. It generates a great deal of confusion, because only supplemental all-*trans*-β-carotene in oil or gelatin beadlets is efficiently absorbed in the intestine. Using the same conversion factor for carotenoids in plant food causes enormous sixfold overestimation of their vitamin A activity. The U.S. Department of Agriculture (USDA) only recently published an updated vitamin A activity database, expressed in RAE per common measure (average serving) and per 100 g of edible portion (Table 11.1).

Preformed vitamin A is found in animal products, fortified foods and supplements. The liver is the richest source of this vitamin, but significant amounts are also found in butter, milk, cheese and other dairy products, as well as in egg yolk. Margarine is usually fortified with retinyl palmitate to a level of 730 RAE/100 g. Fat droplets of milk naturally contain retinyl esters, but nonfat milk, fat-free cheese, reduced-fat dairy products and egg substitute are fortified to provide standard amounts of vitamin A. Preformed vitamin A is also added to many breakfast cereals.

Multivitamin formulas usually contain retinyl acetate or palmitate, and sometimes also β-carotene (5–100% of total vitamin A content). The standard amount of 5000 IU, or 100% of the daily value, listed on the supplement label, may be twice the currently recommended dietary allowance (RDA)

TABLE 11.1
Vitamin A Content of Foods Expressed in Retinol Activity Equivalents (RAE)

Provitamin A Sources		Preformed Vitamin A Sources	
Food Description	RAE/100g	Food Description	RAE/100g
Fruits		*Milk and Milk Products*	
Apricot, raw	131	Milk, nonfat, fluid, added vitamin A	61
Apricot, dry	180	Milk, low fat, 1%	59
Cantaloupe, cubes	160	Milk, reduced fat, 2%	56
Mango, raw	195	Butter	711
Tangerine	42	Margarine	731
		Margarine-like spread	729
Vegetables		Cottage cheese	44
Broccoli, cooked	69	Cheddar cheese	265
Carrots, raw	1406	Mozzarella cheese	205
Carrots, baby, raw	750	Swiss cheese	233
Collard greens, frozen, cooked	299	Cream cheese, fat free	282
Mustard greens	152	Cream, light whipping	287
Peppers, sweet, red, raw	285	Sour cream, reduced fat	107
Pumpkin, canned	1103	Cream, fluid, half and half	100
Pumpkin pie	426	Ice cream, vanilla	182
Spinach, frozen, cooked	389		
Spinach, canned	439	*Meat and Poultry Products*	
Sweet potato, baked	1091	Beef liver	7744
Butternut squash, cooked	167	Braunschweiger, pork	4221
Winter squash, baked	178	Chicken liver	4827
Turnip greens, frozen, cooked	399	Egg, large	192
		Egg yolk	584
		Egg substitute, liquid	108
		Other	
		Complete Bran Flakes, Kellogg	1293
		Cereals, fortified, oats, instant	256

Source: Adapted from USDA Nutrient Database for Standard Reference, Release 17 (2004).

for women,[4] but many multivitamins contain smaller doses of vitamin A (2500, 3000, or 3500 IU). Vitamin A is also available without prescription as a single supplement containing 1250–8000 IU per capsule (575–2400 μg retinol), and cod liver oil can be purchased as a liquid delivering 4000 IU (1200 μg retinol) per teaspoon. Single supplements of β-carotene usually contain 15 mg of this carotenoid, which is equivalent to 7500 μg RAE, because supplemental β-carotene is more bioavailable than dietary β-carotene from plant food (1 RAE = 2 μg of supplemental all-*trans*-β-carotene).[4]

III. ABSORPTION AND METABOLISM OF VITAMIN A

The absorption of carotenoids, vitamin A precursors, from dietary sources requires sufficient digestion of food to release carotenoids, and the formation of mixed micelles in the small intestine, aided by the presence of dietary fat and secretion of bile.[10] Processing of fruits and vegetables (cooking and mashing)[11] and addition of oily dressing to salads[12] greatly improves carotenoids bioavailability.

Preformed vitamin A is usually ingested in the form of retinyl esters. These esters are hydrolyzed in the intestinal lumen together with triglycerides by various pancreatic ester hydrolases,[13] and the resulting retinal is very efficiently absorbed by the intestinal mucosa. Inside enterocytes, provitamin A carotenoids are partially converted to retinal by central cleavage enzyme (15,15'-monooxygenase) or asymmetrically degraded to retinal by other enzymes.[14,15] These enzymes may be also expressed in other tissues (liver, kidney, testes), possibly producing limited amounts of vitamin A from locally stored carotenoids.[16] Retinal is immediately reduced to retinol, but a small percentage may be oxidized to retinoic acid. In the intestinal cell, both the absorbed and the newly formed retinol form a common pool, rapidly esterified by long-chain fatty acids and incorporated into chylomicrons. Chylomicron particles, composed mainly of triglycerides, transport retinyl esters and the unconverted carotenoids through the lymphatic system into the blood stream, and are taken up by the liver. Hepatic cells hydrolyze retinyl esters and repackage retinol for circulation in plasma as a complex with retinol-binding protein (RBP) and transthyretin. Excess retinol is reesterified and stored in stellate cells of the liver, which maintain steady-state levels of circulating retinol and buffer changes in dietary supply or tissue utilization. Within the tissues, the cells contain cellular retinol-binding protein (CRBP) and cellular retinoic acid-binding proteins (CRABP-I and II), as well as specific nuclear retinoid receptors, which allow various forms of vitamin A to fulfill their important functions in cell differentiation.

IV. FUNCTIONS OF VITAMIN A

Vitamin A constitutes a vital part of our visual system.[2] Photoreceptors of the retina in the eye (rods) contain rhodopsin, a photo-sensitive pigment composed of 11-*cis*-retinal and a protein, opsin. Visual impulse is produced when 11-cis-retinal absorbs a photon, changes to all-*trans*-retinal, and disengages from opsin. For continuous vision, rhodopsin must be regenerated by isomerization of all-*trans*-retinol to 11-*cis*-retinol and the oxidation of the latter to 11-*cis*-retinal. These reactions proceed in retinal pigment epithelium (RPE), which contains a local pool of retinyl esters and the specific enzymes. The visual cycle continues because 11-*cis*-retinal is transported back to the rods to combine with opsin. The first symptom of vitamin A deficiency is an impaired dark adaptation, which develops into night blindness.

Vitamin A, oxidized irreversibly to retinoic acid, is required for differentiation of epithelial tissues,[17] including cornea and conjunctival membranes of the eye. Progressive deficiency of vitamin A causes xerophthalmia and eventually destruction of the cornea, resulting in total blindness. Other epithelial tissues (skin, respiratory pathways, urogenital tract) also become hyperkeratinized — thickened, dry and scaly — which prevents their normal function and facilitates infections. In addition, retinoic acid is involved in normal immune function, maintaining proper numbers of white blood cells (natural killer cells, various classes of lymphocytes).[18] This role of retinoic acid is connected with the regulation of cell differentiation and proliferation, which leads to vitamin A involvement in normal reproduction, fetal development and growth. Retinoic acid regulates the expression of various genes encoding for important enzymes, structural proteins, transporters, receptors and growth factors. Specific patterns involving retinoic acid, retinoid receptors and retinoid-binding proteins were found to direct the embryonic development of vertebrae, spinal cord, limbs, viscera, eyes and ears, in timely and spatially appropriate sequence.[19]

Vitamin A deficiency symptoms are rare in the United States, but may include impaired dark adaptation, follicular hyperkeratosis and dryness of skin,[20] loss of appetite, and increased susceptibility to infections. Therefore, it was important to set estimated average requirement (EAR) for various age groups, based on average body weight and designed to maintain minimal acceptable liver reserves of vitamin A.[4] The RDA is designed to cover the needs of 97–98 % of the considered population, and in case of vitamin A, it exceeds EAR by 40 % (Table 11.2).

While it is very important to ingest adequate amounts to maintain optimal health, serious adverse effects are associated with excessive intake of preformed vitamin A. The tolerable upper

---

TABLE 11.2
Vitamin A Requirements and Recommendations (μg RAE/day)

Group (age)	EAR	RDA
Boys (14–18 y)	630	900
Girls (14–18 y)	485	700
Men (>18 y)	625	900
Women (>18 y)	500	700
Pregnant women	550	770
Lactating women	900	1300

Source: Adapted from Food and Nutrition Board, 2001[4].

---

intake level (UL) for adolescent boys and girls (14–18 y) is set at 2,800 μg retinol per day, and for adults at 3000 μg/day. Routine consumption of higher doses from animal products or retinol supplements may lead to chronic hypervitaminosis A. The long-term intakes above 1500 μg retinol/day have been associated with decreased bone mineral density and increased risk of hip fractures in older men and women.[21–23] A comparatively mild hypervitaminosis A may produce teratogenic effects in the fetus while not causing overt toxicity in the mother. Women who ingested more than 4,500 μg retinol/day were at greater risk to deliver a child with a cleft lip or palate than those consuming less than 1500 μg/day.[24] Chronic toxicity, usually associated with doses greater than 30,000 μg/day, is manifested by liver abnormalities, bone and joint pain, skin redness and desquamation, loss of hair, headache, irritability and loss of appetite. The most complete skeleton of *Homo erectus* discovered in Kenya shows pathological changes related to excessive intake of vitamin A, probably from carnivore livers.[25] Unfortunately, many athletes greatly exceed RDA by supplementation. Body builders take 18,000 μg retinol/day over a period of 4–6 weeks before a competition.[26] An adolescent soccer player experienced a strong leg pain after consuming at least 30,000 μg/day for 2 months.[27] The acute poisoning, after ingestion of more than 150 mg retinol by adults, causes an increase in cerebrospinal fluid pressure with resulting severe headache, disorientation, vomiting, blurred vision and loss of muscular coordination. Fatal cases were noted among polar explorers who ingested large amounts of polar bear, seal or husky-dog liver.[28,29]

In contrast to preformed vitamin A, large intakes of dietary provitamin A carotenoids do not cause hypervitaminosis A or exert any toxic effects. However, supplements of β-carotene are not recommended, especially among smokers and alcohol drinkers, because they may increase risk of cancer.[30–32] It is also not advisable to consume excessive amounts of any single food, be it a vegetable or animal product. Such a case was described in Japan, where a young woman consumed mainly pumpkin, liver and laver (a kind of edible seaweed), excluding other foods.[33] She developed hepatic injury, dry skin and limb edema, but recovered on a normal diet.

V. EVALUATION OF VITAMIN A INTAKE AMONG ATHLETES

A great majority of the available studies reported total vitamin A intake without specifying the proportion obtained from animal and plant sources, and many used International Units, which only added to the confusion when reporting total vitamin A intake from mixed foods and supplements. Recently introduced new conversion factors for vitamin A activity of carotenoids[4] render all previous reports inaccurate, because of the overestimated contribution from plant sources.

Adult athletes are usually well nourished in respect to the total vitamin A content of their diet. The cyclists of the Tour de France consumed adequate amounts of vitamin A (1.3 ± 0.4 mg daily) during the race.[34] However, individual variations can be quite large. Two elite U.S. male cyclists participating in an endurance ride (10 days, 2050 miles, 3300 km) had very different intake levels[35] — one consumed 87 % and the other 163% of the RDA, when all their food was measured and recorded by trained dietitians. A 4-year study at Syracuse University, New York[36] revealed enormous range of vitamin A total dietary intake among men's and women's teams across all sport disciplines. A Vitamin A-poor diet was consumed by 17% of the women in this study (< 66% RDA). Some men also had a low vitamin A diet, even among football players, and one wrestler had clinical signs of vitamin A deficiency (impaired dark adaptation, drying of mucous membranes). A smaller study of 30 field athletes (throwers) participating in South African national championships in 1988 (20 males, 10 females) found more than adequate vitamin A intake in a majority of the participants.[37] On the average, the men exceeded RDA by 380%, because some of them consumed large quantities of liver. However, 15% of the men had moderate intake of less than 100% but more than 67% RDA. The mean intake of women was 68% higher than RDA, with 30% of women falling into the moderate category. In a study of female collegiate heavyweight rowers, the women met 100% of the RDA for vitamin A.[38] Male cross-country runners had an average intake of twice the RDA.[39]

As can be seen from the above-mentioned studies, men are more likely to meet and exceed vitamin A requirements than women athletes, due to the higher amount of food consumed and the preference for animal products. Women are more likely to consume excessive amounts of raw vegetables and less fat, which can result in amenorrhea (cessation of menses). In a study of nutritional intakes of highly trained women marathon-runners,[40] the amenorrheic subjects had exceptionally high intakes of total vitamin A (20,359 IU ± 7688 IU), most of it probably in the form of dietary β-carotene, which was also indicated by the high correlation between the vitamin A activity and fiber (r = 0.94, P = 0.001). No such correlation was found in eumenorrheic (normal menses) runners, who selected more animal products, consumed more preformed vitamin A and significantly more fat. More than 30% of vitamin A in this group was provided by supplemental vitamin A in the form of retinol. These studies exemplify the paradoxical state of total vitamin A intake estimates, which do not reflect individual vitamin A status. High amounts of provitamin A carotenoids in the diet were converted by researchers to IU vitamin A activity according to the previously overestimated guidelines, while the amount of ingested preformed vitamin A was usually not reported.

Adolescent athletes may be at a greater risk of inadequate or overabundant vitamin A intake than adults, because of their attitudes, poor knowledge of nutrition and the continuing growth and development of their bodies. A group of 27 female high school athletes (13–17 y) averaged 102 ± 95% RDA for total dietary vitamin A,[41] slightly better than other teenage girls in the U.S, but, although 81% of the subjects were aware of foods high in vitamin A, only 42% of them met the allowance. Male high school football athletes (12–18 y, n = 134) on the average exceeded RDA,[42] but 20% of junior high school and 32% of senior high school boys had intakes below 70% RDA for vitamin A activity. Very young Turkish female gymnasts (11.5 ± 0.5 y) were reported to meet 87% of RDA for total vitamin A.[43] Italian adolescent female athletes (gymnasts, tennis, fencing, n = 119, 14–18 y) had better knowledge of nutrition and significantly higher intake of total vitamin A (805 ± 500 RE) than a control group of age-matched non-athletes (612 ± 408 RE).[44] The elite rhythmic gymnasts of the same age group (n = 20) had even higher total vitamin A diet (1027 ± 569 RE).[45] The wide ranges of intake registered in these studies indicate that many adolescent athletes do not meet their recommendations, and a plausible average should not invalidate the necessary vigilance and attention to the individual diet of each young competitor.

Although many of the described studies mention the use of vitamin supplements among the athletes, the amount and form of vitamin A is usually not specified and not included in the total estimate of vitamin A intake. It is a very important issue because the supplements usually deliver 100% of RDA in one dose, often as retinyl esters, and it is easy to exceed the upper tolerance level of vitamin A intake by taking multiple doses or high-potency supplements in addition to a diet rich in animal products. The supplement use among University of Nebraska-Lincoln athletes (n = 411) was investigated in 1997 and found to be quite prevalent (57% of subjects).[46] Most supplement users were taking multivitamins and minerals, but 10 male subjects reported taking vitamin A supplements. African American males used vitamin A much more frequently than other ethnic groups (P < 0.001). The use of dietary supplements is also higher among former top-level athletes than in the general population. A large study of former male athletes (n = 1282) in Finland found that 9.2% of them used vitamin A supplements,[47] as compared with 5.0% of age-matched controls (P = 0.003). The habit of taking vitamin supplements may have persisted in the athletes from the time of their athletic careers (1920–1965), with possible detrimental effects for their risk of osteoporosis,[21–23] Among the U.S. high school students, greater knowledge about supplements was associated with less use.[48] Nevertheless, 42% of all students used multivitamins and 13% used vitamin A supplements; 34% did not know that taking high doses of vitamin A can be harmful.

VI. VITAMIN A STATUS AND EXERCISE PHYSIOLOGY

The best available assessment of vitamin A status is obtained from analysis of serum or plasma by high-performance liquid chromatography (HPLC)[49] after extraction with organic solvents. The method separates retinol, the major form of vitamin A in plasma, from retinyl esters, which are usually absent in samples from fasting subjects. High amounts of retinyl esters in plasma indicate recent intake of preformed vitamin A (diet or supplement) or excessive habitual consumption, with possible toxicity and liver overload. The high levels may also be a symptom of liver disease due to alcoholism.[50]

Plasma retinol concentration below 0.7 μmol/L (20 μg/dL) indicates a deficient vitamin A status, while the levels between 0.7 and 1.05 μmol/L (20–30 μg/dL) are marginal and predict low liver stores.[51] The normal range of plasma retinol in adults appears to be highly regulated within the range of 1.1–2.8 μmol/L (30–80 μg/dL). Levels above this range indicate excessive intake of preformed vitamin A with possible consequences of increased bone fragility and other symptoms of vitamin A toxicity. The mean serum retinol concentration in U.S. population is 1.92 μmol/L according to NHANES III (1988–1994) with only 5% below 1.1 μmol/L, but close to 10% above 2.8 μmol/L.[52]

In the U.S. and other developed countries, the excessive intake of vitamin A is more prevalent than vitamin A deficiency, but both conditions could be very detrimental to the health and performance of athletes at any age. When serum levels of retinol were tested in German national teams, none of the athletes (n = 24) exhibited vitamin A inadequacy (1.7 to 3.2 μmol/L), and some could be considered above the recommended limit.[26] Highly trained Spanish athletes (n = 38) had significantly higher plasma retinol than the sedentary control subjects (1.9 ± 0.3 versus 1.5 ± 0.3 μmol/L, P < 0.05).[53] Top soccer (n = 21) and basketball (n = 9) players in Belgium had even higher levels of plasma vitamin A, 2.6 ± 0.5 and 2.8 ± 0.2 μmol/L, respectively, after 4 months of regular training and competition.[54] Physically active older women in the Netherlands (n = 25, 60–80y) had an average of 3.0 ± 0.4 μmol/L, practically identical to their sedentary controls, despite higher consumption of fruits and vegetables in the active group, and of milk and meat in the controls.[55] Similar results were obtained from a study of physically active male veterans (n = 26, 69 ± 7y) participating in Golden Age Games in the U.S.[56] Serum concentrations of retinol were 2.3 ± 0.8 μmol/L, nearly the same as in sedentary controls, although their intake of β-carotene significantly exceeded that of controls. These data confirm that provitamin A carotenoid intake has little effect on the levels of circulating retinol, and will not produce vitamin A toxicity.

Strenuous exercise may raise oxygen consumption and increase free radical production, leading to lipid peroxidation and possible tissue damage.[57] Vitamin A, although not a strong antioxidant, is probably required for tissue repair, therefore an increased turnover of vitamin A may be expected under conditions of increased physical activity. The effects of vitamin A supplementation on physical performance are not well investigated. No decrease of ability to perform hard exercise was noted in men maintained on a vitamin A-deficient diet for 6 months and it did not improve after 6 weeks of high supplementation.[58] However, the subjects consumed a daily supplement of 22,500 μg vitamin A for one month before the study and probably had ample liver stores.

A few older studies observed transient changes in serum vitamin A immediately after exercise. A group of young athletes (n = 12) exhibited a striking 43% increase of serum vitamin A following strenuous physical activity consisting of a 15 min warm-up and five or six 220-yard (201-m) dashes at full speed at intervals of 5 min.[59] Similar results were found in another study of 14 males performing a step-up test.[60] Both studies used an old colorimetric assay of vitamin A, which was prone to inconsistent results. However, a more recent study of seven trained athletes also found a significant 18% increase in plasma retinol concentration after completing a half-marathon, as measured by HPLC assay, which was not explained by dehydration (6% decrease in plasma volume).[61] Another investigation of amateur and professional cyclists[62] observed no differences in plasma retinol of both groups, before and after prolonged exercise tests and a mountain stage (170-km) of cycling competition. The well-trained amateur cyclists were submitted to the maximal and submaximal tests on cycloergometer, the professional cyclists participated in the Volta Ciclisto a Mallorca race. Their basal values of plasma retinol were all very close, averaging 2.0 μmol/L. A quite different effect of exercise on plasma retinol was noted in volunteers from the U.S. Marine Corps (n = 40) undergoing strenuous training for 24 days in a cold environment,[63] resulting in an average loss of 5 kg body weight. Retinol levels decreased from 1.7 to 1.4 μmol/L (P < 0.005) in the control group (n = 19) and from 1.7 to 1.6 μmol/L in the treatment group (n = 21) receiving antioxidant supplements, which included 24 mg β-carotene/day, vitamins C and E, selenium, catechin, but not preformed vitamin A.

Because the liver contains 90% of body vitamin A,[64] the body stores of vitamin A are best assessed by liver biopsy, which is too invasive for healthy subjects. Indirect approaches include isotope dilution technique, relative dose response and modified relative dose response. These methods involve administering an oral dose of stable-isotope-labeled vitamin A, an unlabeled vitamin A, or vitamin A_2 (dehydroretinol), respectively. Blood samples are taken after a specified period of equilibration or prescribed interval, and the results are used to assess adequacy of liver stores. Unfortunately, these techniques were not used in studies of athletes or other human subjects performing heavy physical exercise. Studies with laboratory rats indicated a significant decrease in liver vitamin A content after 12 days of daily 90-min exercise on a moving track at 20 m/min.[65] Shorter sessions of exercise elicited a proportionately smaller effect. Kidney levels of vitamin A remained stable, as did plasma levels. These results could indicate a significant mobilization of vitamin A stores from the liver during strenuous exercise if the subject remains on a vitamin A-deficient diet. The assessment of plasma retinol may not reveal any deficiency until liver stores are severely depleted; indeed, plasma levels may even be elevated by exercise. However, another study of rats found a significantly lower concentration of retinol in plasma of animals subjected to training exercise (40 min/d, 5 d/week for 8 weeks at 70% of their VO_2max) compared with sedentary animals.[66] The mitochondrial membranes from liver and skeletal muscle of exercised animals contained significantly more vitamin A than those of sedentary rats. The differences were more pronounced in animals exercised to exhaustion just before sacrifice, and the effect was not cancelled by 30 min rest after the acute exercise session. A study of trained sled dogs[67] found a very significant rise in serum retinyl esters after a 7.5-km race (18–28 min), suggesting their mobilization from liver and adipose tissue. Dogs and many other carnivores have high levels of plasma retinyl esters, even while fasting, because of unspecific transport in plasma lipoprotein fraction.

The equivocal results of the described human and animal intervention studies stem from differences in physiology and methodology. The researchers used different tests, different intensities and varying duration of exercise, but nevertheless the outcomes indicate that sustained physical labor may increase mobilization and utilization of vitamin A.

VII. SUMMARY

Because of its role in cellular differentiation, optimal intake of vitamin A is crucial for general health, athletic performance and the recovery from strenuous exercise. Recent recommendations limit the optimal intake to 900 μg RAE for males and 700 μg RAE for women of any age above

14 years. The tolerable upper intake level should not exceed 2800 µg retinol for adolescents (14–18 years) and 3000 µg retinol for all adults. High levels of vitamin A supplementation will not improve athletic condition, and may cause direct toxicity symptoms, including bone pain, headaches or peeling of skin (desquamation). Even a relatively mild oversupply of vitamin A might induce teratogenic effects in fetal development and increase the risk of osteoporosis in older men and women. Estimates of vitamin A dietary intake among athletes in developed countries indicate adequate nutrition, but suffer from methodological problems of inaccurate reporting by subjects, changing and confusing rules of vitamin A activity conversion for carotenoids in plant based foods and the habit of reporting vitamin A from all sources together, without specifying the proportion from animal sources, fortified foods and supplements on one side, and provitamin A carotenoids on the other. The dietary interview is not sufficient to determine vitamin A status, which should be confirmed by serum analysis, measuring retinol, retinyl esters and individual carotenoids. If serum retinol values are found to be below 1.05 µmol/L (30 µg/dL), it is helpful to perform a noninvasive test of liver stores of vitamin A using the relative dose response procedure or the dark adaptation test.

In general, to avoid possible toxicity, no supplements of preformed vitamin A should be used by athletes. However, an intake of 900 µg preformed vitamin A daily from animal or fortified food products should probably be recommended to all strenuously exercising athletes, since it is uncertain how much (if any) vitamin A is produced by conversion from carotenoids. The current recommendation of 2.5 cups of vegetables and 2 cups of fruits, preferably red, orange and dark green, for a reference 2000 kcal daily intake[68] should be followed to provide carotenoids and other healthful phytochemicals but not as a means of obtaining necessary vitamin A.

The review points to the great need of more accurate assessment of dietary intake and concomitant physiological vitamin A status of athletes, together with measurements of their athletic performance. However, to help athletes to select the best diet and preserve their health, the best available research methodology and recent nutrition guidelines[68] should be universally accepted and used to produce more precise data.

REFERENCES

1. Goodman, D.S. and Blaner, W.S., Biosynthesis, absorption, and hepatic metabolism of retinol, in *The Retinoids*, vol. 2, Sporn, M.B., Roberts, A.B., Goodman, D.S., Eds., Academic Press, New York, 1984, 4.
2. Saari, J.C., Retinoids in photosensitive systems, in *The Retinoids: Biology, Chemistry, and Medicine*, 2nd ed , Sporn, M.B., Roberts, A.B., Goodman, D.S., Eds., New York: Raven Press, 1994, 351.
3. Britton, G., Liaaen-Jensen, S., and Pfander, H., Carotenoids today and challenges for the future, in *Carotenoids*, Vol. 1A, Isolation and Analysis, Birkhauser-Verlag, Basel, 1995, 15.
4. Food and Nutrition Board, Institute of Medicine, Dietary Reference Intakes for Vitamin A, Vitamin K, Arsenic, Boron, Chromium, Copper, Iodine, Iron, Manganese, Molybdenum, Nickel, Silicon, Vanadium, and Zinc, National Academy Press, Washington, D.C., 2001, 82.
5. Stacewicz-Sapuntzakis, M., and Diwadkar-Navsariwala, V., Carotenoids, in *Nutritional Ergogenic Aids*, Wolinsky, I., and Driskell, J.A. Eds., CRC Press, Washington D.C., 2004, 325.
6. van Lieshout, M., West, C.E., Muhilal, P.D., Wang, Y., Xu, X., van Breeman, R.B., Creemers, A.F.L., Verhoeven, M.A., and Lugtenburg, J., Bioefficacy of β-carotene dissolved in oil studied in children in Indonesia, *Am. J. Clin. Nutr.*, 73, 949, 2001.
7. Food and Agriculture Organization / World Health Organization, Requirements of Vitamin A, Thiamin, Riboflavin and Niacin, Report of a Joint FAO and WHO Expert Group, FAO Nutrition Meeting Report Series no. 41, and Technical Series WHO no. 362, Geneva, 1967.
8. Tang, G., Qin, J., Dolnikowski, G.G., Russell, R.M., and Grusak, M.A., Vitamin A value of spinach and carrots as assessed using a stable isotope reference method in adults, *FASEB J.*, 18, A157, 2004.
9. West, C.E., Eilander, A., and van Lieshout, M., Consequences of revised estimates of carotenoid bioefficacy for the dietary control of vitamin A deficiency in developing countries, *J. Nutr.*, 132, 2920S, 2002.
10. Furr, H.C., and Clark, R.M., Intestinal absorption and tissue distribution of carotenoids, *J. Nutr. Biochem.*, 8, 364,1997.

11. Stahl, W., and Sies, H., Uptake of lycopene and its geometrical isomers is greater from heat-processed than from unprocessed tomato juice in humans, *J. Nutr.*, 122, 2161, 1992.

12. Brown, M., Ferruzzi, M.G., Nguyen, M.L., Cooper, D.A., Eldridge, A.L., Schwartz, S.J., and White, W.S., The bioavailability of carotenoids is higher in salad ingested with full-fat versus fat-reduced salad dressings as measured by using electrochemical detection, *Am. J. Clin. Nutr.*, 80, 396, 2004.

13. Harrison, E.H., Enzymes catalyzing the hydrolysis of retinyl esters, *Biochim. Biophys.* Acta, 99, 1170, 1993.

14. Krinsky, N.I., Wang, X.D., Tang, G., and Russell, R.M., Mechanism of carotenoid cleavage to retinoids, *Ann. NY Acad. Sci.*, 167, 691, 1993.

15. Yeum, K. J., and Russell, R., Carotenoid bioavailability and bioconversion, *Ann. Rev. Nutr.*, 22, 483, 2002.

16. Wyss, A., Carotene oxygenases: a new family of double bond cleavage enzymes, *J. Nutr.*, 134, 246S, 2004.

17. Gudas, L.J., Sporn, M.B., and Roberts, A.B., Cellular biology and biochemistry of the retinoids, in *The Retinoids: Biology, Chemistry, and Medicine*, 2nd ed, Sporn, M.B., Roberts, A.B., Goodman, D.S., Eds., New York: Raven Press, 1994, 443.

18. Zhao, Z., and Ross, A.C., Retinoic acid repletion restores the number of leukocytes and their subsets and stimulates natural cytotoxicity in vitamin A-deficient rats, *J. Nutr.*, 125, 2064, 1995.

19. Morriss-Kay, G.M., and Sokolova, N., Embryonic development and pattern formation, *FASEB J.*, 10, 961, 1996.

20. Sauberlich, H.E., Hodges, H.E., Wallace, D.L., Kolder, H., Canham, J.E., Hood, J., Raica, N., Lowry, L.K., Vitamin A metabolism and requirements in the humans studied with the use of labeled retinol, *Vitam. Horm.*, 32, 251, 1974.

21. Melhus, H., Michaelsson, K., Kindmark, A., Excessive dietary intake of vitamin A is associated with reduced bone mineral density and increased risk for hip fracture, *Ann. Intern. Med.*, 129, 1998, 770.

22. Feskanich, D., Singh, V., Willett, W.C., and Colditz, G.A., Vitamin A intake and hip fractures among postmenopausal women, *J. Am. Med. Assoc.*, 287, 47, 2002.

23. Michaelsson, K., Lithell, H., Vessby, B., and Melhus, H., Serum retinol levels and the risk of fracture, *N. Eng. J. Med.*, 348, 287, 2003.

24. Rothman, K.J., Moore, L.L., Singer, M.R., Nguygen, U.D.T., Mannino, S., and Milunsky, B., Teratogenicity of high vitamin A intake, *N. Engl. J. Med.*, 333, 1369, 1995.

25. Walker, A., Zimmerman, M.R., and Leakey, R.E.F., A possible case of hypervitaminosis A in Homo erectus, *Nature*, 296, 248, 1982.

26. Rokitzki, L., Berg, A., and Keul, J., Blood and serum status of water and fat soluble vitamins in athletes and non-athletes, in *Elevated Dosages of Vitamins*, Walteer, P., Brubacher, G., and Stahelin, H., Eds., Hans Huber Publishers, Lewiston, NY, 1989, 192.

27. Fumich, R., and Essig, G., Hypervitaminosis: A case report on an adolescent soccer player, *Am. J. Sports Med.*, 11, 37, 1983.

28. Gerber, A., Raab, A.P., and Sobel, A.E., Vitamin A poisoning in adults; with description of a case, *Am. J. Med.*, 16, 729, 1954.

29. Shearman, D.J.C., Vitamin A and Sir Douglas Mawson, *Br. Med. J.*, 1, 283, 1978.

30. Albanes, D., Heinonen, O.P., Taylor, P.R., Virtamo, J., Edwards, B.K., Rautalahti, M., Hartman, A.M., Palmgren, J., Freedman, L.S., Haapokaski, J., Barrett, M.J., Pietinen, P., Malila, N., Tala, E., Liippo, K., Salomaa, E.R., Tangrea, J.A., Teppo, L., Askin, F.B., Taskinen, E., Erozan, Y., Greenwald, P., and Huttunen, J.K., α-Tocopherol and β- carotene supplements and lung cancer incidence in the Alpha-Tocopherol Beta-Carotene Prevention Study: effects of baseline characteristics and study compliance, *J. Natl Cancer Inst.*, 88, 1560, 1996.

31. Omenn, G.S., Goodman, G.E., Thornquist, M.D., Balmes, J., Cullen, M.R., Glass, A., Keogh, J.P., Jr., Meyskens, F.L., Jr., Valanis, B., Williams, J.H., Jr., Barnhart, S., Cherniack, M.G., Brodkin, C.A., and Hammar, S., Risk factors for lung cancer and for intervention effects in CARET, the Beta-Carotene and Retinol Efficacy Trial, *J. Natl. Cancer Inst.*, 88, 1550, 1996.

32. Baron, J.A., Cole, B.F., Mott, L., Haile, R., Grau, M., Church, T.R., Beck, G.J., and Greenberg, E.R., Neoplastic and antineoplastic effects of β-carotene on colorectal adenoma recurrence: results of a randomized trial, *J. Natl Cancer Inst.*, 95, 717, 2003.

33. Nagai, K., Hosaka, H., Kubo, S., Nakabayashi, T., Amagasaki, Y., and Nakamura, N., Vitamin A toxicity secondary to excessive intake of yellow-green vegetables, liver and laver, *J. Hepatol.*, 31, 142, 1999.

34. Saris, W.H.M., Schrijver, J.V., Erp Baart, M.A., and Brouns, F., Adequacy of vitamin supply under maximal sustained workloads: The Tour de France, in *Elevated Dosages of Vitamins*, Walter, P., Brubacher, G., and Stahelin, H., Eds., Hans Huber Publishers, Lewiston, NY, 205, 1989.

35. Gabel, K.A., Aldous, A., and Edgington, C., Dietary intake of two elite male cyclists during 10-day, 2050 mile ride, *Int. J. Sport Nutr.*, 5, 56, 1995.

36. Short, S.H., and Short, W.R., Four year study of university athletes dietary intake, *J. Am. Diet. Assoc.*, 82, 632, 1983.

37. Faber, M., and Spinnler Benade, A.J., Mineral and vitamin intake in field athletes (discus-, hammer-, javelin-throwers and shotputters), *Int. J. Sports Med.*, 12, 324, 1991.

38. Nelson, S.S., Mayer, K., Brownell, K.D., and Wadden, T.A., Dietary intake of female collegiate heavyweight rowers, *Int. J. Sport Nutr.*, 5, 225, 1995.

39. Niekamp, R.A., and Baer, J.T., In-season dietary adequacy of trained male cross-country runners, *Int. J. Sport Nutr.*, 5, 45, 1995.

40. Deuster, P.A., Kyle, S.B., Vigersky, R.A., Singh, A., and Schoomaker, E.B., Nutritional intakes and status of highly trained amenorrheic and eumenorrheic women runners, *Fertil. Steril.*, 46, 636, 1986.

41. Perron, M., and Endres, J., Knowledge, attitudes, and dietary practices of female athletes, *J. Am. Diet. Assoc.*, 85, 573, 1985.

42. Hickson, J.H., Jr., Duke, M.A., Johnson, C.W., and Stockton, J.E., Nutritional intake from food sources of high school football athletes, *J. Am. Diet. Assoc.*, 87, 1656, 1987.

43. Ersoy, G., Dietary status and anthropometric assessment of child gymnasts, *J. Sports Med. Phys. Fitness*, 31, 577, 1991.

44. Cupisti, A., D'Alessandro, C., Castrogiovanni, S., Barale, A., and Morelli, E., Nutrition knowledge and dietary composition in Italian adolescent female athletes and non-athletes, *Int. J. Sport Nutr. Exerc. Metab.*, 12, 207, 2002.

45. Cupisti, A., D'Alessandro, S., Castrogiovanni, A., and Barale, M.E., Nutrition survey in elite rhythmic gymnasts, *J. Sports Med. Phys. Fitness*, 40, 350, 2000.

46. Krumbach, C.J., Ellis, D.R., and Driskell, J.A., A report of vitamin and mineral supplement use among university athletes in a division I institution, *Int. J. Sport Nutr.*, 9, 416, 1999.

47. Kujala, U.M., Sarna, S., and Kaprio, J., Use of medications and dietary supplements in later years among male former top-level athletes, *Arch. Intern. Med.*, 163, 1064, 2003.

48. Massad, S.J., Shier, N.W., Koceja, D.M., and Elliss, N.T., High school athletes and nutritional supplements: A study of knowledge and use, *Int. J. Sport Nutr.*, 5, 232, 1995.

49. Stacewicz-Sapuntzakis, M., Bowen, P.E., Kikendall, J.W., and Burgess, M., Simultaneous determination of serum retinol and various carotenoids: their distribution in middle-aged men and women, *J. Micronutr. Anal.*, 3, 27, 1987.

50. Mobarhan, S., Seitz, H.K., Russel, R.M., Mehta, R., Hupert, J., Friedman H., Layden, T.J., Meydani, M., and Langenberg, P., Age-related effects of chronic ethanol intake on vitamin A status in Fisher 344 rats, *J. Nutr.*, 121, 150, 1991.

51. Underwood B.A., Hypervitaminosis A: International programmatic issues, *J. Nutr.*, 124, 1467S, 1994.

52. Bollew, C., Bowmen, B.A., Sowell, A.L., and Gillespie, C., Serum retinol distributions in residents of the United States: Third National Health and Nutrition Examination Survey, 1988–1994, *Am. J. Clin. Nutr.*, 73, 586, 2001.

53. Sanchez-Quesada, J.L., Ortega, H., Payes-Romero, A., Serrat-Serrat, J., Gonzalez-Sastre, F., Lasuncion, M.A., and Ordonez-Llanos, J., LDL from aerobically trained subjects shows higher resistance to oxidative modification than LDL from sedentary subjects, *Atherosclerosis*, 132, 207, 1997.

54. Pincemail, J., Lecomte, J., Castiau, J.P., Collard, E., Vasankari, T., Cheramy-Bien, J.P., Limet, R., and Defraigne, J.O., Evaluation of autoantibodies against oxidized LDL and antioxidant status in top soccer and basketball players after 4 months of competition, *Free Rad. Biol. Med.*, 28, 559 2000.

55. Voorrips, L.E., van Staveren, W.A., and Hautvast, J.G.A.J., Are physically active elderly women in a better nutritional condition than their sedentary peers?, *Eur. J. Clin. Nutr.*, 45, 545, 1991.

56. Kazi, N., Murphy, P.A., Connor, E.S., Bowen, P.E., Stacewicz-Sapuntzakis, M., and Iber, F.L., Serum antioxidant and retinol levels in physically active vs. physically inactive elderly veterans, in *National Veterans Golden Age Games Research Monograph*, Langbein, W.E., Wyman, D.J., and Osis, A., Eds., Edward Hines, Jr., VA Hospital, Hines, IL, 1995, 50.

57. Kanter, M.M., Free radicals, exercise, and antioxidant supplementation, *Int. J. Sport Nutr.*, 4, 205, 1994.

58. Wald, G., Brouha, L., and Johnson, R., Experimental human vitamin A deficiency and ability to perform muscular exercise, *Am. J. Physiol.*, 137, 551, 1942.
59. James, W.H., and El Gindi, I.M., Effect of strenuous physical activity on blood vitamin A and carotene in young men, *Science*, 118, 629, 1953.
60. Hillman, R.W., and Rosner, M.C., Effects of exercise on blood (plasma) concentrations of vitamin A, carotene and tocopherols, *J. Nutr.*, 64, 605, 1958.
61. Duthie, G.G., Robertson, J.D., Maugham, R.J., and Morrice, P.C., Blood antioxidant status and erythrocyte lipid peroxidation following distance running, *Arch. Biochem. Biophys.*, 282, 78, 1990.
62. Aguilo, A., Tauler, P., Pilar, G. M., Villa, G., Cordova, A., Tur, J.A., and Pons, A., Effect of exercise intensity and training on antioxidants and cholesterol profile in cyclists, *J. Nutr. Biochem.*, 14, 319, 2003.
63. Schmidt, M.C., Askew, E.W., Roberts, D.E., Prior, R.L., Ensign, W.Y., and Hesslink, R.E., Oxidative stress in humans training in a cold, moderate altitude environment and their response to a phytochemical antioxidant supplement, *Wilderness Environ. Med.*, 13, 94, 2002.
64. Olson, J.A., Recommended dietary intakes (RDI) of vitamin A in humans, *Am. J. Clin. Nutr.*, 45, 704, 1987.
65. Kobylinski, Z., Gronowska-Senger, A., and Swabula, D., Effect of exercise on vitamin A utilization by rat organism (in Polish), *Rocz. Panstw. Zakl. Hig.*, 41, 247, 1990.
66. Quiles, J.L., Huertas, J.R., Manas, M., Ochoa, J.J., Battino, M., and Mataix, J., Oxidative stress induced by exercise and dietary fat modulates the coenzyme Q and vitamin A balance between plasma and mitochondria, *Int. J. Vitam. Nutr. Res.*, 69, 243, 1999.
67. Raila, J., Stohrer, M. Forterre, S., Stangassinger, M., Schweigert, F.J., Effect of exercise on the mobilization of retinol and retinyl esters in plasma of sled dogs, *J. Anim. Physiol. Anim. Nutr.*, 88, 234, 2004.
68. U.S. Department of Health and Human Services, U.S Department of Agriculture, Dietary Guidelines for Americans 2005, www.healthierus.gov/dietaryguidelines, 2005.

12 Vitamins D and K

Douglas S. Kalman

CONTENTS

Vitamin D

I. INTRODUCTION

Vitamin D was classified by scientists as any substance that possessed an anti-rickets property almost 100 years ago. As this was first stated in the 20th century, we have since learned that vitamin D has many functions in the body. For the most part, vitamin D is associated with deficiency states and is not viewed as a true ergogenic substance.

Vitamin D occurs in many different forms within the body. Its active form is $1,25(OH)_2D_3$, otherwise known as calcitriol. Calcitriol is a steroid hormone, thus vitamin D can be considered a prohormone.[1–3] Calcitriol is a hormone that is released by the kidney and taken up by other organs throughout the body. It acts upon the heart, brain, stomach, intestines, bones and within the kidneys.

Calcitriol is transported throughout the body in the blood via an alpha-2-globulin, known as a vitamin D-binding protein.

II. METABOLISM

Vitamin D is a fat-soluble vitamin that is primarily absorbed through the intestinal tract (small intestine) via the inclusion of chylomicrons from transport through the lymphatic system.[4] Calcitriol, an active steroid hormone, is created when stimulation of parathyroid hormone (PTH) occurs. The stimulated PTH will cause a downstream effect of stimulating 1-hydroxylase activity in the kidney so that the vitamin D precursor 25 hydroxyvitamin D_3 (25-OH D_3) is produced. The 25-OH D_3 is converted into active calcitriol.

$1,25(OH)_2D_3$ can be formed from compounds in the skin (via exposure to sunlight). Seven-dehydrocholesterol (7-dehydrocholesterol) is formed in the liver and stored in the skin, where it is converted by "previtamin D_3" via the ultraviolet rays of the sun or other UV light source. The vitamin D_3 ultimately is converted into $1,25(OH)_2D_3$ through hydroxylation reactions in the kidneys and liver as the dietary vitamin D_3 form is hydroxylated.

III. FUNCTION

The primary role of vitamin D is to maintain homeostasis of calcium and phosphorus to maintain bone formation and maintenance, neuromuscular function and other cellular processes.

The primary site of calcitriol's action is within the intestinal tract. Specifically, calcitriol acts upon target tissue to spur the uptake of calcium and phosphorus.[2] Calcitriol will interact with receptors within the enterocyte, where it is carried to the nucleus interacting with specific genes that encode the proteins that are specifically involved in calcium transport.[5] Calcium is extracted from the enterocyte via plasma transport, where it helps to maintain serum calcium concentrations. Calcitriol also affects the activity of alkaline phosphatase so that a greater hydrolyzation of phosphate-ester bonds occurs, allowing for greater phosphorus absorption.

Calcitriol directly affects the mobilization of both calcium and phosphorus from the bone to the bloodstream. Osteoclast activity is enhanced, while also affecting osteocalcin, a protein found in bone that also positively affects bone formation. It is also now thought that calcitriol initiates the differentiation of stem cells to osteoclasts, which aid in bone resorption and release of calcium into the bloodstream.

Besides calcitriol's interactions with calcium and phosphorus, there are also vitamin–vitamin and vitamin–mineral interactions with vitamin K and iron. Iron deficiency will also cause a concomitant decrease in vitamin D absorption.

A recent study evaluated the chemoequivalaence of vitamins D_2 and D_3. Twenty healthy male volunteers were given 50,000 international units (IUs) of each of the respective calciferols over a period of 28 days. The objective was to evaluate the relative potencies of vitamins D_2 and D_3. The two calciferols produced similar rises in serum concentration of the respective vitamins, indicating a probable equivalent absorption. However, when examining the time-course changes and differences between the two forms of vitamin D, it became apparent that by day 14, the serum concentration of D_2, but not D_3 peaked (started to fall, while D_3 remained elevated). In fact, when examining the pharmacokinetic data, it appears that vitamin D_3 has a far greater therapeutic value (about a 9.5 : 1 ratio) than vitamin D_2. The conclusion has meaning for those who deal with the therapeutic treatment of vitamin deficiencies (or malnutrition). Vitamin D_2 has a shorter duration of activity and is of lower potency than an equidose of vitamin D_3.[6]

As it is essential that calcium be present in the sarcoplasmic reticulum for the muscle to contract, it may be possible that $1,25 (OH)_2D_3$ can affect the uptake of calcium through enhancing uptake in high-voltage calcium channels. Theoretically, if one can enhance calcium uptake via a stimulated sarcoplasmic reticulum, it may be possible that strength or muscle contractions can be enhanced.

IV. EXERCISE RELATED RESEARCH—ANIMALS

No current published studies are specific for examining the effect of vitamin D on performance, recovery, muscle strength or frailty.

V. EXERCISE RELATED RESEARCH—HUMANS

There has not been much interest in vitamin D within the sports nutrition or exercise physiology community. Early studies examining the effects of vitamin D supplementation of physical working capacity were conducted in young children. The study utilized a range of doses of the vitamin, with none demonstrating any ergogenic effect.[7]

As humans age, there is a concurrent lost of muscle mass. This loss of muscle mass (sarcopenia) may be mitigated to a great degree if the aging individual engages in resistance training. However, it is not known whether receptors that are located within muscle tissue also decrease with age. Bischoff-Ferrari et al. examined intracellular 1,25-dihydroxyvitamin D receptor expression (VDR). In fact, in this study, where older women had biopsies of their gluteus medius or transversospinalis taken, it was found that all were receptor positive for vitamin D. However, increased age was associated with decreased VDR expression.[8] The importance of this finding of decreased vitamin D receptor expression becomes apparent when examining the effects of genetics of muscle strength. Grundberg and Berven from Sweden examined genetic variation in human vitamin D receptor and its association with vital markers of health in Swedish women. This study of 175 healthy women examined the genetic variation in VDR and its association with muscle strength, fat mass and body weight. Utilizing polymer chain reaction (PCR) to identify polymorphic regions in the VDR gene, these scientists were able to provide us with some interesting findings. VDR polymorphisms also appear to lead to osteoporosis. Reduced serum 25-hydroxyvitamin D at levels below 30 nmol/l is associated with decreased muscle strength.[9] Namely, that there is a strong genetic component of muscular strength, fat mass and body weight and that these anthropometric markers are associated with the vitamin D receptor.[10]

The cost of healthcare for individuals appears to increase with age. In fact, the use of medical services, including allied health care, may be higher for people above 60 years of age as compared with their younger counterparts. Possibly, if older adults were to experience greater lower body strength and function, they would have a reduced number of falls and broken bones. Thus, since there are specific vitamin D receptors in muscle tissue, there might be an association between vitamin D concentrations and lower-extremity function. In a population-based survey study, 4100 people were enrolled and tested for vitamin D concentrations along with a specific walking and sit-stand test. The researchers stratified the results by using the serum vitamin D levels. The results strongly indicated that older adults who have blood levels of vitamin D in the range of 40 to 94 nmol/L are associated with better musculoskeletal function than those with levels < 40nmol/L.[11] While there are no intervention trials with vitamin D in the athletic population, the evidence is mounting that supplementation with this vitamin (and the calcitriol metabolite) can reduce the number of falls in the elderly by 30–40%.[12] The exact mechanism of action still needs elucidation.

There are no current studies in the athletic population, including both the aerobic and anaerobic trained or untrained athlete.

VI. DEFICIENCY

Adequate exposure to sunlight and ingestion of dietary sources of vitamin D are typically sufficient to avoid a deficiency. Rickets, the failure of the bone to properly mineralize, is one type of vitamin D deficiency. The physical symptoms in infants and children include bow-shaped legs, knock knees, abnormal curvature of the spine and deformed thoracic and pelvic regions. In adults, the deficiency results in impaired calcium status. Phosphorus metabolism may also be impaired.[2] Calcium interacts with PTH and if calcium is deficient, mineral metabolism can be affected. Elevated PTH in the presence of vitamin D deficiency can lead to a normal bone matrix turnover, leading to poor mineralization. This condition manifests itself as bone pain and osteomalacia.

Impaired vitamin D metabolism may occur with tropical sprue, or Crohn's disease, as well as parathyroid, liver and kidney disease. Anticonvulsant medications and aging can also negatively affect vitamin D status.

The Vitamin D Council believes that deficiency of this micronutrient may have importance in most major illnesses. Heart disease, hypertension, arthritis, chronic pain, depression, hypertension, inflammatory bowel disease, obesity, premenstrual syndrome, muscle weakness, fibromyalgia, Crohn's disease, multiple sclerosis and various other autoimmune are also implicated by recent research (www.vitamindcouncil.com).

VII. TOXICITY

The risk of vitamin D toxicity is related to the underlying potential cause. Excessive sunlight does not lead to vitamin D toxicity (however, skin cancer is a real risk from exposure to the sun). Overindulging in oral sources (dietary supplements) of vitamin D in infants can lead to anorexia, nausea, renal insufficiency and failure to thrive. In adults, excessive vitamin D intake can lead to hypercalcemia and possible calcification of soft tissue.[13]

Certain people who live in areas where they are not exposed to more than a minimal amount of sun or who are agoraphobic may benefit from dietary supplementation with vitamin D. Vitamin D is found in fatty fish, meats, liver, butter and fortified foods. The recommended daily intake for men and women is 5 μg/d. The upper limit for safe intake is 50 μg/d.[14] Currently, there appears to be no benefit, no ergogenic effect of vitamin D deficiency. Toxicity appears to occur at doses > 40,000 IU (http://www.cholecalciferol-council.com/toxicity.pdf).

VIII. SALES

While there is no direct evidence or publication of the financial value or impact of vitamin D, one can note that the sales of various vitamin classes also encompass vitamin D. In fact, in 2003, the category of multivitamins resulted in $1.2 billion in sales.[14] Many calcium supplements also include vitamin D; the calcium category in 2003 resulted in $451 million in sales. Thus, we can see that vitamin D is often part of various vitamin or mineral completes that generate millions of dollars in sales each year.

IX. AN OVERVIEW OF ATHLETIC USES (REAL AND POTENTIAL)

Currently, there appears to be no benefit, no ergogenic effect of vitamin D deficiency. There also appears to be insufficient data to make any speculation or conclusions regarding optimal levels of vitamin D intake (from all sources) and its effect on exercise performance or body composition.

X. RECOMMENDATIONS AND FUTURE RESEARCH DIRECTIONS

Scientists should possibly evaluate whether there is a synergistic effect of supplemental vitamin D and calcium on muscular strength or performance in the athletic population. Geriatricians may want to do similar studies in the elderly. Research is also needed in the athletic populations that consume low-calorie diets (i.e., dancers, gymnasts, wrestlers) to determine whether these athletes consume adequate vitamin D.

XI. SUMMARY

Vitamin D is a steroid hormone. It is obtained via exposure to the sunlight and from select dietary sources. Supplemental intake might have benefit for those over 60 years of age, but there is no current support for use in the athletic population.

Vitamin K

XII. INTRODUCTION

Vitamin K, discovered in 1929, is made up of many compounds that all contain a 2-methyl-1, 4-napthoquinone ring. The three biologically active sources of vitamin K are phylloquinone, menaquinone and menadione.[15] Phylloquinone is found in the diet, menaquinone is synthesized by the intestinal flora and menadione is synthetic and, when administered to man, is metabolized into phylloquinone.

XIII. METABOLISM

Vitamin K is a fat-soluble vitamin that is absorbed through the small intestine. It is incorporated in chylomicrons for lymphatic transport, and is transported via β-lipoproteins in the liver (entero-hepatic circulation).

IX. FUNCTION

Vitamin K is best known for its role in the clotting of blood. Specifically, vitamin K is necessary for the post-translational carboxylation of specific glutamic acid residues to form γ-carboxyglutarate for normal coagulation of the blood. The clotting factors II, VII, IX and X need vitamin K for the ultimate formation of thrombin, which plays a role in blood clotting via enhancing or facilitating the conversion of fibrinogen to soluble fibrin. Prothrombin activity is dependent upon vitamin K.

Other vitamin K-dependent proteins exist. These include osteocalcin, which is used in the formation of bone. These proteins (those found within osteocalcin) are also found in cartilage, dentin and bone. These proteins are partially dependent on vitamin D. Thus, vitamin D and vitamin K have vitamin–vitamin interactions that are important for bone health and blood clot formation. Young athletes who are still in the formative years or peak years for bone density may be of prime concern to a sports nutritionist for their dietary intake of both vitamins D and K.

Vitamin K interacts with other fat-soluble vitamins. Both vitamins A and E are antagonistic to vitamin K. Vitamin E is thought to block the formation of vitamin K from its reduced state (regeneration). Since both vitamin D and K interact with calcium, it is thought that an interrelationship exists, especially at the level of the kidney, however, this has yet to be elucidated.[16]

XV. EXERCISE RELATED RESEARCH—ANIMALS AND HUMANS

As the primary use of vitamin K in medicine is for the treatment of elevated clotting times (PTT/APTT) or as a treatment for overt vitamin K deficiency, there appears to be no reason to believe that this vitamin would have an ergogenic benefit for the athlete. No current published studies exist examining vitamin K as an ergogenic aid in any model that is of athletic origin.

XVI. DEFICIENCY

A deficiency of this vitamin is unlikely. Those at greatest risk for a deficiency include newborn infants, individuals with renal insufficiency and those who are treated with long-term antibiotics. Case reports exist documenting vitamin K deficiency in patients who have been on long-term home parenteral nutrition (intravenous feeding). Fat malabsorption disorders, biliary fistulas, obstructive jaundice, steatorrhea, chronic diarrhea, intestinal bypass surgery, pancreatitis and liver disease all increase the risk of a vitamin K deficiency.

Symptoms of a vitamin K deficiency include bruising and hemorrhaging.[17] No human studies demonstrate that a vitamin K deficiency affects bone mineralization.

XVII. TOXICITY

Natural vitamin K (phylloquinine) has not been associated with toxicity (no UL for safety). The synthetic vitamin K (menadione) in high doses has been associated with hemolytic anemia, hyper-bilirubinemia and jaundice.[18]

XVIII. SALES

There is no information on the sales of natural or synthetic vitamin K. Thus, the financial impact of this vitamin cannot be estimated at this time.

XIX. AN OVERVIEW OF ATHLETIC USES (REAL AND POTENTIAL)

No studies have been conducted in any semblance of an athletic population with this vitamin. There does not seem to be a reason to study its potential to have an ergogenic benefit in the athletic or active populace. There is a basis for evaluating the supplemental use of this vitamin in the healing of bone fractures, but there is also no evidence that the deficiency of this vitamin negatively impacts bone formation.

XX. RECOMMENDATIONS AND FUTURE RESEARCH DIRECTIONS

At this time, there appears to be no reason to study the effects of this vitamin in an interventional-type study in the athletic population. There is no real or theoretical basis to believe that vitamin K would have any ergogenic value.

XXI. SUMMARY

Vitamin K exists in three forms. It can be synthesized by the gastrointestinal tract by bacteria and is found in spinach, broccoli, kale, Brussels sprouts, cabbage and various lettuces. Dark green leafy vegetables are considered the best dietary source of vitamin K. The recommended daily intake is 80 µg/day for males and 65 µg/day for females. An intake of 1 µg/kg for adults and 0.15 µg/kg body weight for children is recommended to maintain optimal clotting time.

No evidence exists for an ergogenic effect of this vitamin.

REFERENCES

1. Combs GF. *The Vitamins.* New York: Academy Press, 1992, 179–203.
2. Groff JL, Gropper SS, Hunt SM. *Advanced Nutrition and Human Metabolism.* 2nd ed. St. Paul, MN: West Publishing, 1995, 299–306.

3. Holick MF. Vitamin D. In: Shils ME, Olson JA, Shike M, Eds. *Modern Nutrition in Health and Disease*. 8th ed. Philadelphia: Lea and Febiger, 1994, 308–325.

4. Holick MF. Vitamin D: Biosynthesis, Metabolism, and Mode of Action, in *Endocrinology* Vol 2. DeGroot LJ. Ed. Grune & Straton, New York, 1989, 902–926.

5. Haussler MR. Vitamin D. In: Shils ME, Olson JA, Shike M Eds. *Modern Nutrition in Health and Disease*. 8th ed. Philadelphia: Lea and Febiger, 1994, 308–325.

6. Armas LAG, Hollis BW, Heaney RP. Vitamin D_2 is much less effective than vitamin D_3 in humans. *J Clin Endocrin Metab* 2004;89(11):5387–5391.

7. Berven H. The physical working capacity of healthy children: seasonal variation and effects of ultraviolet irradiation and vitamin D supply. *Acta Pediatr* 1963;148:1–22.

8. Bischoff-Ferrari HA, Borchers M, Gudat F, Durmuller U, Stahelin HB, Dick W. Vitamin D receptor expression in human muscle tissue decreases with age. J Bone Miner Res 2004;19(2):265–269.

9. Pfeifer M, Begerow B, Minne HW. Vitamin D and muscle function. *Osteoporosis Int.* 2003;13(3): 187–194.

10. Grundberg E, Brandstrom H, Ribom EL, Ljunggren O, Mallmin H, Kindmark A. Genetic variation in the human vitamin D receptor is associated with muscle strength, fat mass and body weight in Swedish women. *Eur J Endocrinol* 2004;150(3):323–328.

11. Bischoff-Ferrari HA, Dietrich T, Orav EJ, Hu FB, Zhang Y, Karison EW, Dawson-Hughes B. Higher 25-hydroxyvitamin D concentrations are associated with better lower-extremity function in both active and inactive persons aged $\geq$ 60 y. *Amer J Clin Nutr* 2004;80(3):752–758.

12. Gallagher JC. The effects of calcitriol on falls and fractures and physical performance tests. *J Steroid Biochem Mol Biol.* 2004;89–90(1–5):497–501.

13. Council on Scientific Affairs, American Medical Association. Vitamin preparations as dietary supplements and as therapeutic agents. *JAMA* 1987;257:1929–1936.

14. Madley Wright R. Vitamins and minerals: Update. *Nutraceuticals World*, May 2004:56–64.

15. Grandjean A. Vitamin/mineral supplements and athletics. *Strength and Cond J* 2003;25:76–78.

16. Kalman D. In Antonio J, Stout J Eds., *Sports Supplements*. Baltimore, MD. Lippincott: Williams and Wilkens, 2001, pp 137–159.

17. Price PA. Role of vitamin K dependent proteins in bone metabolism. *Ann Rev Nutr* 1988;8:565–583.

18. Van der Meer J, Hemker HC, Loeliger EA. Pharmacological aspects of vitamin K: A clinical and experimental study in man. *Thrombos Diathes Haemorrh Supp F.K.* Schattaeur-Verlag, Stuttgart, 1968, chap. 6.

19. Combs GF. *The Vitamins*. New York: Academy Press, 1992, 205–222.

13 Vitamin E

Angela Mastaloudis and Maret G. Traber

CONTENTS

I. INTRODUCTION

Despite the many known health benefits of exercise, including cardiovascular fitness, blood glucose control, maintenance of lean body mass and positive effects on the lipid profile,[1] there is a wide body of evidence suggesting that exercise results in oxidative damage. This phenomenon is often referred to as the "paradox of exercise." At rest, the body continuously produces reactive oxygen species (ROS) and in healthy individuals at rest, these ROS are produced at levels well within the capacity of the body's antioxidant defense system. Exercise elicits oxidative stress as production of ROS outpaces antioxidant defenses.[2] Hypothetically, supplementation with vitamin E, a potent lipid-soluble antioxidant, could alleviate exercise-induced oxidative stress. This chapter will describe vitamin E structures, functions and interactions with other antioxidants, as these factors relate to exercise and vitamin E status.

II. CHEMICAL STRUCTURE AND ISOMERS

The term "vitamin E" refers to the group of eight molecules having antioxidant activity, including four tocopherols, α, β, γ, δ; and four tocotrienols, α, β, γ, δ (Figure 13.1).[3] The four tocopherols share a common saturated phytyl tail, but differ in the number of methyl groups on the chromanol ring. The tocotrienols differ from the tocopherols in that they have an unsaturated tail. Of these eight naturally occurring forms, α-tocopherol has the greatest antioxidant activity and is the most prevalent form found in the body.[3] Synthetic vitamin E consists of eight α-tocopherol stereoisomers that are distinct due to differences at the three chiral centers of the phytyl tail.[4]

III. FUNCTION

A. Antioxidant Activity of α-Tocopherol

Vitamin E (α-tocopherol) is a potent peroxyl scavenger that acts to protect polyunsaturated fatty acids (PUFAs) against lipid peroxidation.[5] α-Tocopherol can quench peroxyl radicals (ROO•), these

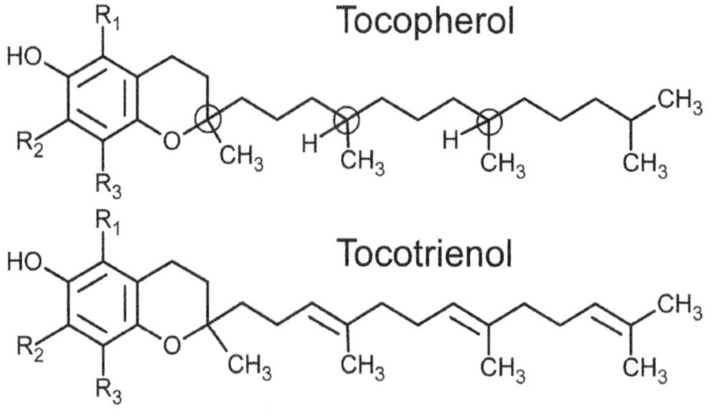

FIGURE 13.1 Structures of tocopherols and tocotrienols. There are eight naturally occurring forms of vitamin E. *RRR*-α-tocopherol is the naturally occurring form, but when vitamin E is chemically synthesized, the three chiral centers (each shown with a circle) give rise to eight different stereoisomers because each can be R or S in the racemic mixture (*all rac*-α-tocopherol). These are: *RRR-, RRS-, RSR-, RSS-, SRR-, SSR-, SRS-, SSS*-α-tocopherols. The dramatic structural difference where the tail and rings are joined (the 2 position) explains why only 2R-α-tocopherols, not 2S-α-tocopherols meet the human vitamin E requirement.

react 1000 times faster with vitamin E (Vit E-OH) than with PUFA (RH).[6] The hydroxyl group of tocopherol reacts with the peroxyl radical to form a hydroperoxide (ROOH) and the tocopheroxyl radical (Vit E-O.):

In the presence of vitamin E: ROO• + Vit E-OH → ROOH + Vit E-O•
In the absence of vitamin E: ROO• + RH → ROOH + R•
R• + O_2 →ROO•

This reaction, however, does not terminate the chain reaction because Vit E-O• is formed in this process. Although Vit E-O• is less reactive than the peroxyl radical,[7] it still can potentially cause damage.
Possible fates of Vit E-O• include:

- The radical can be further oxidized to a quinone (two electron oxidation).
- The radical can react with a PUFA to form a peroxyl radical (pro-oxidant activity).
- The radical can react with another radical to form an adduct.
- Two α-tocopheroxyl radicals can react with each other to form an inactive dimer.

The radical can be reduced back to its active form by another antioxidant, such as ascorbate.

B. NON-ANTIOXIDATIVE FUNCTIONS

In addition to its antioxidant function, α-tocopherol is believed to have anti-atherogenic and anti-inflammatory effects through its modulation of some molecular signaling pathways.[8] Specifically, α-tocopherol modulates cellular proliferation and differentiation through inhibition of protein kinase C activity.[8] Enhanced expression of phospholipase A2 and cyclooxygenase-1 by α-tocopherol increases vasodilation and inhibits platelet aggregation in humans.[6] Furthermore, α-tocopherol has been demonstrated to counter the pro-inflammatory activity of monocytes and improve endothelial function.[9] However, these functions have largely been demonstrated *in vitro*. Non-antioxidant α-tocopherol-functions are an active area of research in the vitamin E field.

IV. BIOAVAILABILITY

A. ABSORPTION AND LIPOPROTEIN TRANSPORT

Vitamin E is fat-soluble and as such, its absorption is dependent on the digestion and absorption of dietary fat. Vitamin E is absorbed into intestinal cells and incorporated by the cells into chylomicrons, which transport dietary fat into the circulation. Some vitamin E is then delivered along with fats to peripheral tissues, but most of the dietary vitamin E is taken up into the liver as part of the chylomicron remnants.[10]
    The liver is the site of vitamin E regulation. In the liver, only α-tocopherol of the dietary vitamin E forms absorbed is repackaged into lipoproteins by the α-tocopherol transfer protein (α-TTP).[5] While *RRR*-α-tocopherol and *all-rac*-α-tocopherol are absorbed at the intestine and carried to the liver via chylomicrons in a non-discriminate manner, *RRR*-α-tocopherol has twice the biological activity of the synthetic form[6] due to the preferential incorporation of *RRR*-α-tocopherol into very low-density lipoproteins (VLDL) by α-TTP.[4,11] Consequently, double the proportion of *RRR*-α-tocopherol as compared to *all rac* is delivered to peripheral tissues by lipoproteins.[4]

B. EXCRETION AND METABOLISM

In the liver, excess vitamin E can be excreted in the bile.[5] Alternatively, it can be metabolized to form the water-soluble compounds (a- or gz-tetramethyl- carboxyethyl-hydroxychromans (CEHCs)) that are then excreted in bile or urine. Production of CEHCs increases with supplementation.[12] The regulation of vitamin E metabolism is a very active area of study. It is of interest because unlike other fat-soluble vitamins, vitamin E does not accumulate to toxic levels in the body.

V. DIETARY AND SUPPLEMENTAL SOURCES

Sources of vitamin E in the diet include: vegetable oils, especially wheat germ, safflower, sunflower, olive, soybean and corn oils; as well as almonds and other nuts, sunflower seeds and whole grains.[5,6,8] Although the Recommended Dietary Allowance for vitamin E for normal healthy adults is 15 mg/day,[6] no specific recommendations were made for athletes.

Larger doses of vitamin E are popular in the U.S. in the form of dietary supplements.[5] The Food and Nutrition Board in its latest dietary reference intakes for vitamin E set tolerable upper intake level (UL) for adults at 1000 mg, which is equivalent to 1500 IU of natural or 1100 IU of synthetic vitamin E.[6] Supplemental doses in exercise studies have varied considerably, from 13.5[13] to 1200 mg per day.[14] Studies evaluating vitamin E in chronic disease resulted in conflicting outcomes: beneficial effects,[15-17] limited effects,[18] no benefit[19] and possible harm.[20-22] The latest meta-analysis of 19 intervention studies with vitamin E suggested that high doses of vitamin E might increase the risk of all-cause mortality.[23] However, the causes of death were not reported and the plethora of data on the safety of vitamin E makes it difficult to speculate on a mechanism for the observation. In general, the meta-analysis included studies that gave vitamin E doses well above the UL. It is therefore recommended that the athlete consider that 400 IU vitamin E (300 mg *RRR*-α-tocopherol) has been shown to decrease markers of lipid peroxidation in athletes replete with vitamin C.[24] Therefore, it is unlikely that higher doses would have additional benefit; moreover intakes should always be below the UL.

Supplements can contain the naturally occurring single stereoisomeric form, *RRR*-α-tocopherol (d-α-tocopherol), or synthetic *all-rac*-α-tocopherol (dl-α-tocopherol), which contains eight different stereoisomers. Supplements are typically sold as either acetate or succinate esters[4] because esterification prevents oxidation, thus extending shelf life.[6] α-Tocopheryl esters are hydrolyzed and absorbed in the gut with similar efficiencies.[5]

According to the U.S. Pharmacopoeia (USP), 1 international unit (IU) of vitamin E equals 1 mg *all rac*-α-tocopheryl acetate, 0.67 mg *RRR*-α-tocopherol, or 0.74 mg *RRR*-α-tocopheryl acetate.[25] These conversions are based on the relative "biologic activities" in the rat fetal resorption assay for vitamin E deficiency. IUs are currently used in labeling vitamin E supplements. It should be noted that the current RDA does not use vitamin E USP units, but rather the recommendation for adults is set at 15 mg of *RRR*-α-tocopherol or 2R-α-tocopherols. To convert 1 IU of *RRR*-α-tocopherol to mg multiply by 0.67 and to convert 1 IU of *all rac*-α-tocopherol multiply by 0.45 to obtain mg 2R-α-tocopherol.

VI. EXERCISE-MEDIATED CHANGES IN VITAMIN E STATUS

A. PLASMA VITAMIN E RESPONSE TO EXERCISE

Most,[26-30] but not all,[13,31-33] of the studies investigating the response of plasma vitamin E to exercise reported increases in plasma α-tocopherol concentration post-exercise, regardless of treatment (supplemented vs. non-supplemented). However, some studies have reported decreased plasma α-tocopherol concentrations post-exercise.[34,35] Whether increased α-tocopherol concentrations can be attributed to increased rates of lipoprotein secretion during exercise remains under investigation. An increase in total plasma α-tocopherol in response to endurance exercise may be due to increased output of α-tocopherol from the liver, perhaps as a result of increased VLDL production, but might also be an oxidative stress-dependent response. With some exception,[13] plasma α-tocopherol consistently increases post-exercise in response to ultra-endurance exercise,[27-30] whereas plasma α-tocopherol levels do not appear to increase in response to shorter-duration exercise,[31–35] again with some exception.[26]

A lack of reporting of plasma α-tocopherol responses to supplementation is a major limitation of studies investigating the efficacy of vitamin E supplementation to influence performance and exercise-induced damage, inflammation and oxidative stress. Studies that fail to measure or report plasma α-tocopherol concentrations following supplementation leave doubt as to the effectiveness of the supplementation protocol; therefore, findings from these studies should be interpreted with caution.

B. Plasma Vitamin E Kinetics

Studies using deuterium-labeled tocopherols have demonstrated that the various forms of vitamin E are absorbed and secreted similarly in the gut, but that *RRR*-α-tocopherol is preferentially secreted in the liver as a result of the activity of the α-TTP.[4,11] Mastaloudis et al.[30] applied deuterium-labeled tocopherols to study α-tocopherol utilization during exercise. By calculating the fractional rate of deuterium-labeled α-tocopherol disappearance during exercise compared with a sedentary period in the same individuals, it was demonstrated that vitamin E utilization is increased during endurance exercise,[30] indicating that runners may have a larger requirement for vitamin E than sedentary individuals.

VII. OXIDATIVE STRESS AND DAMAGE

In response to endurance exercise, oxygen (O_2) consumption increases 10- to 20-fold systemically and as much as 100- to 200-fold at the level of the skeletal muscle, resulting in substantially increased mitochondrial electron flux.[36] Vigorous exercise results in increased lipid peroxidation,[30] DNA damage[37] and protein oxidation.[38]

Leakage of electrons from the mitochondrial electron transport chain is considered a main source of ROS during exercise.[2] Other potential ROS sources include enhanced purine oxidation, damage to iron-containing proteins, disruption of Ca^{2+} homeostasis[39] and neutrophil activation.[40]

A. Protein Oxidation

The effects of vitamin E supplementation on exercise-induced protein oxidation have not been well studied and remain an important area for future research.

B. DNA Damage

Several studies have demonstrated exercise-induced DNA damage in individuals of all training levels: sedentary,[41] recreationally active[14,42,43] and trained athletes,[41,44,45] with some evidence that sedentary individuals experience greater damage than trained subjects.[41] Furthermore, exercise of varying intensity and duration has been demonstrated to cause similar amounts of damage.[14,41–45] Due to the potential involvement of oxidative DNA damage in cancer development and age-related degenerative diseases,[46] the ability of antioxidant vitamins like vitamin E to prevent such damage has been investigated.

To test whether vitamin E supplementation could inhibit exercise-induced DNA damage, Hartmann et al.[14] studied five men in response to a total of four consecutive maximal exercise bouts (average run time 15 min: maximum running time 18.4 min). The four trials included:

1. No supplement (test I)
2. A multivitamin supplement (test II)
3. 800 mg vitamin E 2 h before and 22 h following exercise
4. 1200 mg vitamin E for 14 days prior to the exercise bout (test IV)

The three supplement regimens inhibited DNA damage, but the protocol providing 1200 mg vitamin E for 14 days prior to the exercise bout (test IV) had the greatest effect, suggesting that vitamin E can prevent exercise-induced DNA damage. In contrast, Mastaloudis et al. [37] reported that in trained subjects, prior supplementation with vitamins E and C (300 mg vitamin E and 1000 mg vitamin C for 6 weeks) did not attenuate the increase in DNA damage following an ultramarathon run, although there was an indication of an increased recovery rate in the women runners taking antioxidants. Likely, the training status of the subjects, the exercise duration and the amount of vitamin E all were factors that influenced study outcomes.

C. Lipid Peroxidation

Results from studies investigating supplementation with vitamin E alone or in combination with other antioxidants in the protection against exercise-induced lipid peroxidation have been generally inconclusive, with results varying from reduced lipid peroxidation[13,24,35,47–52] to no effect.[27,28,53,54]

Phospholipids, which are integral components of cell membranes, are essential for membrane fluidity and transport. They generally contain multiple PUFAs (fatty acids containing two or more double bonds), which are most susceptible to lipid peroxidation because of their chemical structure, which includes bis-allylic hydrogens. These hydrogens are located on a carbon that has double bonds on either side, e.g. $-CH=CH-CH2-CH=CH-$, making the bonds weaker and thus more susceptible to abstraction. Oxidizability of PUFAs increases proportionally with increases in the number of double bonds.[55]

Lipid peroxidation is a chain reaction initiated by abstraction of a hydrogen from a carbon forming a carbon-centered radical ($R^\bullet$). The $R^\bullet$ undergoes a conformational change to form the more stable conjugated diene structure.[2] In an aerobic environment, the most likely fate of $R^\bullet$ is reaction with molecular oxygen to form an $ROO^\bullet$.[2] $ROO^\bullet$ can readily abstract a bis-allylic hydrogen of a PUFA, creating both a lipid hydroperoxide (R-OO-H) and an $R^\bullet$, thus perpetuating a chain reaction. Termination may occur when two radicals react with one another,[7] forming an inactive dimer: $R^\bullet + R^\bullet = R - R$; non-radical antioxidants, such as α-tocopherol, may limit the chain reaction.

Damaging effects of lipid peroxidation include impairment of membrane fluidity, disruption of membrane-bound proteins and disruption of active transport of molecules and ions across cell membranes.[56] Additionally, lipid peroxidation products may initiate gene transcription or apoptosis, stimulate the immune response, cause inflammation, initiate fibrosis or inactivate enzymes.[57]

VIII. ASSESSMENT OF LIPID PEROXIDATION IN ENDURANCE EXERCISE

A. Malondialdehyde

Malondialdehyde (MDA), a PUFA oxidation product, has been the most commonly used marker for lipid peroxidation in human exercise trials and is often measured indirectly by the thiobarbituric acid reactive species (TBARS) assay.[58] MDA, formed during lipid peroxidation, can be measured in the plasma using a simple colorimetric assay where MDA is combined with thiobarbituric acid (TBA) under acidic conditions to form a pink substance that absorbs UV light at ~532 nm.[2] Despite its broad use, there are a number of problems with the TBARs assay. Unfortunately, most TBARs are generated during the assay and results differ depending on the assay conditions.[2] Another problem with the assay that leads to artifact is that a number of non-TBARs products absorb at or near 532 nm.[2] Finally, the assay is non-specific in that thiobarbituric acid reacts with compounds other than MDA.[2]

More recently, researchers have begun combining the TBARS assay with high pressure liquid chromatography (HPLC) separation in an effort to increase sensitivity of the assay.[2] First,

TBA-MDA conjugates are separated from non-specific TBA forms by HPLC, followed by detection of TBA-MDA conjugates.[2] However, this method does not release any MDA bound to proteins, leading to an underestimation of MDA.[2] HPLC separation has been used in an effort to reduce artifact, but due to the non-specific nature of the assay, it remains an unreliable tool for measuring lipid peroxidation in complex mixtures such as body fluids and tissues.[2]

B. BREATH PENTANE

Breath pentane is another marker of lipid peroxidation but it has been used infrequently in exercise studies. This assay is based on the concept that hydrocarbon gases formed during lipid peroxidation can be measured as they are exhaled in the breath.[2] Unfortunately, this assay is also susceptible to artifact, hydrocarbons are only a minor end-product of lipid peroxidation, their formation can be influenced by diet and thus breath pentane is not considered a reliable marker.[2]

C. CONJUGATED DIENES

Conjugated dienes, another PUFA oxidation product, have been used to assess oxidative stress resulting from exercise. The assay utilizes the unique characteristic of these structures to absorb ultraviolet light (UV).[2] The sensitivity and reliability of this assay can be increased if a separation technique is utilized to remove other interfering substances.[2] A more useful conjugated dienes assay is to assess the susceptibility of low-density lipoproteins (LDL) to oxidation *in vitro*,[58] but results must be interpreted with caution, as LDL are susceptible to oxidation during the long centrifugation time required for isolation.[58]

D. F_2-ISOPROSTANES

F_2-Isoprostanes (F_2-IsoPs) are unique, chemically stable, prostaglandin-like compounds that are specific end-products of the cyclooxygenase independent free-radical catalyzed oxidation of arachidonic acid (20:4 n-6), a long chain PUFA.[59] F_2-IsoPs are a sensitive and reliable measure of *in vivo* lipid peroxidation.[60] Additional advantages of this biomarker are that they remain stable frozen at $-70°$ C for up to 6 months, have a lower limit of detection in the picogram range and physiological levels are not affected by dietary lipid levels.[61,62] F_2-IsoPs have demonstrated pro-atherogenic biological activity, including vasoconstriction, opposition to nitric oxide and activation of platelet aggregation,[61–63] and they are known to recruit pro-atherogenic monocytes and induce monocyte adhesion.

IX. VITAMIN E SUPPLEMENTATION IN EXERCISE

A. VITAMIN E AND LIPID PEROXIDATION

In a number of studies, vitamin E supplementation has been demonstrated to reduce steady state concentrations of lipid peroxidation markers without affecting exercise-induced increases in oxidative stress.[47,49,54,64] Compared with pre-supplementation, resting concentrations of breath pentane and plasma MDA were significantly reduced by 6 weeks' supplementation with 600 mg α-tocopherol, 1000 mg ascorbic acid and 30 mg β-carotene at rest, prior to and during a 30 min run.[54] In trained cyclists, 400 IU vitamin E for 3 weeks reduced resting MDA levels by nearly half, but did not attenuate the increase in MDA caused by 90 min of cycling.[64] Schroder et al.[47] reported that supplementation with 600 mg vitamin E, 1000 mg vitamin C and 32 mg β-carotene for 31 days of a regular competition basketball season resulted in significant decreases in resting plasma lipoperoxide levels compared with the placebo group, suggesting that an antioxidant mixture might be helpful in preventing accumulation of oxidative stress during habitual exercise training.

In a sedentary elderly population (70–85 yrs), supplementation with 800 IU vitamin E for 16 weeks reduced resting plasma lipid hydroperoxide levels and blood pressure whether or not subjects participated in an exercise training program.[49] Subjects taking placebos who participated in the exercise training program demonstrated similar improvements in oxidative stress markers and blood pressure.[49] Somewhat surprisingly, sedentary subjects taking 800 IU vitamin E gained improvements in oxidative stress markers and blood pressure that were similar to subjects participating in an exercise program.[49]

Taken together, studies examining the effects of vitamin E supplementation on exercise-induced lipid peroxidation demonstrate a trend for protection by vitamin E.[35,48,50–52] However, Meydani et al.[65] reported that 7 weeks of supplementation with 800 IU dl-α-tocopherol had no effect on urinary TBARS in the 72 h following a 45 min downhill run in subjects with sedentary lifestyles. Itoh et al.,[50] on the other hand, reported that in moderately trained subjects 4 weeks of supplementation with 1200 IU α-tocopherol attenuated the increase in plasma TBARS following 6 consecutive days of running (~50 min/day) compared with the placebo group. Importantly, supplementation with vitamin E attenuated increases in markers of exercise-induced muscle damage (CK and lactate dehydrogenase).[50] Using an alternative marker of lipid peroxidation, Sacheck et al.[66] reported differential effects of supplementation with 1000 IU *RRR*-α-tocopherol for 12 weeks prior to a 45 min downhill run in young and elderly men. Vitamin E attenuated the increase in plasma F_2-IsoPs in the elderly men at 24 h post-exercise, but not at 72 h post exercise. In the young men, supplementation prevented any increases in plasma F_2-IsoPs, but the group initially had higher levels at baseline than the placebo group, making interpretation of the results difficult. Furthermore, MDA levels were attenuated at 72 h post-exercise with supplementation in the young men, but they were actually increased 24 and 72 h post-exercise in the elderly men supplemented with vitamin E.[66] Since F_2-IsoPs were not measured immediately post-exercise, comparison with other studies in which F_2-IsoPs peaked at post-exercise,[24,30] is not possible.

With regard to cycling, Sumida et al.[48] reported that 4 weeks of supplementation with 300 mg d-α-tocopherol inhibited serum MDA formation after a cycle ergometer test to volitional exhaustion and supplementation with vitamin E for 20 weeks attenuated the MDA response in trained cyclists.[51] Similarly, 3 weeks daily supplementation with 300 IU dl-α-tocopherol reduced LDL susceptibility to oxidation following 1 hour of cycling at 70%VO_2max.[35]

Vitamin E supplementation has also been demonstrated to be protective during exercise at altitude. Supplementation with 400 mg/day vitamin E during a 10-week expedition at 8000–9000 m altitude helped prevent increases in breath pentane observed in the placebo group.[52]

The effects of vitamin E supplementation on resistance (strength) training have not been thoroughly studied. Three weeks' supplementation with 1200 IU vitamin E in untrained men was ineffective in preventing increases in MDA following repeated bouts of resistance training.[53] Because resistance training is primarily anaerobic, it is not surprising that the exercise-induced increases in lipid peroxidation were not dramatic and that vitamin E had no apparent effect.[53]

Overall, vitamin E supplementation appears to be effective in attenuating lipid peroxidation induced by aerobic/endurance type exercise, but not strength training.

B.   CO-SUPPLEMENTATION WITH VITAMINS E
AND OTHER ANTIOXIDANTS

Studies examining the effects of antioxidant combinations on exercise-induced oxidative stress have yielded inconsistent results: protection,[13,24] no effect [27] or mixed results.[67–69] Studies at high altitude especially have produced mixed results. Pfeiffer et al.[67] supplemented military recruits with 300 mg α-tocopherol, 500 mg ascorbic acid, 20,000 IU β–carotene, 100 μg selenium and 30 mg zinc during 14 days of winter high altitude training. They reported no effect of supplementation on exercise-induced increases in urinary markers of oxidative stress: TBARS, 8-OHdG (8-hydroxy-2′-deoxyguanosine) or

HNE (4-hydroxy-2-nonenal), but plasma lipid hydroperoxides increased only in the placebo group, suggestive of protection in the supplemented group.[67] Chao et al.,[68] in a similar study of military recruits, reported that supplementation with 440 α-tocopherol equivalents (α-TE), 500 mg ascorbic acid, 2000 retinol equivalents (RE) β–carotene, 100 μg selenium and 30 mg zinc during 14 days prior to 28 days of winter altitude training attenuated increases in breath pentane observed in the placebo group, but had no effect on plasma TBARS. In a follow-up study, investigators studied the effects of a phytochemical antioxidant supplement containing 650 IU α-, β-, γ- and δ-tocopherols, 330 mg ascorbic acid, 20,050 IU β–carotene, 167 μg selenium, 13.2 mg catechins, 500 μg lutein and 100 μg lycopene, 181 mg N-acetyl 1-cysteine and 5 mg pomegranate extract, in addition to 100 mg of a vegetable blend concentrate (lutein, zeaxanthin, β-carotene and lycopene) during 24 days of winter altitude training.[69] The phytochemical antioxidant mixture had no apparent effect on serum lipid hydroperoxides or urinary MDA[69] after 24 days of field training. Of note, subjects with initially low plasma antioxidant levels did appear to benefit from the supplementation by exhibiting reduced oxidative stress levels compared with baseline.[69] These studies highlight the differing results obtained by using oxidative stress markers that lack sensitivity or are prone to artifact.

Studies carried out at sea level have also shown conflicting results. Kaikkonen et al.[13] demonstrated that LDL from subjects supplemented with only 13.5 mg/day d-α-tocopherol and 90 mg coenzyme Q10 for 3 weeks had a 17% lower susceptibility to oxidation following a marathon run than LDL from the placebo group. In contrast, supplementation with 294 mg vitamin E, 1000 mg vitamin C and 60 mg coenzyme Q10 daily for 4 weeks had no effect on the exercise-induced increases in conjugated dienes following a 31 km run in trained endurance athletes.[27] Mastaloudis et al.[24] supplemented runners with placebos or 300 mg vitamin E and 500 mg vitamin C twice a day (total of 1000 mg) (Figure 13.2). Lipid peroxidation as assessed by F_2-IsoPs increased dramatically in the placebo group following the 50 km ultramarathon, but the increase was

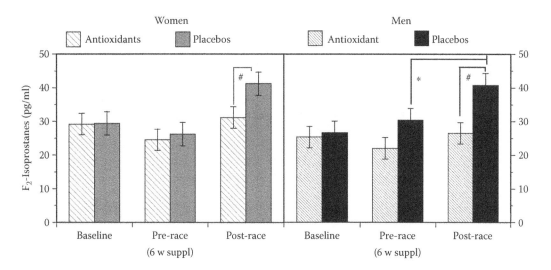

FIGURE 13.2 Antioxidant supplementation (300 mg vitamin E and 1000 mg vitamin C for 6 weeks) prevented increases in plasma F_2-Isoprostane concentrations following a 50 km ultramarathon. There were no statistically significant differences detected between sexes or treatment groups in F_2-Isoprostane concentrations (mean ± SE) at baseline or following 6 weeks daily supplementation with vitamin E and vitamin C (AO) or placebos (PL).[24] At post-race, F_2- Isoprostane concentrations were elevated in the PL group (compared with pre-race, p < 0.001), but not in the AO group and were significantly higher in the PL group compared with the AO treatment group (p < 0.01; * = compared with pre-race; # = AO vs. PL group). (A) In women, F_2- Isoprostane concentrations were elevated in the PL group compared with the AO group at post-race (p < 0.01). (B) In men, F_2- Isoprostane concentrations were higher in the PL group compared with the AO group at post-, 2h post- and 1, 2, 3, 4 and 6 days post-race (these latter time points are not shown, p < 0.03).

completely prevented in the supplementation group,[24] indicating that the antioxidant supplementation protocol conferred protection against lipid peroxidation in these runners.

X. ERGOGENIC EFFECTS OF VITAMIN E

A. Performance

Although many researchers have examined the effects of vitamin E supplementation on athletic performance, there is little evidence of an ergogenic effect. Aerobic capacity as measured by maximal oxygen consumption (VO_2max) increases in response to training, but not in response to vitamin E supplementation.[34,48–50] Similarly, vitamin E supplementation does not appear to improve cycling work capacity[35,64] or marathon run time.[28,29] Finally, there is no evidence that vitamin E supplementation improves strength training parameters including maximal strength, explosive power and muscular endurance.[53]

B. Muscle Damage, Fatigue and Recovery

Exercise can cause damage to active muscles. Damage has been demonstrated by visualization of the ultrastructural disruption of the sarcomere,[70] increased release of muscular enzymes into the plasma[70] and substantial impairment in maximal torque production.[71] The practical implications of this damage have been reviewed[72] and include decreased joint range of motion, increased fatigability, decreased shortening velocity and prolonged strength loss. A 20–30% loss in torque production of the knee extensors has been reported following endurance running.[71,73]

While exercise-induced damage could be the result of ultrastructural damage, impaired excitation–contraction uncoupling[72] or central fatigue,[71] evidence that oxidative damage by ROS mediates skeletal muscle damage is accumulating.[70,74] Damage to skeletal muscle cell membranes by ROS, specifically lipid peroxidation, can impair cell viability, leading to necrosis and an acute-phase inflammatory response.[74,75] ROS may play a central role in the etiology of skeletal muscle damage via oxidation of ion transport systems, leading to disruption Ca^{2+} homeostasis, impaired mitochondrial respiratory control, distortions in signal transduction pathways and ultimately cell dysfunction.[76] Therefore, protection from ROS by antioxidants such as vitamin E could abrogate muscle damage caused by exercise.

However, the decrease in torque production following endurance exercise may be more a result of central fatigue than damage at the level of the skeletal muscle. Millet et al.[73] reported that the 30% decrease in isometric maximal voluntary contractior (MVC) of the knee extensors following a 65 km ultramarathon was due primarily to a decrease in maximal voluntary activation. It is unknown whether ROS are involved in central fatigue.

Vitamin E was reported to have no protective effect against muscle damage in a moderate exercise protocol, 60 min of box-stepping exercise.[77] One week of prior supplementation with 400 mg vitamin E had no effect on recovery of maximal voluntary contraction (MVC) torque deficit.[77] Notably, plasma vitamin E was not substantially increased in the short supplementation period (3 weeks prior to and 1 week post-exercise).[77] When vitamin E was supplemented for a longer time period at a higher dose (1200 IU for 3 weeks) and plasma vitamin E levels were more than doubled, supplementation still had no effect on exercise-induced concentric torque deficits following a short anaerobic muscle-damaging exercise protocol.[78] Similarly, supplementation with 1200 IU/day vitamin E for 3 weeks was ineffective in preventing losses in maximal strength, explosive power and muscular endurance following repeated bouts of resistance exercise.[53] More recently, Mastaloudis et al.[79] reported that the combination of vitamins E and C for 6 weeks had no protective effect against the loss of torque and power generating capacity following endurance running. Taken together, it appears that vitamin E is ineffective in protecting against exercise-induced muscle force deficit in either trained[77,79] or untrained[53,78] individuals.

Explanations for the lack of vitamin E efficacy include the possibility that supplementation was too short for vitamin E to effectively increase in the tissue where muscle damage is occurring, that the damage is so extensive as to overwhelm the protective capability of vitamin E or that ROS are not the cause of the impairment in muscle performance and therefore vitamin E should not be expected to be beneficial.

Creatine kinase (CK) is an intramuscular enzyme that is markedly increased in the plasma following damaging exercise including both prolonged and eccentric activity.[80] Due to the invasive nature of muscle biopsies, CK serves as an effective indirect marker of muscle damage.[81] Increased plasma CK levels are the result of muscle damage, including disruption of muscle cell membrane, causing increased cellular permeability.[81] A major role of vitamin E is to stabilize cellular membranes; therefore it has been proposed that vitamin E may attenuate CK efflux into the plasma and thus play a protective role against muscle damage. The majority of studies investigating the CK responses have reported no protective effect of supplementation with vitamin E alone[70,77,82] or in combination with other antioxidants.[13,29,31,79] There are, however, a number of exceptions. For example, 2-week α-tocopherol supplementation (1200 IU/day) attenuated the CK increase in trained subjects performing resistance exercise compared with those in the placebo group.[83] Furthermore, vitamin E appeared to enhance the rate of recovery as CK returned to baseline levels by 48 h in the treatment group, but not in the placebo group. Beaton et al.[78] also reported an attenuation of the CK increase response to resistance exercise with 3-week α-tocopherol supplementation (1200 IU/day); however, muscle biopsies revealed that ultrastructural muscle damage was similar between groups. These results indicate that CK may be more representative of muscle membrane disruption than damage to the ultrastructure. With regard to endurance exercise, Itoh et al.[50] observed that 4-week α-tocopherol supplementation (1200 IU/day) attenuated CK increases following 6 successive days of running, whereas Kaikkonen et al.[13] reported no positive effect on the plasma CK response when they supplemented with only 13.5 mg/day for 3 weeks prior to a marathon. Rokitzki et al.[28] reported that 4.5-week supplementation with 400 IU vitamin E and 200 mg vitamin C attenuated CK increases following a 90 km ultramarathon. Finally, supplementation with vitamin E for 20 weeks attenuated the CK response in trained cyclists.[51] In contrast, combined supplementation with 300 mg vitamin E and 1000 mg vitamin C for 6 weeks had no effect on increases in CK following a 50 km run.[79]

The efficacy of vitamin E supplementation to attenuate exercise-induced impairment in muscle function or increases in muscle damage markers remains unclear due to conflicting results from various studies. Results appear to be influenced by amount and duration of dose and the type of antioxidant supplemented, as well as intensity, duration and type of exercise; clearly, further research is needed in this area.

C. Inflammation

Endurance or damaging exercise elicits a stress response analogous to the acute phase immune response.[75] A local response to a stressor such as tissue injury or ROS stimulates production of a group of low molecular weight regulatory proteins, called cytokines, which regulate the inflammatory cascade.[75,84,85] In parallel with the local response, a systemic inflammatory response characterized by fever, leukocytosis, production of acute phase proteins and transfer of extracellular iron to intracellular stores occurs.[75]

It has been postulated that ROS may stimulate cytokine production at the level of the skeletal muscle in response to exercise and that vitamin E supplementation may attenuate this stress response.[86] The few studies examining the effects of vitamin E supplementation on exercise-stimulated cytokine production have generated mixed results. Singh et al.[87] reported that vitamin E supplementation (400 IU for 4 days) had no effect on the cytokine response to 1.5 h of treadmill running. Similarly, two weeks of supplementation with antioxidants (400 mg vitamin E and 500 mg vitamin C) had no apparent effect on exercise-induced inflammation following a 1.5 h run.[31] While both of these studies were carried out in trained subjects, in a group of untrained subjects, Niess et al.[82] reported that vitamin E supplementation (500 IU for 8 days) had no effect on the cytokine response to 30 min of exhaustive treadmill running.

It may be that a longer period of vitamin E administration is required to influence the inflammatory response. Cannon et al.[88] reported an attenuation of the increase in the cytokine IL-1β following 48 days vitamin E supplementation (400 IU/day) and Vassilakopoulos et al.[86] reported that increases in cytokines were prevented with an antioxidant cocktail that included vitamins E, A and C (200 mg, 50,000 IU and 1000 mg, respectively) for 60 days; both studies involved untrained subjects and a 45-min moderate-intensity running protocol. In a follow-up study, Cannon et al.[89] demonstrated that 48 days vitamin E supplementation (800 IU/day) attenuated IL-1β and IL-6 secretion, but not TNF-α following a 45-min run. These results reveal that vitamin E supplementation may influence individual cytokines differently, and this should be considered when selecting a limited group of cytokines to represent the inflammatory response.

Most recently, Mastaloudis et al.[24] reported that in trained subjects, vitamins E and C (300 mg vitamin E and 1000 mg vitamin C for 6 weeks) had no apparent effect on inflammatory markers (IL-1β, IL-6, TNF-α and C-reactive protein) following a 50 km (7 h) ultramarathon run. Therefore, the effectiveness of vitamin E to prevent exercise-induced oxidative stress appears to be influenced by the duration of supplementation, the training status of the individual and the duration of the exercise protocol.

XI. CONSIDERATIONS AND FUTURE RECOMMENDATIONS

There are a number of explanations for the inconsistent findings with regard to antioxidant protection in exercise. In addition to differences in the modes, duration and intensity of exercise, there were large discrepancies in the types and amounts of antioxidant supplements provided and in the duration of supplementation. Probably the most important explanation for the inconsistent results in the oxidative stress studies, especially in those with similar protocols, is the different assays used to assess lipid peroxidation. As discussed previously, assays such as TBARS (MDA), breath pentane and conjugated dienes are susceptible to artifact and are often not specific enough to accurately assess lipid peroxidation in complex mixtures such as plasma.[2] F_2-IsoPs, on the other hand, are chemically stable, specific end-products of free-radical catalyzed lipid peroxidation.[59] When handled appropriately (samples flash frozen in liquid nitrogen immediately and stored at $-70°$ C) F_2-IsoPs are a sensitive and reliable measure of in vivo lipid peroxidation.[60]

Regarding the study of exercise-induced inflammation, vitamin E supplementation may influence individual cytokines differently and this should be considered when selecting a limited group of cytokines to represent the inflammatory response.[89] As training status also impacts the inflammatory response, this too should be taken into consideration when designing studies examining the efficacy of vitamin E and other antioxidants to prevent inflammation.

The effect of vitamin E supplementation on exercise-induced protein oxidation has not been well studied and remains an important area for future research.

CK response may not be the best marker for evaluation of muscle damage because, in many cases, CK has not been well correlated with the extent of muscle damage assessed using histological techniques.[90] Therefore, the use of muscle biopsy techniques in addition to plasma markers may offer a more comprehensive picture of the exercise-induced muscle damage response directly at the level of the skeletal muscle.

XII. RECOMMENDATIONS

While vitamin E has no apparent effect on exercise performance, it has been demonstrated that its utilization increases during endurance exercise;[30] therefore, endurance athletes may have a higher requirement for vitamin E. There is also evidence that those participating in repeated bouts of exercise on the same day or consecutive days may benefit from vitamin E supplementation by reducing resting concentrations of oxidative stress markers.[47,50] Persons participating in physical activity, especially those adhering to a low-fat, high-carbohydrate diet, are specifically at risk for consuming inadequate amounts of vitamin E and therefore might consider supplementation. Elderly subjects may also benefit from supplementation, not only by reducing resting concentrations of oxidative stress markers, but also by reducing blood pressure.[49] There is a good indication that vitamin E supplementation prevents, or at least alleviates, exercise-induced increases in lipid peroxidation in those participating in aerobic exercise,[24,35,48,50,51] but not necessarily weight training.[53] However, the long-term health benefits of lowering oxidative stress levels related to exercise have not been well elucidated and remain an important area for future research.

XIII. SUMMARY AND CONCLUSIONS

Despite the apparent increased requirement for vitamin E during endurance exercise,[30] there is little evidence for an ergogenic effect of vitamin E. Supplementation has no apparent effect on VO_2 max,[34,48–50] cycling work capacity[35,64] or marathon run time.[28,29] There is also little support for vitamin E supplementation on strength training parameters including maximal strength, explosive power and muscular endurance.[53]

Vitamin E also has no demonstrated effect on functional parameters of muscle damage such as MVC and muscle soreness in either trained[77,79] or untrained[53,78] individuals. However, there is some evidence that supplementation decreases leakage of CK into the plasma,[28,50,51,78,83] likely due to the ability of vitamin E to stabilize the muscle cell membrane. Nonetheless, the efficacy of vitamin E supplementation to attenuate exercise-induced impairment in muscle function or increases in muscle damage markers remains unclear, due to conflicting results from various studies.

Chronic vitamin E supplementation appears to attenuate the inflammatory response in untrained subjects participating in moderate intensity exercise.[82,86,88] Supplementation appears to be less effective in trained subjects participating in endurance exercise,[24,31,87] possibly due to an enhanced ability to modulate the inflammatory response following training that is independent of supplementation.

Very few studies have tested whether vitamin E supplementation could inhibit exercise-induced DNA damage.[14,37] Results to date suggest that vitamin E may prevent exercise-induced DNA damage[14] or at least increase the rate of recovery in some individuals;[37] obviously, more research is needed to substantiate these results.

While supplementation with vitamin E alone appears to be effective in attenuating lipid peroxidation induced by aerobic/endurance type exercise,[35,48–52] its effects on strength training seem to be limited.[53]

The effects of vitamin E in combination with other antioxidants on exercise-induced oxidative stress are less conclusive. A primary influence on results of these studies has been differences in the assays used to assess lipid peroxidation. Using the most reliable lipid peroxidation marker available, F_2-IsoPs, supplementation with vitamins E and C clearly prevented increases in lipid peroxidation observed in the placebo group following a 50 km ultramarathon.[24] On the other hand, studies using LDL susceptibility to oxidation as a marker of oxidative stress have yielded conflicting results: protection[13] or no effect.[27] Studies at high altitude have involved more complex antioxidant cocktails and have yielded mixed results due to the use of multiple lipid peroxidation assays of varying sensitivity and reliability within each study.[67–69] The use of antioxidant combinations to prevent exercise-induced oxidative stress has not been well studied and more research is needed in this area to determine whether these nutrient cocktails are protective, ineffective or even detrimental.

ACKNOWLEDGMENTS

This work was supported in part by grants from NIH ES11536 (NIEHS) and DK59576 (NIDDK).

REFERENCES

1. Fletcher, G., Balady, G., Blair, S., Blumenthal, J., Caspersen, C., Chaitman, B., Epstein, S., Froelicher, E., Froelicher, V., Pina, I. and Pollock, M., Statement on exercise: benefits and recommendations for physical activity programs for all Americans, *Circulation* 94, 857–862, 1996.
2. Halliwell, B. and Gutteridge, J.M.C., *Free Radicals in Biology and Medicine,* 3rd ed. Oxford University Press Inc., New York, 1999.
3. Brigelius-Flohe, R. and Traber, M.G., Vitamin E: function and metabolism, *FASEB J.* 13, 1145–1155, 1999.
4. Burton, G., Traber, M. and Acuff, R., Human plasma and tissue α-tocopherol concentrations in response to supplementation with deuterated natural and synthetic vitamin E, *Am. J. Clin. Nutr.* 67, 669–684, 1998.
5. Traber, M.G., Vitamin E, in *Modern Nutrition in Health and Disease,* 9th ed., Shils, Olsen, Shike and Ross Williams and Wilkens, Baltimore, 1999, pp. 347–362.
6. Food and Nutrition Board and Institute of Medicine, Dietary reference intakes for vitamin C, vitamin E, selenium and carotenoids, National Academy Press, Washington D.C, 2000.
7. Kehrer, J. and Smith, C., Free radicals in biology: Sources, reactivities and roles in the etiology of human disease, in *Natural Antioxidants in Human Health and Disease,* Academic Press, Inc, 1994, pp. 25–56.
8. Meydani, M., Vitamin E, *Lancet* 345, 170–175, 1995.
9. Kaul, N., Devaraj, S. and Jialal, I., α-Tocopherol and Atherosclerosis, *Exp. Biol. Med.* 226, 5–12, 2001.
10. Traber, M.G. and Sies, H., Vitamin E in humans: Demand and delivery, *Annu. Rev. Nutr.* 16, 321–347, 1996.
11. Traber, M., Ramakrishnan, R. and Kayden, H., Human plasma vitamin E kinetics demonstrate rapid recycling of plasma *RRR*-α-tocopherol, *Proc. Natl. Acad. Sci. USA* 91, 10005–10008, 1994.
12. Schultz, M., Leist, M., Petrzika, M., Gassmann, B. and Brigelius-Flohe, R., Novel urinary metabolite of α-tocopherol, 2,5,7,8-tetramethyl-2(2′-carboxyethyl)-6-hydroxychroman, as an indicator of an adequate vitamin E supply?, *Am. J. Clin. Nutr.* 62, 1527S–34S, 1995.
13. Kaikkonen, J., Kosonen, L., Nyyssonen, K., Porkkala-Sarataho, E., Salonen, R., Dorpela, H. and Salonen, J., Effect of combined coenzyme Q10 and d-a-tocopheryl acetate supplementation on exercise-induced lipid peroxidation and muscular damage: A placebo-controlled double-blind study in marathon runners, *Free Radic. Res.* 29, 85–92, 1998.
14. Hartmann, A., Niess, A., Grunert-Fuchs, M., Poch, B. and Speit, G., Vitamin E prevents exercise-induced DNA damage, *Mutat. Res.* 346, 195–202, 1995.
15. Stephens, N.G., Parsons, A., Schofield, P.M., Kelly, F., Cheeseman, K. and Mitchinson, M.J., Randomised controlled trial of vitamin E in patients with coronary disease: Cambridge Heart Antioxidant Study (CHAOS). *Lancet* 347, 781–6, 1996.
16. Boaz, M., Smetana, S., Weinstein, T., Matas, Z., Gafter, U., Iaina, A., Knecht, A., Weissgarten, Y., Brunner, D., Fainaru, M. and Green, M.S., Secondary prevention with antioxidants of cardiovascular disease in endstage renal disease (SPACE): Randomised placebo-controlled trial, *Lancet* 356, 1213–1218, 2000.
17. Salonen, R.M., Nyyssonen, K., Kaikkonen, J., Porkkala-Sarataho, E., Voutilainen, S., Rissanen, T.H., Tuomainen, T.P., Valkonen, V.P., Ristonmaa, U., Lakka, H.M., Vanharanta, M., Salonen, J.T. and Poulsen, H.E., Six-year effect of combined vitamin C and E supplementation on atherosclerotic progression: The Antioxidant Supplementation in Atherosclerosis Prevention (ASAP) Study, *Circulation* 107, 947–53, 2003.
18. Gruppo Italiano per lo Studio della Streptochinasi nell'Infarcto Miocardico, Dietary supplementation with n-3 polyunsaturated fatty acids and vitamin E after myocardial infarction: results of the GISSI-Prevenzione trial., *Lancet* 354, 447–55, 1999.
19. Yusuf, S., Dagenais, G., Pogue, J., Bosch, J. and Sleight, P., Vitamin E supplementation and cardiovascular events in high-risk patients. The Heart Outcomes Prevention Evaluation Study Investigators, *N. Engl. J. Med.* 342, 154–60, 2000.
20. Cheung, M.C., Zhao, X.Q., Chait, A., Albers, J.J. and Brown, B.G., Antioxidant supplements block the response of HDL to simvastatin-niacin therapy in patients with coronary artery disease and low HDL, *Arterioscler. Thromb. Vasc. Biol.* 21, 1320–6, 2001.

21. Brown, B.G., Zhao, X.Q., Chait, A., Fisher, L.D., Cheung, M.C., Morse, J.S., Dowdy, A.A., Marino, E.K., Bolson, E.L., Alaupovic, P., Frohlich, J. and Albers, J.J., Simvastatin and niacin, antioxidant vitamins, or the combination for the prevention of coronary disease, *N. Engl J. Med.* 345, 1583–92, 2001.
22. Waters, D.D., Alderman, E.L., Hsia, J., Howard, B.V., Cobb, F.R., Rogers, W.J., Ouyang, P., Thompson, P., Tardif, J.C., Higginson, L., Bittner, V., Steffes, M., Gordon, D.J., Proschan, M., Younes, N. and Verter, J.I., Effects of hormone replacement therapy and antioxidant vitamin supplements on coronary atherosclerosis in postmenopausal women: A randomized controlled trial, *JAMA* 288, 2432–40, 2002.
23. Miller, E.R., III, Paston-Barriuso, R., Dalal, D., Riemersma, R.A., Appel, L.J. and Guallar, E., Meta-analysis: High-dosage vitamin E supplementation may increase all-cause mortality, *Ann. Intern. Med.* 142, 2004.
24. Mastaloudis, A., Morrow, J., Hopkins, D., Devaraj, S. and Traber, M., Antioxidant supplementation prevents exercise-induced lipid peroxidation, but not inflammation, in ultramarathon runners, *Free Radic. Biol. Med.* 36, 1329–1341, 2004.
25. United States Pharmacopeia, Vitamin E, in The United States Pharmacopeia, 20th ed. United States Pharmacopeia Convention, Inc., Rockville, 1980, pp. 846–848.
26. Pincemail, J., Deby, C., Camus, G., Pirnay, F., Bouchez, R., Massaux, L. and Goutier, R., Tocopherol mobilization during intensive exercise, *Eur. J. Appl. Physiol. Occup. Physiol.* 57, 189–191, 1988.
27. Vasankari, T.J., Kujala, U.M., Vasankari, T.M., Vuorimaa, T. and Ahotupa, M., Increased serum and low-density-lipoprotein antioxidant potential after antioxidant supplementation in endurance athletes, *Am. J. Clin. Nutr.* 65, 1052–6, 1997.
28. Rokitski, L., Logemann, E., Sagredos, A., Murphy, M., Wetzel-Roth, W. and Keul, J., Lipid peroxidation and antioxidative vitamins under extreme endurance stress, *Acta Physiol. Scand.* 151, 149–158, 1994.
29. Buchman, A., Killip, D., Ou, C., Rognerud, C., Pownall, H., Dennis, K. and Dunn, J., Short-term vitamin E supplementation before marathon running: A placebo-controlled trial, *Nutrition* 15, 278–283, 1999.
30. Mastaloudis, A., Leonard, S. and Traber, M., Oxidative stress in athletes during extreme endurance exercise, *Free Radic. Biol. Med.* 31, 911–922, 2001.
31. Petersen, E., Ostrowski, K., Ibfelt, T., Richelle, M., Offord, E., Halkjaer-Kristensen, J. and Pedersen, B.K., Effect of vitamin supplementation on cytokine response and on muscle damage after strenuous exercise, *Am. J. Physiol.* 280, C1570–C1575, 2001.
32. Viguie, C., Frei, B., Shigenaga, M., Ames, B., Packer, L. and Brooks, G., Antioxidant status and indexes of oxidative stress during consecutive days of exercise, *J. Appl. Physiol.* 75, 566–572, 1993.
33. Duthie, G.G., Robertson, J.D., Maughan, R.J. and Morrice, P.C., Blood antioxidant status and erythrocyte lipid peroxidation following distance running, *Arch. Biochem. Biophys.* 282, 78–83, 1990.
34. Kawai, Y., Shimomitsu, T., Takanami, Y., Murase, N., Katsumura, T. and Maruyama, C., Vitamin E level changes in serum and red blood cells due to acute exhaustive exercise in collegiate women, *J. Nutr. Sci. Vitaminol.* 46, 119–124, 2000.
35. Oostenbrug, G., Mensink, R., Hardeman, M., De Vries, T., Brouns, F. and Hornstra, G., Exercise performance, red blood cell deformability and lipid peroxidation: effects of fish oil and vitamin E, *J. Appl. Physiol.* 83, 746–752, 1997.
36. Child, R.B., Wilkinson, D.M., Fallowfield, J.L. and Donnelly, A.E., Elevated serum antioxidant capacity and plasma malondialdehyde concentration in response to a simulated half-marathon run, *Med. Sci. Sports Exerc.* 30, 1603–1607, 1998.
37. Mastaloudis, A., Yu, D., Frei, B., Dashwood, R. and Traber, M.G., Endurance exercise results in DNA damage as detected by the comet assay, *Free Radic. Biol. Med.* 36, 966–975, 2004.
38. Saxton, J., Donnelly, A. and Roper, H., Indices of free-radical-mediated damage following maximum voluntary eccentric and concentric muscular work, *Eur. J. Appl. Physiol. Occup. Physiol.* 68, 189–193, 1994.
39. Jackson, M., Exercise and oxygen radical production by muscle, in *Handbook of Oxidants and Antioxidants in Exercise,* Sen, C., Packer, L. and Hanninen, O., Eds., Elsevier, Amsterdam, 2000, pp. 57–68.
40. Hessel, E., Haberland, A., Muller, M., Lerche, D. and Schimke, I., Oxygen radical generation of neutrophils: A reason for oxidative stress during marathon running?, *Clin. Chim. Acta* 298, 145–156, 2000.
41. Niess, A., Hartmann, A., Grunert-Fuchs, M., Poch, B. and Speit, G., DNA damage after exhaustive treadmill running in trained and untrained men, *Int. J. Sports Med.* 17, 397–403, 1996.

42. Niess, A., Baumann, M., Roecker, K., Horstmann, T., Mayer, F. and Dickhuth, H.H., Effects of intensive endurance exercise on DNA damage in leucocytes, *J. Sports Med. Phys. Fitness* 38, 111–115, 1998.

43. Mars, M., Govender, S., Weston, A., Naicker, V. and Chuturgoon, A., High intensity exercise: A cause of lymphocyte apoptosis?, *Biochem. Biophys. Res. Commun.* 249, 366–370, 1998.

44. Tsai, K., Hsu, T.-G., Hsu, K.-M., Cheng, H., Liu, T.-Y., Hsu, C.-F. and Kong, C.-W., Oxidative DNA damage in human peripheral leukocytes induced by massive aerobic exercise, *Free Radic. Biol. Med.* 31, 1465–1472, 2001.

45. Hartmann, A., Pfuhler, S., Dennog, C., Germadnik, D., Pilger, A. and Speit, G., Exercise-induced DNA effects in human leukocytes are not accompanied by increased formation of 8-hydroxy-2′-deoxyguanosine or induction of micronuclei, *Free Radic. Biol. Med.* 24, 245–251, 1998.

46. Hartmann, A. and Niess, A., Oxidative DNA damage in exercise, in *Handbook of Oxidants and Antioxidants in Exercise,* Sen, C., Packer, L. and Hanninen, O., Eds., Elsevier, Amsterdam, 2000, pp. 195–217.

47. Schroder, H., Navarro, E., Tramullas, A., Mora, J. and Galiano, D., Nutrition antioxidant status and oxidative stress in professional basketball players: Effects of a three compound antioxidative supplement, *Nutrition* 21, 146–150, 2000.

48. Sumida, S., Tanaka, Kitao, H. and Nakadomo, F., Exercise-induced lipid peroxidation and leakage of enzymes before and after vitamin E supplementation, *Intl. J. Biochem.* 21, 835–838, 1989.

49. Jessup, J., Horne, C., Yarandi, H. and Quindry, J., The effects of endurance exercise and vitamin E on oxidative stress in the elderly, *Biol. Res. Nurs.* 5, 47–55, 2003.

50. Itoh, H., Ohkuwa, T., Yamazaki, Y., Shimoda, T., Wakayama, A., Tamura, S., Yamamoto, T., Sato, Y. and Miyamura, M., Vitamin E supplementation attenuates leakage of enzymes following 6 successive days of running training, *Int. J. Sports Med.* 21, 369–374, 2000.

51. Rokitzki, L., Logemann, E., Huber, G., Keck, E. and Keul, J., alpha-Tocopherol supplementation in racing cyclists during extreme endurance training, *Int. J. Sport Nutr.* 4, 253–264, 1994.

52. Simon-Schnass, I. and Pabst, H., Influence of vitamin E on physical performance, *Intl. J. Vitam. Nutr. Res.* 58, 245–251, 1988.

53. Avery, N., Kaiser, J., Sharman, M., Scheett, T., Barnes, D., Gomez, A., Kraemer, W. and Volek, J. S., Effects of vitamin E supplementation on recovery from repeated bouts of resistance exercise, *J. Strength Cond. Res.* 17, 801–809, 2003.

54. Kanter, M., Nolte, L. and Holloszy, J., Effects of an antioxidant vitamin mixture on lipid peroxidation at rest and postexercise, *J. Appl. Physiol.* 74, 965–969, 1993.

55. Pryor, W., Oxidants and Antioxidants, in *Natural Antioxidants in Human Health and Disease,* Frei, B., Ed., Academic Press, San Diego, 1994, pp. 1–24.

56. Alessio, H.M., Exercise-induced oxidative stress, *Med. Sci. Sports Exerc.* 25, 218–224, 1993.

57. Moore, K. and Roberts, J., Measurement of lipid peroxidation, *Free Radic. Res.* 28, 659–671, 1998.

58. Han, D., Loukianoff, S. and McLaughlin, L., Oxidative stress indices: Analytical aspects and significance, in *Handbook of Oxidants and Antioxidants in Exercise,* 1st ed., Sen, C., Packer, L. and Hanninen, O., Eds., Elsevier, Amsterdam, 2000, pp. 433–485.

59. Morrow, J., Hill, K., Burk, R., Nammour, T., Badr, K. and Roberts, J., A series of prostaglandin F_2-like compounds are produced *in vivo* in humans by a non-cyclooxygenase, free radical catalyzed mechanism, *Proc. Natl. Acad. Sci. USA* 87, 9383–9387, 1990.

60. Roberts, J., The generation and actions of isoprostanes, *Biochim. Biophys. Acta* 1345, 1997.

61. Morrow, J. and Roberts, L., The isoprostanes: Unique bioactive products of lipid peroxidation, *Prog. Lipid Res.* 36, 1–22, 1997.

62. Roberts, J.I. and Morrow, J.D., Measurement of F_2-isoprostanes as an index of oxidative stress *in vivo, Free Radic. Biol. Med.* 28, 505–513, 2000.

63. Minuz, P. andrioli, G., Degan, M., Gaino, S., Ortolani, R., Tommasoli, R., Zuliani, V., Lechi, A. and Lechi, C., The F_2-isoprostane 8-epiprostaglandin $F_2\alpha$ increases platelet adhesion and reduces the antiadhesive and antiaggregatory effects of NO, *Arterioscler. Thromb. Vasc. Biol.* 18, 1248–1256, 1998.

64. Bryant, R., Ryder, J., Martino, P., Kim, J. and Craig, B., Effects of vitamin E and C supplementation either alone or in combination on exercise-induced lipid peroxidation, *J. Strength Cond. Res.* 17, 792–800, 2003.

65. Meydani, M., Evans, W., Handelman, G., Biddle, L., Fielding, R., Meydani, S., Burrill, J., Fiatarone, M., Blumber, J. and Cannon, J., Protective effect of vitamin E on exercise-induced oxidative damage in young and older adults, *Am. J. Physiol.* 33, R992–998, 1993.

66. Sacheck, J.M., Milbury, P., Cannon, J.G., Roubenoff, R. and Blumberg, J.B., Effect of vitamin E and eccentric exercise on selected biomarkers of oxidative stress in young and elderly men, *Free Radic. Biol. Med.* 34, 1575–1588, 2003.

67. Pfeiffer, J., Askew, E., Roberts, D., Wood, S., Benson, J., Johnson, S. and Freedman, M., Effect of antioxidant supplementation on urine and blood markers of oxidative stress during extended moderate-altitude training, *Wilderness Environ. Med.* 10, 66–74, 1999.

68. Chao, W., Askew, E., Roberts, D., Wood, S. and Perkins, J., Oxidative stress in humans during work at moderate altitude, *J. Nutr.* 129, 2009–2012, 1999.

69. Schmidt, M., Askew, E., Roberts, D., Prior, R., Ensign, W., Jr, and Hesslink R., Jr, Oxidative stress in humans training in cold, moderate altitude environment and their response to a phytochemical antioxidant supplement, *Wilderness Environ. Med.* 13, 94–105, 2002.

70. Maxwell, S., Jakeman, P., Thomason, J., Leguen, C. and Thorpe, G., Changes in plasma antioxidant status during eccentric exercise and the effect of vitamin supplementation, *Free Radic. Res.* 19, 191–202, 1993.

71. Millet, G.Y., Martin, V., Lattier, G. and Ballay, Y., Mechanisms contributing to knee extensor strength loss after prolonged running exercise, *J. Appl. Physiol.* 94, 193–198, 2003.

72. Warren, G., Ingalls, C., Lowe, D. and Armstrong, R., Excitation-contraction uncoupling: Major role of contraction-induced muscle injury, *Exerc. Sport Sci. Rev.* 29, 82–87, 2001.

73. Millet, G.Y., Lepers, R., Maffiuletti, N.A., Babault, N., Martin, V. and Lattier, G., Alterations of neuromuscular function after an ultramarathon, *J. Appl. Physiol.* 92, 486–92, 2002.

74. Sjodin, B., Hellsten Westing, Y. and Apple, F., Biochemical mechanisms for oxygen free radical formation during exercise, *Sports Med.* 10, 236–254, 1990.

75. Cannon, J.G. and Blumberg, J.B., Acute phase immune responses in exercise, in *Handbook of Oxidants and Antioxidants in Exercise,* Sen, C., Packer, L. and Hanninen, O. Elsevier, New York, 2000, pp. 177–194.

76. Kourie, J., Interaction of reactive oxygen species with ion transport mechanisms, *Am. J. Physiol.* 275, C1–C24, 1998.

77. Jakeman, P. and Maxwell, S., Effect of antioxidant vitamin supplementation on muscle function after eccentric exercise, *Eur. J. Appl. Physiol. Occup. Physiol.* 67, 426–30, 1993.

78. Beaton, L.J., Allan, D.A., Tarnopolsky, M.A., Tiidus, P.M. and Phillips, S.M., Contraction-induced muscle damage is unaffected by vitamin E supplementation, *Med. Sci. Sports Exerc.* 34, 798–805, 2002.

79. Mastaloudis, A., Traber, M., Carstensen, K. and Widrick, J., Antioxidants do not prevent muscle damage in response to an ultramarathon run, *Med. Sci. Sports Exerc.* in press, 2005.

80. Appell, H.J., Soares, J.M. and Duarte, J.A., Exercise, muscle damage and fatigue, *Sports Med.* 13, 108–15, 1992.

81. Armstrong, R., Muscle damage and endurance events, *Sports Med.* 3, 370–381, 1986.

82. Niess, A.M., Sommer, M., Schneider, M., Angres, C., Tschositsch, K., Golly, I. C., Battenfeld, N., Northoff, H., Biesalski, H.K., Dickhuth, H.H. and Fehrenbach, E., Physical exercise-induced expression of inducible nitric oxide synthase and heme oxygenase-1 in human leukocytes: effects of *RRR*-α-tocopherol supplementation, *Antioxid. Redox Signal.* 2, 113–126, 2000.

83. McBride, J.M., Kraemer, W.J., Triplett-McBride, T. and Sebastianelli, W., Effect of resistance exercise on free radical production, *Med. Sci. Sports Exerc.* 30, 67–72, 1998.

84. Pedersen, B.K., Ostrowski, K., Rohde, T. and Bruunsgaard, H., The cytokine response to strenuous exercise, *Can. J. Physiol. Pharmacol.* 76, 505–11, 1998.

85. Pedersen, B.K., Bruunsgaard, H., Ostrowski, K., Krabbe, K., Hansen, H., Krzywkowski, K., Toft, A., Sondergaard, S.R., Petersen, E.W., Ibfelt, T. and Schjerling, P., Cytokines in aging and exercise, *Int. J. Sports Med.* 21 Suppl 1, S4–9, 2000.

86. Vassilakopoulos, T., Karatza, M., Katsaounou, P., Kollintza, A., Zakynthinos, S. and Roussos, C., Antioxidants attenuate the plasma cytokine response to exercise in humans, *J. Appl. Physiol.* 94, 1025–1032, 2003.

87. Singh, A., Papanicolaou, D.A., Lawrence, L.L., Howell, E.A., Chrousos, G.P. and Deuster, P.A., Neuroendocrine responses to running in women after zinc and vitamin E supplementation, *Med. Sci. Sports Exerc.* 31, 536–42, 1999.

88. Cannon, J., Orencole, S., Fielding, R., Meydani, M., Meydani, S., Fiatarone, M., Blumberg, J. and Evans, W., Acute phase response in exercise: interaction of age and vitamin E on neutrophils and muscle enzyme release, *Am. J. Physiol.* 259, R1214–R1219, 1990.
89. Cannon, J., Meydani, S., Fielding, R., Fiatarone, M., Meydani, M., Farhangmehr, M., Orencole, S., Blumberg, J. and Evans, W., Acute phase response in exercise. II. Associations between vitamin E, cytokines and muscle proteolysis, *Am. J. Physiol.* 260, R1235–R1240, 1991.
90. Stupka, N., Lowther, S., Chorneyko, K., Bourgeois, J., Hogben, C. and Tarnopolsky, M., Gender differences in muscle inflammation after eccentric exercise, *J. Appl. Physiol.* 89, 2325–2332, 2000.

Section Three

Trace Elements

14 Iron

Emily M. Haymes

CONTENTS

I. INTRODUCTION

Iron is the trace mineral found in the greatest amount in the body, about 3–5 grams in adults. Most of this iron is found inside hemoglobin molecules, where it plays a critical role in transporting oxygen from the lungs to the cells. Because very little oxygen dissolves in the plasma, most oxygen molecules must bind to the iron atoms in hemoglobin molecules for transport in the blood. Other iron-containing proteins play important roles in aerobic metabolism, including the cytochromes of the electron transport system and myoglobin, the oxygen-binding protein found in muscles. Iron deficiency anemia, the most common nutritional deficiency in the world, reduces the amount of oxygen available for aerobic metabolism and limits a person's endurance. Thus, iron is an important nutrient in sports that require endurance for success.

II. IRON METABOLISM

A. IRON IN THE HUMAN BODY

Almost all of the iron found in the body is bound to proteins. These include heme proteins (e.g., hemoglobin, myoglobin, cytochromes), storage and transport proteins (e.g., ferritin, hemosiderin, transferrin), iron-sulfur enzymes (e.g, flavoproteins) and other enzymes (nonheme enzymes). Because iron exists in both the ferric (+3) and ferrous (+2) oxidation states, it can serve as a catalyst for Haber-Weiss reactions by receiving and donating electrons when it is in an unbound state.[1]

Iron is stored in the body primarily in the red bone marrow, the liver and the spleen. In the liver, iron is stored in hepatocytes and reticuloendothelial cells, while in the spleen and bone marrow, iron stores are in reticuloendothelial cells. Most of the iron is stored as the iron-containing proteins ferritin and hemosiderin. Men normally have greater iron stores (1000 mg) than women (300 mg).[2]

Two thirds of the body's iron is incorporated in the heme group of the hemoglobin molecules found inside erythrocytes. Each hemoglobin molecule contains four heme groups with an iron atom in its center. The number of hemoglobin molecules found in each erythrocyte is about 250,000. One oxygen molecule can reversibly bind to each iron atom. Therefore, each erythrocyte may carry up to 1 million oxygen molecules in the arterial blood. Because the average man has a greater hemoglobin concentration (144–154 g per liter of blood) than the average woman (132–135 g/L),[1] men have a greater capacity to carry oxygen in the blood than women.

Small amounts of iron are found inside all cells in the cytochrome proteins and in muscle fibers as part of the myoglobin protein. Myoglobin assists the transfer of oxygen through muscle cells to the mitochondria, while the cytochromes are involved in the transfer of electrons in the electron transport system. The end result of this electron transport, called oxidative phosphorylation, is the resynthesis of ATP molecules and the formation of water.

Included among the many iron containing enzymes are aconitase, NADH dehydrogenase and succinate dehydrogenase found in the mitochondria and the heme-containing enzymes lecithin cholesterol acyl transferase, catalase and peroxidase that protect against peroxidation. Enzymes containing iron make up approximately 3% of the total body iron.

B. IRON HOMEOSTASIS

1. Absorption

Absorption of iron occurs in the upper part of the small intestine. Two forms of iron are found in foods, heme iron and non-heme iron. Heme iron is found in meat, fish and poultry and nonheme iron is found in plants and dairy products. More than 80% of the dietary iron in the American diet is nonheme iron. Before absorption can occur, nonheme iron must be converted from the ferric to the ferrous state. Nonheme iron appears to be transported across the duodenal cell membrane by a divalent metal transporter protein (DMT1). Synthesis of DMT1 is inversely proportional to the mucosal cell iron content.[1]

Heme iron absorption is two to three times greater than nonheme iron. However, less than 15% of the dietary iron is heme iron. At present, a specific transporter protein through the duodenal cell membrane has not been identified for heme iron in humans

2. Transport

Iron is transported in the blood bound to transferrin, a plasma transport protein. Transferrin binding sites located on the surface of the protein can bind to two iron atoms. Iron absorbed through the gastrointestinal tract and stored in the liver and spleen is transported via transferrin to the red bone marrow and other cells that are forming iron-containing proteins. The percentage of iron bound to transferrin, known as the transferrin saturation, is used clinically in the diagnosis of iron deficiency.

Transferrin receptors (TfR) located on the plasma membrane of cells will bind to transferrin-iron complex that will be taken up by the cell via endocytosis. When cells are iron deficient or have a high requirement for iron, the number of TfR on the cell surface increases. Conversely, when iron stores are filled, the number of TfR on the cell surface decreases. Serum TfR concentration correlates highly with the cell membrane transferrin receptor number and is used as an indicator of tissue iron deficiency.[3]

3. Excretion

Excretion of iron occurs through four main avenues: the gastrointestinal tract, urinary tract, dermal cell desquamation and sweating, and menstrual blood loss in females. In adults, the average daily iron loss from the gastrointestinal tract including mucosal cell desquamation and hemoglobin is 0.51 mg/d.[4] Most (74%) of the fecal iron is due to blood loss in the gastrointestinal tract. Mucosal iron loss averages 0.14 mg/d.[4]

Urinary iron loss averages approximately 0.1 mg per day.[4] Dermal cell iron loss calculated from the uptake of radioactive iron (Fe^{55}) by the skin from the plasma averaged 0.24 mg/day.[4] Additional iron is lost in the sweat. Whole-body sweat loss measurements for 24 hours in men averaged 0.33 mg of iron/d.[5] It is likely that the whole-body sweat contained desquamated skin cells as well as sweat.

Blood loss in the menses is a major source of iron loss in females between menarche and menopause. Average iron loss in the menses is 0.6 mg/d.[6] However, about 10% of women lose more than 1.4 mg of iron per day in the menses.[6] Total iron loss in menstruating females averages 1.4 mg/d. It is estimated that the mean iron loss in men and in women who are postmenopausal is 0.9 mg/d.[1]

III.   ASSESSMENT OF IRON STATUS

Iron status of an individual can be assessed using several biomarkers in blood. Three stages of iron deficiency are defined: iron depletion, iron-deficient erythropoiesis, and iron deficiency anemia. The amount of iron stored is proportional to the serum ferritin concentration. When the stores are depleted, serum ferritin concentrations will be <12 µg/l.[2,7] Bone marrow biopsies with only traces or no iron also indicate depletion of the bone marrow iron stores.

Once the bone marrow iron stores are depleted, the iron needed for hemoglobin formation must be provided from the absorbed dietary iron and iron recycled by the reticuloendothelial cells. Iron absorption increases when iron stores are depleted, but may not meet the need for hemoglobin formation. When hemoglobin formation decreases, the protoporphyrin used in heme formation will be released into the blood. The increase in this free erythrocyte protoporphyrin (FEP) is one indicator of iron deficient erythropoiesis. Transferrin, the plasma protein that transports iron, will increase in concentration; however, the percentage of iron bound to transferrin will decrease. As the iron content in cells decreases, the number of transferrin receptors on the cells increases. The concentration of serum transferrin receptors (sTfR) will increase proportionally. Criteria used to diagnose iron deficient erythropoiesis are transferrin saturation <16%, FEP >70 µg/dL erythrocytes, and sTfR >8.5 mg/L.[1,2]

Iron deficiency anemia occurs when the hemoglobin concentration falls below normal. Hemoglobin concentrations below 120 g/l in women and 130 g/l in men are defined as anemia. In pregnant women, anemia is defined as a hemoglobin concentration less than 110 g/l. Iron deficiency anemia is characterized by low ferritin concentration and transferrin saturation, and elevated FEP and serum transferrin concentration. Erythrocytes will be smaller than normal (microcytic) and low in iron concentration (hypochromic).

IV.   IRON STATUS OF PHYSICALLY ACTIVE INDIVIDUALS

A.   Iron Status of Athletes

Numerous studies have examined the iron status of female and male athletes. Low ferritin concentrations have been reported in many female athletes engaged in endurance training (Table 14.1). Compared with age-matched control subjects, some studies found no significant differences in serum ferritin concentrations between female runners and controls.[8,9] The percentage of women

TABLE 14.1
Hematologic and Iron Status of Male and Female Athletes

Sport	Gender	Low Ferritin (%)	Iron Deficiency (%)	Anemia (%)	Reference
Runners	Women	25	—	5.4	8
	Men	8	—	5.7	
Runners	Women	28	—	0	14
	Men	3.5	—	1.2	
Runners	Women	35	—	—	11
Runners	Women	30	9	0	9
Runners	Women	20	—	2.8	10
Runners	Men	8	8	0	15
Runners	Girls	—	34	5.7	17
	Boys	—	8	—	
Skiers	Women	21	—	7	12
	Men	13		0	
Skiers	Women	20	20	0	13
	Men	11	0	0	
Swimmers	Girls	47	—	0	18
	Boys	0	—	0	
Variety	Women	31	18	7	21
Track	Girls	44	—	12.5	16
U.S. Population	Girls	24.5	14.2	5.9	2,19,23
	Women	21.3	9.6	5.8	
	Boys	11.9	0.1	2.6	
	Men	1.7	0.6	2.9	

runners who were iron depleted ranged from 20–35%,[10,11] women cross-country skies averaged 20%,[12,13] men runners ranged from 3.5–8%,[8,14,15] and men cross-country skiers averaged 12%.[12,13] Somewhat higher percentages of adolescent female runners and swimmers were reported to be iron depleted.[16–18] Other investigators have used higher ferritin concentrations (<20 µg/l) as their criteria for iron depletion.[10] The prevalence of serum ferritin <12 µg/l in women ages 18–44 yr in the U.S. is 21.3%.[19] Fogelholm[20] concluded from his review of studies measuring serum ferritin that female athletes had lower serum ferritin concentrations than male athletes and a higher prevalence of iron depletion (37%) compared with age-matched female controls (23%).

Anemia is much less common in athletes than iron depletion. Several investigators reported 5–7% of their female athletes had iron deficiency anemia,[8,12,17,21] while others reported anemia in less than 3% of female athletes.[9,14,22] The prevalence of anemia in adolescent girls and women in the U.S. is 5.9% and 5.8–7.5%, respectively.[19,23] Few studies have reported anemia in male runners (1.2–5.7%) and adolescent swimmers (6.7%).[8,14,18] Prevalence of anemia in men and adolescent boys in the U.S. is 2.9% and 2.6%, respectively.[23]

Eichner[24] suggests that low hemoglobin and serum ferritin concentrations in athletes may be due to expansion of plasma volume during training. Plasma volume increases during the first few weeks of training by 15%.[25] Dilution of hemoglobin or serum ferritin concentrations by 15% could be due to plasma volume changes. Several studies found significant decreases in ferritin concentration with training,[26–20] while others found no significant change.[12,31–33]

Several recent studies have examined the effects of resistance training on iron status. Two studies reported significant decreases in serum ferritin in young men and another found ferritin decreased in men with normal ferritin levels, but not in women or men with low ferritin levels after resistance training.[34–36] Decreased hemoglobin concentrations that might have been due to intravascular hemolysis[34] or plasma volume expansion during training were found in men and women following 12 weeks of resistance training.[36]

Following prolonged distance races (e.g., marathons, triathlons) serum ferritin concentrations were increased and serum iron was decreased for 2–3 days.[31,37] Taylor and colleagues[37] suggest the changes in ferritin and serum iron were due to an acute phase response during inflammation. Acute phase responses to infection and inflammation are accompanied by a sequestering of serum iron and an increase in acute phase proteins like ferritin. Decreases in serum iron during intense training may also be due to an acute phase response.[32]

Depletion of iron stores during sports training occurs because of negative iron balance — iron is removed from storage at a faster rate than it is replaced. Negative iron balance could be due to increased iron excretion during exercise or inadequate iron intake — or a combination of both.

B. IRON EXCRETION

1. Gastrointestinal Bleeding

Iron losses in athletes may be greater than that of the average man (0.8 mg/d) and woman (1.4 mg/d). Several studies have examined gastrointestinal bleeding in runners and reported the prevalence varied from 8% to 83%.[38–42] Two of the studies used quantitative techniques to measure the amount of fecal hemoglobin. Following running, fecal hemoglobin increased from 1 to 2.25 mg/g of stool[42] and from 1 to 1.51 mg/g of stool in runners who did not take analgesic drugs.[41] Estimated fecal iron loss is 0.75 mg for runners who did not take drugs and 0.9 mg for runners using analgesic drugs. Iron loss through the gastrointestinal tract would be 50–80% greater than the estimated 0.5 mg/d for the average person.

Possible reasons for the increased bleeding during running include use of analgesic drugs,[41] failure of mechanisms to protect the mucosa from gastric acid[43] and vasoconstriction of splanchnic blood vessels during higher-intensity exercise. Blood flow is shunted away from the gastrointestinal tract at higher intensities, leading to ischemia of the intestinal lining. After the runner stops running, reperfusion of damaged gut vessels could be responsible for the blood loss. Both Robertson[41] and McMahon[40] found bleeding in higher-intensity running.

2. Sweat Iron

Iron loss through sweating is another possible avenue of increased iron loss during exercise. Estimates of the iron content of whole-body cell-rich sweat in resting individuals have ranged from 0.12–0.41 mg/l of sweat.[44,45] Lower iron concentrations (0.02–0.30 mg/l) were found in the cell-free sweat. Brune and colleagues[44] found sweat iron concentration decreased with repeated heat exposures and suggested that much of the iron lost in the early sweat may be due to cellular debris in the sweat pores and contamination from the external environment.

Use of whole-body techniques for measuring sweat iron during exercise is less practical because of the need to prevent environmental contamination of the samples. Both Consolazio et al.[46] and Wheeler et al.[47] included exercise bouts of 30 min and 2 hours, respectively, in more prolonged sweat collection periods. Cell-free sweat iron was 0.33 mg/l from the arm[46] and 0.16 mg/l from the whole body.[47] Paulev et al.[48] took serial sweat samples from the back during 30 min of running and found sweat iron concentration decreased from 0.20 mg/l–0.13 mg/l.

Recent studies found cell-free sweat iron concentration continues to decrease over the first 60–90 min of exercise. Waller and Haymes[49] found significantly lower arm sweat iron concentrations at 60 min compared with 30 min. Also, sweat iron concentrations were lower in the heat (35°C) compared with a neutral environment (25°C), but the total amount of sweat iron lost was the same in both environments.. DeRuisseau et al.[50] found sweat iron concentration from the arm plateaus during the second hour of exercise. Sweat iron loss during the first hour of exercise (0.06 mg/m²/h) was significantly higher than the second hour (0.04 mg/m²/h).

3. Urinary Iron Loss

Few studies have reported urinary iron loss in athletes. Magnusson and colleagues[51] found mean urinary iron was 0.18 mg/d in male distance runners. No difference in urinary iron loss was found between runners who were iron deficient and those with normal iron status. Hematuria has been found in many runners following distance races (e.g., marathons).[52,53]

Hemoglobin may be present in urine due to intravascular hemolysis. Erythrocytes can be damaged mechanically during running.[54] When damaged cells release hemoglobin into the plasma, haptoglobin forms a complex with the hemoglobin and is removed by the liver. Significant decreases in serum haptogloin concentrations have been found following running.[54-56] If excessive hemoglobin is released due to hemolysis, the hemoglobin concentration in plasma will increase. Increased plasma hemoglobin concentrations have been observed following both cycling and running, but the increase was much greater after running.[56]

4. Menstrual Blood Loss

Mean blood loss in menstruating women is 30 ml/cycle (0.6 mg iron/d), however, 25% of menstruating women lose more than 52 ml/cycle (>0.9 mg iron/d).[57] Excessive blood loss in the menses can deplete body iron stores. It is possible that some female athletes are iron depleted because of excessive iron loss through the menses.

Deuster and colleagues[58] compared serum ferritin concentrations between amenorrheic and eumenorrheic distance runners. Although no difference in serum ferritin was found between the two groups, a higher percentage of amenorrheic runners (46%) were iron depleted than the eumenorrheic runners (31%). Serum ferritin was significantly correlated with the amenorrheic runner's iron intake but not the eumenorrheic runner's intake of iron. The results suggest low dietary iron intake was a probable cause of the amenorrheic runners iron depletion.

C. DIETARY IRON INTAKE

Low dietary iron intake is a likely cause of depleted iron stores in some athletes, particularly females. The 2001 recommended dietary allowance (RDA) for iron for women 19–50 yr is 18 mg/d and for older adolescent girls, 14–18 yr, is 15 mg/d.[1] Corresponding RDA for men, >18 yr, is 8 mg/d and for older adolescent boys is 11 mg/d. Many studies have examined iron intakes of female and male athletes and almost all have reported male athletes consume adequate amounts of iron in their diets.

In contrast, few studies of adult female athlete have reported mean iron intakes that meet or exceed the current RDA. Elite women marathon runners reported mean iron intakes of 41.9 mg/d[11] and elite women cross-country skiers had mean iron intakes of 19.2 mg/d.[59] Other studies of women distance runners found mean iron intakes were less than 16 mg/d.[9,10,60] Many female college athletes participating in team sports, including basketball, field hockey, lacrosse, swimming and volleyball, also do not meet RDA for iron.[26,61,62] Other women athletes reported to have lower iron intakes than the RDA include ballet dancers,[63] body builders,[64] field athletes[65] and karate and team handball athletes.[66]

Among adolescent female athletes, low iron intakes (<15 mg/d) have been reported for ballet dancers, gymnasts, and runners.[67-69] Only elite adolescent female swimmers had mean iron intakes (18.3 mg/d) that exceeded the RDA.[70]

Because dietary iron absorption is greater for heme iron than nonheme iron, several studies have examined the bioavailability of the dietary iron intake in female athletes. Snyder and colleagues[71] found that women runners who had meat in their diets had higher serum ferritin concentrations than runners consuming vegetarian diets. Pate and colleagues[10] also found that women distance runners who had low ferritin concentrations consumed less meat (7.4 servings/week) than sedentary women (12.3 servings/wk). Women distance runners who had lower serum ferritin levels consumed significantly less heme iron than their teammates who were sprinters and had higher ferritin concentrations.[9] These studies suggest that low intake of foods containing heme iron may be a contributing factor to depletion of iron stores.

V. IRON SUPPLEMENTATION

A. IMPROVING IRON STORES

Iron supplements are routinely used to treat iron deficiency anemia. The amount of iron in the supplement prescribed by physicians is usually large (e.g., 325 mg of ferrous sulfate)[24] and consumed until normal hemoglobin status is restored. Approximately 24% of women and 16% of men 18–44 yr in the U.S. routinely take supplements that contain iron.[1] The amount of iron contained in these supplements can vary widely from 10–50 mg. Iron supplements also are widely used by athletes. Several studies have examined the effectiveness of iron supplements in improving iron status of athletes (Table 14.2).

Most iron supplementation studies of athletes have used subjects who were iron depleted but not necessarily anemic. Significant increases in serum ferritin were observed if the subjects had low ferritin levels prior to supplementation.[72–84] However, very few of these studies found significant increases in hemoglobin concentration following iron supplementation. If the subjects were mildly anemic (<130 g Hb/l) prior to supplementation, significant increases in hemoglobin concentration were observed.[75,77,81]

Several recent studies have examined the effects of iron supplementation on the serum transferrin receptor (sTfR). Zhu and Haas[85] found 45 mg iron taken three times per day for 8 weeks significantly reduced sTfR (pre 6.40 ± 1.93 mg/l, post 4.51 ± 1.50 mg/l) in non-anemic, iron depleted, physically active women compared with the placebo group (pre 6.04 ± 3.51 mg/l, post

---

TABLE 14.2
Effects of Iron Supplementation on Hemoglobin and Ferritin Concentrations

Study	Fe Supplement (mg/d)	Hemoglobin Increase	Ferritin Increase
Haymes[13]	18	No	No
Hinton[84]	20	No	Yes
Matter[72]	50	No	Yes
Nickerson[73]	60	Yes	Yes
Yoshida[74]	60	No	Yes
Lamanca[75]	100	Yes	Yes
Newhouse[76]	100	No	Yes
Klingshirn[79]	100	No	Yes
Fogelholm[78]	100	No	Yes
Clement[77]	100	No	Yes
Zhu[83]	135	No	Yes
Pattini[80]	160	Yes*	Yes
Clement[77]	200	Yes	Yes
Schoene[81]	270	Yes	Yes
Rowland[82]	300	No	Yes

*Significant increases in supplement and control groups

5.83 ± 2.95 mg/l). Brownlie and colleagues[86] used a smaller amount of iron, 10 mg iron two times per day for 6 weeks, and found no significant change in sTfR in the iron (pre 7.92 ± 0.87 mg/l, post 6.78 ± 0.42 mg/l) or placebo groups (pre 7.94 ± 0.73 mg/l, post 7.93 ± 0.77 mg/l).

B. Performance Enhancement Effects

The effects of iron deficiency anemia on aerobic endurance are well documented.[87–89] Reductions in maximal oxygen intake (VO_2max), physical work capacity, and exercise endurance are found in anemic individuals due to the reduction in oxygen transported in the blood to the tissues. Iron supplementation in anemic individuals significantly increases hemoglobin concentration and oxygen transport and reduces heart rate and blood lactate.[90,91] Celsing and colleagues[89] examined the effects of repeated phlebotomies until subjects became anemic on VO_2max and endurance. Both were significantly decreased and blood lactate concentration during exercise was significantly increased. When the subjects' own erythrocytes were retransfused, the hemoglobin concentrations were restored to normal levels and VO_2max, endurance, and blood lactate returned to the pre-phlebotomy levels.

Many studies have examined the effects of iron supplementation on exercise performance and most did not find significant improvements in endurance among non-anemic iron-depleted women.[72,75,76,78,79,81] However, Rowland and colleagues[82] found increased endurance in adolescent female runners after iron supplementation for 4 weeks. Yoshida and colleagues[74] found faster 3,000 m time trial times among women distance runners and Hinton et al.[84] found faster 15 km cycling time trial times following iron supplementation accompanied by lower blood lactate.

Schoene et al.[81] found significant reductions in maximal blood lactate but no significant change in VO_2max after 2 weeks of iron supplements, while LaManca and Haymes[75] found a significantly increased VO_2max and decreased blood lactate during submaximal exercise after 8 weeks. The women athletes in both of these studies were mildly anemic prior to supplementation, and hemoglobin also increased. Zhu and Haas[83] found time to complete a 15 km cycling time trial and blood lactate were negatively correlated to hemoglobin concentration following 8 weeks of iron supplements. More recently, Brownlie and collegues[86] found improved 15 km time trial performance in women with elevated sTfR (>8.0 mg/l) after iron supplementation but not in women with lower sTfR (<8.0 mg/l). Greater improvements in VO_2max were found following training in women who received iron supplements compared with the placebo group.[92] In the placebo group subjects with elevated sTfR, no improvement in VO_2max was observed after training.

C. Risk of Iron Overload

In the 2001 dietary reference intake for iron, a tolerable upper intake level (UL) for adults was set at 45 mg/d.[1] This is the highest daily "intake that is likely to pose no risk of adverse health effects for almost all individuals." Elevated iron intake, especially from supplements, can have adverse effects including reduced zinc absorption, constipation and other gastrointestinal complaints. Because excretion of iron is limited, an excessive amount of it can be stored. Several epidemiological studies have reported an association between elevated serum ferritin concentrations and increased risk of myocardial infarction in men[93,04] but other studies did not find an increased risk.[95,96]

Hereditary hemochromatosis affects between two and five persons per 1000 in the U.S., with a higher prevalence in white than black populations.[97] In hemochromatosis, iron absorption is elevated, leading to abnormally high iron stores that can damage the liver. Elevated transferrin saturation (>60%) is used to initially screen individuals for hemochromatosis.[98] Periodic phlebotomy is used to treat patients with hemochromatosis.

Aruoma and colleagues[99] found untreated hemochroatosis patients have elevated free (unbound) iron in the plasma. Because iron is a transition metal, unbound iron can serve as a catalyst for lipid peroxidation. Transferrin acts as an antioxidant when it binds unbound iron. Following phlebotomy treatments, unbound iron decreased significantly in direct proportion to the decline in plasma ferritin.[99]

Iron can be toxic if taken in large amounts such as an overdose of iron supplements. Among young children in the U.S., iron poisoning is a leading cause of death.[1] Early symptoms of iron toxicity are diarrhea and vomiting. As more iron accumulates in the body, organ damage occurs, leading to metabolic acidosis, shock, and defects in blood coagulation.[3]

VI. DIETARY IRON

A. FOOD SOURCES

The richest food sources of iron are meat, fish and poultry, because they contain both heme and nonheme iron. Cereals, breads and grain products are very good sources of nonheme iron. Iron is added to flour and grain products in the enrichment process. Some cereals are fortified with additional iron. Other good sources of nonheme iron are legumes and vegetables, especially green leafy vegetables.

Approximately one third of dietary iron intake in the U.S. diet is from meat, fish, and poultry and one third is from cereals and grain products. Vegetables and fruits provide about 15% of the dietary iron intake, with lesser amounts from eggs and legumes, fats, sweets, drinks and milk and dairy products.[100]

B. IRON BIOAVAILABILITY

The bioavailability of heme iron is 2–3 times greater than that of nonheme iron. Average heme iron absorption is 23%. Heme iron absorption is affected by the amount of stored iron and is greatest when iron stores are depleted. Not all of the iron in meat, poultry and fish is heme iron. Liver, pork and fish iron will be approximately 30–40% heme iron and chicken, beef and lamb are about 50–60% heme iron.[101] The remaining iron in meat, poultry and fish is nonheme iron.

Nonheme iron bioavailability is much lower and quite variable, ranging from 2–8% of the food iron. It is enhanced by factors found in meat, fish and poultry that are present in the same meal with the nonheme iron. For example, the presence of ascorbic acid in the same meal will enhance the bioavailability of nonheme iron. Absorption of nonheme iron will be greatest when iron stores are depleted and decreases as the body iron stores increase.

Several inhibitors of iron absorption reduce the bioavailability of food iron. Phytic acid, found in whole grains and legumes, reduces the absorption of iron from these sources. When flour is milled, the iron and phytate contents are reduced and the bioavailability of iron increased.[1] Tannic acid, found in tea and coffee, in a meal reduces nonheme iron absorption by up to 60%.[102] Absorption of iron also is inhibited by the presence of calcium in the same meal. The larger the dose of calcium, especially in supplements, the greater the reduction of both heme and nonheme iron absorption.[1]

C. RECOMMENDATIONS

Male athletes appear to have little trouble meeting the RDA of 8 mg/d for iron, and the prevalence of iron depletion and iron deficiency anemia is very low among men. Because iron status tends to be low and many women athletes do not meet the RDA for iron of 18 mg/d, some women athletes may benefit from taking a small iron supplement (18 mg/d) on a regular basis. Women athletes should be encouraged to include foods containing heme iron in their daily food intake. Athletes at greatest risk of becoming iron depleted are those following a vegetarian diet and those who restrict their energy intake to maintain a lower body weight. Iron supplements that exceed the upper limit for iron (>45 mg) should be used only when an athlete has been diagnosed as iron depleted, iron deficient without anemia, or iron deficiency anemia. Such athletes should be monitored on a regular basis and supplementation discontinued when hemoglobin or iron stores reach the normal range.

Future research should examine the effects of iron supplementation on serum transferrin receptor concentration in endurance athletes. Improvement in performance may be linked to low tissue iron status. Changes in sTfR following iron supplements may explain why some nonanemic athletes increase in endurance. Inclusion of sTfR measurements during training studies with athletes should provide further insight about depletion of iron stores and tissue iron deficiency.

VII. SUMMARY

The prevalence of low ferritin levels corresponding to depleted iron stores (<12 µg/l) is slightly higher in female endurance athletes than in the U.S. population. However, the prevalence of iron deficiency anemia is no greater than found in the general population. Low intake of dietary iron along with low heme iron intake appears to be the most likely reason for low iron stores. Other potential causes of depleted iron stores are gastrointestinal bleeding and, in women, elevated menstrual blood loss.

Most studies of iron supplementation among athletes with low iron stores have found significant increases in serum ferritin following supplementation. If the female athletes had marginal hemoglobin concentrations (<130 g/l), iron supplements increased hemoglobin concentration as well. Several studies also found significant improvements in exercise performance or reduced blood lactate concentrations after supplementation. While increased hemoglobin may be responsible for the improvement, change in tissue iron status may be involved. Future studies should include sTfR to examine changes in tissue iron status in athletes during training and during iron supplementation.

REFERENCES

1. Food and Nutrition Board, Institute of Medicine. Dietary Reference Intakes for Vitamin A, Vitamin K, Arsenic, Boron, Chromium, Copper, Iodine, Iron, Manganese, Molybdenum, Nickel, Silicon, Vanadium and Zinc. Washington: National Academy Press, 2001.
2. Expert Scientific Working Group. Summary of a report on assessment of the iron nutritional status of the United States population. *Am. J. Clin. Nutr.* 42, 1318, 1985.
3. Yip, R. and Dallman, P.R. *Iron in Present Knowledge of Nutrition* 7th ed. International Life Sciences Institute. Washington, D.C., 1996. chap. 28.
4. Green, R., Charlton, R., Seftel, H., Bothwell, T., Mayet, F., Adams, B. and Finch, C. Body iron excretion in man. *Am. J. Med.* 45, 336, 1968.
5. Jacob, R.A., Sandstead, M.D., Munoz, J.M., Klevay, L.M. and Milne, D.B. Whole body surface loss of trace metals in normal males. *Am. J. Clin. Nutr.* 34, 1379, 1981.
6. Hallberg, L. and Rossander-Hulten, L. Iron requirements in menstruating women. *Am. J. Clin. Nutr.* 54, 1047, 1991.
7. Cook, J.D. and Finch, C.A. Assessing iron status of a population. *Am. J. Clin. Nutr.* 32, 2115, 1979.
8. Balaban, E.P., Cox, J.V., Snell, P., Vaughan, R.H. and Frenkel, E.P. The frequency of anemia and iron deficiency in the runner. *Med. Sci. Sports Exer.*, 21, 643, 1989.
9. Haymes, E.M. and Spillman, D.M. Iron status of women distance runners. *Int. J. Sports Med.* 10, 430, 1989.
10. Pate, R.R., Miller, B.J., Davis, J.M., Slentz, C.A. and Klingshirn, L.A. Iron status of female runners. *Int. J. Sport Nutr.* 3, 222, 1993.
11. Deuster, P.A., Kyle, S.B., Moser, P.B., Vigersky, R.A., Singh, A. and Schoonmakers, E.B. Nutritional survey of highly trained women runners. *Am. J. Clin. Nutr.*, 45, 954, 1986.
12. Clement, D.B., Lloyd-Smith, D.R., MacIntyre, J.G., Matheson, G.O., Brock, R. and DuPont, M. Iron status in winter Olympic sports. *J. Sports Sci.*, 5, 261, 1987.
13. Haymes, E.M., Puhl, J.L. and Temples, T.E. Training for cross-country skiing and iron status. *Med. Sci. Sports Exer.*, 18, 162, 1986.
14. Colt, E. and Heyman, B. Low ferritin in runners. *J. Sports Med. Phys. Fitness*, 24, 13, 1989.
15. Robertson, J.D., Maughan, R.J., Milne, A.C. and Davidson, R.J.L. Hematological status of male runners in relation to the extent of physical training. *Int. J. Sport Nutr.*, 2, 366, 1992.

16. Brown, R.T., McIntosh, S.M., Seabolt, V.R. and Daniel, W.A. Iron status of adolescent female athletes. *J. Adolesc. Health Care*, 6, 349, 1985.

17. Nickerson, H.J., Holubets, M.C., Weller, B.R., Haas, R.G., Schwarz, S. and Ellefson, M.E. Causes of iron deficiency in adolescent athletes. *J. Pediatr*, 114, 657, 1989.

18. Rowland, T.W. and Kelleher, J.F. Iron deficiency in athletes: insights from high school swimmers. *Am. J. Dis. Child*, 142, 197, 1989.

19. Cook, J.D., Skikne, B.S., Lynch, S.R. and Reusser, M.E. Estimates of iron sufficiency in the U.S. population. *Blood*, 68, 726, 1986.

20. Fogelholm, M. Indicators of vitamin and mineral staus in athletes' blood: A review. *Int. J. Sport Nutr.*, 5, 267, 1995.

21. Risser, W.L., Lee, E.J., Poindexter, H.B.W., West, M.S., Pivarnik, J.M., Risser, J.M.H. and Hickson, J.F. Iron deficiency in female athletes: Its prevalence and impact on performance. *Med. Sci. Sports Exer.*, 20, 116, 1988.

22. Pate, R.R., Dover, V., Goodyear, L., Jun-Zong, P. and Lambert, M. Iron storage in female runners. In *Sport, Health and Nutrition*, Katch, F.I. Ed. Human Kinetics, Champaign, IL, 1986, chap. 9.

23. Dallman, P., Yip, R. and Johnson, C. Prevalence and causes of anemia in the United States, 1976 to 1980. *Am. J. Clin. Nutr.*, 39, 437, 1984.

24. Eichner, E.R. Minerals: Iron. In: *Nutrition and Exercise*. Maughan, R.J. Ed. Blackwell Science, Oxford. 2000, chap. 24.

25. Schmidt, W., Maassen, N., Tegtbur, U. and Braumann, K.M. Changes in plasma volume and red cell formation after a marathon competition. *Eur. J. Appl. Physiol.*, 58, 453, 1989.

26. Diehl, D.M., Lohman, T.G., Smith, S.C. and Kertzer, R. Effects of physical training and competition on the iron status of female field hockey players. *Int. J. Sports Med.*, 7, 264, 1986.

27. Blum, S.M., Sherman, A.R. and Bioleau, R.A. The effects of fitness-type exercise on iron status in adult women. *Am. J. Clin. Nutr.*, 43, 456, 1986.

28. Nickerson, H.J., Holubets, M., Tripp, A.D. and Pierce, W.E. Decreased iron stores in high school female runners. *Am. J. Dis. Child.*, 139, 1115, 1985.

29. Roberts, D. and Smith, D. Serum ferritin values in elite speed and synchronized swimmers and speed skaters. *J. Lab. Clin. Med.*, 116, 661, 1990.

30. Lyle, R.M., Weaver, C.M., Sedlock, D.A., Rajaram, S., Martin, B. and Melby, C.L. Iron status in exercising women: the effects of oral iron therapy vs. Increased consumption of muscle foods. *Am. J. Clin. Nutr.*, 56, 1049, 1992.

31. Lampe, J.W., Slavin, J.L. and Apple, F.S. Poor iron status of women runners training for a marathon. *Int. J. Sports Med.*, 7, 111, 1986.

32. Moore, R.J., Friedl, K.E., Tulley, R.T. and Askew, E.W. Maintenance of iron status in healthy men during an extended period of stress and physical activity. *Am. J. Clin. Nutr.*, 58, 923, 1993.

33. Pratt, C.A., Woo, V. and Chrisley, B. The effects of exercise on iron status and aerobic capacity in moderately exercising adult women. *Nutr. Res.*, 16, 23, 1996.

34. Schobersberger, W., Tschann, M., Hasibeder, W., Steidl, M., Herold, M., Nachbauer, W. and Koller, A. Consequences of 6 weeks of strength training on red cell O_2 transport and iron status, *Eur. J. Appl. Physiol.*, 60, 163, 1990.

35. Lukaski, H.C., Bolonchuk, W.W., Siders, W.A. and Milne, D.B. Chromium supplementation and resistance training: effects on body composition, strength and trace element status of men. *Am. J. Clin. Nutr.*, 63, 954, 1996.

36. DeRuisseau, K.C., Roberts, L.M., Kushnick, M.R., Evans, A.M., Austin, K. and Haymes, E.M. Iron status of young males and females performing weight-training exercise. *Med. Sci. Sports Exer.*, 36, 241, 2004.

37. Taylor, C., Rogers, G., Goodman, C., Baynes, R.D., Bothwell, T.H., Bexwoda, W.R., Kramer, F. and Hattingh, J. Hematologic, iron-related and acute-phase protein responses to sustained strenuous exercise. *J. Appl. Physiol.*, 62, 464, 1987.

38. Porter, A.M.W. Do some marathon runners bleed into the gut? *Br. Med. J.* 1983, 287, 1427.

39. McCabe, M.E., Peura, D.A., Kadakia, S.C., Bocek, Z. and Johnson, L.F. Gastorintestinal blood loss associated with running a marathon. *Dig. Dis. Sci.* 31, 1229, 1986.

40. McMahon, L.F., Ryan, M.J., Larson, D. and Fisher, R.L. Occult gastrointestinal blood loss in marathon runners. *Ann. Intern. Med.* 100, 846, 1984.

41. Robertson, J.D., Maughan, R.J. and Davidson, R.J.L. Fecal blood loss in response to exercise. *Br. Med. J.*, 295, 303, 1987.

42. Stewart, J.D., Ahlquist, D.A., McGill, D.B., Ilstrup, D.M. and Schwartz, S. Gastrointestinal blood loss and anemia in runners. *Ann. Intern. Med.*, 100, 843, 1984.

43. Cooper, B.T., Douglas, S.A., Firth, L.A., Hannagan, J.A. and Chadwick, V.S. Erosive gastritis and gastrointestinal bleeding in a female runner. *Gastroenterology*, 92, 2019, 1987.

44. Brune, M., Magnusson, B., Persson, H. and Hallberg, L. Iron losses in sweat. *Am. J. Clin. Nutr.*, 43, 438, 1986.

45. Vellar, O.D. Studies on sweat losses of nutrients. I. Iron content of whole body sweat and its association with other sweat constituents, serum iron levels, hematological indices, body surface area and sweat rate. *Scand. J. Clin. Lab. Invest.*, 21, 157, 1968.

46. Consolazio, D.F., Matoush, L.G., Nelson, R.A., Harding, R.S. and Canham, J.E. Excretion of sodium, potassium, magnesium and iron in human sweat and the relation of each to balance and requirements. *J. Nutr.*, 79, 407, 1963.

47. Wheeler, E.F., El-Neil, H., Willson, J.O. and Weiner, J.S. The effect of work level and dietary intake on water balance and the excretion of sodium, potassium and iron in a hot climate. *Br. J. Nutr.*, 30, 127, 1973.

48. Paulev, P.E., Jordal, R. and Pedersen, N.S. Dermal excretion of iron in intensely training athletes. *Clin. Chim.* Acta, 127, 19, 1983.

49. Waller, M.F. and Haymes, E.M. The effects of heat and exercise on sweat iron loss. *Med. Sci. Sports Exer.*, 28, 197, 1996.

50. DeRuisseau, K.C., Cheuvront, S.N., Haymes, E.M. and Sharp, R.G. Sweat iron and zinc losses during prolonged exercise. *Int. J. Sport Nutr. Exer. Metab.* 12, 428, 2002.

51. Magnusson, B., Hallberg, L., Rossander, L. and Swolin, B. Iron metabolism and "sports anemia." I. A study of several iron parameters in elite runners with differences in iron status. *Acta Med. Scand.*, 216, 149, 1984.

52. Boileau, M., Fuchs, E., Barry, J.M. and Hodges, C.V. Stress hematuria: athletic pseudonephritis in marathoners. *Urology*, 15, 471, 1980.

53. Siegal, A.J., Hennekens, C.H., Solomon, H.S. and Van Boekel, B. Exercise-related hematuria: findings in a group of marathon runners. *J. Am. Med. Assoc.*, 241, 391, 1979.

54. Miller, B.J., Pate, R.R. and Burgess, W. Foot impact force and intravascular hemolysis during distance running. *Int. J. Sport Med.*, 9, 56, 1988.

55. Falsetti, H.L., Burke, E.R., Feld, R.D., Frederick, E.D. and Ratering, D. Hematological variations after endurance running with hard- and soft-soled running shoes. *Phys. Sportsmed.*, 11, 118, 1983.

56. Telford, R.D., Sly, G.J., Hahn, A.G., Cunningham, R.B., Bryant, C. and Smith, J.A. Footstrike is the major cause of hemolysis during running. *J. Appl. Physiol.*, 94, 38, 2003.

57. Hallberg, L., Hogdahl, A.M., Nilsson, L. and Rybo, G. Menstrual blood loss and iron deficiency. *Acta Med. Scand.*, 180, 639, 1966.

58. Deuster, P.A., Kyle, S.B., Moser, P.B., Vigersky, R.A., Singh, A. and Schoonmaker, E.B. Nutritional intakes and status of highly trained amenorrheic and eumenorrheic women runners. *Fert. Steril.*, 46, 636, 1986.

59. Ellsworth, N.B., Hewitt, H.F., and Haskell, W.L. Nutrient intake of elite male and female Nordic skiers. *Phys. Sportsmed.*, 13, 78, 1985.

60. LaManca, J.J., Haymes, E.M., Daly, J.A., Moffatt, R.J. and Waller, M.F. Sweat iron loss of male and female runners during exercise. *Int. J. Sports Med.*, 9, 52, 1988.

61. Short, S.A. and Short, W.R. Four-year study of university athletes' dietary intake. *J. Am. Diet. Assoc.*, 83, 632, 1983.

62. Lukaski, H.C., Hoverson, B.S., Gallagher, S.K. and Bolonchuk, W.W. Physical training and copper, iron and zinc status of swimmers. *Am. J. Clin. Nutr.*, 51, 1093, 1990.

63. Cohen, J.L., Patosnak, L., Frank, O. and Baker, H. A nutritional and hematologic assessment of elite ballet dancers. *Phys. Sportsmed.*, 13, 43, 1985.

64. Kleiner, S.M., Bazzarre, T.L. and Ainsworth, B.E. Nutritional status of nationally ranked elite body-builders. *Int. J. Sport Nutr.*, 4, 54, 1994.

65. Faber, M. and Benade, A.J. Mineral and vitamin intake in field athletes (discus, hammer, javelin-throwers and shotputters). *Int. J. Sports Med.*, 12, 324, 1991.

66. Nuviala, R.J., Castillo, M.C., Lapienza, M.G. and Escanero, J.F. Iron nutritional status in female karatekas, handball and basketball players and runners. *Physiol. Behav.*, 59, 449, 1996.

67. Benson, J., Gillien, D.M., Bourdet, K. and Loosli, A.R. Inadequate nutrition and chronic caloric restriction in adolescent ballerinas. *Phys. Sportsmed.*, 13, 79, 1985.

68. Moffatt, R.J. Dietary status of elite high school gymnasts: Inadequacy of vitamin and mineral intake. *J. Am. Diet. Assoc.*, 84, 1361, 1984.

69. Moen, S.M., Sanborn, C.F. and Dimarco, N. Dietary habits and body composition in adolescent female runners. *WomenSport Phys. Act. J.*, 1, 85, 1992.

70. Berning, J.R., Troup, J.P., Van Handel, P.J., Daniels, J. and Daniels, N. The nutritional habits of young adolescent swimmers. *Int. J. Sport Nutr.*, 1, 240, 1991.

71. Snyder, A.C., Dvorak, L.L. and Roepke, J.B. Influence of dietary iron source on measures of iron status among female runners. *Med. Sci. Exer. Sport*, 28, 197, 1996.

72. Matter, M., Stittfall, t., Graves, J., Myburgh, K., Adams, B., Jacobs, P. and Noakes, T.D. The effect of iron and folate therapy on maximal exercise performance in female marathon runners with iron and folate deficiency. *Clin. Sci.*, 72, 415, 1987.

73. Nickerson, H.J. and Tripp, A.D. Iron deficiency in adolescent cross-country runners. *Phys. Sportsmed.*, 11, 60, 1983.

74. Yoshida, T., Udo, M., Chida, M., Ichioka, M. and Makiguchi, K. Dietary iron supplement during severe physical training in competitive distance runners. *Sport Train. Med. Rehab.*, 1, 279, 1990.

75. Lamanca, J.J. and Haymes, E.M. Effects of iron repletion on VO_2max, endurance and blood lactate. *Med. Sci. Sports Exer.*, 25, 1386, 1993.

76. Newhouse, I.J., Clement, D.B., Taunton, J.E. and McKenzie, D.C. The effects of prelatent/latent iron deficiency on work capacity. *Med. Sci. Sports Exer.*, 21, 263, 1989.

77. Clement, D.B., Taunton, J.E., McKenzie, D.C., Sawchuk, L.L and Wiley, J.P. High- and low-dosage iron-supplementation in iron-deficient, endurance trained females. In *Sport, Health and Nutrition*, Katch, F.I., Ed., Human Kinetics, Champaign, IL, 1986, chap. 6.

78. Fogelholm, M., Jaakkola, L and Lammpisjarvi, T. Effects of iron supplementation in female athletes with low serum ferritin concentration. *Int. J. Sports Med.*, 13, 158, 1992.

79. Klingshirn, L.A., Pate, R.R., Bourque, S.P, Davis, J.M. and Sargemt, R.G. Effect of iron supplementation on endurance capacity in iron-depleted female runners. *Med. Sci. Sports Exer.*, 24, 819, 1992.

80. Pattini, A. and Schena, F. Effects of training and iron supplementation on iron status of cross-country skiers. *J. Sports Med. Phys. Fitness*, 30, 347, 1990.

81. Schoene, R.B., Escourrous, P., Robertson, H.T., Nilson, K.L., Parsons, J.R. and Smith, N.J. Iron repletion decreases maximal exercise lactate concentrations in female athletes with minimal iron-deficiency anemia. *J. Lab. Clin. Med.*, 102, 306, 1983.

82. Rowland, T.W., Deisroth, M.B., Green, G.M. and Kelleher, J.F. The effect of iron therapy on exercise capacity of nonanemic iron-deficient adolescent runners. *Am. J. Dis. Child.*, 142, 165, 1988.

83. Zhu, Y.I. and Haas, J.D. Altered metabolic response of iron-depleted nonanemic women during a 15-km time trial. *J. Appl. Physiol.*, 84, 1768, 1998.

84. Hinton, P.S., Giordano, C., Brownlie, T. and Haas, J.D. Iron supplementation improves endurance after training in iron-depleted, nonanemic women. *J. Appl. Physiol.*, 88, 1103, 2000.

85. Zhu, Y.I. and Haas, J.D. Response of serum transferrin receptor to iron supplementation in iron-depleted, nonanemic women. *Am. J. Clin. Nutr.*, 67, 271, 1998.

86. Brownlie, T., Utermohlen, V., Hinton, P.S. and Haas, J.D. Tissue iron deficiency without anemia impairs adaptation in endurance capacity after aerobic training in previously untrained women. *Am. J. Clin. Nutr.*, 79, 437, 2004.

87. Gardner, G.W., Edgerton, V.R., Senewiratne, B., Barnard, R.J. and Ohira, Y. Physical work capacity and metabolic stress in subjects with iron deficiency anemia. *Am. J. Clin. Nutr.*, 30, 910, 1977.

88. Edgerton, V.R., Ohira, Y., Hettiarachchi, J., Senewiratne, B., Gardner, G.W. and Barnard, R.J. Elevation of hemoglobin and work tolerance in iron deficient subjects. *J. Nutr. Sci. Vit.*, 27, 77, 1981.

89. Celsing, F., Blomstrand, E., Werner, B., Pihlstedt, P. and Ekblom, B. Effects of iron deficiency on endurance and muscle enzyme activity in man. *Med. Sci. Sports Exer.*, 18, 156, 1986.

90. Gardner, G.W., Edgerton, V.R., Barnard, R.J. and Bernauer, E.M. Cardiorespiratory, hematological and physical performance responses of anemic subjects to iron treatment. *Am. J. Clin. Nutr.*, 28, 982, 1975.

91. Ohira, Y., Edgerton, V.R., Gardner, G.W., Senewiratne, B., Barnard, R.J. and Simpson. D.R. Work capacity, heart rate and blood lactate responses to iron treatment. *Br. J. Haematol.*, 41, 365, 1979.

92. Brownie, T., Utermohlen, V., Hinton, P.S., Giordano, C. and Haas, J.D. Marginal iron deficiency without anemia impairs aerobic adaptation among previously untrained women. *Am. J. Clin. Nutr.*, 75, 734, 2002.

93. Salonen, J.T., Nyssonen, K., Korpela, H., Tuomileehto, J., Seppanen, R. and Salonen, R. High stored iron levels are associated with excess risk of myocardial infarction in eastern Finnish men. *Circulation*, 86, 803, 1992.

94. Salonen, J.T., Nyssonen, K. and Salonen, R. Body iron stores and the risk of coronary heart disease. *N. Engl. J. Med.* 331, 1159, 1994.

95. Magnusson, M.K., Sigfusson, N., Sigvaldason, H., Johanneson, G.M., Magnusson, S. and Thorgeirsson, G. Low iron-binding capacity as a risk factor for myocardial infarction. *Circulation*, 89, 102, 1994.

96. Stampfer, M.J., Grodstein, F., Rosenberg, I., Willett, W. and Hennekens, C. A prospective study of plasma ferritin and risk of myocardial infarction in U.S. physicians. *Circulation*, 87, 688, 1993.

97. Cogswell, M.E., McDonnell, S.M., Khoury, M.J., Franks, A.L., Burke, W. and Brittenham, G. Iron overload, public health and genetics: evaluating the evidence for hemochromatosis screening. *Ann. Intern. Med.*, 129, 971, 1998.

98. Looker, A.C. and Johnson, C.L. Prevalence of elevated serum transferrin saturation in adults in the United States. *Ann. Intern. Med.*, 129, 940, 1998.

99. Aruoma, O.L, Bomford, A., Oiksib, R.J. and Halliwell, B. Nontransferrin-bound iron in plasma from hemochromatosis patients: effect of phlebotomy therapy. *Blood*, 72, 1416, 1988.

100. National Research Council, Committee on Diet and Health. *Diet and Health: Implications for Reducing Chronic Disease Risk.* Washington: National Academy Press, 1989, chap. 3.

101. Monsen, E.R., Hallberg, L., Layrisse, M., Hegsted, D.M., Cook, J.D., Mertz, W. and Finch, C.A. Estimation of available dietary iron. Am. J. Clin. Nutr., 31, 134, 1978.

102. Hallberg, L. Bioavailability of dietary iron in man. *Ann. Rev. Nutr.* 1, 123, 1981.

15 ZINC

Henry C. Lukaski

CONTENTS

I. INTRODUCTION

The growing awareness of the synergy between diet and physical activity to promote health and boost performance fuels an expanding interest in the role that micronutrients can play in attaining one's genetic potential. Although the public press emphasizes the value of certain foods and nutritional products for

Mention of a trademark or proprietary product does not constitute a guarantee of the product by the United States Department of Agriculture and does not imply its approval to the exclusion of other products that may also be suitable.

    U.S. Department of Agriculture, Agricultural Research Service, Northern Plains Area is an equal opportunity/affirmative action employer and all agency services are available without discrimination.

health and fitness enhancement, the findings from valid scientific studies to support these claims are limited. Information about the needs of mineral elements, particularly zinc (Zn), for physically active individuals is accumulating.[1] Data from epidemiological surveys reveal that many adults and children may not consume adequate dietary Zn, with the mean Zn intake of the U.S. population less than one half of the recommended amount.[2] Furthermore, low Zn intake is common among individuals who regularly participate in aerobic activities,[3,4] including those recommended to promote health and well-being.[5]

As a transition element, Zn has the ability to form stable complexes with side chains of proteins and nucleotides, with a specific affinity for thiol and hydroxyl groups and for ligands containing nitrogen; Zn generally forms complexes with a tetrahedral arrangement of ligands around the metal. Thus, the Zn ion acts as a good electron acceptor, but does not participate in direct oxidation-reduction reactions. These characteristics serve to explain the principal biological function of Zn, that is, its varied roles in regulation of body metabolism.

Zn is essential for the function of more than 200 enzymes in various species.[6] At least one Zn-containing enzyme is found in each of the six major categories of enzymes designated by the International Union of Biochemistry Commission on Enzyme Nomenclature.[6,7]

Zn has several recognized functions in Zn-metalloenzymes, including catalytic, structural and regulatory roles.[7] Catalytic function specifies that Zn participates directly in facilitating the action of the enzyme. If the Zn is removed by chelates or other agents, the enzyme becomes inactive. Carbonic anhydrase is an enzyme in which Zn plays a catalytic role.[8]

In a structural role, Zn atoms are required to stabilize the quaternary structure of the enzyme protein and to maintain the integrity of the complex enzyme molecules, but not impact enzyme activity. Zn plays a structural role in the enzymes superoxide dismutase and protein kinase c.[6]

The importance of Zn in biological systems is reflected by the numerous functions and activities on which Zn exerts a regulatory role.[9] Zn is involved extensively in macronutrient metabolism. It is required for nucleic acid and protein metabolism and, hence, the fundamental processes of cell differentiation, particularly replication. Similarly, Zn is needed for glucose utilization and the secretion of insulin. Because of this role in glucose homeostasis, Zn also affects lipid metabolism; Zn-deficient animals display decreased *de novo* lipid synthesis.[10] Thus, Zn status impacts energy substrate utilization.

Zn exerts regulatory actions in various aspects of hormone metabolisms.[9] Zn is required for the production, storage and secretion of individual hormones, including growth and thyroid hormones, gonadotrophins and sex hormones, prolactin and corticosteroids. Zn status also regulates the effectiveness of the interaction of some hormones at receptor sites and end-organ responsiveness.

Integrated biological systems also require Zn for optimal function.[11] Adequate dietary Zn is necessary for proper taste perception, reproduction, immuno-competence, skin integrity, wound healing, skeletal development, brain development, behavior, vision and gastrointestinal function in humans. It is apparent, therefore, that Zn is a nutrient that regulates many physiological and psychological functions and is required to promote human health and well-being.

II. ZINC METABOLISM

A. ZINC IN THE HUMAN BODY

Zn is present in all organs, tissues, fluids and secretions of the body. More than 95% of Zn in the body is found within cells. Zn is associated with all organelles of the cell but only 60 to 80% of cellular Zn is localized in the cytosol; the remainder has been shown to be specifically bound to membranes that may be important in defining the effects of Zn deficiency on cellular function.[12] The concentration of Zn in extracellular fluids is very low; plasma Zn concentration is approximately 0.65 μmol/l. If the body plasma concentration is 45 ml/kg body weight,[13] then a 70-kg man has about 3 l of plasma, which contains only 3 mg of Zn, or about 0.1% of the body Zn content.

The Zn concentration in various organs and tissues of the body is variable (Table 15.1). Although the concentration of Zn in skeletal muscle is not large, the substantial mass of skeletal muscle

TABLE 15.1

Approximate Zinc Concentration and Content of Some Organs and Tissues in a Healthy Adult Man (70/kg)

Tissue or Organ	Zinc Concentration		Total Zinc Content		Percentage of Body Zinc
	$(\mu mol/g)^a$	$(\mu g/g)^a$	(nmol)	(g)	
Skeletal muscle	0.78	51	24	1.53	57.0
Bone	1.54	100	12	0.77	29.0
Skin	0.49	32	2	0.16	6.0
Liver	0.89	58	2	0.13	0
Brain	0.17	11	0.6	0.04	1.5
Kidneys	0.85	55	0.3	0.02	0.7
Heart	0.35	23	0.15	0.01	0.4
Hair	2.30	150	<0.15	<0.01	0.1
Plasma	0.02	1	<0.15	<0.01	0.1

Source: Adapted from International Commission on Radiological Protection, Report on the Task Group of Reference Man.[9]

[a] Wet weight

makes it the principal reservoir of Zn in the body. Bone and skeletal muscle account for almost 90% of the body's Zn content.

The Zn concentration in muscles varies with their metabolic functions. The highest Zn concentrations are found in skeletal muscles, which are highly oxidative, with a large proportion of slow-twitch fibers.[14] The rat soleus muscle, composed of 63% slow-twitch fibers, contains about 300 μg Zn per gram dry weight. Conversely, the extensor digitorum longus, which is primarily a fast-twitch glycolytic muscle, has only 100 μg Zn per gram dry weight.[15] The Zn concentration of skeletal muscles generally is not reduced with restricted dietary Zn, except for small decreases (~5%) in the soleus. The size and number of various types of muscle fibers, however, may be reduced and their relative distribution altered, with a characteristic decrease of the slow-twitch oxidative and an increase in the fast-twitch glycolytic fibers.[14,15] Thus, skeletal muscle is relatively unresponsive to changes in dietary Zn.

Because the concentration of Zn in bone is quite large relative to other body tissues and organs, and the amount of bone is very substantial, the skeleton is the major depot of Zn (Table 15.1). Bone Zn is impacted adversely by dietary Zn restriction, particularly in growing animals. The decline in bone Zn is more responsive to dietary Zn intake than that of other tissues and may better reflect the gradual decline in overall Zn status of the body than plasma Zn concentration. Studies in growing rats fed Zn-deficient diets found a 50% reduction in bone Zn; short-term Zn supplementation of Zn-deficient rats significantly increased bone Zn.[16] In adult male rats, however, bone Zn responded only to a minor degree to dietary Zn.[9]

B.   ZINC HOMEOSTASIS

1.   Absorption

The amount of Zn in the body represents a dynamic balance between the Zn intake and losses (Figure 15.1). Zn is absorbed principally along the small intestine, with only negligible amounts absorbed in the stomach and the large intestine. The quantity of Zn in the intestines is a combination of dietary Zn and Zn-containing endogenous secretions that aid in digestion. Pancreatic secretions are a major source of endogenous Zn. Other sources include biliary and gastro-duodenal secretions, transepithelial flux of Zn from mucosal cells into the small intestine and mucosal cells sloughed

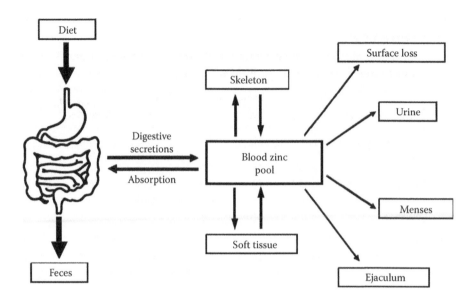

FIGURE 15.1 Components of human zinc metabolism.

into the gut.[9] Thus, the amount of Zn in the lumen of the small intestine after a meal exceeds the quantity of Zn from the meal because of endogenous secretions.

During digestion, secreted enzymes release Zn from the food and endogenous Zn from various ligands. The free Zn can form coordination complexes with various exogenous and endogenous ligands such as amino acids, organic acids and phosphates.[17] The amino acids, histidine and cysteine, are preferred amino acid ligands. It has been shown that Zn-histidine complexes are very efficiently absorbed, more so than Zn sulfate.[18] Other compounds such as iron and phytate, found in the intestinal milieu, can compete with Zn for mucosal binding sites or form insoluble complexes that inhibit Zn absorption.[19]

Zn enters mucosal cells by a mechanism that is not well understood.[20] It is thought that Zn enters the mucosal cell by a carrier-mediated process, saturable at higher luminal Zn concentrations and by diffusion. Within the mucosal cell, Zn is released at the serosal surface and into the blood, where it binds with albumin then is transported by the portal blood to the liver.

Functional evidence reveals that at least 24 specific transporters are responsible for either Zn influx or efflux in mammalian cells. These transporters are designated as two gene families: the ZnT proteins and the Zip family.[21] ZnT transporters reduce intracellular Zn availability by promoting Zn efflux from cells, whereas Zip transporters increase intracellular Zn availability by promoting extracellular uptake of Zn. Information about the actions of these transporters in muscle or other tissues in response to physical activity is lacking.

The total body content of Zn is partially controlled by the regulation of the efficiency of intestinal absorption of Zn. Numerous studies in animals and humans have reported an inverse relationship between Zn intake and absorption.[22] Thus, the regulation of Zn absorption by the mucosal cell provides a general control of total body Zn.

2. Excretion

Control of Zn excretion in feces represents another regulatory mechanism for maintenance of body Zn. In normal dietary circumstances, the feces are the major route of Zn excretion. In healthy humans with an average intake of 10 to 14 mg of Zn per day, more than 90% of dietary Zn is excreted in the feces.[9] Some of the Zn in the feces is from endogenous secretions. Studies indicate that 2.5 to 5 mg of Zn are secreted into the duodenum after a meal.[19] Much of the Zn secreted into the lumen of the gut is absorbed and returned to the body. The amount of Zn secreted into the gut varies with the Zn content of the meal. Endogenous fecal Zn excretion is directly related to dietary Zn intake.[22] In humans, endogenous fecal Zn losses may range from 1 mg/d with very low Zn intakes to more than 5 mg/d with extremely large Zn intakes.[23,24] In contrast to absorption, endogenous fecal Zn excretion represents a sensitive control to balance Zn retention to metabolic needs.

Other routes of Zn excretion are present in humans (Figure 15.1). About 0.4 to 0.5 mg of Zn are excreted daily in the urine.[9] Urinary Zn originates from the ultrafilterable portion of plasma Zn and represents a fraction of previously absorbed dietary Zn. Dietary Zn affects urinary Zn losses only under conditions of extreme intakes and results in corresponding changes in Zn output in the urine.[9]

Zn also is lost from the skin and in various secretions. Surface losses, which include sloughing of the skin, sweat and hair, contribute up to 1 mg of Zn loss daily. Surface losses range from 0.3–0.4 to 0.4–0.5 and 0.7–0.8 mg at intakes of 3–4, 8–9 and 33–34 mg/d, respectively.[26] A marked change in Zn intake results in parallel changes in surface Zn loss.[25] Other sources of Zn loss include seminal and menstrual secretions. An ejaculum of semen includes about 1 mg of Zn.[23] Total menstrual losses of Zn may reach 0.5 mg per menstrual period.[27]

The elimination of absorbed Zn from the body has been modeled with a two-component model.[9] In humans, an initial or rapid phase has a half-life of 12.5 d and a slower turnover phase of about 300 d. The initial rapid phase represents liver uptake of circulating Zn and its quick release into the circulation. The slower turnover rate reflects the different rates of turnover in various organs, excluding the liver. The most rapid rates of Zn uptake and turnover are found in the pancreas, liver, kidney and spleen, with slower rates in erythrocytes and muscle. Zn turnover is slowest in bone and the central nervous system.

Manipulation of dietary Zn impacts zinc turnover. In rats, dietary Zn restrictions promote retention of Zn in soft tissues and organs but not in bone.[28] In humans, the turnover of the slow Zn pool is increased by ingestion of pharmacologic amounts (100 mg) of Zn.[29] These homeostatic actions maintain soft tissue Zn concentrations despite variations in dietary Zn.

3. Transport

Distribution of absorbed Zn to the extrahepatic tissues occurs primarily in the plasma, which contains approximately 3 mg of Zn or about 0.1% of total body Zn.[30] Zn is partitioned among α_2-macroglobulin (40%), albumin (57%) and amino acids (3%) in plasma. Zn is bound loosely to albumin and amino acids; these fractions are responsible for transport of Zn from the liver to tissues. The amino acid-bound Zn constitutes the ultrafilterable fraction that is filtered at the kidneys and excreted in the urine. Because the total amount of Zn present in tissue is far greater than the Zn in the plasma, relatively small changes in tissue Zn content, such as in the liver, can have striking effects on the plasma Zn concentration. Importantly, because all absorbed Zn is transported from the plasma to tissues, the exchange of Zn from plasma into tissues is very rapid to maintain relatively constant plasma Zn concentrations (Figure 15.1).

III. ASSESSMENT OF HUMAN ZINC NUTRITIONAL STATUS

A deficiency of Zn progresses in a pattern that is different from that for most nutrients.[31] In general, an insufficient intake of a nutrient initially induces a mobilization of body stores or functional reserves. As depletion persists, tissue nutrient concentrations decrease, which results in deterioration in one or more nutrient-dependent metabolic functions. Therefore, growth reduction is a late manifestation of the nutritional deficiency. In contrast, when dietary Zn is decreased, the initial response is a reduction in growth by children and a decrease in endogenous losses of Zn as a means to conserve tissue Zn. If the dietary deficiency is mild, homeostasis may be reestablished after adjusting growth and Zn excretion, with no further impairment of function or biochemical changes. When dietary Zn is severely restricted, however, the body cannot restore homeostasis by adjusting endogenous losses and growth, consequently generalized impairment of organ and tissue function develops quickly.

Although severe dietary Zn deficiency can be induced in animals, it is rarely present in humans, with the exception of infants and children with acrodermatitis enteropathica, patients fed total parenteral nutrition solutions lacking Zn and experimental human Zn depletion. Evidence of moderate or mild Zn deficiency is difficult to demonstrate because of the lack of a sensitive and specific indicator of human Zn nutriture.[32]

Two general approaches have been used to assess human Zn status. One strategy has been to measure static indices, including concentrations of Zn in tissues or body fluids or measurements of biochemical surrogates for Zn nutriture in the form of Zn-containing enzymes and proteins. Another approach involves the measurement of dynamic indices that reflect the biological performance of Zn-dependent physiological or psychological functions.

Although frequently measured, plasma and serum Zn concentrations have been shown to be relatively insensitive to modest changes in dietary and body Zn.[33] Because whole-body Zn content is conserved in Zn deficiency, plasma and serum Zn are not reliable indicators of human Zn status. Further, plasma Zn is unresponsive to changes in dietary Zn unless the Zn intake is low and homeostasis cannot be reestablished. It is more realistic to describe plasma Zn as a component of a labile, nutritionally available pool of total body Zn.[33] Any decrease in plasma Zn concentration, therefore, should be interpreted as a decrease in the size of the labile Zn pool. Use of this concept is limited, however, by the findings that metabolic factors also influence the labile Zn pool. Infection, food intake, stress, brief-duration fasting and hormonal status can alter the distribution of Zn among the tissues and thus influence the amount of Zn in the plasma.[30]

Other static indices of human Zn status have failed to be useful. Red blood cell (RBC) Zn concentration is relatively unresponsive to mild or moderate Zn deficiency.[32] The Zn concentration in various populations of leukocytes also is not sensitive to changes in Zn status.[34] Timed urinary Zn excretion rates are decreased in severe Zn deficiency but are not responsive to more moderate changes in dietary Zn.[33] Therefore, current biochemical methods of assessment of human Zn status remain a limitation for routine clinical evaluation of Zn nutritional status.

IV. ZINC NUTRITURE OF PHYSICALLY ACTIVE ADULTS

Attempts to evaluate the Zn status of physically active individuals have been complicated by the use of different experimental designs and reliance on indirect indices of Zn nutritional status. The lack of an integrated assessment of factors affecting Zn homeostasis contributes to the deficit of knowledge about Zn requirements during periods of increased physical activity.

A. PLASMA ZINC CONCENTRATION

Awareness of potentially adverse effects of physical activity on human Zn nutritional status began with the observation that some endurance runners had significantly decreased serum Zn concentrations as compared with non-training men.[4] About 25% of 76 competitive male runners had serum Zn concentrations less than 11 µmol/l, the lower limit designated for the range of normal values. Importantly, serum Zn concentration was inversely related to weekly training distance. The investigators speculated that dietary habits, including avoidance of animal products and consumption of carbohydrate-rich foods, which are low in Zn, and possible increased losses of Zn in sweat, may have predisposed the runners to hypozincemia.

Similar findings of reduced plasma Zn concentrations have been reported for some, but not all, groups of highly trained athletes. In a survey of elite German athletes,[35] there was no difference between mean serum Zn concentrations of athletes and sex-matched non-athletes. Hypozincemia, defined as serum Zn concentration less than 11 µmol/l, was observed in about 25% of the athletes. Among female marathon runners, plasma Zn values were clustered at the low end of the range of

TABLE 15.2
Zinc Intake and Plasma Zinc Concentrations of Athletes and Control Subjects

Study	Activity	Sex	Dietary Zinc (mg/d)	Plasma Zinc (µmol/l)
Lukaski et al.[38]	Football, basketball, hockey, track & field	Male	16.3 ± 1.5[a]	13.3 ± 1.1
	Untrained	Male	13.7 ± 1.7	13.1 ± 1.2
Deuster et al.[41]	Running	Female	10.3 ± 0.7	10.1 ± 0.4
	Untrained	Female	10.0 ± 0.7	11.1 ± 0.4
Lukaski et al.[39]	Swimming	Female	12.4 ± 0.8	12.6 ± 0.5
	Untrained	Female	9.8 ± 0.9	12.8 ± 0.4
	Swimming	Male	17.9 ± 1.0	14.3 ± 0.5
	Untrained	Male	15.2 ± 1.0	12.8 ± 0.5
Fogelholm et al.[96]	Endurance	Male	17.7[b]	13.6[b]
	Untrained	Male	14.1[b]	13.8[b]
Fogelholm et al.[44]	Skiing	Female	15.8[b]	12.7[b]
	Untrained	Female	10.5[b]	12.6[b]
	Skiing	Male	21 .9[b]	14.1[b]
	Untrained	Male	14.1[b]	14.3[b]

[a] Mean ± SE
[b] Mean

normal values, with 22% of the values less than 11 µmol/l.[36,37] In contrast, no differences in plasma Zn concentrations were found in comparisons of male and female collegiate athletes with age-matched non-training students.[38,39] One explanation for these divergent results is that Zn intake may have been inadequate in the athletes with decreased circulating Zn concentrations.

B. DIETARY ZINC

Based on self-reported food and beverage consumption (Table 15.2), athletes generally consume Zn in amounts exceeding the estimated average requirement (EAR)[40] of 9.4 and 6.8 mg/d for men and women, respectively. However, a significant proportion of participants in some activities, including long-distance running and gymnastics, may consume less than 10 mg of Zn daily. Marginal intake is more widespread among female, as compared with male, athletes who restrict food intake. This behavior is characteristic among groups of athletes who participate in activities in which physical appearance is a component of performance evaluation.[41-43]

A general relationship between dietary Zn and plasma Zn in athletes is evident. On the average, athletes who consume at least the EAR for Zn have plasma Zn concentrations within the range of normal values (Table 15.2). This observation is independent of sex and sporting activity. Thus, if an individual consumes adequate dietary Zn, regardless of activity status, plasma Zn is within normal values.[44] Conversely, if dietary Zn is marginal, then plasma Zn concentration declines;[36,41] the apparent threshold for plasma Zn to decline is 4 mg of Zn/d.[45,46] Thus, low dietary Zn is associated with a reduced labile pool of Zn in the plasma and reflects impaired Zn status.

C. ZINC LOSSES

1. Surface Loss

Exercise is a stressor that can perturb body Zn homeostasis because it increases Zn loss. Estimates of whole-body Zn loss in sweat in men consuming controlled dietary Zn at 12.7 mg/d and not involved in vigorous activity were variable at 0.8 ± 0.2 (mean ± SE) mg/d and represented about

5% of daily Zn intake.[47] When acute bouts of submaximal exercise (30 min/d) were coupled with daily heat exposure (7.5 h at 37.8°C) for 18 d, Zn loss estimated from measurements of arm sweat of three men decreased appreciably after the first 4 days of acclimatization from 13.7 to 2.2 mg/d, which represented about 18% of the daily Zn intake of 12.5 mg.[48]

The concentration of Zn in sweat depends on the location from which sweat is collected during exercise and the ambient temperature. Zn concentration in sweat collected from 12 men during 30–40 min of strenuous ergocycle work ranged from 12.7 μmol/l at the abdomen as compared with about 7 μmol/l at the arm, chest and back.[49] Variation in sweat Zn concentration by site was considerable, ranging from 50 to 100% among the participants. Arm sweat Zn concentration after 1 h of low-intensity ergocycle work was lower at 35°C than at 25°C (0.8 vs. 1.3 μmol/l) but sweat Zn losses were similar (1.15 vs. 1.06 μg/min) in male and female athletes during submaximal ergocycle exercise, indicating that differences in rate of sweating tend to normalize surface Zn losses.[50] Exercise intensity and duration, therefore, contribute to differences in estimates of Zn loss in sweat. Furthermore, the large variability in estimates of surface loss of Zn suggests contamination of samples may be a problem when evaluating the reported magnitude of Zn lost during exercise.

Increased excretion of Zn in sweat during exercise coincides with moderate reductions in circulating Zn. Men and women exposed to heat for 1 week have decreased serum Zn concentrations.[51] Similarly, men participating in a 20-d marathon road race demonstrated a tendency toward a decrease in serum Zn concentration.[52] It is unclear whether the slight reductions in serum Zn reflect differences in dietary Zn or a modest expansion of plasma volume as an adaptation to chronic exposure to a stressor.

2. Urinary Excretion

Increased Zn excretion in the urine with exercise also has been reported. Studies of untrained men participating in short-duration activity (10 min of stair climbing to exhaustion) or trained men participating in a 10-mi road race observed a 50–60% increase in urinary Zn loss during the first hour after exercise as compared with a similar period of time before the exercise.[53] Similarly, Anderson et al.[54] reported a 50% increase in urinary Zn excretion on the day of exercise as compared with the day before in men performing a 6-mi run. In contrast, another study[55] found no differences in urinary Zn output when trained and untrained men performed high-intensity (90% peak work capacity), brief-duration bouts of treadmill running (30 s run followed by 30 s rest). Urinary Zn excretion, however, returns to pre-exercise values on the day following the exercise bouts.[54] Thus, acute increases in urinary Zn excretion are homeostatically regulated, with commensurate reductions in urinary Zn on the day following the exercise bout.

D. ZINC REDISTRIBUTION DURING EXERCISE

Exercise is a potent stressor that influences circulating Zn concentrations in the blood. In general, short-duration, high-intensity activities induce an immediate increase in plasma and serum Zn concentrations.[45,53,56] Longer-duration activities, such as distance runs or skiing, tend to have no immediate effect on plasma or serum Zn, but decreases have been observed in the hours after the activity.[53,54] These changes in circulating Zn have been interpreted as evidence of redistribution of Zn in the body despite no reports of Zn intake.

Limited data support the hypothesis that exercise induces Zn redistribution. Plasma Zn concentrations, determined before and immediately after progressive peak ergocycle work-capacity tests, changed in response to dietary Zn.[45] Although pre-exercise plasma Zn concentration values (15 μmol/l) were within the range of normal values, they decreased significantly (10.2 μmol/l) when dietary Zn was reduced and increased significantly (16.3 μmol/l) when dietary Zn was increased. Post-exercise plasma Zn concentrations increased significantly after exercise; they responded similarly to the pre-exercise values to changes in dietary Zn. As compared with the control period, when dietary Zn was adequate, the change in plasma Zn concentration in response to exercise was significantly smaller (8%) when dietary Zn was restricted and significantly larger (19%) when dietary Zn was increased. To correct for the effects of hemoconcentration, plasma Zn concentrations were adjusted for changes in hematocrit and hemoglobin to yield values of change in plasma Zn content. The adjusted values, which were positive (+1%) when dietary Zn was adequate and negative (−8%) when Zn intake was low, have been interpreted to indicate altered Zn mobilization, presumably a release of Zn from muscle Zn stores in association with exercise-induced catabolism when dietary Zn was inadequate.[45] This postulated explanation is consistent with data from animal studies in which slow-twitch muscle Zn was reduced in response to restricted Zn intake.[15]

Alternatively, exercise-induced changes in plasma Zn may be explained by release of Zn from erythrocytes. Ohno et al.[56] found that red blood cell Zn concentration decreased immediately after short-duration, high-intensity ergocycle exercise and returned to pre-exercise values within 1 h. A significant correlation was reported between erythrocyte Zn and $\alpha2$-macroglobulin Zn in plasma after exercise. Thus, brief physical exercise apparently induces the movement of Zn into the plasma.

Although it is clear that a transient redistribution of Zn occurs during exercise, the mechanism is unclear. Immune factors, such as cytokines, have been shown to change circulating Zn concentrations of rats.[57] Acute exercise induces metallothionein expression in liver and exerts small but significant increases in hepatic Zn with concomitant decreases in plasma Zn.[58]

V. ZINC SUPPLEMENTATION

Zn supplements are used by some athletes to improve performance. Singh et al.[37] found that 21% of elite female runners, despite consuming diet adequate in Zn, consumed Zn supplements to enhance their performance. Although there is evidence that Zn is needed for optimal muscle function,[59] the effects of supplemental Zn on performance are equivocal.

A. PERFORMANCE-ENHANCING EFFECTS

Ex vivo studies of frog skeletal muscle found that Zn added to the media increased muscle strength.[60] This ergogenic effect was associated with increased tension without tetanus and prolonged contraction and relaxation periods of the muscle twitch. The effects of supplemental Zn on muscle function were examined in adult male rats fed a chow-based diet and supplemented with Zn (2 or 4 mg/d) dissolved in water for 30 days.[61] Rats supplemented with 4, as compared with 2 mg Zn, had a greater time to fatigue (19.8 ± 1.0 vs. 16.2 ± 0.8 s). These findings should be viewed with caution because there is no indication that the observed change in performance resulted from an improvement in Zn status or increased activity of Zn-dependent enzymes.

There is limited information about the effects of Zn supplementation on human muscle strength and endurance. Sixteen middle-aged women received a Zn supplement (30 mg/d) and a placebo in a double-blind cross-over design study for 14-d periods.[62] Muscle strength and endurance were measured with an isokinetic one-leg exercise test using a standardized dynamometer before and after each treatment. As compared with placebo, Zn supplementation significantly increased dynamic isokinetic strength and isometric endurance. Because these types of muscular strength and endurance require recruitment of fast-twitch glycolytic muscle fibers, it can be hypothesized that Zn supplementation enhanced activity of the Zn-containing enzyme lactate dehydrogenase. Neither dietary Zn nor Zn status was determined. Thus, it is unclear that Zn supplementation had a physiological or pharmacological effect on the measured indices of performance.

The effects of graded dietary Zn on physical performance also have been evaluated. In untrained men fed diets containing variable Zn contents (3.6, 8.6 and 33.6 mg Zn daily), Zn status indicators and peak oxygen uptake were not affected.[45] Rats fed diets containing 5 compared with 50 mg Zn/kg of diet for 3 wk had significantly reduced serum Zn concentrations (10 vs 19 µmol/l) but no decrease in time to exhaustion during treadmill running at a constant speed and elevation.[63] The lack of an effect on physical performance may be explained by the some limitations in experimental design. The brief duration of the experiment might have impacted only circulating but not tissue Zn, particularly the activities of Zn-containing enzymes. The conditions of the endurance test could have favored the rats fed the lower Zn diet if they had significantly reduced body weight, because the intensity of the exercise would have been reduced, thus enabling longer duration of exercise before exhaustion.

In contrast, recent research shows that low Zn status was associated with decrements in physical performance. Men fed a formula-based diet severely low compared with adequate in zinc content (1 vs. 12 mg/d) had significantly decreased serum zinc associated with significant decreases in knee and shoulder extensor and flexor muscle strength.[64] Also, men fed whole-food diets low in zinc (3–4 mg/d) that were consistent with zinc intakes of endurance athletes,[65] demonstrated significantly increased ventilation rates and decreased oxygen uptake, carbon dioxide output and respiratory exchange ratio during prolonged submaximal ergocycle exercise.[46] The low-Zn diet was associated with significantly decreased serum Zn concentration and decreased Zn retention. RBC Zn concentration and the activity of carbonic anhydrase, a Zn-dependent enzyme, decreased significantly when the low-Zn diet was consumed. The attenuated oxygen uptake and carbon dioxide elimination, as well as the decreased respiratory exchange ratio, are consistent with previous findings in Zn-deficient men.[66] Thus, Zn deficiency, evidenced by decreased concentrations of blood biochemical measures of Zn nutritional status, adversely affects muscle strength and cardiorespiratory function.

B. ANTIOXIDANT EFFECTS

Recent studies support the hypothesis that Zn possesses antioxidant properties.[67] Results from some human studies indicate that Zn supplementation may benefit only individuals with impaired Zn status. Insulin-dependent diabetic patients with low plasma Zn concentrations supplemented with 30 mg Zn (as Zn gluconate) daily for 3 months had significant increases in plasma Zn and selenium-dependent glutathione peroxidase, and reductions in plasma thiobarbituric acid reactants and plasma copper.[68] In contrast, Zn supplementation (50 mg/d as Zn sulfate for 28 d) of healthy men with normal serum Zn concentrations increased serum Zn with no measurable changes on *in vitro* low-density lipoprotein oxidation.[69] Beneficial effects of Zn supplementation on physiological function are manifest, therefore, only when Zn status is reduced.

C. ADVERSE EFFECTS OF ZINC SUPPLEMENTATION

Zn supplements are consumed by 20–25% of athletes,[70] which is similar to the estimate of the rate of use by the general population.[40,71] There is concern that Zn supplements should be used with caution and under the guidance of a physician or a registered dietitian. Copper absorption is impaired by Zn supplements providing 22.5 mg/d,[72] even when the supplement is taken independently of meals.[73] RBC superoxide dismutase activity, an index of copper status, is decreased within 12 days of ingesting 50 mg of supplemental Zn daily.[74] Larger doses of Zn supplements, 160 mg/d, taken for 16 weeks, reduce high-density lipoprotein (HDL) concentrations.[66] It has been suggested that use of Zn supplements ranging from 17 to 50 mg/d is sufficient to prevent an exercise-induced increase in HDL concentration.[75]

Recent evidence shows that Zn supplementation at a pharmacological dose (80 mg Zn as Zn oxide) with copper (Cu; 2 mg) for 5 yr to prevent macular degeneration had no adverse effect on hematocrit, Cu or lipids.[76] This level of supplementation was accompanied by dietary Zn intakes of 10 mg/d, which is similar to the general population.[40,71] Thus, the adverse effects of high-dose Zn supplementation on hematology and lipids is offset with adequate Cu intake.

D. Supplementation and Performance Trials

Generalized trials of the effects of vitamin and mineral supplementation on human physical performance have reported negligible results. A group of 30 male, trained long-distance runners participated in a 9-month cross-over design experiment in which supplements or placebos were consumed for 3 months, followed by a 3-month period in which no experimental treatment was given; then the treatments were reversed for the final 3 months.[77,78] On the basis of laboratory and field performance tests, there was no measurable ergogenic effect of multiple vitamin and mineral supplementation. Analyses of self-reported dietary records indicated that nutrient intakes, exclusive of supplements, were adequate based on recommended dietary intake values. Blood biochemical measurements of nutritional status were within ranges of normal values.

Similar results were reported in other studies[79,80] of 86 competitive Australian athletes (50 men and 36 women) training in basketball, gymnastics, swimming and rowing, and receiving either a placebo or a commercially prepared vitamin and mineral supplement designed for athletes. During the 7–8-month experimental period there was no significant change in serum Zn concentration in either the supplemented or the placebo group (17.1 and 17.8 μmol/l, respectively). Dietary Zn, exclusive of supplementation, was consistent with recommended dietary intake for Australians. Performance, as assessed with a battery of general and sport-specific tests, was not impacted by the supplementation. Therefore, the results of these well-controlled and extensive trials[77-80] clearly indicate that general supplementation of individuals with adequate dietary intake of Zn provides no measurable improvement of Zn status or physical performance.

VI. DIETARY ZINC

A. Zinc in Foods

Zn content is a major determinant of the adequacy of various foods as sources of Zn for an individual planning a healthful diet.[81,82] Commonly consumed foods in the U.S. have a highly variable content of Zn (Table 15.3). Animal products (meat, fish and poultry) have the greatest concentration of Zn and provide the principal source of Zn in the U.S. diet.[83] Oysters are the richest source of Zn. Meat from fish has a smaller concentration of Zn than most animal muscle meats. Milk and milk products are important sources of Zn, particularly for infants and children and contribute 19% of the daily Zn intake. Importantly, adipose tissue or fat in animal and dairy products has negligible Zn content. The content of Zn consequently is high in cheese and low in butter and cream.

Cereals represent significant sources of energy and Zn in many areas throughout the world. Large differences in the Zn content, depending on the cereal type and including the variety, class and location of production have been reported. For example, the Zn content of wheat has been found to range from 15–102 mg/kg depending on the strain and from 219–61 mg/kg for the same variety of wheat grown in different locations and different years.[84] Cereal and grain products provide about 13% of the dietary Zn in the U.S.[83] Data for the Zn content of legumes consumed by humans are limited. As with cereals, factors such as variety, strain and growing location impact the Zn content of legumes.

Fruits and vegetables have modest contents of Zn (1–8 mg/kg) because of the high water content of the produce. Because these products provide limited energy intake, their contribution to total daily Zn intake is minimal.

TABLE 15.3
Content and Estimated Contribution to Meeting the Zn Needs of an Individual [%RDA of Zn] in Selected Foods

Foods	Serving Size[a]	Zinc (mg)[b,c]	% RDA[d] Men	% RDA[d] Women
Meats and fish				
Chuck blade roast, braised	3 oz (85 g)	8.7	79	108
Beef, ground lean, broiled	3 oz (85 g)	5.3	48	66
Steak, T-bone	3 oz (85 g)	4.6	42	58
Beef, eye of round, roasted	3 oz (85 g)	4.0	36	50
Pork shoulder blade, broiled	3 oz (85 g)	4.3	39	53
Pork loin chop, broiled	3 oz (85 g)	1.9	17	24
Chicken, drumstick, fried	3 oz (85 g)	2.7	25	33
Chicken, dark meat, fried	3 oz (85 g)	1.8	16	23
Chicken, breast meat, fried	3 oz (85 g)	0.9	8	11
Turkey, dark meat, roasted	3 oz (85 g)	3.8	35	47
Turkey, light meat, roasted	3 oz (85 g)	1.7	15	21
Tuna, canned in oil	3 oz (85 g)	0.8	7	10
Haddock, breaded, fried	3 oz (85 g)	0.5	4	6
Lobster, cooked moist heat	3 oz (85 g)	2.5	23	31
Shrimp, boiled	3 oz (85 g)	1.3	12	16
Dairy products				
Yogurt, nonfat/fruit flavored	6 oz (170 g)	1.3	12	16
Milk, lowfat, 2%	1 cup (244 g)	0.9	8	11
Cottage cheese lowfat, 2%	1/2 cup (113 g)	0.5	4	6
Cereals				
Raisin bran	3/4 cup (38 g)	1.1	10	14
Corn flakes	1 cup (25 g)	0.1	1	1
Grains				
Bagel, whole wheat	3 in (55 g)	1.3	12	16
Whole wheat bread	1 slice (28 g)	0.5	4	6
Macaroni, boiled	1/2 cup (70 g)	0.4	4	5
Fruits				
Banana	8 3/4 in (114 g)	0.2	2	3
Orange, raw	medium (131 g)	0.1	1	1
Vegetables				
Spinach, boiled, drained	1/2 cup (90 g)	0.7	6	9
Potato, white, baked w/skin	2–3 in (122 g)	0.4	4	5
Broccoli, chopped, raw	1/2 cup (44 g)	0.2	2	3
Carrots, raw	7.5 in (72 g)	0.2	2	3
Tomato	2 in (76 g)	0.1	1	1
Beans and Legumes				
Pork and beans	1/2 cup (126 g)	7.4	67	93
Kidney beans	1/2 cup (86 g)	1.0	9	13

TABLE 15.3 (*Continued*)
**Content and Estimated Contribution to Meeting the Zn Needs of an
Individual [%RDA of Zn] in Selected Foods**

Foods	Serving Size[a]	Zinc (mg)[b,c]	% RDA[d]	
			Men	Women
Mixed dishes				
Beef cheeseburger, bun	4 oz (95 g)	6.8	62	85
Chile con carne	1 cup (253 g)	3.6	33	45
Lasagna	1 cup (250 g)	3.3	30	41
Spaghetti, meatball and tomato sauce	1 cup (248 g)	2.6	24	33
Macaroni and cheese, prepared from box	3/4 cup (147 g)	1.3	12	16

[a] English units with metric units in parentheses.
[b,c] Values estimated by using data provided by U.S. Department of Agriculture[81,82]
[d] RDA for ages 19–70 y; men = 11mg, women = 8 mg[40]

B. Processing and Preparation of Foods

The amount of Zn present in foods is affected by how the fresh product is processed and prepared. Unfortunately, knowledge of nutrient losses during food processing and preparation is limited and generally restricted to vitamins.

The food process that has a major impact on Zn intake is refinement of cereals and grains. Because Zn is located in the outer layers, the germ and bran of grain and cereal kernels, large losses of Zn occur during milling and extraction. For example, about 80% of Zn in wheat is lost during the milling process.[85] Similar losses occur during the polishing of rice and in the refining of sugar.

Other pretreatments of foods before cooking or consumption, and cooking procedures themselves, can influence the Zn content of a meal. Use of galvanized cookware and storage of foods in Zn oxide-lined cans adds Zn to foods.[86] Zn losses into the storage media may be significant (20%) from foods prepared in water and from foods stored in cans.[87]

C. Zinc Bioavailability

The quantity of dietary Zn that is absorbed by a human is a function of the Zn status of the individual, the amount of Zn ingested and the bioavailability of the Zn from the meal. Bioavailability refers to the combined effects of various promoters and inhibitors of Zn absorption in the foods present in a meal.[17] Various nutrients and food components impact human Zn bioavailability.

The amount and type of protein affects human Zn absorption, which is positively related to the amount of protein in a meal, and Zn bioavailability is generally better from foods of animal than plant origin.[22] Factors that impact Zn bioavailability from plant foods are fiber and phytic acid.

Fiber in the form of bran has been found to reduce Zn absorption[88,89] or to have no effect.[90] Differences in particle size of the bran has been suggested to be a factor in these conflicting results.[90] In humans, Zn absorption from whole-meal bread was less than half (17%) of that from white bread (38%), but the Zn content of the whole-meal bread was three times greater than that of the white bread, so the total Zn absorbed was greater from the whole-meal bread.[91]

Phytic acid also has been shown to interfere with human Zn absorption. Stable isotope studies in humans showed a 50% reduction in Zn absorption when 3 g/d of sodium phytate was added to the diet.[92]

Zn absorption is inhibited in humans by the presence of excesses of certain minerals. When inorganic salts of iron and Zn are given, Zn absorption is decreased.[93] Zn absorption from food was not affected by large amounts of heme iron.[94,95]

VII. RESEARCH NEEDS

Specific aspects of the interaction between Zn nutrition and physical activity merit additional study. Because low Zn intakes are common among children and adolescents, and low Zn status is associated with impaired growth and development, future research should focus on determination of relationships among Zn status (intake and blood markers) and physical and mental function. Surveys and Zn supplementation trials of children and adolescents are needed to establish appropriate Zn intakes for optimal physiological and psychological function, and thus contribute to development of a recommendation for Zn in this segment of the population.

Previous studies examining the effect of increasing physical activity on Zn status markers are hampered by reliance on static measures of Zn status (e.g., plasma or serum Zn). There is a need to evaluate the specificity and sensitivity of newer biochemical indicators in this model. For example, studies of responsiveness of Zn-containing enzymes, including carbonic anhydrase and lactate dehydrogenase, are needed, particularly in association with determinations of metabolites affected by these enzymes.

The need to determine the interaction between dietary Zn and metabolic pools of Zn in response to increasing and decreasing physical activity is obvious. Although limited evidence suggests that the metabolizeable Zn pool is affected by dietary Zn restriction, it is unknown whether this pool is impacted by increasing physical activity or different types of exercise (e.g., aerobic vs. strength training).

These proposed investigations are needed to clearly determine whether current dietary recommendations for Zn are appropriate for the growing segment of the population thath is initiating and continuing physical activity to promote health and well-being. In addition, fundamental studies to determine whether excretory losses of Zn (sweat, surface, urine and feces) are affected by physical activity are needed.

VIII. CONCLUSIONS

Zn has biological roles in protein, carbohydrate and lipid metabolism and, hence, is needed for health and optimal performance. Experimental evidence describing the interaction of dietary Zn and physical activity in humans is limited. Recent evidence indicates that restricted Zn intake reduces Zn status indicators (serum and RBC Zn and Zn retention), decreases muscle strength and endurance and impairs cardiorespiratory function. Athletes who consume adequate amounts of dietary Zn have plasma or serum Zn concentrations that are within the range of normal values. Conversely, athletes who restrict food intake and concomitantly dietary Zn, have low concentrations of Zn in the circulation. As compared with nonexercise conditions, exercise induces increased losses of Zn in the sweat and urine that represent a small and perhaps significant percentage of daily Zn intake. Because the body tends to maintain the Zn content by selectively adjusting absorption and endogenous excretion of Zn, and an adaptation in urinary Zn output occurs on the day following a bout of exercise, the losses of Zn associated with heavy exercise probably are compensated. Proper selection of a variety of foods with varied Zn content, including animal products, unprocessed grains and cereals, will ensure an adequate Zn intake. Unequivocal evidence of beneficial effects of Zn supplementation on physical performance of humans is lacking if Zn intake meets population recommendations.

Consumption of Zn supplements by individuals with adequate Zn status might cause harm by inducing copper deficiency. Without biochemical or physical evidence of altered Zn status, individuals should avoid the use of Zn supplements in amounts exceeding 15 mg/d. Consumption of supplemental Zn in amounts of 50–150 mg/d can lead to impaired copper absorption and decreased HDL cholesterol, unless Cu supplements are consumed concomitantly. Because Zn impacts many diverse biological functions, physically active people should attempt to consume a balanced diet to ensure an adequate Zn intake and thus optimize health and physical performance.

REFERENCES

1. Lukaski, H.C., Micronutrients (magnesium, Zn and copper): are mineral supplements needed for athletes? *Int. J. Sport Nutr.* 5 Suppl, S74–S83, 1995.
2. Briefel, R.R., Bialostosky, K., Kennedy-Stephenson, J., McDowell, M.A., Ervin, R.B. and Wright, J.D., Zinc intake of the U.S. population: Findings from the third National Health and Nutrition Examination Survey, 1988–1994, *J. Nutr* 130, 1367S–1373S, 2000.
3. Dressendorfer, R.H. and Sockolov, R., HyperZnemia in runners, *Phys. Sportsmed.* 8, 97–100, 1980.
4. Lukaski, H.C., Vitamin and mineral status: effects on physical performance, *Nutrition* 20, 632–644, 2004.
5. World Health Organization, Obesity: Preventing and managing the global epidemic. World Health Organization, Geneva, 2000.
6. Vallee, B.L. and Falchuk, K.H., The biochemical basis of Zn physiology, *Physiol. Rev.* 73, 79–118, 1993.
7. Vallee, B.L. and Auld, D.S., Active Zn binding sites of zinc metalloenzymes, *Matrix Suppl.* 1, 5–19, 1992.
8. Vallee, B.L. and Auld, D.S., Zinc coordination, function and structure of zinc enzymes and other proteins, *Biochemistry* 29, 5647–5659, 1990.
9. Hambidge, K.M., Casey, C.E. and Krebs, N.F., Zinc, in *Trace Elements in Human and Animal Nutrition*, Mertz, W. and Underwood, E.J., Eds., Academic Press, Orlando, 1986, 1.
10. Reeves, P.G. and O'Dell, B.L., The effect of zinc deficiency on glucose metabolism in meal-fed rats, *Br. J. Nutr* 49, 441–452, 1983.
11. Mills, C.F., *Zinc in Human Biology.* Springer-Verlag, London, 1989, 1.
12. Bettger, W.J. and O'Dell, B.L., A critical physiological role of Zn in the structure and function of biomembranes, *Life Sci.* 28, 1425–1438, 1981.
13. International Comission on Radiological Protection, Report No. 23, Report of the Task Group on Reference Man. Pergamon Press, Oxford, 1975.
14. Maltin, C.A., Duncan, L., Wilson, A.B. and Hesketh, J.E., Effect of zinc deficiency on muscle fibre type frequencies in the post-weanling rat, *Br. J. Nutr.* 50, 597–604, 1983.
15. O'Leary, M.J., McClain, C.J. and Hegarty, P.V., Effect of Zn deficiency on the weight, cellularity and zinc concentration of different skeletal muscles in the post-weanling rat, *Br. J. Nutr.* 42, 487–495, 1979.
16. Jackson, M.J., Jones, D.A. and Edwards, R.H., Tissue zinc levels as an index of body zinc status, *Clin. Physiol.* 2, 333–343, 1982.
17. Sandstrom, B. and Lonnerdal, B., Promoters and antagonists of zinc absorption, in *Zinc in Human Biology,* Mills, C.F., Ed., Springer-Verlag, London, 1989, 57.
18. Scholmerich, J., Freudemann, A., Kottgen, E., Wietholtz, H., Steiert, B., Lohle, E., Haussinger, D. and Gerok, W., Bioavailability of zinc from zinc-histidine complexes. I. Comparison with zinc sulfate in healthy men, *Am. J. Clin. Nutr.* 45, 1480–1486, 1987.
19. Dibley, M.J.C., Zinc, in Present knowledge in nutrition, Bowman, B.A. and Russell, R.M., Eds., ILSI Press, Washington, D.C., 2001, 329.
20. Cousins, R.J., Absorption, transport and hepatic metabolism of copper and zinc: special reference to metallothionein and ceruloplasmin, *Physiol. Rev.* 65, 238–309, 1985.
21. Liuzzi, J.P. and Cousins, R.J., Mammalian zinc transporters, *Annu. Rev. Nutr* 24, 151–172, 2004.
22. Johnson, P.E., Zinc absorption and excretion in humans and animals, in *Copper and Zinc in Inflammation*, Milanino, R., Rainsford, K.D. and Velo, G.P., Eds., Kluwer Academic, Dordrecht, 1989, 103.
23. Baer, M.T. and King, J.C., Tissue zinc levels and zinc excretion during experimental zinc depletion in young men, *Am. J. Clin. Nutr.* 39, 556–570, 1984.
24. Jackson, M.J., Jones, D.A., Edwards, R.H., Swainbank, I.G. and Coleman, M.L., Zinc homeostasis in man: studies using a new stable isotope-dilution technique, *Br. J. Nutr.* 51, 199–208, 1984.
25. Prasad, A.S. and Schulbert, A.R., Zinc, iron and nitrogen content of sweat in normal and zinc-deficient men, *J. Lab. Clin. Med.* 62, 84–89, 1963.
26. Milne, D.B., Canfield, W.K., Mahalko, J.R. and Sandstead, H.H., Effect of dietary zinc on whole body surface loss of zinc: impact on estimation of zinc retention by balance method, *Am. J. Clin. Nutr.* 38, 181–186, 1983.
27. Hess, F.M., King, J.C. and Margen, S., Zinc excretion in young women on low zinc intakes and oral contraceptive agents, *J. Nutr* 107, 1610–1620, 1977.

28. Coppen, D.E. and Davies, N.T., Studies on the effects of dietary zinc dose on ^{65}zinc absorption *in vivo* and on the effects of zinc status on ^{65}zinc absorption and body loss in young rats, *Br. J. Nutr.* 57, 35–44, 1987.

29. Aamodt, R.L., Rumble, W.F., Babcock, A.K., Foster, D.M. and Henkin, R.I., Effects of oral zinc loading on zinc metabolism in humans — I: Experimental studies, *Metabolism* 31, 326–334, 1982.

30. Cousins, R.J., Systemic transport of zinc, in *Zinc in Human Biology,* Mills, C.F., Ed., Springer-Verlag, London, 1989, 79.

31. Golden, M.H.N., The diagnosis of zinc deficiency, in *Zinc in Human Biology,* Mills, C.F., Ed., Springer-Verlag, London, 1989, 323.

32. Solomons, N.W., On the assessment of zinc and copper nutriture in man, *Am. J. Clin. Nutr.* 32, 856–871, 1979.

33. King, J.C., Assessment of zinc status, *J. Nutr* 120 Suppl 11, 1474–1479, 1990.

34. Milne, D.B., Ralston, N.V. and Wallwork, J.C., Zinc content of cellular components of blood: methods for cell separation and analysis evaluated, *Clin. Chem.* 31, 65–69, 1985.

35. Haralambie, G., Serum zinc in athletes in training, *Int. J. Sports Med.* 2, 135–138, 1981.

36. Deuster, P.A., Kyle, S.B., Moser, P.B., Vigersky, R.A., Singh, A. and Schoomaker, E.B., Nutritional survey of highly trained women runners, *Am. J. Clin. Nutr.* 44, 954–962, 1986.

37. Singh, A., Deuster, P.A. and Moser, P.B., Zinc and copper status in women by physical activity and menstrual status, *J. Sports Med. Phys. Fitness* 30, 29–36, 1990.

38. Lukaski, H.C., Bolonchuk, W.W., Klevay, L.M., Milne, D.B. and Sandstead, H.H., Maximal oxygen consumption as related to magnesium, copper and zinc nutriture, *Am. J. Clin. Nutr.* 37, 407–415, 1983.

39. Lukaski, H.C., Hoverson, B.S., Gallagher, S.K. and Bolonchuk, W.W., Physical training and copper, iron and zinc status of swimmers, *Am. J. Clin. Nutr.* 51, 1093–1099, 1990.

40. Institute of Medicine, Dietary reference intakes for vitamin A, vitamin K, arsenic, boron, chromium, copper, iodine, iron, manganese, molybdenum, nickel, silicon, vanadium and zinc, National Academy Press, Washington, D.C., 2001, 442.

41. Deuster, P.A., Day, B.A., Singh, A., Douglass, L. and Moser-Veillon, P.B., Zinc status of highly trained women runners and untrained women, *Am. J. Clin. Nutr.* 49, 1295–1301, 1989.

42. Benson, J., Gillien, D.M., Bourdet, K. and Loosli, A.R., Inadequate nutrition and chronic calorie restriction in adolescent ballerinas, *Phys. Sportsmed.* 13, 79–90, 1985.

43. Loosli, A.R., Benson, J., Gillien, D.M. and Bourdet, K., Nutrition habits and knowledge in competitive adolescent female gymnasts, *Phys. Sportsmed.* 14, 118–130, 1986.

44. Fogelholm, M., Rehunen, S., Gref, C.G., Laakso, J.T., Lehto, J., Ruokonen, I. and Himberg, J.J., Dietary intake and thiamin, iron and zinc status in elite Nordic skiers during different training periods, *Int. J. Sport Nutr.* 2, 351–365, 1992.

45. Lukaski, H.C., Bolonchuk, W.W., Klevay, L.M., Milne, D.B. and Sandstead, H.H., Changes in plasma zinc content after exercise in men fed a low-zinc diet, *Am. J. Physiol.* 247, E88–E93, 1984.

46. Lukaski, H.C., Low dietary zinc decreases erythrocyte carbonic anhydrase activities and impairs cardiorespiratory function in men during exercise, *Am. J. Clin. Nutr.* (in review), 2004.

47. Jacob, R.A., Sandstead, H.H., Munoz, J.M., Klevay, L.M. and Milne, D.B., Whole body surface loss of trace metals in normal males, *Am. J. Clin. Nutr.* 34, 1379–1383, 1981.

48. Consolazio, C.F., Nutrition and performance, *Prog. Food. Nutr. Sci.* 7, 1–187, 1983.

49. Aruoma, O.I., Reilly, T., MacLaren, D. and Halliwell, B., Iron, copper and zinc concentrations in human sweat and plasma; the effect of exercise, *Clin. Chim. Acta* 177, 81–87, 1988.

50. Tipton, K., Green, N.R., Waller, M. and Haymes, E.M., Mineral losses from sweat in athletes exercising at two different temperatures, *FASEB J.* 6, A768, 1991.

51. Uhari, M., Pakarinen, A., Hietala, J., Nurmi, T. and Kouvalainen, K., Serum iron, copper, zinc, ferritin and ceruloplasmin after intense heat exposure, *Eur. J. App. Physiol. Occup. Physiol.* 51, 331–335, 1983.

52. Dressendorfer, R.H., Wade, C.E., Keen, C.L. and Scaff, J.H., Plasma mineral levels in marathon runners during a 20-day road race, *Phys. Sportsmed.* 10, 113–118, 1982.

53. van Rij, A.M., Hall, M.T., Dohm, G.L., Bray, J. and Pories, W.J., Changes in zinc metabolism following exercise in human subjects, *Biol. Trace Elem. Res.* 10, 99–105, 1986.

54. Anderson, R.A., Polansky, M.M. and Bryden, N.A., Strenuous running. Acute effects on chromium, copper, zinc and selected clinical variables in urine and serum of male runners, *Biol. Trace Elem. Res.* 6, 327–336, 1984.

55. Anderson, R.A., Bryden, N.A., Polansky, M.M. and Deuster, P.A., Acute exercise effects on urinary losses and serum concentrations of copper and zinc of moderately trained and untrained men consuming a controlled diet, *Analyst* 120, 867–870, 1995.

56. Ohno, H., Yamashita, K., Doi, R., Yamamura, K., Kondo, T. and Taniguchi, N., Exercise-induced changes in blood zinc and related proteins in humans, *J. Appl. Physiol.* 58, 1453–1458, 1985.

57. Cannon, J.G. and Kluger, M.J., Endogenous pyrogen activity in human plasma after exercise, *Science* 220, 617–619, 1983.

58. Oh, S.H., Deagen, J.T., Whanger, P.D. and Weswig, P.H., Biological function of metallothionein. V. Its induction in rats by various stresses, *Am. J. Physiol.* 234, E282–E285, 1978.

59. Wang, J. and Pierson, R.N., Jr., Distribution of zinc in skeletal muscle and liver tissue in normal and dietary controlled alcoholic rats, *J. Lab. Clin. Med.* 85, 50–58, 1975.

60. Isaacson, A. and Sandow, A., Effects of zinc on responses of skeletal muscle, *J. Gen. Physiol.* 46, 655–677, 1963.

61. Richardson, J.H. and Drake, P.D., The effects of zinc on fatigue of striated muscle, *J. Sports Med. Phys. Fitness* 19, 133–134, 1979.

62. Krotkiewski, M., Gudmundsson, M., Backstrom, P. and Mandroukas, K., Zinc and muscle strength and endurance, *Acta Physiol Scand* 116, 309–311, 1982.

63. McDonald, R. and Keen, C.L., Iron, zinc and magnesium nutrition and athletic performance, *Sports Med.* 5, 171–184, 1988.

64. Van Loan, M.D., Sutherland, B., Lowe, N.M., Turnlund, J.R. and King, J.C., The effects of zinc depletion on peak force and total work of knee and shoulder extensor and flexor muscles, *Int. J. Sport Nutr.* 9, 125–135, 1999.

65. Micheletti, A., Rossi, R. and Rufini, S., Zinc status in athletes: Relation to diet and exercise, *Sports Med.* 31, 577–582, 2001.

66. Wada, L. and King, J.C., Effect of low zinc intakes on basal metabolic rate, thyroid hormones and protein utilization in adult men, *J. Nutr* 116, 1045–1053, 1986.

67. Bray, T.M. and Bettger, W.J., The physiological role of zinc as an antioxidant, *Free Radic. Biol. Med.* 8, 281–291, 1990.

68. Faure, P., Benhamou, P.Y., Perard, A., Halimi, S. and Roussel, A.M., Lipid peroxidation in insulin-dependent diabetic patients with early retina degenerative lesions: effects of an oral zinc supplementation, *Eur. J. Clin. Nutr.* 49, 282–288, 1995.

69. Gatto, L.M. and Samman, S., The effect of zinc supplementation on plasma lipids and low-density lipoprotein oxidation in males, *Free Radic. Biol. Med.* 19, 517–521, 1995.

70. Schwenk, T.L. and Costley, C.D., When food becomes a drug: nonanabolic nutritional supplement use in athletes, *Am. J. Sports Med.* 30, 907–916, 2002.

71. National Research Council, Recommended dietary allowances. National Academy Press, Washington, D.C., 1989, 30.

72. Hackman, R.M. and Keen, C.L., Changes in serum zinc and copper levels after zinc supplementation in running and non-running men, in *Sport, Health and Nutrition*, Katch, F.I., Ed., Human Kinetics Publishers, Champaign, Ill., 1986, 89.

73. Van den Hamer, C.J.A., Hoogeraad, T.U. and Klompjan, E.R.K., Persistence of the antagonistic effect of zinc on copper absorption after cessation of zinc supplementation for more than five days, *Biol. Trace Elem. Res.* 1, 99, 1984.

74. Abdallah, S.M. and Samman, S., The effect of increasing dietary zinc on the activity of superoxide dismutase and zinc concentration in erythrocytes of healthy female subjects, *Eur. J. Clin. Nutr.* 47, 327–332, 1993.

75. Goodwin, J.S., Hunt, W.C., Hooper, P. and Garry, P.J., Relationship between zinc intake, physical activity and blood levels of high-density lipoprotein cholesterol in a healthy elderly population, *Metabolism* 34, 519–523, 1985.

76. Age-Related Eye Disease Study Research Group, The effect of five-year zinc supplementation on serum zinc, serum cholesterol and hematocrit in persons randomly assigned to treatment group in the age-related eye disease study: AREDS Report No. 7, *J. Nutr* 132, 697–702, 2002.

77. Weight, L.M., Noakes, T.D., Labadarios, D., Graves, J., Jacobs, P. and Berman, P.A., Vitamin and mineral status of trained athletes including the effects of supplementation, *Am. J. Clin. Nutr.* 47, 186–191, 1988.

78. Weight, L.M., Myburgh, K.H. and Noakes, T.D., Vitamin and mineral supplementation: effect on the running performance of trained athletes, *Am. J. Clin. Nutr.* 47, 192–195, 1988.
79. Telford, R.D., Catchpole, E.A., Deakin, V., McLeay, A.C. and Plank, A.W., The effect of 7 to 8 months of vitamin/mineral supplementation on the vitamin and mineral status of athletes, *Int. J. Sport Nutr.* 2, 123–134, 1992.
80. Telford, R.D., Catchpole, E.A., Deakin, V., Hahn, A.G. and Plank, A.W., The effect of 7 to 8 months of vitamin/mineral supplementation on athletic performance, *Int. J. Sport Nutr.* 2, 135–153, 1992.
81. USDA, Consumer Nutrition Data Set 456-3. U.S. Dept. of Agriculture, Hyattsville, MD, 1977.
82. USDA, Composition of foods: Agriculture handbook 8.1–12. U.S. Dept. of Agriculture, Hyattsville, MD, 1984.
83. USDA, Nutrition monitoring in the United States: The directory of federal nutrition monitoring activities. U.S. Dept. of Health and Human Services, Public Health Service, Hyattsville, MD., 1989.
84. Davis, K.R., Peters, L.J., Cain, R.F., LeTourneau, D. and McGinnis, J., Evaluation of the nutrient composition of wheat. III. Minerals, *Cereal Foods World* 29, 246–248, 1984.
85. Schroeder, H.A., Losses of vitamins and trace minerals resulting from processing and preservation of foods, *Am. J. Clin. Nutr.* 24, 562–573, 1971.
86. Henriksen, L.K., Mahalko, J.R. and Johnson, L.K., Canned foods: appropriate in trace element studies? *J. Am. Diet. Assoc.* 85, 563–568, 1985.
87. Schmitt, H.A. and Weaver, C.M., Effects of laboratory scale processing on chromium and zinc in vegetables, *J. Food Sci.* 47, 1693–1694, 1982.
88. Sandberg, A.S., Hasselblad, C., Hasselblad, K. and Hulten, L., The effect of wheat bran on the absorption of minerals in the small intestine, *Br. J. Nutr.* 48, 185–191, 1982.
89. Schwartz, R., Apgar, B.J. and Wien, E.M., Apparent absorption and retention of Ca, Cu, Mg, Mn and Zn from a diet containing bran, *Am. J. Clin. Nutr.* 43, 444–455, 1986.
90. Van Dokkum, W., Wesstra, A. and Schippers, F.A., Physiological effects of fibre-rich types of bread. 1. The effect of dietary fibre from bread on the mineral balance of young men, *Br. J. Nutr.* 47, 451–460, 1982.
91. Sandstrom, B., Arvidsson, B., Cederblad, A. and Bjorn-Rasmussen, E., Zinc absorption from composite meals. I. The significance of wheat extraction rate, zinc, calcium and protein content in meals based on bread, *Am. J. Clin. Nutr.* 33, 739–745, 1980.
92. Turnlund, J.R., King, J.C., Keyes, W.R., Gong, B. and Michel, M.C., A stable isotope study of zinc absorption in young men: effects of phytate and alpha-cellulose, *Am. J. Clin. Nutr.* 40, 1071–1077, 1984.
93. Solomons, N.W. and Jacob, R.A., Studies on the bioavailability of zinc in humans: effects of heme and nonheme iron on the absorption of zinc, *Am. J. Clin. Nutr.* 34, 475–482, 1981.
94. Solomons, N.W., Pineda, O., Viteri, F. and Sandstead, H.H., Studies on the bioavailability of zinc in humans: mechanism of the intestinal interaction of nonheme iron and zinc, *J. Nutr* 113, 337–349, 1983.
95. Valberg, L.S., Flanagan, P.R. and Chamberlain, M.J., Effects of iron, tin and copper on zinc absorption in humans, *Am. J. Clin. Nutr.* 40, 536–541, 1984.
96. Fogelholm, M., Laakso, J., Lehto, J. and Ruokonen, I., Dietary intake and indicators of magnesium and zinc status in male athletes, *Nutr. Res* 11, 1111–1118, 1991.

16 Copper

Philip G. Reeves and W. Thomas Johnson

CONTENTS

I. INTRODUCTION

Over the past few years, a sustained interest has developed in trace element nutrition and metabolism as it relates to athletic performance. The current beliefs are that athletes require more minerals than a more sedentary individual, that athletes do not eat a balanced diet and that low consumption of some trace elements will worsen performance. Whether these beliefs have substance in fact is an ongoing debate. Of all the minerals covered in this volume concerned with athletic conditioning and performance, copper (Cu) may be one of the most important. It serves as an essential component of oxygen utilization and the antioxidant system, but at the same time, it can be toxic by initiating free-radical generation.

Cu is a transition metal that has valence states of +1 and +2. It is highly reactive in oxidation-reduction reactions and, because of this property, nature has devised means to assure that very little free Cu is present in living tissues. Most of the Cu is bound to organic ligands such as proteins, peptides and amino acids. Ninety-three percent of Cu in plasma is bound to the ceruloplasmin (Cp) protein. Cu can interact with other metals near it in the periodic table, which include iron, zinc and cadmium. These interactions often involve the substitution of the other metal in the active site of the

Mention of a trademark or proprietary product does not constitute a guarantee of the product by the United States Department of Agriculture and does not imply its approval to the exclusion of other products that may also be suitable.

U.S. Department of Agriculture, Agricultural Research Service, Northern Plains Area is an equal opportunity/affirmative action employer and all agency services are available without discrimination.

Cu enzyme, or in a metal transport site normally reserved for Cu, and inhibit the function of Cu at that site. Sometimes the reverse occurs, where Cu interferes with the metabolism of the other metals.

Cu is involved in many chemical reactions in the body that may be more prominently involved with oxygen consumption and stress—conditions that become exaggerated during participation in vigorous exercise. For example, Cu is essential for maximal activity of cytochrome c oxidase, the enzyme in a chain of reactions that transfer electrons from cytochrome c to oxygen during metabolism, which leads to the production of high-energy phosphate bonds (ATP) and water. Cu is an active component of Cu, Zn-superoxide dismutase (SOD1), an enzyme involved in free-radical quenching and elimination, thus lessening free-radical damage in tissues. Cu is required for iron (Fe) absorption, and blood cell and hemoglobin formation, which prevents anemia. Cu plays a major role in the acute phase response to stress situations.

Cu also is involved in cardiovascular and neuronal development and function. Cu is an active component of enzymes that cross-link collagen and elastin in the vascular system, lungs and other organs. Cu deficiency in young animals causes lung damage, with clinical signs similar to emphysema. The trace element is intimately involved in enzyme systems that generate brain and somatic neurotransmitters where, in young animals, a Cu deficiency produces a Parkinson-like syndrome.

On the other hand, Cu can be toxic. Free Cu can participate in the superoxide-driven Fenton reaction to produce the free radical $HO^{\bullet}$ from hydrogen peroxide. This radical is strongly reactive at the site of formation. Cu is more reactive than iron in causing DNA damage, which suggests that the free Cu concentrations in the body should be carefully controlled.

The preceding describes the broad involvement of Cu in metabolism and the following review will go into more detail about how Cu is obtained from the diet, how it is absorbed into the body, how much is in the body, how Cu functions biochemically and physiologically, and what are the dietary requirements for Cu. This chapter attempts to relate each point to athletic training and performance where applicable. For in-depth reviews of the biochemistry of Cu and its metabolism, please refer to Mason[1], O'Dell[2], Linder[3] and the DRI manual.[4]

II. COPPER IN FOOD AND ITS DIETARY REQUIREMENT

Of all the minerals known to have a physiological function in the body, Cu was at one time considered one of the most limiting in the human diet. In 1980, the Food and Nutrition Board (FNB) of the National Research Council (NRC) of the U.S. National Academy of Sciences[5] could not agree on a recommended dietary allowance (RDA) for Cu. Instead, a value called "the estimated safe and adequate daily dietary intake" (ESADDI) was established for Cu that ranged from 2.0 to 3.0 mg/day for individuals over the age of 11. In 1989, the FNB again could not agree on an RDA for Cu, even though much more data had accumulated over the ensuing 9 years. The board instead lowered the ESADDI to 1.5 to 3 mg/day.[6] In the meantime, the Canadian estimate for an adequate intake of Cu was held at 1.0 to 2.0 mg/day.[7] During the most recent deliberations of the Institute of Medicine of the FNB, it was finally agreed to set the recommended Cu intake at 0.9 mg/day for individuals of age 19 and over.[4]

Before the FNB established the RDA for Cu, the normal intake was relatively low when compared with the ESADDI. Klevay et al.[8] chemically analyzed Cu in 849 individual western-type diets consisting of foods from Belgium, Canada, the U.K. and the U.S. They found that the mean intake of Cu per day was 1.48 mg, with 95% of the values falling between 0.46 and 3.64, and 32% of the diets providing less than 1.01 mg of Cu per day. Pang et al.[9] measured daily Cu intakes of 68 individuals in a single geographic area of the U.S. in a 1-year period and found that about 65% consumed near or below the RDA for Cu. However, the Third National Health and Nutrition Examination Survey (NHANES III, 1988–1994) estimated Cu intakes based on dietary recall and found that only 25% of the population sampled fell near or below the RDA for Cu.[10] Johnson et al.[11] reported intakes of 1.3 mg of Cu/day for men and 0.95 mg/day for women between the ages of 19 and 40 who consumed self-selected diets. However, when intakes were expressed on a caloric density basis, women consumed about 15% more Cu than men. Depending on which standard is used for assessing adequate intakes of Cu, a large portion of the population might experience low Cu status. Selecting a diet with less than the RDA for Cu could be easy for an individual in the Western world if the diets are not balanced with a variety of foods.

Staple foods including breads, rice, vegetables, fruits or even meats do not contain a large amount of Cu (Table 16.1). Lawler and Klevay[12] suggest that foods containing more than 2 mg of

TABLE 16.1
Content and Estimated Percent of the RDA for Cu in Selected Foods by Serving Size

	Serving size	Cu (mg)[a]	% RDA[b]
Meats and fish			
Liver, cooked	3 oz.(85 g)	3.842	427
Oysters, Pacific, cooked	3 oz.(85 g)	2.279	253
Oysters, Atlantic, cooked	3 oz.(85 g)	1.220	136
Trout, broiled	3 oz.(85 g)	0.204	23
Duck, roasted w/skin	3 oz.(85 g)	0.193	21
Beef, sirloin roast	3 oz.(85 g)	0.105	12
Whitefish, broiled	3 oz.(85 g)	0.078	9
Salmon, Coho, broiled	3 oz.(85 g)	0.076	8
Pork loin, roasted	3 oz.(85 g)	0.069	8
Chicken, roasted	3 oz.(85 g)	0.068	8
Fruits and vegetables			
Potato, white, baked, w/skins	1 med (173 g)	0.616	68
White beans, boiled	1 cup (179 g)	0.514	57
Lentils, boiled	1 cup (198 g)	0.497	55
Avocado, raw	1 med (201 g)	0.460	51
Kidney beans, boiled	1 cup (177 g)	0.428	48
Asparagus tips, steamed	1 cup (90 g)	0.308	34
Potato, white, boiled, wo/skins	1 med (167 g)	0.261	29
Sweet potato, baked	1 sml (60 g)	0.237	26
Mushrooms, raw	1/2 cup (48 g)	0.172	19
Green beans, snap, boiled	1 cup (125 g)	0.070	8
Nuts, grains and seeds			
Sunflower kernels, dry roasted	2 oz.(57 g)	1.037	115
Walnuts, fresh	2 oz.(57 g)	0.787	87
Almonds, dry roasted	2 oz.(57 g)	0.694	77
Wheat germ	1/2 cup (58 g)	0.458	51
Peanuts, dry roasted	2 oz.(56.7 g)	0.381	42
Wild rice, cooked	1 cup (164 g)	0.200	22
Brown rice, cooked	1 cup (195 g)	0.195	22
Whole wheat bread	2 slices (56 g)	0.172	19
Barley, cooked	1 cup (157 g)	0.165	18
Oatmeal, cooked	1 cup (234 g)	0.129	14
White bread	2 slices (50 g)	0.126	14
White rice, cooked	1 cup (158 g)	0.108	12
Milk, 1% fat	1 cup (240 mL)	0.025	3
Brewer's yeast	1/2 oz.(14.2 g)	0.700	78
Molasses, brown	1 fl.oz.(32 mL)	0.225	25

[a] Values were generated from nutrition data set, version SR17 provided by the U.S.Department of Agriculture, which can be accessed through the website: http://www.nal.usda.gov/fnic/foodcomp/Data/SR17/sr17.html
[b] Based on the RDA of 0.9 mg Cu /day[4]

Cu/kg of edible portions are good sources of dietary Cu. Table 16.1 lists some common foods and their Cu concentrations.[13] Some fruits and vegetables have moderate quantities of Cu, with potatoes and beans having the highest amount. Nuts and seeds have high amounts of Cu compared with other foods, and seeds such as sunflower kernels are excellent sources of Cu. However, these foods also contain high concentration of polyunsaturated fats, up to 40%.

The foods containing the highest amount of Cu are liver and Pacific oysters. A person could obtain more than 100% of the RDA with a 1-oz. (28.4 g) serving of liver or a 1.5-oz. (42.5 g) serving of oysters. In contrast, other meats and fish have low concentrations of Cu. It seems an unfortunate quirk of nature to have the highest amount of Cu in foods that are the most expensive (oysters), that contain high fat (nuts and seed) or are disliked by most of the U.S. and Canadian public (liver). However, clever disguises of the latter or substitutions of these foods for others in combination dishes would not only improve one's nutritional Cu status but would provide a host of other required nutrients as well. Wheat flour is low in Cu; however, wild rice, if eaten regularly, could provide a moderate amount of Cu in the diet.

III. COPPER INTAKES IN ATHLETES

Nutritionist are often concerned that persons undergoing strenuous exercise or prolonged training and sports competition are not consuming enough of the required nutrients to sustain nutritional status, thus jeopardizing performance. The Australian Institute of Sports undertook a study to determine whether vitamin/mineral supplementation of a normal diet would affect the vitamin and mineral status of athletes.[14] There were 86 athletes, men and women, who participated in various sports activities for 8 months. One half of the group consumed a supplement that contained 13 known essential vitamins and 8 essential minerals (Cu was not included). After eight months of training and participation, none of the mineral supplements changed the overall mineral status of the athletes when measured as a change in blood concentration and compared with those not receiving the supplements. Of the vitamins supplemented, only thiamine, B6 and B12 in blood were elevated. Before sports activities began, only 7% of the participants were considered below the laboratory acceptable range for blood Cu concentration. However, at the end of the sports activities, no participant was below normal whether he or she took the supplements or did not. Throughout the study, personal and group dietary counseling sessions were carried out to ensure that each athlete maintained a well-balanced diet. Therefore, one could interpret the results of this study to mean that if athletes maintain a well-balanced diet of a variety of foods, they do not require extra supplementation with vitamins and minerals. In addition, a corresponding study using the same subjects showed that the vitamin and mineral supplementation had no significant effects on performance.[14]

Another study observed dietary patterns and assessed the nutritional knowledge of recreational triathletes.[15] They found that, over an 11-week training period, women consumed an average ± SD of 1.5 ± 0.5 mg of Cu/day and men 1.8 ± 0.7 mg/day. These values represent 167 and 200% of the current RDA, respectively. Therefore, it is unlikely that any of these athletes suffered from low or marginal Cu status.

In a well-controlled study, Lukaski et al.[16] found no correlation between Cu intakes of men and women swimmers and control non-swimmers and Cu status indicators measured before and after extensive training. The daily intakes of Cu averaged 1.15 ± 0.36 mg/day for women non-swimmers and 1.35 ± 0.40 for women swimmers. Men averaged about 1.7 ± 0.54 mg Cu/day for both swimmers and non-swimmers; this was significantly higher than for women. However, when intakes were calculated on the basis of caloric intake, there were no significant differences in intake between men and women. Plasma concentrations of Cu ranged from 13.8 ± 3.2 to 15.9 ± 5.2 μmol/L for women and 13.2 ± 1.6 to 14.3 ± 2.0 for men, whether they were swimmers or not. In another study by Lukaski et al.,[17] collegiate men and women free-style swimmers reported intakes of Cu of 1.8 ± 0.2 and 1.3 ± 0.2 mg/day, respectively. Serum Cu concentrations were 13.9 ± 1.3 μmol/L for men and 15.9 ± 2.5 for women. Based on these studies reported 6 years apart, it seems that Cu intakes and serum Cu concentrations are very consistently controlled among young athletes.

Rigorously controlled studies at the Grand Forks Human Nutrition Research Center were performed on non-athletic women volunteers ages 18 to 36.[18] Half of the group consumed natural-ingredient diets with as little as 0.65 ± 0.05 mg Cu/day while the other half consumed similar diets with 1.45 mg Cu/day for 7 weeks. Those consuming the low Cu diets had plasma Cu concentrations and Cp activities that were 9 and 19% lower than the control volunteers, respectively. The volunteers fed the low Cu diets also were in negative balance with respect to Cu. When supplemented with 2.65 mg Cu/day for 5.5 weeks, they came back into Cu balance. These data suggest that the basal Cu requirement for non-athletic women is higher than 0.65 mg/day, but lower than 1.5 mg/day. Studies from this laboratory in the 1980s suggested that the requirement for adult human males is about 1.6 mg/day when body surface losses of Cu are considered.[19] Please note that this value is nearly 1.5 times higher than the current RDA. However, the concentration of dietary Cu at which signs of low status might develop would depend on the length of time volunteers were consuming a particular amount of Cu. Therefore, in studies such as these, the experimental periods may be too short to find an indication of low status.

IV. COPPER BIOAVAILABILITY

The bioavailability of a nutrient is defined as that amount absorbed from the diet and how well it is utilized in metabolic processes; however, in many studies, this term may refer only to absorption. In humans as well as other mammals, the amount of Cu absorbed from the gut varies with the amount of Cu in the diet. On a percentage basis, there is an inverse relationship between dietary Cu concentration and absorption. However, the net amount of Cu absorbed actually increases as dietary Cu increases, up to a point. With data referred to by Turnlund et al.,[20,21] it can be predicted by using a hyperbolic curve fit analysis of Cu absorbed vs. Cu intakes over a range of 0.4 to 7.5 mg/day that the maximal rate of Cu absorbed will be approximately 1.2 mg/day, with the half maximal rate at 1.0 mg Cu intake/day. This suggests that a person consuming the RDA of 0.9 mg would absorb only about 0.5 mg of Cu.

Although some foods may contain moderate amounts of Cu, the availability of the Cu for absorption and utilization may not be realized because of other factors in the food. Some of the inhibiting factors include fructose, ascorbic acid, iron and zinc. Phytate, a common component of most plant foods, is an enhancing factor. For the most part, the RDA accounts for the effects of other dietary components on Cu absorption.

A. EFFECT OF DIETARY CARBOHYDRATES ON COPPER ABSORPTION

It has been known for years that dietary sucrose or fructose intensifies the effects of low dietary Cu intakes in laboratory animals such as the rat.[22–24] Some evidence suggests that dietary fructose reduces the absorption of Cu from the gut of rats by lowering the solubility of Cu in the gut lumen.[25–27] Fructose is a reducing agent, and other reducing factors such as ascorbic acid have been found to lower Cu absorption as well.[28] The detrimental effects of fructose on Cu metabolism have not been successfully demonstrated for other species including the pig or human.[29–31] Nonetheless, with the ever-increasing use of high-fructose syrups in foods, including some sports beverages, there may be some concern in the future about the effects of long-term use of this carbohydrate on Cu metabolism in athletes.

B. EFFECT OF DIETARY REDUCING AGENTS ON COPPER ABSORPTION

Van Campen and Gross[32] were the first to show that dietary ascorbic acid (vitamin C) attenuates the absorption of Cu from the gut of mammals. The mechanism is probably related to the chemical reduction of Cu from +2 to +1 oxidation state by the acid, which is a strong reducing agent.

However, recent studies suggest that Cu^{+1} is the form favored by the specific Cu transporter, Ctr1, in the duodenal enterocyte.[33,34] Van den Berg's group[28] did extensive work on the effects of ascorbic acid on Cu absorption and showed that the acid lowered the amount of soluble Cu in the small intestine of rats, which subsequently impaired Cu absorption. Finley and Cerklewski[35] found that young men fed 500 mg of ascorbic acid three times/day showed a gradual decrease in plasma Cu and Cp activity over 64 days of treatment. When the ascorbic acid supplement was removed, both parameters rebounded within 20 days. Milne et al.[36] demonstrated a negative effect of dietary ascorbic acid on Cu status of non-human primates, but did not find an effect on Cu status when adult women were given 1500 mg of ascorbic acid and only 0.6 mg of Cu/day for 42 days. Another study showed that feeding 1500 mg of ascorbic acid and 0.67 mg Cu/day to women for 135 days had no effect on Cu balance; however, Cp activity was lower.[18] Based on these studies, it seems likely that short-term consumption of high amounts of ascorbic acid will have little effect on Cu status if the consumption of Cu is normal; however, information is not available to state conclusively that long-term consumption of the vitamin would not have a negative effect on Cu absorption, especially if dietary Cu intakes were low.

C. EFFECT OF DIETARY MINERALS ON COPPER ABSORPTION

The mineral components of the diet affect Cu availability. Mineral elements with similar electronic structures are likely to be antagonistic; for example, both Zn and Cu are d^{10} elements and are antagonistic. Van Campen and Scaife[37] were the first to demonstrate that high dietary Zn reduces the absorption of Cu from the gut of rats. Since then, many studies with laboratory animals and cultured cells have shown this effect of Zn.[38–41] Although not studied as extensively as in animals, there is ample evidence that Zn is antagonistic to Cu in humans as well. Patterson et al.[42] demonstrated sideroblastic anemia and low Cu status in a patient who had consumed as much as 450 mg Zn/day for 2 years. Others have shown similar effects.[43,44] In addition, high oral Zn therapy has been used successfully to treat Wilson's disease patients who, because of a genetic defect in Cu metabolism, accumulate toxic amounts of Cu. Cu status also can be affected by more normal concentrations of dietary Zn.[45,46] Studies have suggested that a dietary Zn:Cu molar ratio of greater than 16:1 may have a negative effect on physiological parameters associated with Cu metabolism. Dietary intakes of Zn as low as 25 and 50 mg/day for up to 10 weeks have produced small changes in Cu status in both men and women.[47–51] Balance studies have shown that the amount of dietary Cu required to maintain Cu equilibrium is directly proportional to the amount of Zn in the diet.[52] It is not recommended that supplementations of Zn much greater than the RDA (8–11 mg/day) be taken unless the Cu intake is relatively high, also.

V. COPPER CONCENTRATIONS IN BLOOD
AND BODY ORGANS

The human body contains about 1.6 mg of Cu/kg of body weight with variable distributions in various organs and blood. Examples of Cu concentrations in various tissues include kidney, 12 mg/kg; liver, 6 mg/kg; brain, 5 mg/kg; heart, 5 mg/kg; bone, 4 mg/kg; and muscle 0.9 mg/kg. Bone contains 40% of body Cu, the highest percentage of any other organ; muscle is second at about 23%. These organs also make up the greatest percentages of the body mass. Blood contains about 6% of total body Cu. The Cu concentration of RBC is approximately 16.1 ± 2.0 μmol/L of packed cells and plasma has an average concentration of 16.5 ± 2.5 μmol/L for men and 18.3 ± 2.5 μmol/L for women. The normal range of red blood cell (RBC) Cu for both men and women is 12.5 to 23.6 μmol/L, whereas the normal range for plasma Cu is 8.8 to 17.5 μmol/L for men and 10.8 to 26.6 μmol/L for women. However, plasma values consistently as low as 8.8 μmol/L might be considered a sign of low Cu status.

About 93% of Cu in plasma is covalently bound to Cp, while the remainder is in ionic arrangement with amino acids and albumin. Cp is synthesized in the liver and released into the blood, where its amine oxidase activity in plasma is proportional to the amount of Cu present. The activity of this enzyme is often used as an indicator of Cu status; however, pinpointing this as a specific indicator is difficult because certain stress and inflammatory conditions cause plasma Cp activity to increase, which could result in a false indication of Cu status.

Reports show that Cu concentrations and Cp activity in serum, and Cu concentrations in blood and plasma change when a person engages in various types of vigorous exercise and sports activities. Haralambie[53] was the first to report that serum Cp activity was elevated in human volunteers after they engaged in physical training. However, Dowdy and Burt[54] reported that Cp activity declined after 8 weeks of training and remained constant for the remainder of the study. Lukaski et al.[55] found that plasma Cu concentrations were 11% higher in trained male collegiate athletes compared with non-athletes in the same age group. Studies with laboratory animals also have shown an elevation in serum or plasma Cu when the animals were exercised to exhaustion.[56,57] This led to speculation that intensive exercise or physical training might alter Cu status.

Other studies have shown variable results. Resina et al.[58] found that male runners who trained for 6 weeks had 35% lower serum Cu concentrations than control subjects who did not train. However, the change in serum Cu did not affect Cp activity. On the other hand, Marrella et al.[59] found a small increase in plasma Cu of runners after a marathon when compared with values from the same subjects before the race. A total blood cell (TBC) Cu concentration, most of which was from red cells, was 30% lower in pre-marathon runners than in non-runner controls. TBC Cu did not change in runners immediately after the race; however, at 24 and 72 hours after the race, the Cu values were reduced and significantly different from values found immediately afterward. Cu concentrations were elevated in moderately trained and untrained volunteers immediately following acute exercise to exhaustion.[60] Lukaski[61] showed that the Cu concentration and Cp activity of young women swimmers were unchanged during a competitive swimming season. In addition, no differences were found between swimmers and controls who were non-swimmers.

The inconsistencies among different studies are confusing and may be caused partly by the different types of exercise or training, duration and intensity of the exercise, nutritional status of the subjects at the beginning of the program and the age and sex of the volunteers. Nevertheless, the change in serum Cu concentrations shown in some athletes does not necessarily mean that they have an altered Cu status. It could mean that the changes observed are nothing more than normal adaptive responses to strenuous exercise that result in a redistribution of Cu among various tissues and organs, with no detrimental effects on the athlete.

VI. COPPER METABOLISM

A. ROLE OF COPPER IN IRON ABSORPTION AND UTILIZATION

The metal iron (Fe) is a required nutrient in the diet of all mammals including humans, and Fe deficiency anemia is one of the world's most prominent health problems. For the most part, the deficiency is caused by a low intake or low bioavailability of dietary Fe. However, other factors may be involved. For example, there is a direct link between the Cu status of individuals and their ability to absorb and utilize dietary Fe.[62] It was known as early as the mid 19th century that Cu was associated with the cure of certain types of Fe-resistant anemia. In the early and mid 20th century, it was found through animal studies that dietary Fe or Fe injections would not prevent Cu deficiency-induced anemia in the rat model.[63–65] It was then discovered that a Cu-dependent ferroxidase, Cp, was required to move Fe out of cells. However, not until the age of molecular biology, in the late 1990s and early 2000s, was it discovered that a Cu-dependent ferroxidase, hephaestin, similar to Cp resides in the enterocytes of the small intestine, aided the absorption of Fe from the diet.[66–69] Thus, Cu affects Fe metabolism, and low Cu status can reduce Fe absorption and hamper Fe utilization in the body. Although most of the research so far has been done with animal models, it is likely that similar results will be found in humans. Because of these discoveries, it is recommended that no studies on iron requirements be attempted without first assuring that the Cu status of the study population is adequate. Individuals presenting with anemia that is unresponsive to iron therapy probably should have a Cu status assessment performed. Athletes are especially sensitive to the effects of anemia, because exercise performance depends on maximal efficiency of oxygen carrying capacity and oxygen utilization in the active muscles. As discussed later in this chapter, Cu along with Fe is closely involved in oxygen utilization.

B. ROLE OF COPPER IN BLOOD CELL FORMATION AND FUNCTION

Although knowledge of the exact role of Cu in blood cell formation is limited, observations in Cu-deficient animals and humans show prominent connections between Cu status and blood cell production, survivability and function. These functions could be compromised during strenuous exercise. In both animals and humans, Cu deficiency presents with a reduced population of RBCs that are smaller than normal and with a reduced hemoglobin concentration. Although the signs mimic Fe deficiency, supplemental Fe by diet or injections will not reverse them. Neutropenia also is a key sign of Cu deficiency in humans,[70,71] and in severe cases, the bone marrow will show morphologic characteristics typical of myelodysplastic syndrome with ringed sideroblasts.[72] All of these Cu deficiency signs can be reversed by supplementing the diet with Cu.

Although the neutropenia associated with copper deficiency is well characterized from a cellular viewpoint, the underlying causative mechanism is unknown. Several reports show that patients receiving total parenteral nutrition develop anemia and neutropenia as a result of copper deficiency when the parenteral solutions do not contain copper.[70,72–78] Morphologic findings from bone marrow assessment of these patients show several general characteristics including myeloid and erythroid precursors with cytoplasmic vacuoles, increased numbers of ringed sideroblasts, reduced numbers of mature granulocytes and increased numbers of promyelocytes.

The increase in the ratio of immature cells to mature granulocytes in the bone marrow of copper-deficient patients suggests that copper deficiency arrests the differentiation of neutrophils. Neutrophils and all other blood cells arise from a common parent cell, the pluripotent hematopoietic stem cell, in the bone marrow. The pluripotent stem cell differentiates into a myeloid progenitor cell called the colony forming unit-GEMM (CFU-GEMM) that further differentiates into colony forming units for erythrocytes (CFU-E), platelets (CFU-MEG), granulocytes (CFU-GM) and monocytes (CFU-M). The CFU-GM gives rise to the myeloblast that further differentiates into the promyelocyte, which becomes either the neutrophilic myelocyte, the eosinophilic myelocyte, or the basophilic myelocyte. Neutrophilic myelocytes differentiate through a pathway that has several stages that give rise to the metamyelocyte, the banded neutrophil and the segmented neutrophil. Presently, there are only a few reports showing that copper deficiency perturbs this pathway for neutrophil differentiation.

In one study, examination by using a granulocyte colony formation assay in bone marrow from a copper-deficient subject showed that neutrophil differentiation was abnormal.[73] In this study, the subject's bone marrow cells produced fewer granulocyte colonies when they were cultured in the subject's copper-deficient serum than when they were cultured in normocupric serum. However, bone marrow cells from a normal subject produced a normal number of granulocyte colonies when they were cultured in serum from the copper-deficient subject. These findings indicate that progenitor cells from the bone marrow of the copper-deficient subject were impaired in their ability to differentiate into mature granulocytes. In another study, researchers found that the bone marrow of a copper-deficient subject had a normal number of colony-forming units but a low number of mature neutrophils.[79] When the progenitor cells from the subject's marrow were stimulated to differentiate with the colony-stimulating factor or erythropoietin, they produced a normal number of colony-forming units. It was concluded from this study that the copper-deficient patient had a sufficient number of progenitor cells for neutrophil differentiation, but for some reason neutrophil maturation was arrested in the bone marrow. Collectively, these studies indicate that copper is essential for normal neutrophil differentiation in the bone marrow

A role for copper in neutrophil differentiation is also supported by a cell culture model using HL-60 cells, which are promyelocytic leukemia cells that can be induced to differentiate along the neutrophil lineage. It was reported that copper supplementation of HL-60 cells induced to differentiate with retinoic acid increased the number of cells that differentiated into banded and segmented neutrophils.[80] Even in the absence of retinoic acid, copper supplementation of the HL-60 cells resulted in fewer cells at the promyelocyte stage and more at the myelocyte stage. Results from this study strongly suggest that copper can promote the differentiation of progenitor cells into neutrophils.

Several factors may contribute to the biochemical mechanisms for neutropenia caused by copper deficiency. It was found that SOD1 activity was significantly reduced in the erythrocytes of a copper-deficient subject with anemia and neutropenia.[70] Furthermore, the half-life of the subject's erythrocytes was only 19 days compared with a normal half-life of 28–40 days. This suggests that the low level of SOD1 activity promoted oxidative damage to the erythrocytes that shortened their circulating life span and contributed to the subject's anemia. SOD1 activity was not measured in the neutrophils, but if the activity was sufficiently reduced, then oxidative damage may have contributed to the subject's neutropenia by shortening the lifetime of the neutrophils in the bone marrow or in the circulation. A recent study shows that copper-deficient HL-60 cells are more susceptible to cell death when presented with an oxidant challenge.[81] HL-60 cells are a promyelocytic cell line, and the finding that oxidative stress caused by copper deficiency can increase their susceptibility to cell death suggests that copper deficiency may arrest neutrophil maturation in bone marrow by increasing the susceptibility of promyelocytes, or more differentiated progenitor cells, to cell death triggered by oxidative stress. Another study showed that patients with severe or moderate nutritional copper deficiency produce anti-neutrophil antibodies, a condition that could be partially responsible for neutropenia.[82,83] Thus, several factors are capable of contributing to neutropenia induced by copper deficiency and further research is needed to clarify the biochemical mechanisms through which copper deficiency impairs the process of blood cell maturation in the bone marrow, and the viability of blood cells in the bone marrow and in the circulation.

The primary function of erythrocytes is to transport oxygen from the lungs to other tissues. Physiological oxygen deficit associated with physical endurance exercise leads to increased expression of the hematopoietic hormone, erythropoietin that results in elevated erythropoiesis and oxygen capacity of the blood. However, the formation of erythrocytes depends on the maturation of colony-forming units in the bone marrow. Copper clearly has a role in the maturation of blood cells in bone marrow and low dietary copper intakes may impair the formation of erythrocytes in response to the oxygen deficit created by endurance exercise. Although dietary copper requirements for optimal physical performance have not been thoroughly investigated, intakes at the RDA for copper are recommended to assure proper erythrocyte maturation in the bone marrow in response to exercise training.

C. ANTIOXIDANT FUNCTIONS OF COPPER

Reductions in SOD1 by low dietary Cu intake may significantly compromise the body's defense against damage caused by reactive oxygen species (ROS). Lipids, proteins and DNA are intracellular targets for attack by ROS and several lines of evidence indicate that these biomolecules are oxidatively modified when dietary Cu intakes are low. It has been shown in laboratory animals that consuming Cu-deficient diets increases the lipid hydroperoxide content of hepatic microsomes and mitochondria,[84] increases the production of breath ethane[85] and increases the susceptibility of tissues to lipid peroxidation.[86,87] Lipid hydroperoxides and ethane are byproducts of lipid oxidation and the results of these studies indicate that lipids in membranous cellular components are subject to increased oxidation during Cu deficiency. Cu deficiency also increases the carbonyl content of the alpha and beta subunits of spectrin in erythrocyte membranes in rats[88] and proteins with molecular weights of 90 kDa and 100 kDa in mitochondria of HL-60 cells grown in culture.[89] Oxidation of proteins converts some of their amino acid side chains to carbonyl derivatives, and the presence of carbonyls is a marker of ROS-induced protein oxidation.[90] Thus, the increase in protein carbonyl content is evidence that Cu deficiency increases the susceptibility of intracellular proteins to oxidative modifications by ROS. Low dietary Cu intake in rats has also been shown to increase the activity of hepatic nuclear DNA repair enzymes,[91] suggesting that Cu deficiency increases DNA damage. Direct assessment of DNA damage by the Comet assay has shown that Cu deficiency increases DNA damage in cattle[92] and that DNA in Cu-deficient Jurkat T-lymphocytes is more susceptible to oxidative damage by hydrogen peroxide.[93] These studies indicate that Cu deficiency leads to nuclear DNA damage and imply that the damage is caused by ROS. Collectively, these studies demonstrate that Cu deficiency weakens the antioxidant defenses and leads to oxidative damage to cellular lipids, proteins and nuclear DNA. They also emphasize the importance of Cu as an antioxidant nutrient.

D. ROLE OF COPPER IN CARDIOVASCULAR AND NEUROLOGIC FUNCTIONS

Adequate Cu intake during pregnancy and the postpartum period is very important for proper brain development and maturation in neonates. When low Cu concentrations occur in the developing brain of laboratory animals before terminal differentiation occurs, the concentration tends to remain persistently low in several regions of the brain even after Cu deficiency is corrected by supplying adequate Cu in the diet.[94] The persistence of low Cu content in the brain may have long-term consequences on physical performance, as indicated by a recent study showing that Cu deficiency during brain development has persistent consequences on motor function in rats after 6 months of Cu repletion.[95]

Results from a diet survey indicate that young women may be at particular risk for low Cu intakes. It has been estimated that the Cu intakes for 14–16-year-old women and 25–30-year-old women are 0.76 mg/day and 0.94 mg/day, respectively.[96] These Cu intakes are below the RDA of 1.0 mg/day for pregnant women and the RDA of 1.3 mg/day for lactating women in these age groups. Although marginal to low Cu intakes may occur in a substantial number of young women, it is not known whether the low intakes have effects on brain development that lead to permanent impairment of motor function in their offspring. However, judging by the results from the animal studies described above, it is prudent for pregnant and lactating women to consume at least 1.5 mg Cu/day to ensure normal development of the central nervous system and motor functions of their children.

E. COPPER AND MITOCHONDRIAL OXIDATIVE STRESS

Four oligomeric enzymes, NADH:ubiquinone oxidoreductase (complex I), succinate:ubiquinone oxidoreductase (complex II), ubiquinol:cytochrome c oxidoreductase (complex III) and ferrocytochrome c:oxygen oxidoreductase (complex IV), compose the mitochondrial electron transport chain located in the inner mitochondrial membrane. Electrochemical energy derived from the transfer of electrons between these enzymes to molecular oxygen drives the vectorial translocation of protons across the inner mitochondrial membrane that provides the energy required for ATP synthesis. Although electron transport accounts for about 85–90% of the oxygen utilized by cells, not all of the oxygen consumed by the electron transport chain is converted to water; about 1–5% is converted to superoxide.[97–99] Thus, a 70-kg adult who uses about 14.7 moles of O_2/day would produce about

0.15–0.74 moles of mitochondria-generated superoxide on a daily basis. Much of the superoxide ($O_2^{\cdot-}$) formed is converted to hydrogen peroxide (H_2O_2) by a manganese-dependent form of superoxide dismutase (MnSOD) located in the mitochondrial matrix. However, a portion of superoxide generated by the electron transport chain escapes conversion by MnSOD and is available to react with H_2O_2 to form hydroxyl radicals (HO-) by the Haber-Weiss reaction catalyzed by mitochondrial iron (equation 1). H_2O_2 can also react with mitochondrial iron to produce hydroxyl radicals by the Fenton reaction (equation 2).

$$(1)\ O_2^{\cdot-} + H_2O_2 \rightarrow HO^{\cdot} + HO^-$$

$$(2)\ H_2O_2 + Fe^{2+} \rightarrow HO^{\cdot} + HO^- + Fe^{3+}$$

Several lines of evidence indicate that exercise increases the production of ROS. Studies employing electron spin resonance spectroscopy have shown that acute exercise increases free-radical production in skeletal muscle of mice, rats and humans[99] and accumulation in serum of humans.[97] Acute exercise has also been shown to increase ROS production in skeletal muscle of young and old rats in a study where ROS production was monitored by measuring the oxidation of the intracellular probe dichloroflourescin.[98] Another study employing an *in situ* model showed that hydroxyl radical is produced in contracting feline triceps muscle.[100] While these studies provide convincing evidence that exercise increases ROS production in muscle, the sources of ROS production are less clear.

Mitochondria may be a major source of the ROS that become elevated in muscle during exercise. As discussed above, mitochondria convert about 1–5% of the oxygen consumed by the electron transport chain to superoxide. During exercise, oxygen consumption by muscle cells increases substantially, and if the percentage of oxygen that is converted to superoxide remains the same, mitochondrial superoxide generation will increase. However, the experimental evidence for increased mitochondrial ROS production during exercise is problematic. No significant increases in the rate of ROS production were detected in mitochondria isolated from the deep *vastus lateralis* muscle in rats following acute exercise when dichloroflourescin oxidation was measured under conditions promoting state 4 respiration.[98] Also, H_2O_2 production in intermyofibrillar mitochondria and subsarcolemmal mitochondria isolated from oxidative muscle of rats was not affected by voluntary wheel running.[101] However, the stress of exercise on oxygen consumption by the electron transport chain was no longer present because these data were obtained by using isolated mitochondria. As a result, this finding does not necessarily provide definitive evidence that exercise does not enhance mitochondrial ROS production. In contrast, the hypothesis that mitochondria are a major site of ROS production during exercise is supported by indirect evidence of mitochondrial oxidative damage. After a single bout of treadmill running, oxidative enzymes were inactivated and the protein thiol content was lowered in rat skeletal muscle mitochondria.[102] It has also been reported that ortho-tyrosine, meta-tyrosine and o,o'-dityrosine are increased in mitochondrial proteins of heart muscle after acute exercise,[103] indicating that oxidation of mitochondrial proteins by hydroxyl radical was increased during exercise. Several studies have shown that MnSOD is induced in heart and skeletal muscle after acute or short-term exercise training.[104–106] The expression of MnSOD, a mitochondrial matrix enzyme whose genes are encoded in nuclear DNA, is increased by hydrogen peroxide and other oxidants.[107] Due to the proximity of MnSOD to the mitochondrial electron transport chain, its induction during exercise may be directly related to an increase in mitochondria-generated ROS. Collectively, these studies indicate that mitochondrial production of ROS is increased sufficiently during acute and short-term exercise to cause oxidative damage to mitochondrial proteins and induce MnSOD.

While it is likely that mitochondrial generation of ROS contributes to increased production of muscle ROS during exercise, dietary Cu intake may affect the magnitude of the mitochondrial ROS contribution. Cytochrome c oxidase is the terminal complex (complex IV) of the electron transport chain and catalyzes the formation of water through the reduction of molecular oxygen. Cytochrome c oxidase is a cuproenzyme whose activity is reduced in hearts of Cu-deficient rats and mice[108,109] and in muscles of mouse mutants who become Cu-deficient because of a genetic abnormality that impairs Cu homeostasis.[110,111] Mitochondrial ROS production, which is highly dependent on the redox state of the respiratory complexes, is greatest when the complexes are in a highly reduced state.[112] Blockage of electron transport near the terminus of the electron transport chain increases the reducing potential of the respiratory complexes upstream from the blockage and facilitates the formation of superoxide by single electron transfer to molecular oxygen at these upstream sites. This principle has been demonstrated using mitochondria of housefly flight muscle in which partial inhibition of cytochrome c oxidase activity caused a significant increase in the rate of H_2O_2 production.[113] Theoretically, Cu deficiency, by inhibiting cytochrome c oxidase, should increase mitochondrial production of superoxide and related ROS. At present, a single report shows that Cu deficiency in rats increases H_2O_2 production by hepatic mitochondria.[114] However, the hypothesis that Cu deficiency increases mitochondrial ROS production is indirectly supported by the observation that oxidation of mitochondrial proteins and induction of mitochondrial MnSOD are increased in Cu-deficient HL-60 cells.[89] These limited findings suggest that reductions in cytochrome c oxidase activity caused by Cu deficiency could increase ROS production by mitochondria in heart and muscle. Whether low Cu intakes can inhibit cytochrome c oxidase sufficiently to further increase the ROS burden in heart and muscle during exercise remains to be clarified.

VII. COPPER REQUIRMENTS OF ATHLETES

The FNB defines the dietary reference intakes (DRI) as "reference values that are quantitative estimates of nutrient intakes to be used for planning and assessing diets for apparently healthy people. They include not only RDAs but also three other types of reference values."[4] These reference values include the adequate intake (AI), the recommended average daily intake based on experimental determinations or estimates of nutrient intakes by groups of healthy people; the tolerable upper intake level (UL), the highest average daily nutrient intake that is likely to pose no health risk; and the estimated average requirement (EAR), the average daily nutrient intake estimated to meet the requirement of half the healthy individuals in a particular life stage and gender group. Most of these criteria are based on the best estimates gleaned from information gathered from both human and animal experimentation. But generally, the experts do not always agree on the criteria for determining the physiological requirements for nutrients.

What criteria do we use to determine Cu requirements in humans? Because of ethical considerations, only a few methods can be used. In the past, metabolic balance studies have been used to estimate the RDAs for Cu; however, this method is flawed because the rate of Cu absorption varies with intake. This could cause misinterpretation of requirements. In addition, individuals might adapt to a particular intake and begin to regulate the output of Cu so that zero balance is obtained even in the face of possible long-term dietary shortages of the mineral.

Other possible criteria for determining requirement include changes in the Cu concentration or changes in activities of Cu-dependent enzymes in blood. These methods, however, have not been too successful because the values tend to be affected by a variety of conditions not related to the function of Cu. Likewise, accurate assessment of Cu requirements may be hampered because of limitations on the number of invasive and noninvasive tests allowed in studies with human volunteers.

One of the main drawbacks to determining the requirements for any nutrient, including Cu, in humans is the enormous cost involved in conducting controlled experiments. Most human studies in the past have not been of sufficient length to overcome the adaptation responses to low intakes of Cu, or to be able to observe changes in Cu concentrations in blood or in enzyme activities. Longer experimental periods may help solve some of these problems, but may present the additional problem of volunteer compliance. This in turn demands an increase in the number of volunteers, and the cost spirals. Moreover, extending the experimental period to the point of observing frank signs of Cu deficiency might be considered unethical, and the protocol would not meet the requirements of the human studies review boards of most research institutions in the U.S.

Because of these difficulties, the FNB could not assemble sufficient data to establish an RDA for Cu in 1989.[6] Instead, they recommended an ESADDI of 1.5 to 3 mg/day for both men and women over the age of 11. In 1995, a workshop was sponsored by the FNB and the U.S. Department of Agriculture, Agricultural Research Service, to consider new approaches, endpoints and paradigms for the assessment of mineral requirements for humans.[115] Evidence was presented to suggest that the requirement for Cu might be lower than the 1989 ESADDI. Indeed, in the 2001 deliberation of the FNB, the RDA for Cu was set at 0.9 mg/day.[4] This is more in line with the values of 1–2 mg/day set by the Canadian Department of Health and Welfare.[7] The RDA is based on the needs of the general population, but to date, there is no strong evidence to suggest that the Cu requirement for athletes is any different.

VIII. CONCLUSIONS

Cu is a required dietary nutrient. Without an adequate intake of this nutrient, health and physiological function cannot be maintained. There is a need for Cu in enzyme systems that regulate mitochondrial oxygen utilization, cardiovascular function and neurological function. The safe and adequate range of intakes of Cu for the general adult population is 1.5 to 3.0 mg/day; however, the dietary requirement is at least 0.9 mg/day. There are indications that athletes may have concentrations of blood Cu outside the range of normal values and increased losses of Cu in sweat and urine during exercise. Dietary surveys of athletes also indicate that, like the general population, some may consume less than the recommended amount of Cu, especially if the diet is not balanced with a variety of foods. However, there is no convincing evidence that low Cu status exists in athletes who consume a well-balanced diet of a variety of foods. It is highly recommended, therefore, that athletes obtain the required amount of Cu by eating a variety of foods, including those with moderate to high amounts of Cu. They should not rely upon dietary supplementations of Cu or any other nutrient unless they are found to be lacking in the nutrient by clinically recognized tests conducted under the supervision of a qualified nutritionist or physician.

For future work, more comprehensive studies should be performed to determine if indeed the new lower RDA for Cu is adequate with regard to demands on Cu-dependent antioxidant enzyme during very stressful sports activities and exercise that increase oxygen consumption and utilization. With the rediscovery of the close Cu/Fe connection, would the athlete with a higher level of Cu status utilize Fe more efficiently? In addition, recent research has discovered several proteins that serve as chaperones to deliver Cu to enzymes that catalyze important metabolic reactions. Future research needs to be directed toward understanding whether polymorphisms in genes encoding these chaperone proteins can affect dietary Cu requirements for optimal metabolism and performance in athletes by improving or impairing delivery of Cu to these key metabolic enzymes.

ACKNOWLEDGMENTS AND ASSURANCES

The assembly of this review was supported by the U.S. Department of Agriculture CRIS Project Nos. 5450-51000-035-00D and 5450-51000-033-00D. Mention of trade names or commercial products in this article is solely to provide specific information and does not imply recommendation or endorsement by the U.S. Department of Agriculture. In addition, dietary or procedural changes recommended by the authors do not imply that these represent the policies of the U.S. Department of Agriculture.

REFERENCES

1. Mason, K.E., A conspectus of research on copper metabolism and requirements of man, *J. Nutr.,* 109, 1979, 1979.
2. O'Dell, B.L., Copper, *Present Knowledge in Nutrition,* Brown, M.L., Ed., Washington, D.C., International Life Sciences Institute, Nutrition Foundation, 1990, p.261.
3. Linder, M.C., *Biochemistry of Copper,* Plenum Press, New York, 1991.
4. Panel on Micronutrients, Copper, Dietary Reference Intakes for Vitamin A, Vitamin K, Arsenic, Boron, Chromium, Copper, Iodine, Iron, Manganese, Molybdenum, Nickel, Silicon, Vanadium and Zinc, National Research Council, Eds., National Academy Press, Washington, D.C., 2001, p.224.
5. National Research Council, Trace Elements, Recommended Dietary Allowances, National Academy Press, Washington, D.C., 1980, p.151.
6. National Research Council, Trace elements, Recommended Dietary Allowances, National Academy Press, Washington, D.C., 1989, p.224.
7. Health and Welfare Canada, Recommended Nutrient Intakes for Canadians, Department of Health and Welfare, Ottawa, ON, 1983.
8. Klevay, L.M., Buchet, J.-P., Bunker, V.W., Clayton, B.E., Medeiros, D.M., Moser-Veillon, P.B., Patterson, K.Y., Taper, L.J. and Wolf, W.R., Copper in the Western diet (Belgium, Canada, U.K. and USA), *Trace Elements in Man and Animals — TEMA* 8, Anke, M., Meissner, D. and Mills, C.F., Eds., Verlag Media Touristik, Gersdorf, Germany, 1993, p.207.
9. Pang, Y., MacIntosh, D.L. and Ryan, P.B., A longitudinal investigation of aggregate oral intake of copper, *J. Nutr.,* 131, 2171, 2001.
10. Panel on Micronutrients, Appendix C, Table C-15, Dietary Reference Intakes for Vitamin A, Vitamin K, Arsenic, Boron, Chromium, Copper, Iodine, Iron, Manganese, Molybdenum, Nickel, Silicon, Vanadium and Zinc, National Research Council, Eds., National Academy Press, Washington, D.C., 2001, p.622.
11. Johnson, P.E., Milne, D.B. and Lykken, G.I., Effects of age and sex on copper absorption, biological half-life and status in humans, *Am. J. Clin. Nutr.,* 56, 917, 1992.
12. Lawler, M.R. and Klevay, L.M., Copper and zinc in selected foods, *J. Am. Diet Assoc.,* 84, 1028, 1984.
13. USDA Food Database, http://www.nal.usda.gov/fnic/foodcomp/search, 2004.
14. Telford, R.D., Catchpole, E.A., Deakin, V., McLeay, A.C. and Plank, A.W., The effect of 7 to 8 months of vitamin/mineral supplementation on the vitamin and mineral status of athletes, *Int. J. Sport Nutr.,* 2, 123, 1992.
15. Worme, J.D., Doubt, T.J., Singh, A., Ryan, C.J., Moses, F.M. and Deuster, P.A., Dietary patterns, gastrointestinal complaints and nutrition knowledge of recreational triathletes, *Am. J. Clin. Nutr.,* 51, 690, 1990.
16. Lukaski, H.C., Hoverson, B.B., Gallagher, S.K. and Bolonchuk, W.W., Physical training and copper, iron and zinc status of swimmers, *Am. J. Clin. Nutr.,* 51, 1093, 1990.
17. Lukaski, H.C., Siders, W.A., Hoverson, B.B. and Gallagher, S.K., Iron, copper, magnesium and zinc status as predictors of swimming performance, *Int. J. Sports Med.,* 17, 535, 1996.
18. Milne, D.B., Klevay, L.M. and Hunt, J.R., Effects of ascorbic acid supplements and a diet marginal in copper on indices of copper nutriture in women, *Nutr. Res.,* 8, 865, 1988.
19. Klevay, L.M., Reck, S.J., Jacob, R.A., Logan, G.M., Jr., Munoz, J.M. and Sandstead, H.H., The human requirement for copper. I. Healthy men fed conventional American diets, *Am. J. Clin. Nutr.,* 33, 45, 1980.
20. Turnlund, J.R., Keyes, W.R. Anderson, H.L. and Acord, L.L., Copper absorption and retention in young men at three levels of dietary copper by use of the stable isotope ^{65}Cu, *Am. J. Clin. Nutr.,* 49, 870, 1989.
21. Turnlund, J.R., Keyes, W.R., Peiffer, G.L. and Scott, K.C., Copper absorption, excretion and retention by young men consuming low dietary copper determined by using the stable isotope ^{65}Cu, *Am. J. Clin. Nutr.,* 67, 1219, 1998.
22. Fields, M., Ferretti, R.J., Smith, J.C. and Reiser, S., The interaction of type of dietary carbohydrates with copper deficiency, *Am. J. Clin. Nutr.,* 39, 289, 1984.
23. Koh, E.T., Comparison of copper status in rats when dietary fructose is replaced by either cornstarch or glucose, *Proc. Soc. Exp. Biol. Med.,* 194, 108, 1990.

24. Reiser, S., Ferretti, R.J., Fields, M. and Smith, J.C., Jr., Role of dietary fructose in the enhancement of mortality and biochemical changes associated with copper deficiency in rats, *Am. J. Clin. Nutr.,* 38, 222, 1983.

25. Johnson, M.A., Interaction of dietary carbohydrate, ascorbic acid and copper with the development of copper deficiency in rats, *J. Nutr.,* 116, 802, 1986.

26. O'Dell, B.L., Fructose and mineral metabolism, *Am. J. Clin. Nutr.,* 58 Suppl., 771S, 1993.

27. Van den Berg, G.J., Yu, S., Van der Heijden, A., Lemmens, A.G. and Beynen, A.C., Dietary fructose vs. glucose lowers copper solubility in the digesta in the small intestine of rats, *Biol. Trace Elem. Res.,* 38, 107, 1993.

28. Van den Berg, G.J., Yu, S., Lemmens, A.G. and Beynen, A.C., Dietary ascorbic acid lowers the concentration of soluble copper in the small intestinal lumen of rats, *Br. J. Nutr.,* 71, 701, 1994.

29. Schoenemann, H.M., Failla, M.L. and Fields, M., Consequences of copper deficiency are not differentially influenced by carbohydrate source in young pigs fed a dried skim milk-based diet, *Biol. Trace Elem. Res.,* 25, 21, 1990.

30. Holbrook, J.T., Smith, J.C. and Reiser, S., Dietary fructose or starch: Effects on copper, zinc, iron, manganese, calcium and magnesium balances in humans, *Am. J. Clin. Nutr.,* 49, 1290, 2004.

31. Reiser, S., Smith, J.C., Jr., Mertz, W.E., Holbrook, J.T., Scholfield, D.J., Powell, A.S., Canfield, W.K. and Canary, J.J., Indices of copper status in humans consuming a typical American diet containing either fructose or starch, *Am. J. Clin. Nutr.,* 42, 242, 1985.

32. Van Campen, D. and Gross, E., Influence of ascorbic acid on the absorption of copper by rats, *J. Nutr.,* 95, 617, 1968.

33. Lee, J., Marjorette, M., Peña, O., Nose, Y. and Thiele, D.J., Biochemical characterization of the human copper transporter Ctr1, *J. Biol. Chem.,* 277, 4380, 2002.

34. Sharp, P.A., Ctr1 and its role in body copper homeostasis, *Inter. J. Biochem. Cell Biol.,* 35, 288, 2003.

35. Finley, E.B. and Cerklewski, F.L., Influence of ascorbic acid supplementation on copper status in young adult men, *Am. J. Clin. Nutr.,* 37, 553, 1983.

36. Milne, D.B., Omaye, S.T. and Amos, W.H., Jr., Effect of ascorbic acid on copper and cholesterol in adult cynomolgus monkeys fed a diet marginal in copper, *Am. J. Clin. Nutr.,* 34, 2389, 1981.

37. Van Campen, D.R. and Scaife, P.U., Zinc interference with copper absorption in rats, *J. Nutr.,* 91, 473, 1967.

38. Oestreicher, P. and Cousins, R.J., Copper and zinc absorption in the rat: Mechanism of mutual antagonism, *J. Nutr.,* 115, 159, 1985.

39. Ogiso, T., Mariyama, K., Sasaki, S., Ishimura, Y. and Minato, A., Inhibitory effect of high dietary zinc on copper absorption in rats, *Chem. Pharm. Bull.,* 22, 55, 1974.

40. Ogiso, T., Ogawa, N. and Miura, T., Inhibitory effect of high dietary zinc on copper absorption in rats. II. Binding of copper and zinc to cytosol proteins in the intestinal mucosa, *Chem. Pharm. Bull.,* 27, 515, 1979.

41. Reeves, P.G., Briske-Anderson, M. and Newman, S.M., Jr., High zinc concentrations in culture media affect copper uptake and transport in differentiated human colon adenocarcinoma cells, *J. Nutr.,* 126, 1701, 1996.

42. Patterson, W.P., Winkelmann, M. and Perry, M.C., Zinc-induced copper deficiency: megamineral sideroblastic anemia, *Ann. Intern. Med.,* 103, 385, 1985.

43. Fiske, D.N., McCoy, H.E., III and Kitchens, C.S., Zinc-induced sideroblastic anemia: Report of a case, review of the literature and description of the hematologic syndrome, *Am. J. Hematol.,* 46, 147, 1994.

44. Simon, S.R., Branda, R.F. and Tindle, B.F., Copper deficiency and sideroblastic anemia associated with zinc ingestion, *Am. J. Hematol.,* 28, 181, 1988.

45. Hill, G.M., Brewer, G.J., Prasad, A.S., Hydrick, C.R. and Hartmenn, D.E., Treatment of Wilson's disease with zinc: I. Oral zinc therapy regimens, *Hepatology,* 7, 522, 1987.

46. Brewer, G.J., Yuzbasiyan-Gurkan, V. and Lee, D.Y., Use of zinc-copper metabolic interaction in the treatment of Wilson's disease, *J. Am. Coll. Nutr.,* 9, 487, 1990.

47. Festa, M.D. anderson, H.L., Dowdy, R.P. and Ellerseick, M.R., Effect of zinc intake on copper excretion and retention in man, *Am. J. Clin. Nutr.,* 41, 285, 1985.

48. Fischer, P.W.F., Giroux, A. and L'Abbe, M.R., Effect of zinc supplementation on copper status in adult man, *Am. J. Clin. Nutr.,* 40, 743, 1984.

49. Greger, J.L., Zaikis, S.C., Abernathy, R.P., Bennett, O.A. and Huffman, J., Zinc, nitrogen, copper, iron and manganese balance in adolescent females fed two levels of zinc, *J. Nutr.,* 108, 1449, 1978.

50. Taper, W., Hinners, M.L. and Ritchey, S.J., Effects of zinc intake on copper balance in adult females, *Am. J. Clin. Nutr.,* 33, 1077, 1980.

51. Yadrick, M.K., Kenney, M.A. and Winterfeldt, E.A., Iron, copper and zinc status: response to supplementation with zinc or zinc and iron in adult females, *Am. J. Clin. Nutr.,* 49, 145, 1989.

52. Sandstead, H.H., Interactions that influence bioavailability of essential metals to humans, *Metal Speciation: Theory, Analysis and Application,* Kramer, J.R. and Allen, H.E., Eds., Lewis Publications, Chelsea, MI, 1995, p.315.

53. Haralambie, G., Changes in electrolytes and trace minerals during long-lasting exercise, *Metabolic Adaptation to Prolonged Physical Exercise,* Howald, H. and Poortmans, J.R., Eds., Birkhauser Verlag, Basel, 1975, p.340.

54. Dowdy, R.P. and Burt, J., Effect of intensive, long-term training on copper and iron nutriture in men, *Fed. Proc.,* 39, A786, 1980.

55. Lukaski, H.C., Bolonchuk, W.W., Klevay, L.M., Milne, D.B. and Sandstead, H.H., Maximal oxygen consumption as related to magnesium, copper and zinc nutriture, *Am. J. Clin. Nutr.,* 37, 407, 1983.

56. Cordova, A., Gimenez, M. and Escanero, J.F., Changes of plasma zinc and copper at various times of swimming until exhaustion, in the rat, *J. Trace Elem. Electrolytes Health Dis.,* 4, 189, 1990.

57. Cordova, A., Gimenez, M. and Escanero, J.F., Effect of swimming to exhaustion, at low temperatures, on serum Zn, Cu, Mg and Ca in rats, *Physiol. Behav.,* 48, 595, 1990.

58. Resina, A., Fedi, S., Gatteschi, L., Rubenni, M.G., Giamberardino, M.A., Trabassi, E. and Imreh, F., Comparison of some serum copper parameters in trained runners and control subjects, *Int. J. Sports Med.,* 11, 58, 1990.

59. Marrella, M., Guerrini, F., Solero, P.L., Tregnaghi, P.L., Schena, F. and Velo, G.P., Blood copper and zinc changes in runners after a marathon, *J. Trace Elem. Electrolytes Health Dis.,* 7, 248, 1993.

60. Anderson, R.A., Bryden, N.A., Polansky, M.M. and Deuster, P.A., Acute exercise effects on urinary losses and serum concentrations of copper and zinc of moderately trained and untrained men consuming a controlled diet, *Analyst,* 120, 867, 1995.

61. Lukaski, H.C., Effects of exercise training on human copper and zinc nutriture, *Adv. Exp. Med. Biol.,* 258, 163, 1989.

62. Fox, P.L., The copper-iron chronicles: The story of an intimate relationship, *BioMetals,* 16, 9, 2003.

63. Hart, E.B., Steenbock, H., Waddell, J. and Elvehjem, C.A., Iron in Nutrition. VII. Copper as a supplement to iron for hemoglobin building in the rat, *J. Biol. Chem.,* 77, 797, 1928.

64. McHargue, J.S., Healy, D.J. and Hill, E.S., The relation of copper to the hemoglobin content of rat blood, *J. Biol. Chem.,* 78, 637, 1928.

65. Josephs, H.W., Studies on iron metabolism and the influence of copper, *J. Biol. Chem.,* 96, 559, 1932.

66. Vulpe, C.D., Kuo, Y.M., Murphy, T.L., Cowley, L., Askwith, C., Libina, N., Gitschier, J. and Anderson, G.J., Hephaestin, a ceruloplasmin homologue implicated in intestinal iron transport, is defective in the *sla* mouse, *Nat. Genet.,* 21, 195, 1999.

67. Eisenstein, R.S., Discovery of the ceruloplasmin homologue Hephaestin: new insight into the copper/iron connection, *Nutr. Rev.,* 58, 22, 2000.

68. Anderson, G.J., Frazer, D.M., McKie, A.T. and Vulpe, C.D., The ceruloplasmin homolog hephaestin and the control of intestinal iron absorption, *Blood Cells Mol. Dis.,* 29, 367, 2002.

69. Reeves, P.G., DeMars, L.C.S., Johnson, W.T. and Lukaski, H.C., Dietary copper deficiency reduces iron absorption and duodenal enterocyte Hephaestin protein in male and female rats, *J. Nut,* 135, In Press, 2005.

70. Hirase, N., Abe, Y., Sadamura, S., Yufu, Y., Muta, K., Umemura, T., Nishimura, J., Nawata, H. and Ideguchi, H., Anemia and neutropenia in a case of copper deficiency: Role of copper in normal hematopoiesis, *Acta Haematol.,* 87, 195, 1992.

71. Percival, S.S., Neutropenia caused by copper deficiency: Possible mechanisms of action, *Nutr. Rev.,* 53, 59, 1995.

72. Gregg, X.T., Reddy, V. and Prchal, J.T., Copper deficiency masquerading as myelodysplastic syndrome, *Blood,* 100, 1493, 2002.

73. Zidar, B.L., Shadduck, R.K., Zeigler, Z. and Winkelstein, A., Observations on the anemia and neutropenia of human copper deficiency, *Am. J. Hematol.,* 3, 177, 1977.

74. Sriram, K., O'Gara, J.A., Strunk, J.R. and Peterson, J.K., Neutropenia due to copper deficiency in total parenteral nutriton, *J. Parenter. Enteral Nutr.*, 10, 530, 1986.

75. Fujita, M., Itakura, T. and Okada, A., Copper deficiency during total parenteral nutrition: Clinical analysis of three cases, *J. Parenter. Enteral Nutr.*, 13, 421, 1989.

76. Tamura, H., Hirose, S., Watanabe, O., Arai, K., Murakawa, M., Matsumura, O. and Isoda, K., Anemia and neutropenia due to copper deficiency in enteral nutrition, *J. Parenter. Enteral Nutr.*, 18, 185, 1994.

77. Spiegel, J.E. and Willenbucher, R.F., Rapid development of severe copper deficiency in a patient with Crohn's disease receiving parenteral nutrition, *J. Parenter. Enteral Nutr.*, 23, 169, 1999.

78. Fuhrman, M.P., Herrmann, V., Masidonski, P. and Eby, C., Pancytopenia after removal of copper from total parenteral nutrition, *J. Parenter. Enteral Nutr.*, 24, 361, 2000.

79. Dunlap, W.M., James, G.W., III and Hume, D.M., Anemia and neutropenia caused by copper deficiency, *Ann. Int. Med.*, 80, 470, 1974.

80. Bae, B. and Percival, S.S., Retinoic acid-induced HL-60 cell differentiation is augmented by copper supplementation, *J. Nutr.*, 123, 997, 1993.

81. Raymond, L.J. and Johnson, W.T., Supplemental ascorbate or α-tocoperol induces cell death in Cu deficient HL-60 cells, *Exp. Biol. Med.*, 229, 885, 2004.

82. Higuchi, S., Higashi, A., Nakamura, T., Yanabe, Y. and Matsuda, I., Anti-neutrophil antibodies in patients with nutritional copper deficiency, *Eur. J. Pediatr.*, 150, 327, 1991.

83. Higuchi, S., Hirashima, M., Nunoi, H., Higashi, A., Naoe, H. and Matsuda, I., Characterization of antineutrophil antibodies in patients with neutropenia associated with nutritional copper deficiency, *Acta Haematol.*, 94, 192, 1995.

84. Balevska, P.S., Russanov, E.M. and Kassa, T.A., Studies on lipid peroxidation in rat liver by copper deficiency, *Int. J. Biochem.*, 13, 489, 1981.

85. Saari, J.T., Dickerson, F.B. and Habib, M.P., Ethane production in copper-deficient rats, *Proc. Soc. Exp. Biol. Med.*, 195, 30, 1990.

86. Rayssiguier, Y., Gueux, E., Bussiere, L. and Mazur, A., Copper deficiency increases the susceptibility of lipoproteins and tissues to peroxidation in rats, *J. Nutr.*, 123, 1343, 1993.

87. Fields, M., Ferretti, R.J., Smith, J.C., Jr. and Reiser, S., Interaction between dietary carbohydrate and copper nutriture on lipid peroxidation in rat tissues, *Biol. Trace Elem. Res.*, 6, 379, 1984.

88. Sukalski, K.A., LaBerge, T.P. and Johnson, W.T., *In vivo* oxidative modification of erythrocyte membrane proteins in copper deficiency, *Free Radic. Biol. Med.*, 22, 835, 1997.

89. Johnson, W.T. and Thomas, A.C., Copper deprivation potentiates oxidative stress in HL-60 cell mitochondria, *Proc. Soc. Exp. Biol. Med.*, 221, 147, 1999.

90. Berlett, B.S. and Stadtman, E.R., Protein oxidation, aging, disease and oxidative stress, *J. Biol. Chem.*, 272, 20313, 1997.

91. Webster, R.P. and Gawde, M.D., Modulation by dietary copper of aflatoxin B1-induced activity of DNA repair enzymes poly(ADP-ribose) polymerase, DNA polymerase beta and DNA ligase, *In Vitro*, 10, 533, 1996.

92. Picco, S.J., DeLuca, J.C., Mattioli, G. and Dulout, F.N., DNA damage induced by copper deficiency in cattle assessed by the Comet assay, *Mutat. Res.*, 498, 1, 2001.

93. Pan, Y.J. and Loo, G., Effect of copper deficiency on oxidative DNA damage in Jukat T-lymphocytes, *Free Radic. Biol. Med.*, 28, 824, 2000.

94. Prohaska, J.R. and Hoffman, R.G., Auditory startle response is diminished in rats after recovery from perinatal copper deficiency, *J. Nutr.*, 126, 618, 1996.

95. Penland, J.G. and Prohaska, J.R., Abnormal motor function persists following recovery from perinatal copper deficiency in rats, *J. Nutr.*, 134, 1984, 2004.

96. Pennington, J.A. and Young, B.E., Total diet study: Nutritional elements, 1982–1989, *J. Am. Diet. Assoc.*, 91, 179, 1991.

97. Ashton, T., Rowlands, C.C., Jones, E., Young, I.S., Jackson, S.K., Davies, B. and Peters, J.R., Electron spin resonance spectroscopic detection of oxygen-centered radicals in human serum following exhaustive exercise, *Eur. J. Appl. Physiol. Occup. Physiol.*, 77, 498, 1998.

98. Bejma, J. and Ji, L.L., Aging and acute exercise enhance free radical generation in rat skeletal muscle, *J. Appl. Physiol.*, 87, 465, 1999.

99. Jackson, M.J., Edwards, R.H. and Symons, M.C., Electron spin resonance studies of intact mammalian skeletal muscle, *Biochim. Biophys. Acta*, 847, 185, 1985.

100. O'Neill, C.A., Stebbins, C.L., Bonigut, S., Halliwell, B. and Longhurst, J.C., Production of hydroxyl radicals in contracting muscle of cats, *J. Appl. Physiol.*, 81, 1197, 1996.

101. Servais, S., Couturier, K., Koubi, H., Rouanet, J.L., Desplanches, D., Sornay-Mayet, M.H., Sempore, B., Lavoie, J.M. and Favier, R., Effect of voluntary exercise on H2O2 release by subsarcolemmal and intermyofibrillar mitochondria, *Free Radic. Biol. Med.*, 35, 24, 2003.

102. Ji, L.L., Stadtman, F.W. and Lardy, H.A., Enzymatic down regulation with exercise in rat skeletal muscle, *Arch. Biochem. Biophys.*, 263, 137, 1988.

103. Leeuwenburgh, C., Hansen, P.A., Holloszy, J.O. and Heinecke, J.W., Hydroxyl radical generation during exercise increases mitochondrial protein oxidation and levels of urinary dityrosine, *Free Radic. Biol. Med.*, 27, 186, 1999.

104. Navarro-Arévalo, A., Cañavate, C. and Sánchez-del Pino, M.J., Myocardial and skeletal muscle aging and changes in oxidative stress in relationship to rigorous exercise training, *Mech. Ageing Dev.*, 108, 207, 1999.

105. Somani, S.M., Frank, S. and Rybak, L.P., Responses of antioxidant systems to acute and trained exercise in rat subcellular fractions, *Pharmacol. Biochem. Behav.*, 51, 627, 1995.

106. Hamilton, K.L., Powers, S.K., Sugiura, T., Kim, S., Lennin, S., Tumer, N. and Hehta, J.L., Short-term exercise training can improve myocardial tolerance to I/R without elevation of heat shock proteins, *Am. J. Physiol. Heart Circ. Physiol.*, 281, H1346, 2001.

107. Warner, B.B., Stuart, L., Gebb, S. and Wispé, J.R., Redox regulation of manganese superoxide dismutase, *Am. J. Physiol.*, 271, L150, 1996.

108. Prohaska, J.R., Changes in tissue growth, concentrations of copper, iron, cytochrome oxidase and superoxide dismutase subsequent to dietary or genetic copper deficiency in mice, *J. Nutr.*, 113, 2048, 1983.

109. Prohaska, J.R., Changes in Cu,Zn-superoxide dismutase, cytochrome c oxidase, glutathione peroxidase and glutathione transferase activities in copper-deficient mice and rats, *J. Nutr.*, 121, 355, 1991.

110. Phillips, M., Camakaris, J. and Danks, D.M., Comparisons of copper deficiency states in the murine mutants blotchy and brindled. Changes in copper-dependent enzyme activity in 13-day-old mice, *Biochem. J.*, 238, 177, 1986.

111. Kuznetsov, A.V., Clark, J.F., Winkler, K. and Kunz, W.S., Increase of flux control of cytochrome *c* oxidase in copper-deficient mottled brindled mice, *J. Biol. Chem.*, 271, 283, 1996.

112. Freeman, B.A. and Crapo, J.D., Biology of disease: Free radicals and tissue injury, *Lab. Invest.*, 47, 412, 1982.

113. Sohal, R.S., Aging, cytochrome c oxidase activity and hydrogen peroxide release by mitochondria, *Free Radic. Biol. Med.*, 14, 583, 1993.

114. Johnson, W.T. and DeMars, L.C.S., Increased heme oxygenase-1 expression during copper deficiency in rats results from increased mitochondrial generation of hydrogen peroxide, *J. Nutr.*, 134, 1328, 2004.

115. Klevay, L.M. and Medeiros, D.M., Deliberations and evaluations of the approaches, endpoints and paradigms for dietary recommendations about copper, *J. Nutr.*, 126, 2419S, 1996.

17 Iodine

Christine D. Thomson

CONTENTS

I. INTRODUCTION

Iodine was one of the earliest trace elements to be identified as essential. By 2700 BC, the Chinese treated goiter by feeding seaweed, marine animal preparations and burnt sponge (rich in iodine).[1] In the first half of the 19th century, the incidence of goiter was linked with low iodine content of food and drinking water. By the late 19th century, the geographic distribution of endemic goiter and cretinism was recognized to extend around the world.[2] In the 1920s, iodine was shown to be an integral component of the thyroid hormone thyroxine, required for normal growth and metabolism, and later in 1952 of triiodothyronine.

II. FUNCTIONS OF IODINE

Iodine functions as an integral part of the thyroid hormones, the pro-hormone thyroxine (T_4), and the more potent active form 3,5,3'-triiodothyronine (T_3) which is the key regulator of important cell processes.[3] Selenium is essential for normal thyroid hormone metabolism as a component of the iodothyronine 5'-deiodinases that control the synthesis and degradation of the biologically active hormone, T_3.[4] The thyroid hormones are required for normal growth and development of individual tissues such as the central nervous system and maturation of the whole body, and also for energy production and oxygen consumption in cells, thereby maintaining the body's metabolic rate.

The regulation of thyroid hormone synthesis, release and action is a complex process involving the thyroid, the pituitary, the brain and peripheral tissues.[5] The hypothalamus regulates the plasma concentrations of the thyroid hormones by controlling the release from the pituitary of the thyroid-stimulating hormone (TSH) through a feedback mechanism related to the level of T_4 in the blood. If blood T_4 falls, the secretion of TSH is increased, which enhances both thyroid activities and the output of T_4 into the circulation. This fine control of T_4 secretion is essential, because either an excess or a deficit in the hormone will be detrimental to normal function. If the level of circulating T_4 hormone is not maintained because of severe iodine deficiency, TSH remains elevated. Both of these measures are therefore useful in diagnosing hypothyroidism due to iodine deficiency. If thyroid hormone secretion is inadequate, the basal metabolic rate (BMR) is reduced and the general level of activity of the individual is decreased (hypothyroidism), and normal growth and development will be impaired.

III. DEFICIENCY OF IODINE

Iodine deficiency is recognized as a major international public health problem because of the large number of populations living in iodine-deficient environments, characterized primarily by iodine-deficient soils. The term iodine deficiency disorders (IDD) refers to the wide spectrum of effects of iodine deficiency on growth and development.[6] Goiter, a swelling of the thyroid gland, is the most obvious and familiar feature of iodine deficiency.[6] The swelling reflects an attempt by the thyroid to adapt to the increased need to produce hormones. Hyperplasia of the thyroid cells occurs and the thyroid gland increases in size.[5] Other effects are seen at all stages of development of iodine deficiency, but especially during fetal and neonatal periods.

The most damaging consequences of iodine deficiency are on fetal and infant development.[7,8] Thyroid hormones and, therefore, iodine are essential for normal development of the brain, and insufficient levels may result in permanent mental retardation of the fetus or newborn child. Iodine deficiency is the world's greatest single cause of preventable brain damage and mental retardation. The World Health Organization (WHO) estimates that 1.6 billion people are at risk of iodine deficiency, with at least 20 million suffering from mental defects that are preventable by correction of iodine deficiency.[9,10] The most severe effect of fetal iodine deficiency is endemic cretinism,[11] which affects up to 10% of populations living in severely iodine-deficient areas of the world. In general, cretins are mentally defective, with other physical abnormalities. Clinical manifestations may differ with geographical location, and two quite distinct syndromes have been observed. In myxedematous cretinism, hypothyroidism is present during fetal and early post-natal development and results in stunted growth and mental deficiency.[11,12] In the nervous or neurological type of cretinism, which appears to result from iodine deficiency of the mother during fetal development, mental retardation is present as well as hearing and speech defects and characteristic disorders of stance and gait, while hypothyroidism is absent.[11,12]

There are also less obvious detrimental effects of iodine deficiency on mental performance of schoolchildren, which may have considerable social consequences to national development.[13] A meta-analysis of 18 studies in which comparisons were made between iodine-deficient populations and a control population revealed that mean IQ scores for the iodine and non-iodine deficient groups were 13.5 points apart,[14] indicating the effect of iodine deficiency on neuro-psychological development.[7] The effects of mild iodine deficiency are less clear.[15]

The major cause of IDD is inadequate dietary intake of iodine from foods grown in soils that are poor in plant-available iodine.[16] Goiter is usually seen in areas where intakes are less than 50 µg/day, and cretinism where intakes of the mothers are less than 30 µg/day.[12] However, thyroid function may also be impaired after exposure in foods and drugs to anti-thyroid compounds called goitrogens, which prevent the uptake of iodine into the thyroid gland.[6,11] The etiology of myxedematous and nervous cretinism may be influenced by the simultaneous occurrence of selenium deficiency along with iodine deficiency in some areas,[17] because of the role of selenium in thyroid hormone metabolism.[18]

Iodization of salt has been the major method for combating iodine deficiency since the 1920s, when it was first used successfully in Switzerland.[19] The success of iodization, however, depends on the extent to which all salt used is iodized. Acceptability of iodized salt is a problem in some countries.[5] In some Asian countries with poorly developed infrastructure, there are major difficulties in producing, monitoring and distributing iodized salt. Iodized oil by injection has been used in the prevention of endemic goiter in China as well as in South America and Zaire.[16] A single intramuscular injection of iodized oil given to girls and young women can correct severe iodine deficiency for a period of more than 4 years. Because of hazards associated with injection, oral administration of iodized oil has been implemented with evidence of successful prevention of IDD.[5]

IV. METABOLISM OF IODINE

Iodine occurs in the tissues in both inorganic (iodide) and organically bound forms. The adult human body usually contains 15–50 mg iodine, of which 70–80% is in the thyroid gland, which has a remarkable concentrating power for iodine. The remainder is mainly in the circulating blood.[3]

The metabolism of iodine is closely linked to thyroid function, and the only known function for iodine is in the synthesis of thyroid hormones. Iodine is an anionic trace element that is rapidly absorbed from the gastrointestinal tract[1] in the form of iodide and taken up immediately by the thyroid gland, which needs to trap around 60 µg per day to maintain an adequate supply of T_4.[5] Iodide is converted to iodine in the thyroid gland, and bound to tyrosine residues from which the hormones T_3 and T_4 are formed.[20] Excess iodine in the inorganic form is readily excreted in the urine, with smaller amounts in feces and sweat.[11] Since fecal output and losses from the skin are normally small, 24-hour urinary excretion of iodine reflects the dietary intake and hence may be used for estimating the intake. Normally, urine contains more than 90% of all ingested iodine.[21]

A. EFFECT OF EXERCISE ON IODINE METABOLISM

There has been very little study of the effects of exercise on iodine metabolism. Just two studies[22–24] have investigated the iodine in sweat and urine of athletes. In a study of 10 Japanese rowing club students in 1985, the iodine concentration in sweat was close to 37 µg/l regardless of urinary iodine excretion, which was 50–393 (mean 149) µg/day during 6 consecutive days of a summer training camp, similar to that of 40–441 (mean 153) µg/day in five sedentary students,[22] In a subsequent Chinese study of 13 soccer-team players and 100 sedentary students,[23,24] sweat iodine concentration of the 13 physically active male athletes was 37 ± 6.6(SE) µg/l. There was no difference in iodine concentrations in sweat samples collected before and after intake of food high in iodine, nor between those collected before and after 1 hour of strenuous exercise, indicating that iodine concentration in sweat is more stable than that of urine.[23] The sweat lost in 1 hour was estimated at 52 ± 24 (12–100) µg, which may be 50% or more of the total daily intake.[24] Urinary iodine concentration was 59 ± 28 µg/l and the total daily excretion was estimated at 86 ± 42 µg. Thirty-eight percent of the athletes, but only 2% of the sedentary students, had urinary iodine values that were less than 50 µg/g creatinine, which is indicative of moderate iodine deficiency and risk of goiter (see below). In addition, 46% of the athletes had grade 1 goiter, compared with only 1% of sedentary students.

The results of both these studies indicate that profuse sweating in hot climates may result in a substantial loss of iodine, and open up the possibility that exercise may contribute to iodine deficiency.

B. Effect of Exercise on Thyroid Function

Exercise appears to enhance the rate of utilization or disposal of T_4.[25] Evidence for an increase in T_4 metabolism induced by physical activity comes from research, using the radioactive T_4 turnover technique in which the loss of a single injection of T_4 ^{125}I from the plasma was determined as a function of time, in horses[26] and rats,[27,28] as well as in athletes.[29] In athletes, exercise resulted in the degradation of circulating T_4 by 17% per day compared with 10% in the control group.[29] This increased rate of T_4 turnover was quantitatively similar to that found in hyperthyroid individuals, and would require approximately a 75% increase in T_4 secretion rate from the thyroid gland to keep circulating levels unchanged.

There are two possible mechanisms for increased rate of turnover of T_4. First, an increase in serum-free T_4 (fT_4) would result in increased availability of circulating T_4 for uptake by peripheral tissues, and could be the stimulus for greater T_4 degradation in athletes. In support of this, Terjung and Tipton[30] observed an increase in fT_4 in human subjects following exercise on a bicycle ergometer and in exercising animals, and Irvine[29] also noted that fT_4 was higher in exercising athletes than non-athletes. On the other hand, De Nayer and colleagues[31] observed a decrease in fT_4 in 11 male athletes following very strenuous exercise, while Simsch et al.[32] observed no change in highly trained rowers.

Second, an increase in T_4 deiodinating activity of peripheral tissues that would result in increased deiodination, thereby facilitating net rate of disposal of T_4, could be the stimulus. Irvine[29] observed an increased urinary excretion of T_4-derived iodide in both humans and rats, although no changes in T_4 deiodinating activities were observed in liver, kidney or muscle enzymes of rats, which would indicate increased deiodination[28]. Therefore, an increased rate of turnover of T_4 is more likely to be due to increases in fT_4 levels in blood than to the induction of deiodinating enzymes in peripheral tissues, although, at least in some circumstances, both mechanisms might be simultaneously involved.

Increased T_4 turnover is consistent with studies showing approximately half as much iodine in the thyroid glands of exercising rats as in those of non-exercising rats.[33] There was no significant difference in the rate of renewal of thyroidal iodine between these groups, resulting in less storage of iodine in the exercising rats. Endurance training is associated with lower uptake of radio-iodine by the thyroid of humans. Hooper and colleagues[34] observed that human volunteers who ran at least 10 miles per week had lower mean 24-hour thyroid radio-iodine uptake ($8 \pm 3\%$) than non-exercising subjects ($14 \pm 5\%$). In spite of the reduced uptake in these subjects, other thyroid function tests, such as T_3, T_4 and TSH, did not differ significantly, nor did urinary iodine excretion.[34] Khoral[35] also found that the percent uptake of a dose of ^{131}I into thyroids of 16 athletes immediately after exercise was lower than resting values 2 hours later, while Wilson[36] observed 24-hour uptake in 17 men to fall from 30% before exercise conditioning to 24% (not significant) after, and to increase again to 28% 2 weeks after cessation of training. Again, urinary iodine excretion did not differ between the two groups.

Others have investigated the effects of exercise on serum levels of thyroid hormones in human subjects, and most studies indicate a small increase in circulating TSH[32,37,38] or response of TSH to thyroliberin (TRH) stimulation[39,40] during endurance training, which could possibly explain the increase in thyroid hormone secretion rate.[37] Exceptions are the observation of Simsch et al.[32] of a decrease in TSH during resistance training by rowers, that of Pakarinen et al.[41] of a slight decrease in TSH during very strenuous exercise and that of Hooper et al.[34] of no change. Galbo and colleagues[37] reported that serum concentrations of TSH increased with increasing workload in men during graded and prolonged exhaustive treadmill running, along with plasma catecholamine levels, which increased progressively with intensity and duration of exercise. The effects of exercise on T_3 and T_4 are even more variable with either no change,[25,29,34,37,38,42] or small decreases in concentrations.[38, 39,40,41,43]

Taken together, these changes in thyroid hormones are indicative of mild thyroidal impairment during physical training, and may be associated with changes in BMR that occur with physical training, and increases in catecholamines associated with the stress of exercise. Loucks and Heath[44] observed that in untrained women exercising at 70% of aerobic capacity for 4 days, reductions in T_3 and fT_3 occurred when energy intake fell below 25 lean kcal/kg body mass (LBM)/day, indicating that inadequate energy availability may be a factor in impaired thyroid function during exercise.

There does, however, appear to be many inconsistencies in the results of studies on exercise and thyroid hormones. Much of the research was carried out several decades ago and may have suffered from less sensitive methodologies than those currently available. It is likely that factors not taken into account in earlier studies, such as type, duration and intensity of exercise or training regime (acute vs. chronic; endurance vs. resistance) and level of physical fitness of subjects may be involved. Notably, too, the superimposed effect of stress was not taken into account in early studies. Furthermore, Baylor and Hackney[45] observed that 20 weeks of exercise training resulted in two distinct categories of responses among a group of college athletes, with responders (n = 10) showing a decrease in fT_3 and non-responders (n = 7) showing no change. Such factors may account for the apparent inconsistencies in results, especially of earlier studies.

Even though there is an increased turnover of T_4 in athletes to a level seen in hyperthyroid patients, no reports indicate that athletes are functionally hyperthyroid, since there are no significant changes in plasma TSH concentrations.[30,36] The physiological significance of this elevated T_4 degradation, with no clinical manifestation of hyperthyroidism, is not known and requires further investigation. It is possible that the change in T_4 metabolism may simply represent a passive disposal phenomenon introduced by exercise, a passive and transient change associated with hormonal responses to stress, or a response to energy deficit or weight loss. On the other hand, the thyroid hormones may play an important role in some physiological and biochemical responses to exercise, such as in carbohydrate and lipid metabolism. Thyroid hormones are involved in the reduction in cholesterol observed with exercise training, and T_4 is known to increase fatty acid mobilization from adipose tissue and thus may be needed for normal release of fatty acids during exercise.[25] Kudelska and colleagues[46] investigated the rate of glycogen metabolism in different muscle types of rats treated with T_3 and concluded that T_3 markedly affects exercise-induced metabolism of glycogen, suggesting the possible role of thyroid hormones in glycogen metabolism.

Thyroid hormones do not appear to be involved in the increase in mitochondria content in muscle in response to endurance training, nor in other training-induced changes.[47,48] The concentration of T_4 in muscle is not influenced by exercise; rather, the liver appears to be the major site for the increased uptake of T_4 from the blood.[25] Rone et al.,[49] however, observed a positive correlation between aerobic capacity and T_3 metabolism in healthy euthyroid men, which suggested a link between muscle physiology and T_3 activity and a possible physiological role for thyroid in physical conditioning

V. INTERACTIONS OF IODINE WITH DRUGS AND OTHER NUTRIENTS

The utilization of absorbed iodine is influenced by goitrogens, which interfere with the biosynthesis of the hormones.[50] Goitrogens are found in vegetables of the genus brassica (cabbage, turnip, Brussels sprouts and broccoli) and in some staple foods such as cassava, corn and lima beans used in poorer countries. Goitrogens can become a problem where people whose iodine intake is only marginal eat these staple foods, particularly if they are not well cooked. Therefore, where the diet is proportionally high in these foods, the dietary requirement for iodine is likely to be higher.[50] Most goitrogens are inactivated by heat, though those in milk are not affected by pasteurization.[51]

Because selenium has an essential role in thyroid hormone metabolism, it has the potential to play a major part in the outcome of iodine deficiency[4] through two aspects of its biological function. First, the selenium-containing deiodinases regulate the synthesis and degradation of T_3. Second, seleno-peroxidases and possibly thioredoxin reductase protect the thyroid gland from hydrogen peroxide produced during the synthesis of thyroid hormones. Thus, selenium deficiency may exacerbate the hypothyroidism due to iodine deficiency.[4]

VI. ASSESSMENT OF IODINE STATUS

A. Urinary Iodine Excretion

The most widely used method of assessing iodine status is to determine urinary iodide excretion in a 24-hour urine specimen, as daily urinary excretion closely reflects iodine intake.[12,52] Approximately 90% of iodine intake is excreted in the urine. Twenty-four-hour urine collections are preferable, but are not very practical for large field surveys in developing countries where iodine deficiency is being assessed. Non-fasting casual urine specimens are usually obtained in these situations. As there are large day-to-day variations in urinary iodide excretion, more than one urinary analysis should be made for assessment of an individual's iodine status. In populations with adequate general nutrition, urinary iodide concentration correlates well with the iodine/creatinine ratio, so urinary iodide excretion relative to creatinine may be determined on the assumption that creatinine excretion is constant over time. However, the iodine/creatinine ratio may not be suitable in all situations, as creatinine excretion increases with age and physical training due to increases in muscle mass and creatinine production;[53] it is also influenced by malnutrition, strenuous exercise, fever and trauma.[52]

B. Thyroid Hormones

The level of serum T_4 or TSH provides an indirect measure of iodine nutritional status. When supplies of iodine in the diet are limited, stimulation of the thyroid gland by increased plasma TSH may be enough to maintain circulating T_4 and T_3 concentrations. Therefore, plasma TSH concentrations are often elevated when T_4 and T_3 concentrations are within the normal range.[54] In more severe iodine deficiency (moderate deficiency), T_4 concentrations begin to decrease, and only in the severest of iodine deficiency, when median urinary iodine excretion is less than 20 µg/l, do plasma T_3 concentrations decline. TSH is not a particularly useful parameter to determine iodine status in adults, as it does not reflect recent dietary iodine intake and is not particularly sensitive to borderline deficiencies.[6,12] However, neonates exhibit elevated serum TSH more frequently than adults, and therefore appear to be hypersensitive to the effects of iodine deficiency.[54] Another hormone, serum thyroglobulin, changes inversely to iodine intake at all ages and is very sensitive to iodine status. It might be a more sensitive indicator of mild iodine deficiency in children and adults, as levels are elevated in subjects with low iodine excretion while TSH and T_4 levels remain within the normal range.[55–57]

C. Assessment of Thyroid Size and Goiter Rate

In contrast to urinary iodide, the prevalence of goiter reflects a population's history of iodine nutrition but does not properly reflect its present iodine status.[10] Goiter assessment is made by inspection, palpation or more recently, by ultrasonography. Normative values proposed by the WHO and the International Council for the Control of Iodine Deficiency Disorders (ICCIDD) for thyroid volume by ultrasonography are based on data obtained from a large sample of iodine-replete school-age children.[58]

D. Radioactive Iodine Uptake

Radioactive ^{131}I uptake by the thyroid gland is used as a test of thyroid function in clinical settings.[52] The thyroid gland concentrates more radioactive iodine in iodine deficiency and less in iodine excess. Thus, in areas of iodine deficiency, the thyroidal uptake of ^{131}I is much faster and approaches 100%.

E. Assessment of Iodine Deficiency in a Population

The epidemiological assessment of nutritional status of iodine is important in relation to a population or group living in an area or region that is suspected to be iodine deficient. In surveys for assessing iodine deficiency of a population, iodine concentration in casual urine samples from about 40 people is usually adequate.[59] The most important information comes from measurement of the urinary iodide and blood TSH concentrations in neonates and pregnant women. The results of these two measures indicate the severity of the problem, and can also be used to assess the effectiveness of remedial measures.[60]

VII.   REQUIREMENT AND RECOMMENDED DIETARY INTAKES

Goiter occurs when iodine intakes are less than about 50 µg/day, and cretinism when intakes of mothers are 30 µg/day or less.[12] Minimum requirements to prevent goiter are based on the urinary excretion associated with a high incidence of goiter in a population, estimated at 50 µg/g creatinine, and the observation that a minimum intake of 70 µg/day appears to be necessary to avoid signs of goiter. Therefore, the minimum requirement for prevention of goiter is approximately one µg/kg body weight/day.[61] However, recommended dietary intakes are based on physiological requirements, which are in turn based on a number of indicators, including thyroidal radio-iodine accumulation and turnover, iodine balance studies, urinary iodide excretion, thyroid hormones measures and thyroid volume. Physiological requirement is at least equal to the daily amount of hormonal iodine degraded in the peripheral tissues and not recovered by the thyroid. There is an obligatory loss of iodine from the body via urine, feces, and sweat. Fecal iodine loss is relatively constant and is likely to be significant only when iodine intake is very low. Sweat has generally not been considered an important avenue for iodine loss,[62] however, losses may be appreciable in hot climates. Urine, the major excretion pathway for iodine, is related to dietary intake. Individuals over a period of time adapt well to low or high iodine intakes, although the length of this adaptation time is uncertain.[63] The consensus of reviewed studies would appear to be that iodine balance is achievable at intakes over 100 µg/day and not achievable below 40 µg/day.[64] From this physiological requirement of around 100 µg/day, a rather large safety margin is added to give a recommended dietary intake, which for most countries is 150 µg/day.[65] This level is adequate to maintain normal thyroid function, which is essential for growth and development. Requirements may increase if the diets contain goitrogens.

At present, there are no recommendations for iodine intake for athletes. However, reports of high sweat losses during strenuous activity[22–24] in the heat suggest that further investigation of requirements for active individuals should be made.

VIII.   TOXICITY

Most people can tolerate up to 1000 µg iodine daily without adverse effects, but daily intakes of up to 2000 µg are regarded as excessive and potentially harmful.[5] Such intakes are unlikely to be obtained from normal diets of natural foods except where they are exceptionally high in marine fish or seaweed, or where foods are contaminated with iodine from iodine-containing medications or other adventitious sources. The effects of high iodine intake on thyroid function are variable and depend on the health of the thyroid gland. Dietary intakes of up 1000 µg/day have few long-term effects when the thyroid is healthy. Adverse effects include hypothyroidism and elevated TSH, goiter and increased incidence of autoimmune thyroid disease.[66] People who have underlying autoimmune disease such as Grave's Disease or Hashimoto's thyroiditis, or who have previously been iodine deficient, may be more sensitive to iodine.[8] Iodine-induced thyrotoxicosis (Jod-Base-dow) has been described following the iodization programs, particularly in women over 40 years of age who had always been living in a low-iodine environment. Some individuals have thyroid nodules that can start making too much thyroid hormone when dietary iodine increases, which produces a condition called iodine-induced hyperthyroidism. Excess iodine can also cause hypothy-roidism because large amounts of iodine block the thyroid's ability to produce hormones.

Iodine overload may occur in vegans when seaweed and iodine-containing dietary supplements are consumed.[67] The use of kelp supplements is not recommended as these can contain very high but variable amounts of iodine.

There might also be a danger from consumption of thyroid preparations. Scally et al.[68] reported case studies of two physically fit adults who supplemented with tiratricol, an over-the-counter thyroid preparation marketed as a metabolic accelerator and fat loss aid. They presented with lethargy, loss of appetite and muscle weakness, symptoms that were accompanied by low serum TSH and profoundly elevated T_3 concentrations. These cases illustrate the danger of consumption of substances marketed as "nutritional" supplements, but which may have pharmacological effects capable of inducing thyroid abnormalities when consumed inappropriately.

IX. DIETARY AND SUPPLEMENTAL SOURCES

Adequate dietary iodine intakes are around 100–150 µg/day. Foods of marine origin such as sea fish and shell fish, seameal (custard made of ground seaweed) and seaweeds are rich in iodine, reflecting the greater iodine concentration of sea water compared with fresh water.[69] The iodine content of plants and animals depends on the environment in which they grow. Vegetables, fruit and cereals grown in soils with low iodine content are poor sources of iodine.

Because the mammary gland concentrates iodine, dairy products are usually a good source, but only if the cows get enough iodine. In recent years, iodine contamination in dairy products and bread has made a major contribution to the daily intake in some countries. The use of iodophors as sanitizers in the dairy industry has resulted in variable but considerable amounts of residual iodine in milk, cheese and other milk products.[70] The use of these compounds, however, is declining in many countries. Tasmania, Australia, adopted the addition of iodate as a bread improver as an iodine supplement.[71] Other adventitious sources of iodine include kelp tablets and drugs or foods, and beverages containing the iodine-containing coloring erythrosine.

Iodized salt, another source of iodine, has been one of the most efficient means of improving iodine nutrition. The amount added varies widely in different regions. In Canada and the U.S., salt is iodized to a concentration of 77 ppm iodine as potassium iodide so that the daily recommended intake might be obtained from 2 g salt.[8] Most other countries add 10–40 ppm iodide to salt. However, in some countries, both iodized and non-iodized salts are available. In developed countries, much of the salt intake now comes from processed foods; whether such foods contain iodized salt depends on local commercial practice.[8]

Iodine from foods is readily absorbed, as is iodine in supplements. The bioavailability of iodine is assumed to be high,[72] however, the utilization can be influenced by goitrogens, which interfere with the biosynthesis of thyroid hormones.

Iodine intakes vary considerably depending on geographical location, dietary habits and salt iodization. Intakes are usually assessed from urinary excretion rather than direct measurement of food iodine, because of lack of good food composition data in many countries. Only one study has reported the dietary iodine intakes of athletes; intakes of 41 U.S. figure skaters aged 11–18 years were 131 ± 159 (mean ± SD) µg/day in females and 139 ± 138 in males.[73] This study is discussed further in Section X.

X. EFFECT OF DEFICIENCY OR EXCESS ON PHYSICAL PERFORMANCE

Lack of evidence of a significant increase in urinary iodine excretion during exercise suggests that the changes in thyroid hormone metabolism are perhaps transitory and compensated for by feedback mechanisms in the body. Current opinion is that there is no evidence to suggest a greater requirement in physically active individuals, and that iodine intake in athletes is adequate or excessive.[74,75]

This is probably due to, and may be also a reason for, the complete lack of research on the role of iodine in physical performance. The assumption that iodine intakes are adequate may be erroneous, as recent studies indicate less than adequate intake of iodine in a number of countries as a result of changes in dietary patterns, reduction in use of iodized salt and other dietary sources.[76]

The only reported study of iodine intakes of athletes was that of Ziegler et al.[73] who found mean ($\pm$ SD) iodine intakes of 41 U.S. figure skaters aged 11–18 years of 131 ± 159 and 139 ± 138 µg/day for females and males, respectively, which they reported as being below the adult recommended dietary intake (RDA)[66] of 150 µg/day. However, the mean intake was well above the estimated average requirement (EAR) of 95 µg/day[66] and within the normal range of adequate intakes. Furthermore, many of these athletes may have been aged between 11 and 13 years, for whom the EAR is 73 µg/day and the RDA 120 µg/day. There was no comparison with intakes of non-athletes. However, two studies have reported significant losses of iodine in sweat, losses that could be substantial for endurance athletes exercising in the heat,[22–24] suggesting that current recommended dietary intakes may not be appropriate for athletes. There have been no studies to date of the effect of iodine supplementation on physical performance.

A small number of studies have investigated the effects of thyroid hormones on physical performance, but unfortunately, investigation of iodine metabolism was not included in any of these studies. Reed et al.[77] investigated the effect of supplementation with L-thyroxine in 12 subjects working in Antarctica and observed that 4 months of T_4 supplementation attenuated the decline in cognition and mood, but did not prevent decrements in submaximal exercise performance, body temperature or serum T_3 observed during Antarctic residence. L-thyroxine has been shown to improve cardiac and exercise performance in patients with chronic heart failure.[78,79]

Zarzeczny and colleagues[80] studied the effects of thyroid hormone deficit and T_3 treatment on exercise performance, blood concentrations and lactate threshold in trained and untrained rats and showed that both T_3 deficiency and excess reduced maximal exercise performance and shifted blood lactate threshold to lower workloads. Endurance training or administration of T_3 to hypothyroid rats markedly improved their exercise performance. This observation might be associated with the finding of increased mobilization of muscle glycogen during exhaustive exercise in rats treated with T_3.[46]

XI. CONCLUSIONS AND OPPORTUNITIES FOR FUTURE RESEARCH

Although there is little research on the involvement of iodine in exercise performance or recovery from exercise, iodine is essential for the maintenance of normal metabolism and for normal growth and development and, therefore, is likely to take part in various processes of importance to exercising individuals. Given iodine's key functions, it is surprising that more research has not been done in this area. Clearly, there are many questions to be answered. Strenuous activity and endurance training cause some changes in thyroid metabolism, but it is not clear whether these changes are temporary or permanent or whether they have any biological significance. In spite of the increased turnover of T_4, it appears that serum levels of T_4 and T_3 do not change substantially, which leaves a major discrepancy in the reported observations. It is not clear how exercise can cause both decreased iodine uptake and increased thyroid turnover while serum hormone levels remain unaltered.[34] Preliminary research indicates the involvement of thyroid hormones in metabolism of carbohydrates and lipids, although to what extent inadequate or excess iodine affects these processes is not known. Considering the involvement of iodine and thyroid hormones in maintaining BMR, substantial further investigation of the relationship between thyroid metabolism and the observed increase in post-exercise metabolism and in the possible increase in BMR as a result of training is warranted.

The conflicting observations of changes in thyroid hormones during exercise training may result from varying methods and study designs, such as the type and intensity of exercise and timing of observations. Well designed trials and with more sensitive analytical methods are required to answer specific questions and to clarify the confusion. In much of the research on thyroid hormones and exercise, there has been little or no discussion of the role of iodine. Inclusion of assessment of iodine status and metabolism in future studies is highly desirable.

Significant losses of iodine may occur in sweat and these can be substantial in extended exercise in hot conditions.[22-24] Preliminary evidence suggests that sweat losses may be significant enough to cause iodine deficiency and induce clinical changes such as increased thyroid volume.[24] This issue needs further investigation. Athletes may require increased intakes of iodine, especially in light of the inadequate iodine intakes in many developing countries and the decreasing iodine intakes in several developed countries.[76]

REFERENCES

1. Sumar, S. and Ismail, H., Iodine in food and health, *Nutr. Food Sci.*, 97, 175, 1997.
2. Semba, R.D. and Delange, F., Iodine in human milk: Perspectives for infant health, *Nutr. Rev.*, 59, 269, 2001.
3. Freake, H.C., Iodine, in *Biochemical and Physiological Aspects of Human Nutrition*, Stipaunk, M., Ed., W.B. Saunders Company, Philadelphia, 2000, chap 2.
4. Arthur, J.R., Beckett, G.J. and Mitchell, J.H., The interactions between selenium and iodine deficiencies in man and animals, *Nutr. Res. Rev.*, 12, 55, 1999.
5. Hetzel, B.S. and Clugston, G.A., Iodine, in *Modern Nutrition in Health and Disease*, Shils, M.E., Olson, J.A., Shike, M. and Ross, A.C., Eds., Wilson & Wilkie, Baltimore, 1999.
6. Hetzel, B.S., Potter, B.J. and Dulberg, E.M., The iodine deficiency disorders: Nature, pathogenesis and epidemiology, *World Rev. Nutr. Dietet.*, 62, 59, 1990.
7. Hetzel, B.S., Iodine and neurophysical development, *J. Nutr.*, 130, 493S, 2000.
8. Anonymous, Ideal iodine nutrition: A brief nontechnical guide, *IDD Newsletter*, 17, 27, 2001.
9. WHO, UNICEF and ICCIDD, Indicators for Assessing Iodine Deficiency Disorders and Their Control Through Salt Iodization, World Health Organization, Geneva, 1994, 2.
10. Delange, F., de Benoist, B., Pretell, E. and Dunn, J.T., Iodine deficiency in the world: Where do we stand at the turn of the century?, *Thyroid*, 11, 437, 2001.
11. Lamberg, B., Iodine deficiency disorders and goitre, *Eur. J. Clin. Nutr.*, 47, 1, 1993.
12. Hetzel, B.S. and Dunn, J.T., The iodine deficiency disorders: Their nature and prevention, *Ann. Rev. Nutr.*, 9, 21, 1989.
13. Delange, F., The role of iodine in brain development, *Proc. Nutr. Soc.*, 59, 75, 2000.
14. Bleichrodt, N. and Born, M.P., A meta-analysis of research on iodine and its relationship to cognitive development, in *The Damaged Brain of Iodine Deficiency*, Stanbury, J.B., Ed., Cognizant Communication, New York, 1994, 195.
15. Delange, F., Editorial. Iodine deficiency as a cause of brain damage, *Postgrad. Med. J.*, 77, 217, 2001.
16. Maberly, G.F., Iodine deficiency disorders: Contemporary scientific issues, *J. Nutr.*, 124, 1473S, 1994.
17. Vanderpas, J.B., Contempré, B., Duale, N.L., Goossens, W., Bebe, N., Thorpe, R., Ntambue, K., Dumont, J.E., Thilly, C.H. and Diplock, A.T., Iodine and selenium deficiency associated with cretinism in northern Zaire, *Am. J. Clin. Nutr.*, 52, 1087, 1990.
18. Arthur, J.R. and Beckett, G.J., Thyroid function, *Br. Med. Bull.*, 55, 658, 1999.
19. Hetzel, B.S., *The Story of Iodine Deficiency: An International Challenge in Nutrition*, Oxford University Press, Oxford, 1989.
20. Clugston, G.A. and Hetzel, B.S., Iodine, in *Modern Nutrition in Health and Disease*, Shils, M.E., Olson, J.A. and Shike, M., Eds., Lea & Febiger, Malvern, PA, 1994, chap 13.
21. Nath, S.K., Moinier, B., Thuillier, F., Rongier, M. and Desjeux, J.-F., Urinary excretion of iodide and fluoride from supplemented food grade salt, *Int. J. Vit. Nutr. Res.*, 62, 66, 1992.
22. Suzuki, M. and Tamura, T., Iodine uptake of Japanese male university students: Urinary iodine excretion of sedentary and physically active students and sweat iodine excretion during exercise, *J. Nutr. Sci. Vitaminol. (Tokyo)*, 31, 409, 1985.
23. Mao, I-F., Ko, Y-C. and Chen, M-L., The stability of iodine in human sweat, *Jpn. J. Physiol.*, 40, 693, 1990.

24. Mao, I-F., Chen, M-L. and Ko, Y-C., Electrolyte loss in sweat and iodine deficiency in a hot climate, *Arch. Environ. Health,* 56, 271, 2001.
25. Terjung, R.L. and Winder, W.W., Exercise and thyroid function, *Med. Sci. Sport Exer.,* 7, 20, 1975.
26. Irvine, C.H.G., Thyroxine secretion rate in the horse in various physiological states, *J. Endocrinol.,* 39, 313, 1967.
27. Story, J.A. and Griffith, D.R., Effect of exercise on thyroid hormone secretion rate in aging rats, *Horm. Metab. Res.,* 6, 403, 1974.
28. Winder, W.W. and Heninger, R.W., Effect of exercise on degradation of thyroxine in the rat, *Am. J. Physiol.,* 224, 572, 1973.
29. Irvine, C.H.G., Effect of exercise on thyroxine degradation in athletes and non-athletes, *J. Clin. Endocrinol.,* 28, 942, 1968.
30. Terjung, R.L. and Tipton, C.M., Plasma thyroxine and thyroid-stimulating hormone levels during submaximal exercise in humans, *Am. J. Physiol.,* 220, 1840, 1971.
31. De Nayer, P., Malvaux, P., Ostyn, M., Van der Schrieck, H.G., Beckers, C. and De Visscher, M., Serum free thyroxine and binding-proteins after muscular exercise, *J. Clin. Endocrinol.,* 28, 714, 1968.
32. Simsch, C., Lormes, W., Petersen, K.G., Baur, S., Liu, Y., Hackney, A.C., Lehmann, M. and Steinacker, J.M., Training intensity influences leptin and thyroid hormones in highly trained rowers, *Int. J. Sports Med.,* 23, 422, 2002.
33. Rhodes, B.A., Effect of exercise on the thyroid gland, *Nature,* 216, 917, 1967.
34. Hooper, P.L., Rhodes, B.A. and Conway, M.J., Exercise lowers thyroid radioiodine uptake: Concise communication, *J. Nucl. Med.,* 21, 835, 1980.
35. Khoral, I.S., Absorption of ^{131}I by the thyroid gland in athletes during physical exertion, *Bull. Exptl. Biol. Med.,* 54, 962, 1963.
36. Wilson, O., Field study of the effect of cold exposure and increased muscular activity upon metabolic rate and thyroid function in man, *Fed. Proc.,* 25, 1357, 1966.
37. Galbo, H., Hummer, L., Petersen, I.B., Christensen, N.J. and Bie, N., Thyroid and testicular hormone responses to graded and prolonged exercise in man, *Eur. J. Appl. Physiol.,* 36, 101, 1977.
38. Krotkiewski, M., Sjostrom, L., Sullivan, L., Lundberg, P.-A., Lindstedt, G., Wetterqvist, H. and Bjorntorp, P., The effect of acute and chronic exercise on thyroid hormones in obesity, *Acta Med. Scand.,* 216, 269, 1984.
39. Boyden, T.W., Pamenter, R.W., Stanforth, P., Rotkis, T. and Wilmore, J.H., Evidence for mild thyroidal impairment in women undergoing endurance training, *J. Clin. Endocrinol. Metab.,* 54, 53, 1982.
40. Hohtari, H., Pakarinen, A. and Kauppila, A., Serum concentrations of thyrotropin, thyroxine, triiodothyronine and thyroxine binding globulin in female endurance runners and joggers, *Acta Endocrinol.,* 114, 41, 1987.
41. Pakarinen, A., Kakkinen, K. and Alen, M., Serum thyroid hormones, thyrotropin and thyroxine binding globulin in elite athletes during very intense strength training of one week, *J. Sports Med. Phys. Fitness,* 31, 142, 1991.
42. Banfi, G., Pontillo, M., Marinelli, M., Dolci, A. and Roi, G.S., Thyrotropin and free thyroid hormones in athletes during and after ultra-endurance sport performances, *J. Clin. Ligand Assay,* 21, 331, 1998.
43. Tremblay, A., Poehlman, E.T., Despres, J.P., Theriault, G., Danforth, E. and Bouchard, C., Endurance training with constant energy intake in identical twins: Changes over time in energy expenditure and related hormones, *Metabolism: Clin. Exper.,* 46, 499, 1997.
44. Loucks, A.B. and Heath, E.M., Induction of low-T_3 syndrome in exercising women occurs at a threshold of energy availability, *Am. Physiol. Soc.,* R817, 1994.
45. Baylor, L.S. and Hackney, A.C., Resting thyroid and leptin hormone changes in women following intense, prolonged exercise training, *Eur. J. Appl. Physiol.,* 88, 480, 2003.
46. Kudelska, G., Gorski, J., Swiatecka, J. and Gorska, M., Effect of exercise on glycogen metabolism in muscles of triiodothyronine-treated rats, *Eur. J. Appl. Physiol.,* 72, 496, 1996.
47. Winder, W.W. and Heninger, R.W., Effect of exercise on tissue levels of thyroid hormones in the rat, *Am. J. Physiol.,* 221, 1139, 1971.
48. Winder, W.W., Garhart, S.J. and Premachandra, B.N., Peripheral markers of thyroid status unaffected by endurance training in rats, *Eur. J. Physiol.,* 389, 195, 1981.
49. Rone, J.K., Dons, R.F. and Reed, H.L., The effect of endurance training on serum triiodothyronine kinetics in man: Physical conditioning marked by enhanced thyroid hormone metabolism, *Clin. Endocrinol.,* 37, 325, 1992.

50. Gaitan, E., Goitrogens in the etiology of endemic goiter, in *Endemic Goiter and Endemic Cretinism,* Stanbury, J.B. and Hetzel, B.S., Eds., Wiley Medical, New York, 1980.

51. Mahan, L.K. and Escott-Stump, S., *Kraus's Food, Nutrition and Diet Therapy,* W.B. Saunders Company, 1996.

52. Gibson, R., Assessment of iodine status, in *Principles of Nutritional Assessment,* Oxford University Press, New York, 1990, 527.

53. Remer, T. and Manz, F., The inadequacy of the urinary iodine–creatinine ratio for the assessment of iodine status during infancy, childhood and adolescence, *J. Trace Elem. Electrolytes Health Dis.,* 8, 217, 1994.

54. Bourdoux, P.P., Biochemical evaluation of iodine status, in *Iodine Deficiency in Europe: A Continuing Concern,* Delange, F., Dunn, J.T. and Glinoer, D., Eds., Plenum Press, New York, 1993, 119.

55. Mißler, U., Gutekunst, R. and Wood, W.G., Thyroglobulin is a more sensitive indicator of iodine deficiency than thyrotropin: development and evaluation of dry blood spot assays for thyrotropin and thyroglobulin in iodine-deficient geographical areas, *Eur. J. Clin. Chem. Clin. Biochem.,* 32, 137, 1994.

56. Thomson, C.D., Woodruffe, S., Colls, A.J., Joseph, J. and Doyle, T.C., Urinary iodine and thyroid status of New Zealand residents, *Eur. J. Clin. Nutr.,* 55, 387, 2001.

57. Knudsen, N., Bulow, I., Jorgensen, T., Perrild, H., Ovesen, L. and Laurberg, P., Serum Tg—A sensitive marker of thyroid abnormalities and iodine deficiency in epidemiological studies, *J. Clin. Endocrinol. Metab.,* 86, 3599, 2001.

58. Zimmerman, M.B., Molinari, L., Spehl, M., Weidinger-Toth, J., Podoba, J., Hess, S. and Delange, F., Updated provisional WHO/ICCIDD reference values for sonographic thyroid volume in iodine-replete school-age children, *IDD Newsletter,* 17, 12, 2001.

59. Frey, H.M., Rosenlund, B. and Torgersen, J.P., Value of single urine specimens in estimation of 24 hour iodine excretion, *Acta Endocrinol.,* 72, 287, 1973.

60. WHO/FAO/IAEA, Trace Elements in Human Nutrition and Health, World Health Organization, Geneva, 1996, chap 4.

61. National Research Council, Recommended Dietary Allowances 9th rev ed, National Academy of Sciences, Washington D.C., 1980, 147.

62. Consolazio, C., Matoush, R., Nelson, R., Isaac, G. and Canham, J., Comparison of nitrogen, calcium, and iodine excretion in arm and total body sweat, *Am. J. Clin. Nutr.,* 18, 443, 1966.

63. Soto, R., Codevilla, A., Weinstein, M., Rozardos, I., Rabinovich, L. and Goldberg, D., Adaptive mechanisms to iodine deficiency in endemic goiter in Misiones, Argentina, *Metabolism,* 4, 326, 1968.

64. DeGroot, L.J., Kinetic analysis of iodine metabolism, *J. Clin. Endocrinol. Metab.,* 26, 149, 1966.

65. Thomson, C.D., Dietary recommendations for iodine around the world, *IDD Newsletter,* 18, 38, 2002.

66. Food and Nutrition Board and Institute of Medicine, Dietary Reference Intakes for Vitamin A, Vitamin K, Boron, Chromium, Copper, Iodine, Iron, Manganese, Molybdenum, Nickel, Silicon, Vanadium, and Zinc, National Academy Press, Washington, D.C., 2001, chap 8.

67. Lightowler, H.J. and Davies, G.J., Iodine intake and iodine deficiency in vegans as assessed by the duplicate-portion technique and urinary iodine excretion, *Br. J. Nutr.,* 80, 529, 1998.

68. Scally, M.C. and Hodge, A., A report of hypothyroidism induced by an over-the-counter fat loss supplement (Tiratricol), *Int. J. Sport Nutr. Exer. Metab.,* 13, 112, 2003.

69. Kidd, P.S., Trowbridge, G.L., Goldsby, J.B. and Nichman, M.Z., Sources of dietary iodine, *J. Am. Diet. Ass.,* 65, 420, 1974.

70. Joerin, M.M. and Bowering, A., The total iodine content of cow's milk, *N.Z. J. Dairy Sci. Technol.,* 7, 155, 1972.

71. Eastman, C.J., The status of iodine nutrition in Australia, in *Iodine Deficiency in Europe—A Continuing Concern,* Delange, F., Dunn, J.T. and Glinoer, D., Eds., Plenum Press, New York, 1993.

72. Fairweather-Tait, S. and Hurrell, R.F., Bioavailability of minerals and trace elements, *Nutr. Res. Rev.,* 9, 295, 1996.

73. Ziegler, P.J., Nelson, J.A. and Jonnalagadda, S.S., Nutritional and physiological status of US National Figure Skaters, *Int. J. Sport Nutr.,* 9, 345, 1999.

74. Speich, M., Pineau, A. and Ballereau, F., Minerals, trace elements and related biological variables in athletes and during physical activity, *Clin. Chim. Acta,* 312, 1, 2001.

75. Maughan, R.J., Role of micronutrients in sport and physical activity, *Br. Med. Bull.,* 55, 683, 1999.

76. Thomson, C.D., Selenium and iodine intakes and status in New Zealand and Australia, *Br. J. Nutr.*, 91, 661, 2004.

77. Reed, H.L., Reedy, K.R., Palinkas, L.A., Van Do, N., Finney, N.S., Case, H.S., LeMar, H.J., Wright, J. and Thomas, J., Impairment in cognitive and exercise performance during prolonged Antarctic residence: Effect of thyroxine supplementation in the polar triiodothyronine syndrome, *J. Clin. Endocrinol. Metab.*, 86, 110, 2001.

78. Moruzzi, P., Doria, E., Agostoni, P.G., Capacchione, V. and Sganzerle, P., Usefulness of L-thyroxine to improve cardiac and exercise performance in idiopathic dilated cardiomyopathy, *Am. J. Cardiol.*, 73, 374, 1994.

79. Moruzzi, P., Doria, E. and Agostoni, P.G., Medium-term effectiveness of L-thyroxine treatment in idiopathic dilated cardiomyopathy, *Am. J. Med.*, 101, 461, 1996.

80. Zarzeczny, R., Pilis, W., Langfort, J., Kaciuba-Uscilko, H. and Nazar, K., Influence of thyroid hormones on exercise tolerance and lactate threshold in rats, *J. Physiol. Pharmacol.*, 47, 503, 1996

18 Chromium

*Michael G. Bemben, Debra A. Bemben
and Michael J. Hartman*

CONTENTS

I. INTRODUCTION

A. CHEMICAL STRUCTURE

Chromium (Cr), whose atomic number of 24, is known as a transitional element. Cr can exist in a number of oxidative states such as Cr^{+6} bound to oxygen, however, in an acidic environment, like the stomach, Cr^{+6} is reduced to trivalent Cr (Cr^{+3}), the most stable form of Cr.[1]

Cr has been used as a tool for diagnosis and research in hematology, as a label for red blood cells and as a fecal marker.[2] In general, Cr^{+3} complexes are relatively inert, which suggests that it is unlikely to have a function in enzyme systems;[1,3] however, it may play a role in stabilizing or maintaining the structure of proteins and nucleic acids.[4] It seems that Cr's primary function of potentiating the effects of insulin in carbohydrate, fat and protein metabolism acts through a constituent of the glucose tolerance factor (GTF).[3] GTF (Cr in combination with nicotinic acid and glutathione)[5] plays a role in helping to move glucose into the cell by binding to and potentiating the action of insulin.[3]

B. PROPOSED FUNCTIONS

Cr has been thought to be important for increasing muscle mass and reducing body fat relative to body composition and for increasing phosphate stores relative to improved sport performance.[3] It is interesting to note that the supplemental form of Cr, Cr picolinate [Cr(pic)$_3$], is better absorbed than dietary Cr, and most research has focused on this supplement in relation to possible ergogenic effects.[6]

It seems that most research fails to substantiate Cr as an effective supplement[3] and, in fact, recent animal studies suggest that [Cr(pic)$_3$] may actually generate oxidative damage of DNA and lipids and may be mutagenic,[6,7] which may suggest that Cr taken in the form of Cr chloride may be less likely to pose a health risk.[6] However, in a response to an article by Stearns et al.,[7] McCarty suggests that these studies were seriously flawed, which may limit their credibility.[8] Cr has also been suggested to be involved in anabolic protein metabolism by stimulating RNA synthesis and amino acid incorporation in protein.[9]

Davis and Vincent[10] have demonstrated a functional link between Cr and insulin action through a low molecular weight Cr-binding substance, referred to as LMWCr, that activates a phosphotyrosine phosphatase in adipose tissue. Davis et al.[11] suggest that the biological function of LMWCr is as an insulin-signaling amplification mechanism by stimulating insulin receptor protein tyrosine kinase activity after the receptor is activated by insulin binding.

It should be noted that Stearns[12] suggests that there has yet to be a Cr-containing glucose tolerance factor characterized, that the presence of a low molecular weight Cr-binding protein is questionable and that there has been no direct interaction between Cr and insulin that has been found. She bases these opinions on the premise that Cr^{+3} should not be considered a trace essential metal, because it does not satisfy the criterion that essential elements play a role in enzymes and cofactors.

C. ESTIMATED REQUIREMENTS

Cr is a naturally occurring trace mineral element found in a balanced diet.[13] It appears that the body stores around 5 mg of Cr and that approximately 0.5% of the inorganic form (Cr^{+3}) and 1% of the form of GTF is absorbed from the small intestines. Absorption can be enhanced when Cr is consumed with vitamin C[14], although the mechanism of Cr absorption is not completely understood.

Foods such as mushrooms, nuts, whole grains and processed meats, as well as wine and beer, are good sources of Cr. On the other hand, foods high in simple sugars such as fructose are low in Cr content and actually promote Cr losses.[15] In 1989, the National Research Council recommended that the estimated safe and adequate daily dietary intake (ESADDI) for Cr to be between 50 and 200 µg per day.[16] In 2001, the U.S. Food and Nutrition Board of the National Academy of Sciences redefined the daily adequate intake of Cr to 35 µg per day for adult males and 25 µg per day for adult females.[17,18] These guidelines are supported by various research. Anderson and Kozlovsky[18] analyzed the self-selected diets of free-living American adults and determined an average daily intake of Cr of 33 µg for males and 25 µg for females. Additional research by the same researchers[18] reports adults living in the United Kingdom, Canada, Finland and New Zealand also fail to meet the ESADDI minimum requirement of 50 µg of Cr per day. Offenbacher et al.[19] determined healthy adults consuming 35 µg of dietary Cr daily were Cr sufficient. This may suggest that the original recommendation of Cr intake between 50–200 µg/day as being unrealistic and not necessary. It has been suggested that adults consuming a normal diet are not likely to be Cr deficient and as such should receive little if any benefit from Cr supplementation. However, there is little information available on Cr status in athletes and the general recommendation is that athletes consume sufficient Cr to compensate for possible exercise-induced increases in Cr excretion.[13]

Generally, Cr supplements like [Cr(pic)$_3$], provide about 200 to 600 µg per day. The supplement form is also better absorbed (2–5%) so that individuals taking this supplement would be ingesting about 100 times the amounts of Cr compared with individuals on normal diets. It has been estimated that more than 10 million Americans take Cr supplements, which contributes to a 500 million dollar market per year and is the largest selling supplement next to calcium.[6,20,21] However, there appears to be an inverse relationship between dietary intake of Cr and absorption in healthy adults. Research has shown adults consuming 10 µg daily had Cr absorption of 2%,[22] while adults consuming 40 µg/day had only 0.5% absorption.[18] With a dietary intake of 40–240 µg/day, Cr absorption is relatively constant with a range of 0.4–2.0% of daily intake.[23]

Excretion of Cr^{+3} occurs primarily through the kidney, with small amounts lost in hair, sweat and bile.[1] It appears that Cr excretion can be increased by acute bouts of exercise[24] that mobilize Cr stores into the blood in order to facilitate insulin function, but then cannot be re-absorbed, so it is excreted in the urine. Other factors that can enhance the loss of Cr is lactation, diets that are high in simple sugars,[15,25] glucose loading, infection and trauma.[26,27]

II. NUTRITIONAL ASSESSMENT

A. SUPPLEMENTAL SOURCES

Supplemental Cr has been touted as an ergogenic aid and as a means to increase daily Cr intake. Typically, supplemental Cr is presented as [Cr(pic)$_3$]. Picolinate a derivative of the amino acid tryptophan that may increase Cr absorption in the body.[28] Supplement companies market [Cr(pic)$_3$] as a weight-loss agent, muscle builder and even an alternative to anabolic steroids.[29]

1. Effects on Body Composition

Early research supported the notion of [Cr(pic)$_3$] as an effective weight-loss supplement. Studies by Evans[28] using college-aged males suggested an increase in lean body mass (LBM) when using [Cr(pic)$_3$] in conjunction with a weekly exercise program. Both studies randomly assigned subjects to either a supplement group (200 μg of [Cr(pic)$_3$]/day) or a placebo group. All subjects participated in a supervised weight training program. Anthropometric measures (skinfold thickness and limb circumference) were used to determine changes in body composition. Following the experimental procedures, the [Cr(pic)$_3$] group experienced greater increases in LBM and a decrease in percent body fat during the second study, when compared with the placebo group.

These results were published in a review on the potential benefits of Cr supplementation and were, as such, peer reviewed. Moreover, the measures of body composition used in these studies are not considered extremely accurate or sensitive to acute changes in LBM and at best are estimates of LBM.

The results of the Evans studies have been challenged using more stringent supplementation protocols and sensitive measures of body composition. The vast majority of scientific evidence suggests that [Cr(pic)$_3$] is not an essential part of a weight-loss program.[30] Numerous studies involving both males and females have shown no change in body composition following supplementation of [Cr(pic)$_3$].[31–37] Many of these studies used hydrostatic weighing to assess changes in body composition,[32–34,37] with several others utilizing dual energy x-ray absorptiometry.[31,35,36] Dosages of [Cr(pic)$_3$] ranging from 200–1000 μg per day for experimental periods of 6–12 weeks[31–37] have consistently demonstrated no change in body composition. When combined with exercise, supplemental [Cr(pic)$_3$] offers no additional improvement in body composition when compared with exercise alone.[30] As presented in Lukaski,[1] in 1997 the U.S. Federal Trace Commission concluded no basis for claims of [Cr(pic)$_3$] as a weight or fat loss agent in humans.

2. Effects on Physical Performance

The majority of [Cr(pic)$_3$] studies use resistance exercise as an intervention along with the supplementation. Various measures of muscle size and function have been assessed with [Cr(pic)$_3$] supplementation. Hallmark et al.[38] determined no effect on muscle strength in untrained males following 12 weeks of resistance exercise and 200 μg of [Cr(pic)$_3$]/day. Walker et al.[29] found no additional effect of 200 μg of [Cr(pic)$_3$]/day on neuromuscular performance, including muscle strength and peak power, in national-level collegiate wrestlers during 14 weeks of preseason strength and conditioning training. These results have also been confirmed by Livolsi et al.[39] in collegiate female athletes.

Similar results were found by Campbell et al.[32,40] when examining muscle size and function of older adults (54–71 years of age) following [Cr(pic)₃] supplementation and resistance exercise. In two separate studies, 18 older males and 17 older females were given 924 μg of [Cr(pic)₃]/day or a placebo, while participating in 12 weeks of high-intensity resistance exercise. Following the experimental procedures, it was determined that [Cr(pic)₃] had no significant effect on muscle size, strength or power.

In theory, the use of supplemental Cr may benefit endurance performance by improving carbohydrate metabolism by increasing insulin sensitivity during exercise.[15] However, limited studies have been performed examining the effects of Cr on exhaustive aerobic exercise. Davis et al.[41] looked at the effects of [Cr(pic)₃] and 6% carbohydrate solution (CHO) on time to fatigue in eight active males. Subjects were given CHO alone, CHO + [Cr(pic)₃] or a placebo in a random repeated measure design, and time to fatigue was measured during a shuttle run at 55–95% of VO₂max. There was no difference in performance results in the CHO + [Cr(pic)₃] group when compared with the CHO alone group. However, both treatment groups did perform better than the control.

In summary, the use of supplemental Cr appears to have no effect on measures of physical performance when used in association with an exercise program.

3. Effects on Glucose/Insulin and Lipid Metabolism

Early studies that examined animals fed with Cr-depleted diets reported that these animals, most often rats, had impaired glucose tolerance, and that if Cr was added to their diets, glucose tolerance was restored to normal levels.[21,31,42] Improved glucose tolerance in human was also reported with long-term administration of Cr.[43]

Having mentioned this, Hellerstein[21] points out that, 40 years after these early studies, little progress has been made relative to the possible mechanistic actions of Cr.

Early studies involving humans seemed to indicate improved glucose tolerance following Cr supplementation[43–45] but numerous methodological problems existed, like the lack of control or placebo groups, no blinding of the procedures and inconsistent findings. There were two early placebo-controlled, double-blinded studies[46,47] in Type 2 diabetics; however, both failed to demonstrate an effect on glucose tolerance or body weight and had only mixed results regarding an effect on lipid levels. Uusitupa et al.[46] reported no change in serum total cholesterol and triglycerides and in high-density, low-density and very-low-density lipoprotein subfractions, whereas Abraham et al.[47] reported increases in high-density lipoprotein levels and decreases in very-low-density lipoprotein cholesterol levels.

Perhaps the first placebo-controlled study with a fairly large Type 2 diabetic sample that was published was that of Anderson et al.[48] One hundred and eighty Type 2 diabetics were randomized into one of three treatment groups for 4 months — (1) placebo,(2) low-dose Cr (200 μg/day [Cr(pic)₃]) or (3) high-dose Cr (1000 μg/day [Cr(pic)₃]). The researchers reported that Cr supplementation had a pronounced effect on glucose and insulin variables and that the effects were larger and more consistent with the high-dose Cr regimen.

It is interesting to note that a recent meta-analysis[49] of 20 randomized clinical trials of Cr supplementation on glucose and insulin responses indicated that the combined data showed no effect of Cr on glucose or insulin concentrations in non-diabetic subjects, and that the data on diabetics still remain inconclusive and variable.

The data are also conflicting and contradictory when examining the effects of Cr on lipid fractions. A few studies report elevated high-density lipoprotein cholesterol levels and significant decreases for low-density lipoprotein cholesterol and apolipoprotein B (principal protein of the low-density lipoprotein fraction) following supplementation with [Cr(pic)₃],[50] while others report significant improvements in high-density lipoprotein levels — but only for those with insulin resistance but normal glucose tolerance.[51] There is also a sufficient body of literature that reports that Cr supplementation has no effect on lipid levels,[44] or at best shows some mixed results[52] with no change in high-density lipoprotein levels or triglyceride levels but a decreased total cholesterol.

III. TOXICITY

The hexavalent form of Cr (Cr^{6+}), used for industrial purposes such as dyes, leather tanning and chrome plating, is toxic, and exposure to this form has caused short-term effects such as asthma or bronchitis, or long-term carcinogenic effects.[53] Cr^{6+} passes through the cell membrane where it reacts with DNA in the process of being converted to its trivalent form, with the potential for genotoxic effects.[54] One tissue culture study reported that high concentrations of [Cr(pic)$_3$] caused chromosome breakdown; however, the evidence pointed to picolinate rather than Cr as the likely cause of the damage.[54] Iron metabolism may be negatively affected by Cr, as iron deficiency and anemia have been documented in rats treated with Cr and [Cr(pic)$_3$] supplementation in men undergoing a resistance training program resulted in a 30% decrease in transferrin saturation.[1]

Cr toxicity has been investigated in a number of randomized clinical trials, with doses ranging from 175–1000 µg/day for durations of 6–64 weeks with no documented evidence of toxic effects.[54] Also, animal experiments have shown that the trivalent form of Cr is safe at very high doses, i.e., several thousand fold greater than the ESADDI.[55] However, there have been safety concerns raised about the use of [Cr(pic)$_3$].[6]

Negative effects of over-the-counter (OTC) picolinate use such as renal failure,[56,57] liver failure,[56] hemolysis,[56] rhabdomyolysis[58] and allergic contact dermatitis[59] have been reported in case studies. A frequently cited case report by Cerulli et al.[56] described Cr toxicity in a woman who had taken 1200–2400 µg/day of [Cr(pic)$_3$] for 4–5 months. The patient had anemia (hematocrit of 15%) and blood Cr concentrations twice the normal range; she was diagnosed with hemolysis and acute liver and renal failure secondary to Cr toxicity. She was hospitalized for 26 days, requiring blood-product transfusions and hemodialysis. Her laboratory values were within normal limits when re-evaluated 1 year later, indicating a complete recovery. In another case study involving a 24-year-old woman body builder,[58] short-term ingestion (48 hours) of high doses (1200 µg) of [Cr(pic)$_3$] supplements was the suspected cause of rhabdomyolysis, a condition where muscle cells are damaged, causing symptoms of myalgia and elevated creatine kinase laboratory results. These case reports point out the potential for serious side effects associated with high doses of OTC [Cr(pic)$_3$] supplements.

IV. RECOMMENDATIONS

A. GENERAL POPULATION

The overwhelming majority of the well controlled research studies estimate that no additional Cr is needed for adults consuming a balanced diet and that caution should be used with taking OTC [Cr(pic)$_3$] supplements because of potential for serious side effects.

B. EXERCISE AND SPORT PERFORMANCE

Adults participating in strenuous exercise or competitive sports may be candidates for decreased Cr levels. Researchers have determined that Cr loss is associated with stress, including exercise in humans,[1] and have concluded that strenuous exercise (90% of VO_2max) may lead to increased urinary excretion of Cr.[27] Lefavi[60] has theorized that an increase in exercise intensity and duration may increase Cr excretion. Coupled with the fact that adults participating in exercise or sports may be on a restrictive diet, the risk of becoming Cr deficient does exist. Adults participating in strenuous exercise or competitive sport should be aware of the potential threat and consume a balanced diet high in meats, whole grains and vegetables.[13] However, at this time, it appears the need for additional supplemental Cr is not warranted. More research is needed to evaluate the Cr status of athletes as well as on the potential deleterious effects of [Cr(pic)$_3$].

V. SUMMARY

It appears as though [Cr(pic)$_3$] supplementation has no effect on body composition, physical performance and glucose or insulin concentrations in healthy individuals. There may be some benefit for those with Type 2 diabetes with impaired glucose homeostasis, but more research is needed in this area.

The money spent on [Cr(pic)$_3$] supplementation by just those in the United States suggests that there is an enormous market and demand for this supplement. However, individuals should be aware of the potential deleterious effects of this non-regulated nutritional supplement.

REFERENCES

1. Lukaski, H.C. Chromium as a supplement. *Ann. Rev. Nutr.*, 19, 279–302, 1999.
2. Mertz, W. Chromium occurrence and function in biological systems. *Physiol. Rev.*, 49, 163–239, 1969.
3. Haymes, E.M. and Clarkson, P.M. Minerals and trace minerals, in *Nutrition For Sports and Exercise*, 2nd ed., Berning, J.R. and Steen, S.N., Eds., Aspen Publishing, Gaithersburg, MD, 1998, Chapter 5.
4. Mackenzie, R.D., Anwar, R., Byerrum, R.U. and Hoppert, C. Absorption and distribution of 51Cr in the albino rat. *Arch. Biochem.*, 79, 200–205, 1959.
5. Hunt, S.M. and Groff, J.L. *Advance Nutrition and Human Metabolism.* West Publishing, St. Paul, MN, 1990, 273–316.
6. Vincent, J.B. The potential value and toxicity of chromium picolinate as a nutritional supplement, weight loss agent and muscle development agent. *Sports Med.*, 33(3), 213–230, 2003.
7. Stearns, D.M., Belbruno, J.J. and Wetterhahn, K.E. A prediction of chromium (III) accumulation in humans from chromium dietary supplements. *FASEB J.*, 9, 1650–1657, 1995.
8. McCarty, M.F. Chromium (III) picolinate (letter). *FASEB J.*, 10,365–367, 1996.
9. Okada, S., Tsukada, H. and Tezuka, M. Effect of chromium (III) on nucleolar RNA synthesis. *Biol. Trace Elem. Res.*, 21, 35–39, 1989.
10. Davis, C.M. and Vincent, J.B. Chromium oligopeptide activates insulin receptor tyrosine kinase activity. *Biochem.*, 36, 4382–4385, 1997.
11. Davis, C.M., Sumrall, K.H. and Vincent, J.B. A biologically active form of chromium may activate a membrane phosphotyrosine phosphatase. *Biochem.*, 35, 12963–12969, 1996.
12. Stearns, D.M. Is chromium a trace essential metal? *Biofactors*, 11, 149–62, 2000.
13. Clarkson, P.M. and Haymes, E.M. Trace mineral requirements for athletes. *Int. J. Sports Nutr.*, 4, 104–119, 1994.
14. Stoecker, B.J. Cr. In: Ziegler, E.E. and L.J. Filer, Jr., (Eds). *Present Knowledge in Nutrition.* 7th ed., Washington, D.C.: International Life Sciences Institute, 344–353, 1996.
15. Kozlovsky, A.S., Moser, P.B., Reiser, S. and Anderson, R.A. Effects of diets high in simple sugars on urinary chromium losses. *Metabolism*, 35, 515–518, 1986.
16. National Research Council. Recommended Dietary Allowances (10th ed.) National Academy Press, Washington, DC, 241–243, 1989.
17. Trumbo, P., Yates, A.A., Schlicker, S. and Poos, M. Dietary reference intakes: Vitamin A, vitamin K, arsenic, boron, chromium, copper, iodine, iron, manganese, molybdenum, nickel, silicon, vanadium and zinc. *J. Am. Diet. Assoc.*, 101, 294–301, 2001.
18. Anderson, R.A. and Kozlovsky, A.S. Chromium intake, absorption and excretion of subjects consuming self-selected diets. *Am. J. Clin. Nutr.*, 41, 1177–1183, 1985.
19. Offenbacher, E.G., Spencer, H., Dowling, H.J. and Pi-Sunyer, F.X. Metabolic chromium balances in men. *Am. J. Clin. Nutr.*, 44, 77–82, 1986.
20. Nielsen, F.H. Controversial chromium: Does the superstar mineral of the mountebanks receive appropriate attention from clinicians and nutritionists? *Nutr. Today*, 31, 226–233, 1996.
21. Hellerstein, M.K. Is chromium supplementation effective in managing type II diabetes? *Nutr. Rev.*, 56, 302–306, 1998.

22. Anderson, R.A., Polansky, M.M., Bryden, N.A. and Canary, J.J. Supplemental—chromium effects on glucose, insulin, glucagon and urinary chromium losses in subjects consuming controlled low-chromium diets. *Am. J. Clin. Nutr.*, 54, 909–916, 1991.

23. Anderson, R.A. Essentiality of chromium in humans. *The Sci. Total Environ.*, 86, 75–81, 1989.

24. Anderson, R.A., Polansky, M.M., Bryden, N.A., Roginski, E.E., Patterson, K.Y. and Reamer, D.C. Effects of exercise (running) on serum glucose, insulin, glucagon and chromium excretion. *Diabetes*, 31, 212–216, 1982.

25. Anderson, R.A. Dietary chromium intake: Freely chosen diets, institutional diets and individual foods. *Biol. Trace Elem. Res.*, 32,117–121, 1992.

26. Anderson, R.A., Bryden, N.A., Polansky, M.M. and Thorp, J.W. Effects of carbohydrate loading and underwater exercise on circulating cortisol, insulin and urinary losses of chromium and zinc. *Eur. J. Appl. Physiol.*, 63, 146–150, 1991.

27. Anderson, R.A., Bryden, N.A., Polansky, M.M. and Deuster, P.A. Exercise effects on chromium excretion of trained and untrained men consuming a constant diet. *J. Appl. Physiol.*, 64, 249–252, 1988.

28. Evans, G.W. The effect of chromium picolinate on insulin controlled parameters in humans. *Int. J. Bios. Med. Res.*, 11, 163–180, 1989.

29. Walker, L.S., Bemben, M.G., Bemben, D.A. and Knehans, A.W. Chromium picolinate effects on body composition and muscular performance in wrestlers. *Med. Sci. Sports Exerc.*, 30, 1730–1737, 1998.

30. Clarkson, P.M. Effects of exercise on chromium levels: Is supplementation required? *Sports Med.*, 23, 341–349, 1997.

31. Amato, P., Morales, A.J. and Yen, S.S.C. Effects of chromium picolinate supplementation on insulin sensitivity, serum lipids and body composition in healthy, nonobese older men and women. *J. Gerontol. A. Biol. Sci. Med. Sci.*, 55A, M260–M263, 2000.

32. Campbell, W.W., Joseph, L.J.O., Davey, S.L., Cyr-Campbell, D., Anderson, R.A. and Evans, W.J. Effects of resistance training and chromium picolinate on body composition and skeletal muscle in older men. *J. Appl. Physiol.*, 86, 29–39, 1999.

33. Clancy, S.P., Clarkson, P.M., DeCheke, M.E., Nosaka, K., Freedson, P.S., Cunningham, J.J. and Valentine, B. Effects of chromium picolinate supplementation on body composition, strength and urinary chromium loss in football players. *Int. J. Sports Nutr.*, 4, 142–153, 1994.

34. Grant, K.E., Chandler, R.M., Castle, A.L. and Ivy, J.L. Chromium and exercise training: Effect on obese women. *Med. Sci. Sports Exerc.*, 29, 992–998, 1997.

35. Kaats, G.R., Blum, K., Pullin, D., Keith, S.C. and Wood, R. A randomized, double-masked, placebo-controlled study of the effects of chromium picolinate supplementation on body composition: A replication and extension of a previous study. *Curr. Therapeutic Res.*, 59, 379–388, 1998.

36. Lukaski, H.C., Bolonchuk, W.W., Siders, W.A. and Milne, D.B. Chromium supplementation and resistance training: effects of body composition, strength and trace element status of men. *Am. J. Clin. Nutr.*, 63, 954–961, 1996.

37. Volpe, S.L., Huang, H.W., Larpadisorn, K. and Lesser, I.I. Effect of chromium supplementation and exercise on body composition, resting metabolic rate and selected biochemical parameters in moderately obese women following an exercise program. *J. Am. Coll. Nutr.*, 20, 293–306, 2001.

38. Hallmark, M.A, Reynolds, T.H., DeSouza, C.A., Dotson, C.O., Anderson, R.A. and Rogers, M.A. Effects of chromium and resistive training on muscle strength and body composition. *Med. Sci. Sports Exerc.*, 28, 139–144, 1996.

39. Livolsi, J.M., Adams, G.M. and Laguna, P.L. The effect of chromium picolinate on muscular strength and body composition in women athletes. *J. Strength Cond. Res.*, 15, 161–166, 2001.

40. Campbell, W.W., Joseph, L.J.O., Anderson, R.A., Davey, S.L., Hinton, J. and Evans, W.J. Effects of resistance training and chromium picolinate on body composition and skeletal muscle size in older women. *Int. J. Sports Nutr. Exerc. Metabol.*, 12, 125–135, 2002.

41. Davis, J.M., Welsh, R.S. and Alderson, N.A. Effects of carbohydrate and chromium ingestion during intermittent high-intensity exercise to fatigue. *Int. J. Sport Nutr. Exerc. Metab.* 10, 476–85, 2000.

42. Schwartz, K. and Mertz, W. Chromium (III) and the glucose tolerance factor. *Arch. Biochem. Biophys.*, 85, 292–295, 1959.

43. Glinsmann, W.H. and Mertz, W. Effect of trivalent chromium on glucose tolerance. *Metabolism*, 15, 510–519, 1966.

44. Potter, J.F., Levin, P., Anderson, R.A., Freiberg, J.M., Andres, R. and Elahi, D. Glucose metabolism in glucose-tolerant older people during chromium supplementation. *Metab. Clin. Exp.*, 34, 199–204, 1985.

45. Levine, R.A., Streeten, D.H.P. and Doisy, R.J. Effects of oral chromium supplementation on the glucose tolerance of elderly human subjects. *Metab. Clin. Exp.*, 17, 114–125, 1968.

46. Uusitupa, M.I.J., Kumpulainen, J.T., Voutilainen, E., Hersio, K., Sarlund, H., Pyorala, K.P. and Kovistoinen, P.E. Effect of inorganic chromium supplementation on glucose tolerance, insulin response and serum lipids in noninsulin-dependent diabetics. *Am. J. Clin. Nutr.*, 38, 404–410, 1983.

47. Abraham, A.S., Brooks, B.A. and Eylath, U. The effects of chromium supplementation on serum glucose and lipids in patients with and without non-insulin dependent diabetes. *Metabolism*, 41,768–771, 1992.

48. Anderson, R.A., Cheng, N., Bryden, N.A., Polanskey, M., Cheng, N., Chi, J. and Feng, J. Elevated intakes of supplemental chromium improves glucose and insulin variables in individuals with type 2 diabetes. *Diabetes*, 46, 1786–1791, 1997.

49. Althius, M.D., Jordan, N..E, Ludington, E.A. and Wittes, J.T. Glucose and insulin responses to dietary chromium supplements: A meta-analysis. *Am. J. Clin. Nutr.*, 76,148–155, 2002.

50. Press, R.I., Gelle, J. and Evans, G.W. The effect of chromium picolinate on serum cholesterol and apolipoprotein fractions in human subjects. *West. J. Med.*, 152, 41–45, 1990.

51. Riales, R. and Albrink, M.J. Effect of chromium chloride supplementation on glucose tolerance and serum lipids including HDL of adult men. *Am. J. Nutr.*, 34, 2670–2678, 1981.

52. Boyd, S.G., Boone, B.E., Smith, A.R. and Conners, J. Combined dietary chromium picolinate and an exercise program leads to a reduction of serum cholesterol and insulin in college-aged subjects. *J. Nutr. Biochem.*, 9, 471–475, 1998.

53. Katz, S.A. and Salem, H. The toxicology of chromium with respect to its chemical speciation: A review. *J. Appl. Toxicol.*, 13, 217–224, 1993.

54. Jeejeebhoy, K.N. The role of chromium in nutrition and therapeutics and as a potential toxin. Nutr. *Rev.*, 57, 329–335, 1999.

55. Anderson, R.A., Bryden, N.A. and Polansky, M.M. Lack of toxicity of chromium chloride and Cr picolinate in rats. *J. Am. Coll. Nutr.*, 16, 273–279, 1997.

56. Cerulli, J., Grabe, D.W., Gauthier, I., Malone, M. and McGoldrick, M.D. Chromium picolinate toxicity. *Ann. Pharmacother.*, 32, 428–31, 1997.

57. Wasser, W.G. and D'Agati, V.D. Chronic renal failure after ingestion of over-the-counter chromium picolinate [letter]. *Ann. Intern. Med.*, 126, 410, 1997.

58. Martin, W.R. and Fuller, R.E. Suspected chromium picolinate-induced rhabdomyolysis. *Pharmaco-therapy*, 18, 860–862, 1998.

59. Fowler, J.F. Systemic contact dermatitis caused by oral chromium picolinate. *Cutis*, 65, 116, 2000.

60. Lefavi, R.G. Chromium picolinate is an efficacious and safe supplement: response [letter]. *Int. J. Sport Nutr.*, 3, 120–122, 1993.

19 Selenium

L. Mallory Boylan and Julian E. Spallholz

CONTENTS

I. INTRODUCTION

The trace element selenium (Se) is an essential nutrient, but is toxic when consumed in excessive quantities. Selenosis or selenium toxicity signs in animals were described by Marco Polo in 1295 during his travels to China. It was 1934 before Franke[1] identified Se as a toxic agent found in some plant foods. About 20 years later, Schwarz and Foltz[2] demonstrated that, for the rat, Se was an essential dietary element that prevented liver necrosis. Subsequently, Se deficiency syndromes have been identified in animals and humans. Cardiomyopathy, muscle pain and osteoarthropathy are key features of Se deficiency in humans.[3]

In 1973, Rotruck and co-workers[4] discovered that Se, in a selenocysteine residue, was a constituent of the enzyme glutathione peroxidase (GSHPx), an enzyme that converts hydrogen peroxide to water. Most of the research in the area of Se and exercise has centered around the role of Se in this antioxidant enzyme. Strenuous exercise dramatically increases oxygen uptake and production of reactive oxygen species (ROS) including superoxide ($O_2^{\cdot-}$)hydroxyl radical ($\cdot OH$) and hydrogen peroxide (H_2O_2) that may be responsible for biochemical and physiologic changes indicative of oxidative stress induced by exercise.[5,6] Peroxidative injury to tissues is also found in severe Se deficiency due to the depletion of GSHPx activity. It would also seem obvious that in the rare cases of severe Se deficiency that result in arthritis, cardiomyopathy or Se toxicity with nerve damage, athletic ability would be impaired. Research in the area of Se status or supplementation and exercise performance is sparse and results of studies are often contradictory.

II. CHEMICAL STRUCTURES OF SOME SELENIUM-CONTAINING COMPOUNDS

Some common forms of Se in foods and supplements include sodium selenite (Na^2–SeO^4), sodium selenate (Na^2–SeO^3), L-selenomethionine (CH^3–Se–CH^2–CH(NH^2)–COOH) and L-Se- methylselenocysteine (CH^3–Se–CH^2–CH^2–CH(NH^2)–COOH).[7] Other selenocompounds identified in plants include selenocystine, selenohomocysteine, γ-glutamyl-selenocystathionine, selenomethionine selenoxide, selenocyseineselenic acid, Se-proponylselenocysteine, selenoxide, Se-methylselenomethionine selenocystathionine, dimethyl diselenide, selenosinigrin, selenopeptide, selenowax and elemental selenium.[7]

Inorganic forms of Se are generally more toxic than organic forms.[8] Organic forms include selenomethionine, the major form in food and most selenium yeast supplements, and Se-methylselenocysteine, the major Se form in broccoli and garlic grown under high soil selenium conditions.[9]

III. GENERAL PROPERTIES OF SELENIUM

Selenium is a metalloid that can occur in multiple oxidation states, 0, +6, +4 and −2.[3,7] In many ways, it behaves like its sister element sulfur, although it is found in soils and foods to a much lesser extent. Unlike plants, which do not knowingly require Se, Se is required by all other life forms from bacteria all the way through the phylogenic tree to humans. Here, Se replaces the sulfur in amino acids in plants forming the major selenoamino acids, selenomethionine, selenocysteine and Se-methylselenocysteine. Higher animals and humans make only selenocysteine and encode it into proteins from an m-RNA UGA codon. From the human genome sequence, 25 selenoproteins are recognized, with about half of these proteins having been isolated and studied. Most selenoproteins studied are enzymes involved in the various redox pathways for the elimination of the oxidation products of lipids and H_2O_2. The facile catalytic ability of selenium, rather than sulfur, accounts for selenocysteine's inclusion into enzymes such as glutathione peroxidase, phospholipidhydroperoxide glutathione peroxidase, thioredoxin reductase and the deiiodinases. This catalytic property of selenium extends also to the simpler organic forms of selenium and, when in the selenide state, −2, they themselves are catalytic, accounting for toxicity when overingested.

IV. METABOLIC FUNCTIONS OF SELENIUM

Since the discovery of cytosolic GSHPx, other selenoproteins including additional antioxidant enzymes have been identified in mammals. A distinct, glycosylated GSHPx has been found in the plasma and a membrane-associated enzyme, phospholipid hydroperoxide GSHPx (PLGSHPx) has been reported to be widely distributed in tissues.[10,11] While an exact function is not totally clear, selenoprotein-P is found in plasma and tissues and appears to have some antioxidant or selenium transport properties.[10,12] An additional enzyme that contains Se is Type I iodothyronine 5–deiodinase, which is the enzyme that catalyzes the removal of iodine from thyroxine (T_4), converting it to 3,3,5–triiodothyronine (T_3).[10]

The primary task of the Se-containing antioxidant enzymes is to protect cellular components from peroxidation by controlling the H_2O_2 and organic peroxide levels in aerobic cells.[10] According to Ursini and Bindoli,[13] both glutathione peroxidase enzymes will reduce peroxidic substrates such as H_2O_2, linoleic acid hydroperoxide, tert-butyl hydroperoxide and cumene hydroperoxide. Cholesteryl hydroperoxides, some prostaglandin peroxides and peroxidized DNA are also substrates for GSHPx. Additional substrates for PLGSHPx include peroxidized phosphatidyl choline, phosphatidyl ethanolamine and phosphatidyl serine; cardiolipin, phosphatidic acid and peroxidized membranes. An adequate intercellular concentration of reduced glutathione (GSH) is needed as a cofactor for both[14] enzymes. The riboflavin-containing enzyme, glutathione reductase (GR) with flavin adenine dinucleotide (FAD) as its coenzyme and reduced nicotinamide adenine dinucleotide phosphate (NADPH) are the reducing agents that converts oxidized glutathione (GSSG) back to GSH.

A. TISSUE DISTRIBUTION OF GLUTATHIONE PEROXIDASES AND EFFECT OF SELENIUM ON TISSUE ENZYME ACTIVITY LEVELS

Se and GSHPx activity are both widely distributed in animal tissues. Behne and Wolters[15] analyzed the Se content and GSHPx activity in tissues of female rats. The largest percentage of Se was found in muscle (39.8%) and liver (31.7%), with other tissues each containing less than 10% of the remaining Se. The GSHPx activity was greatest in the liver (65.6%), followed by erythrocytes (21.2%) and muscle (6.1%), with other tissues containing 2.1% or less of the remaining GSHPx activity.

Se deficiency results in a decrease in both GSHPx and PLGSHPx activity in tissue[16] as well as an increase in tissue peroxide and signs of peroxidative injury to tissues.[17,18] Results of a study by Weitzel et al.[16] indicated that the two GSHPxs have individual depletion kinetics, as GSHPx activity in liver samples from mice fed a Se-deficient diet decreased by 90% of the control mice, whereas PLGSHPx was depleted by only 45% of control activity. In Se-deficient animals or humans, Se supplementation will induce production of GSHPx. In general, there is a correlation between the dietary Se intake and tissue GSHPx activity in both rats and humans.[19] Over a 20-week period, in rats fed a torula yeast basal diet with no added Se or a diet with 5.0 mg Se/kg, erythrocyte GSHPx steadily increased as Se intake increased. However, when mice were fed a diet containing 1.0 mg Se per kg of diet, liver GSHPx activity levels were lower than for mice fed an adequate 0.2 mg/kg Se diet, although still much higher than the value for mice fed a Se-deficient diet.[20]

In humans who have a hereditary lack of GSHPx in erythrocytes, the ability of the erythrocytes to withstand stress induced by oxidizing agents is impaired and results in a hemolytic crisis.[21] Glutathione peroxidase and PLGSHPx are major enzyme systems responsible for detoxification of H_2O_2 and lipid hydroperoxides. Lack of sufficient quantities of these enzymes from a Se deficiency, as well as from genetic defects or the inability to incorporate dietary Se into GSHPx, leads to signs and symptoms associated with peroxidative tissue damage.

B. SELENIUM DEFICIENCY-RELATED SYNDROMES

Evidence that the endemic cardiomyopathy in China called Keshan disease was linked to poor Se status, and was prevented by selenium supplementation, provided support for the nutritional essentiality of Se in humans.[22] Se was recognized as an essential nutrient and was assigned a Recommended Dietary Allowance (RDA) in 1989.[23] The RDA for Se was set at 55 μg/day for women and 70 μg /day for men. The current RDI (2000) is 55 μg/day for adult men and women.[24] Dietary Se intake in areas of China affected by Keshan disease averages about 7 to 11μg/day of Se, with estimated minimum daily requirements of Se for adult men and women of 19 and 13 μg, respectively.[22]

Se deficiency has been identified as a factor in two human diseases in China — Keshan disease and Kaschin-Beck disease.[22] Keshan disease is a cardiomyopathy that is characterized by multifocal necrosis in the myocardium.[22] Signs and symptoms of Keshan disease include nausea, vomiting, chest discomfort, chills, dyspnea and palpitations on exertion, cardiogenic shock followed by congestive heart failure and arrhythmias. Individuals with Keshan disease have been reported to have significantly lower levels of blood Se and GSHPx activity than normal subjects living in the same area in China.[25] While Se deficiency appears to be a major factor, the etiology of Keshan disease has not been totally elucidated and other factors may be contributing to the disease.[26] Se may have a protective and stabilizing effect on membranes[27,28] due to PLGSHPx, which may lessen membrane susceptibility to environmental pathogenic agents.

Other factors associated with Keshan disease are a Coxsackie virus,[29,30] pathogenic factors from endemic grains,[31] vitamin E deficiency[32] and methionine deficiency.[22] When inoculated with a Coxsackie virus CB-21 isolated from the blood of a Keshan disease patient, mice that had been fed a Se-deficient diet developed significantly more myocardial lesions than mice of normal Se status.[29] Beck et al.[30] reported that Se-deficient mice developed more severe myocardial lesions after infection with Coxsackie B3 virus than did mice with normal Se status, and when the virus was replicated in Se-deficient mice it underwent changes associated with an increased virulence.

In regard to cardiovascular disease other than Keshan disease, there is some epidemiologic evidence associating low blood or dietary Se with increased risk of cardiovascular disease.[33] Pucheu and co-workers[34] reported that plasma Se values of patients with coronary artery disease or myocardial infarction were 80% of the values found in healthy control subjects. Other studies have found no relationship between Se and cardiovascular disease.[35,36] Possible mechanisms by which low selenium status with below normal GSHPx levels could be related to cardiovascular disease include alterations in arachidonic acid metabolites and blood-clotting mechanisms.[37,38]

Kaschin-Beck's disease is an endemic osteoarthropathy characterized by chondronecrosis, which is prevalent in the areas of China and Russia classified as Se-deficient zones.[22,39,40] Signs and symptoms include endochondral ossification, hyaline cartilage necrosis, joint pain and deformity, limited flexion of fingers and elbows and muscular atrophy. [19] Pain in the weight-bearing joints is described as stabbing and is intensified by exposure to cold or exercise. Adjuvant arthritis is more pronounced in Se-deficient rats and their macrophages have lower GSHPx activity and produce higher levels of H_2O_2 when compared with control rats.[41] These factors may lead to peroxidative cell injury and the worsening of arthritis. Se deficiency has also been noted in conjunction with protein energy malnutrition, acquired immunodeficiency syndrome, short bowel syndrome, long-term total parenteral nutrition without Se, alcoholism and the use of formulas for inborn errors of metabolism that had no added Se.[26,42–46] In these conditions, problems related to Se deficiency may include muscle pain, nail changes, cardiomyopathy, fatty liver, poor growth and immunosuppression.

It would appear that severe Se deficiency would have detrimental effects on exercise performance as the cardiovascular system and joints are damaged. Cardiac abnormalities and arthritis are generally not conducive to optimal athletic performance.

V. BODY RESERVES OF SELENIUM

There is a limited body pool of Se in tissue GSHPx and selenomethionine. Using plasma GSHPx as an index of Se status, Yang et al.[22] evaluated the effect of graded doses of Se in the form of selenomethionine on Chinese men with an initial low Se status. After 5 months, plasma GSHPx levels were found to reach a stationary level in groups given 30 μg or more of the Se supplement per day in addition to the approximate 10 μg /day from their diets. As Se needs are related to body weight and Americans tend to be taller and heavier than people from China, and using a safety factor of 1.3 (1.3 × the Chinese dietary intake), the requirement for Se is about 0.87 μg /kg body weight.[23]

In children from a Se-deficient area of China, the plasma Se concentration (mean +/– SD) was 0.16+/–0.03 μmol/L.[47] Supplementation for 8 weeks with selenite and Se-yeast increased plasma Se to plateau values of 1.0+/–0.2 and 1.3+/–0.2 μmol/L, respectively. Se-yeast increased the red blood cell Se level sixfold and selenite threefold as compared with placebo. In regard to the relative bioavailability of Se-yeast and selenite as reflected by plasma, red blood cells and GSHPx activity, GSHPx activity reached maximal levels in plasma and platelets of 300% and 200%, respectively, compared with the placebo group. Red blood cell selenium levels continued to rise for 16 weeks. The authors concluded that either form of Se was effective in raising GSHPx activity, but Se-yeast supplementation resulted in a increased body pool of Se. Waschulewski and Sunde[48] reported that, in the rat, there was an inability of stored selenomethionine to provide Se for GSHPx synthesis over a prolonged period of time and they suggested that selenomethionine may not be an optimal form of Se for supplements.

VI. DIETARY AND SUPPLEMENTAL SOURCES OF SELENIUM

Selenium in food varies with the Se content of the soil in which it was grown.[7] The Se content of grains grown in high-Se soils may contain up to 30 µg Se per gram while those grown in low-Se soils may be less than 0.1 µg per gram. Foods that are generally good sources of selenium include Brazil nuts, tuna, beef, turkey and cereal grains. The major form of Se in plant and animal foods grown under normal conditions is selenomethionine, but there are also small amounts of many other Se compounds. Plants like garlic and broccoli grown under high-Se conditions contain larger amounts of Se-methylselenocysteine.[9]

Selenium in nutritional supplements includes organic forms such as selenomethionine and Se-methylselenocysteine and inorganic forms such as sodium selenite and sodium selenate. Another Se supplement is high-Se broccoli, which contains primarily Se-methylselenocysteine. Selenium-yeast is also used frequently as a Se supplement and the selenocompounds in this product have been reported to vary widely with a selenomethionine content ranging from 16.0–62.6%. There have been efforts to have a standard of 85% of the Se as selenomethionine by some companies.[7] All of the supplements are useful in correcting selenium GSHPx deficiency, but selenomethionine is incorporated in a nonspecific manner into tissue proteins in place of methionine, as methionine-tRNA does not distinguish between the two amino acids.[7] Thus, less Se may be available for cancer chemoprevention or other functions when the Se in supplements is provided predominantly as selenomethionine.

Of these supplement forms, sodium selenite is most toxic.[8] If selenite is in a product containing ascorbic acid, it can be converted to an elemental selenium form with poor bioavailability.[3] Many fortified waters and sports beverages unfortunately contain both ascorbic acid and selenite.

VII. SELENIUM STATUS ASSESSMENTS

Selenium status can be assessed using a variety of methods including measurement of Se in blood, plasma, serum, urine, red blood cells, platelets, hair and nails.[49] Status may also be assessed using a functional test such as blood, plasma, or red blood cell glutathione peroxidases or selenoprotein-P. There are currently no uniformly accepted normal ranges for any selenium status indicators. Each assessment tool has advantages and disadvantages. Plasma or serum Se reflects short-term status while red blood cells, platelets, hair and nails are better indicators of longer-term status. Hair samples may be contaminated by Se-containing shampoos or henna products that contain Se, which would render hair Se levels inaccurate and not reflective of status. According to Thomson,[49] plasma or serum values are considered to be the favored tool for comparing Se status among countries. Selenium-containing proteins or enzymes will rise during supplementation in those with deficiency, but will reach a maximal level. This makes these tests poor indicators of exposure to higher levels of selenium.

VIII. SELENIUM TOXICITY

The Food and Nutrition Board (FNB) has set the tolerable upper level (TUL) for selenium at 400 µg/day for adults.[24] Se toxicity or selenosis occurs in areas of China where dietary intake of Se is about 5 mg/day.[22] A few cases of Se toxicity have also been reported due to consumption of Se supplements such as sodium selenite, with most of the cases occurring in individuals who were taking a supplement which, by the manufacturers error, contained about 23 mg of Se in each tablet.[50] However, some symptoms of Se toxicity were noted in subjects who consumed only 1 mg/day of Se from sodium selenite for 2 years.[22] Se toxicity causes dry, brittle, easily broken hair that is depigmented and lackluster; thick, brittle deformed finger and toenails; skin that is red, swollen, blistered and itchy; nausea, vomiting and abdominal pain; fatigue; a breath garlic odor and neurological abnormalities including peripheral paresthesia, paralysis, hemiplegia, motor disturbances, extremity pain and convulsions.[22,50]

The molecular mechanism that causes Se toxicity appears to be related to reactions between Se and GSH in which oxygen radicals are produced. Se compounds that form selenide (RSe-) anions can oxidize GSH and other cellular thiols, and produce superoxide that in turn initiates a cascade of ROS production.[51–54]

IX. INTERACTION OF SELENIUM WITH OTHER NUTRIENTS

Vitamin E and Se function as synergistic antioxidants, and many of the signs and symptoms of a double deficiency of these two nutrients can be prevented or will be improved by supplementation with either nutrient.[22] Beck et al.[32] reported that vitamin E deficiency increased the cardiac pathology associated with Coxsackie B3 infection in mice, especially in mice fed diets high in menhaden oil as opposed to lard, for dietary fat. Work by Beck et al.[30,32] on the effects of both Se and vitamin E deficiency on myocardial injury from the Coxsackie B3 virus supports the possibility that both nutrients influence the development of Keshan disease.

Selenium also works synergistically with ascorbic acid as an antioxidant. Selenium-dependent thioredoxin reductase helps protect the cell from oxidants and catalyzes the regeneration of ascorbic acid from dehydroascorbic acid. [56] However, in regard to selenium absorption, Robinson et al. reported that when sodium selenite was taken orally, a light meal had little effect on Se absorption; 200 mL of orange juice slightly improved absorption, but the availability of selenite was reduced almost to zero when it was taken with 1 g ascorbic acid.

The effects of iodine deficiency may be exacerbated by selenium deficiency due to selenium's role in iodothyronin deiodinases which convert thyroxine to the active triiodothyronine. Systemic utilization of iodine is impaired in subjects who are deficient in selenium. [57]

Riboflavin as flavin adenine dinucleotide (FAD) is necessary to ensure adequate levels of reduced glutathione for the GSHPx cycle and riboflavin deficient rats have compromised antioxidant defenses.[58] In pigs, a riboflavin supplement caused kidney, muscle, heart and brain GSHPx activity to increase when the pigs were given sodium selenite but not when they were given selenomethionine.[59]

Both selenium and folate may influence one carbon metabolism and cancer risk.[60] In rats fed diets supplemented with selenium (2 mg selenite/kg diet) and deficient in folate, precancerous lesions, plasma homocysteine and liver S-adenosylhomocysteine were higher and plasma folate, liver S-adenosylmethionine and the activity of liver methionine synthase were lower than in control rats or rats with either deficient diet alone. Selenium deficiency was found to decrease some of the effects of folate deficiency and it was speculated that there was a shunting of the accumulation of homocysteine due to folate deficiency to cysteine and glutathione.

X. EFFECTS OF SELENIUM ON ATHLETIC PERFORMANCE

Most research in the area of Se and exercise has focused on the role of Se in the antioxidant enzyme GSHPx which, using GSH, converts H_2O_2 to water. Whole-body and especially muscle oxygen uptake increases sharply during intense physical exercise leading to increased oxidative stress.[61] This oxidative stress may be related to production of ROS such as superoxide in the mitochondria during exercise. Superoxide, when acted on by superoxide dismutase (SOD), produces H_2O_2, which can then be converted to water by GSHPx or catalase. In tissues that experience ischemia during exercise, reperfusion and reoxygenation contribute to a burst of ROS production. When biomembrane polyunsaturated fatty acids are acted on by ROS under aerobic conditions, a peroxidative chain reaction occurs leading to increased excretion of ethane and pentane in expired air and increased levels of malondialdehyde (MDA), conjugated dienes and thiobarbituric acid reactive substances (TBARS) in tissues.[5,62,63]

Only limited animal and very limited human research has been conducted regarding Se and exercise. Types, duration and intensity of exercise and dietary Se levels fed to animals are varied, which may account in part for the lack of continuity in results of acute exercise and training effects on activity levels of GSHPx and indicators of oxidative damage to tissues. One consistent finding is that animals fed a Se-deficient diet have lower tissue levels of GSHPx when compared with values from animals fed adequate selenium.[64–68] Lower Se status is also associated with decreased levels of GSHPx activity in human subjects.

The only human study in which subjects were in less than optimal Se status was conducted by Edwards et al.[69] Subjects also had intermittent claudication in addition to altered Se status. Edwards and co-workers[69] evaluated the effects of treadmill exercise on patients with intermittent claudication due to peripheral vascular disease, and normal controls. Subjects with intermittent claudication were found to have significantly lower plasma Se and GSHPx activity levels than in the 19 control subjects. A group of 11 patients with intermittent claudication and seven controls participated in a treadmill exercise test. Neutrophils were noted to be significantly higher in patients with claudication and these were further elevated by the exercise. Plasma thromboxane, an indicator of platelet activation, and Von Willebrand's factor, a marker of endothelial injury, were also higher in patients with claudication than in controls and both were increased 15 min after exercise in claudicants and controls ($p < 0.05$). Edwards and co-workers[69] speculated that reduced GSHPx activity levels in patients with claudication may contribute to unopposed action of oxygen radicals, resulting in increased damage to the endothelium. No attempt was made to evaluate the effects of a Se supplement in these patients and other antioxidant enzymes were not evaluated in the study. It does appear that in intermittent-claudication patients, lower plasma GSHPx values may be one factor contributing to lack of protection from the oxidative stress of exercise.

In rats that are subjected to acute exercise and fed Se-deficient diets, Brady et al.[68] found no significant effect of exercise on liver, blood or muscle GSHPx activity levels. Lang and co-workers[67] reported decreased GSHPx, increased GSH, decreased vitamin E and increased ubiquinone levels in tissues of Se-deficient rats. Exercise did not cause a significant rise in liver GSHPx in either control or Se-deficient animals. Plasma total GSH and oxidized glutathione were both significantly higher in animals after exercise to exhaustion, with levels in rats fed Se-deficient diets about twice the values found in control rats. While not a significant difference, the Se-deficient rats had a 16% higher mean running time to exhaustion than control rats. Adequate dietary vitamin E levels, residual GSHPx and activation of other antioxidant pathways were suggested as mechanisms that preserved the exercise capacity in the rats fed Se-deficient diets. Ji et al.[65] did find increased levels of catalase and cytosolic SOD in livers of Se-deficient rats after acute exercise and significant increases in manganese SOD in liver and Se-independent GSHPx in muscle after training. Manganese SOD activity was 24% higher in heart mitochondria from Se-deficient rats as compared with controls.[65] Exercised rats fed a Se-deficient diet were reported by Soares et al.[70] to have lower levels of delta-aminolevulenic acid in liver, kidney and muscle than control mice. These thiol enzymes were noted to decrease during exposure to oxidizing agents.

In trained athletes participating in a half marathon, Duthie et al.[71] found no significant differences in erythrocyte GSHPx activity pre-race and up to 120 hr post-race. They also noted no significant change in erythrocyte catalase or SOD, but total GSH and GSH values were significantly lower than pre-race values at 5 min post-race. While plasma creatinine kinase, an index of damage to muscles, was elevated in plasma post-race, conjugated dienes and TBARS, indexes of oxidative damage, were not elevated by the exercise. Erythrocytes were more susceptible to hydrogen peroxide-induced peroxidation after the half marathon, however. Using a cross-over design, Dragan and co-workers[72] evaluated the effect of a 150 μg Se supplement or placebo given before a 2-hour endurance training session on 33 swimmers. No significant differences were noted in alondialdehyde in serum. Also, in another cross-over design experiment, they administered 100 μg Se or placebo for 14 days to swimmers, and in this trial, Se treatment did result in a significantly lower serum level of malondialdehyde.

Acute exercise also results in an increase in exhaled pentane, which is a derivative of omega-6 fatty acid hydroperoxides in expired air.[62] Pentane in expired air is also increased by Se deficiency.[73] Pentane excretion can be reduced in Se-deficient rats by providing them with adequate amounts of vitamin E. Muscle mitochondrial MDA levels are also elevated in untrained rats subjected to acute exercise and in rats with a dietary Se deficiency. [66] So both Se deficiency and acute exercise increase levels of substances that may be considered indicative of oxidative damage to tissues. In a double-blind, placebo-controlled study, Tessier et al.[74] evaluated the effect of Se supplementation (240 µg of an organic Se capsule containing 70% selenomethionine) or placebo on response to acute exercise and training in 24 healthy non-smoking males. The Se-supplemented group had a significant elevation in plasma Se levels, with the supplemented group's mean values 182% of the mean value of the control group. Neither Se supplementation nor training resulted in an elevation of vastus lateralis muscle GSHPx activity levels. Margaritis et al. [75] reported that muscle GSHPx at rest was not altered by an endurance training program or a Se supplement (180 µg selenomethionine) in 24 male subjects. The intensity level of the training was higher in the animal studies, which, in addition to species differences, may account for the contradictory results regarding GSHPx inducement by training in humans vs. animals. In rats, training has been reported to result in an increase in GSHPx in muscle tissue.[76–78] Before training and following a run to exhaustion, muscle GSHPx activity levels were lower than resting levels.[62] After training, the placebo group muscle GSHPx activity declined, but not to as great a degree as in the pre-training exercise test. In the Se-supplemented group, post-training muscle GSHPx activity was increased 64 to 79% after the max aerobic capacity test. In light of the finding by Storz et al.[79] that oxygen radicals induced transcription of messenger RNA that codes for antioxidant enzymes including peroxidases in prokaryotic cells, Tessier et al.[74] speculated that production of oxygen radicals during exercise may be a stimulus to induce higher GSHPx activity in muscle tissues after Se supplementation. In the same group of subjects, Tessier et al.[80] found no effect of the selenium supplement on GSHPx activity levels in resting muscle, but an increase in the muscle GSHPx in the Se supplement group after a bout of acute exercise.

XI. RECOMMENDATION FOR SELENIUM SUPPLEMENTATION

More research is needed before any recommendations for athletes can be made for any deviation from the RDA intake levels for Se. As Se is a toxic mineral when taken in excess, any Se supplement should be used with great caution. If supplements are taken, it would seem best to take one of the less toxic organic forms of Se and definitely do not exceed the TUL.

XII. FUTURE RESEARCH

Many areas regarding selenium and athletic performance are yet to be explored. Most studies in this area have had only a small number of subjects and were short-term studies. There has been virtually no research comparing the various forms of Se in any kind of athletic or exercise scenarios. Most of the current research has not explored effects of varying dosages of Se. There are no long-term studies of the effects of exercise on Se balance.

In some areas, such as the possible effect of training on elevation of muscle GSHPx, a conflict exists between results of animal and human studies. The studies have been of short duration; so while they were sufficiently long to cause a major decline in tissue activity levels of GSHPx, the activity of PLGSHPx, which depletes much more slowly than GSHPx, could have remained very well preserved. No studies reviewed evaluated the effects of any aspect of exercise on tissue activity of PLGSHPx.

XIII. CONCLUSIONS

Data in the area of Se status as a factor in athletic performance are scarce. It does appear that in Se deficiency, compensatory use of many of the body's other antioxidant defense mechanisms come into play to protect the body from ROS stress induced by exercise. However, more research is needed before routine use of Se supplements by athletes can be recommended.

REFERENCES

1. Franke, G., A new toxicant occurring naturally in certain samples of plant foodstuffs, *J. Nutr.*, 8, 597, 1934.
2. Schwarz, K. and Foltz, C., Selenium as an integral part of factor 3 against dietary necrotic liver degeneration, *J. Am. Chem. Soc.*, 79, 3292, 1957.
3. Combs, G. and Combs, S., *The Role of Selenium in Nutrition,* Academic Press, London, 1986.
4. Rotruck, J.T., Pope, A.L., Ganther, H.E., Swanson, A.B., Hafeman, D.G. and Hoekstra, W.G., Selenium: Biochemical role as a component of glutathione peroxidase, *Science*, 179, 588, 1973.
5. Ji, L., Oxidative stress and antioxidant response during exercise, oxidative processes and antioxidants, 13th Ross Laboratories Conference Report, 13,23, Ross Product Division, Abbott Laboratories, Columbus, OH, 1994.
6. Jenkins, R., Free radical chemistry: Relationship to exercise, *Sports Med.*, 5, 156,1988.
7. Whanger, P.D., Selenocompounds in plants and animals and their biological significance, *J. Am. Col. Nutr.*, 21, 223, 2002.
8. Weiller, M., Latta, M., Kresse, M., Lucas, R., Wendel, A. Toxicity of nutritionally available selenium compounds in primary and transformed hepatocytes, *Toxicology,* 201, 21,2004.
9. Finley J.W., Grusak, M.A., Keck, A.S., Gregoire, B.R.. Bioavailability of selenium from meat and broccoli as determined by retention and distribution of ^{75}Se. *Biol. Trace Elem. Res.* 99, 191, 2004.
10. Zachara, B., Mammalian selenoproteins, *J. Trace Elem. Electrol. Health Dis.,* 6, 137,1992.
11. Ursini, F., Malorino, M., Valente, M. and Gregolin, C., Purification from pig liver of a protein which protects liposomes and biomembranes from peroxidative degradation and exhibits glutathione peroxidase activity on phosphatidylcholine hydroperoxides, *Biochem. Biophys. Acta,* 197, 710, 1982.
12. Burk, R., Molecular biology of selenium with implications for its metabolism, *FASEB, J.*, 5, 22, 1991.
13. Ursini, F. and Bindoli, A., Catalysis by selenoglutathione peroxidase, in *Biological Macromolecules and Assemblies,* Jurnaic, F.A. and McPherson, A., Eds., John Wiley & Sons, New York, 1987.
14. Wendel, A., Pilz, W., Ladenstein, R., Sawatzki, G. and Weser, U., Substrate-induced redox change of selenium in glutathione peroxidase studied by X-ray photoelectron spectroscopy, *Biochem. Biophys. Acta,* 377, 211, 1975.
15. Behne, D. and Wolters, W., Distribution of selenium and glutathione peroxidase in the rat, *J. Nutr.,* 113, 456, 1983.
16. Weitzel, F., Ursini, F. and Wendel, A., Different dietary selenium requirement for the two selenoenzymes, glutathione peroxidase and phospholipid hydroperoxide glutathione peroxidase, in the mouse, Abstr., 4th mt. S*ymp. Selenium in Biology and Medicine, Tubingen, West Germany,* Walter de Gruyer, New York, 1989.
17. Baker, S.S. and Cohen, H.J., Increased sensitivity to H_2O_2 in glutathione peroxidase deficient rat granulocytes, *J. Nutr.,* 114, 2003, 1984.
18. Lane, H.W., Shirley, R.L. and Cerda, J.J., Glutathione peroxidase activity in intestinal and liver tissues of rats fed various levels of selenium, sulfur and cs-tocopherol, *J. Nutr.,* 109, 4– 44, 1979.
19. Hafeman, D.G., Sunde, R.A. and Hoekstra, W.G., Effect of dietary selenium on erythrocyte and liver glutathione peroxidase in the rat, *J. Nutr.,* 104, 580, 1974.
20. Boylan, M., Cogan, D., Huffman, N. and Spallholz, J., Behavioral characteristics in open field testing of mice fed selenium deficient and selenium supplemented diets, *J. Trace Elem. Exp. Med.,* 3, 157, 1990.

21. Necheles, T.F, Maldonado, N., Barquet-Chediak, A. and Allen, D.M., Homozygous erythrocyte glutathione peroxidase deficiency: clinical and biochemical studies, *Blood,* 33, 164, 1969.

22. Yang, G., Ge, K., Chan, J. and Chen, X., Selenium-related endemic diseases and the daily selenium requirement of humans, *World Rev. Nutr. Diet.,* 55, 98, 1988.

23. Food and Nutrition Board, Recommended Dietary Allowances, National Academy Press, Washington, D.C., 1989, chap. 10.

24. Institute of Medicine, Food and Nutrition Board. Dietary Reference Intakes: Vitamin C, vitamin E, Selenium and Carotenoids. National Academy Press, Washington, DC, 2000.

25. Luo, X., Wei, H., Yang, C., Xing, J., Liu, X., Qiao, C., Feng, Y., Liu, J., Liu, Y., Wu, Q., Liu, X., Guo, J., Stoecker, B.J., Spallholz, J.E. and Yang, S.P., Bioavailability of selenium to residents in a low selenium area of China, *Am. J. Clin. Nutr.,* 42, 439, 1985.

26. Zumkley, H., Clinical aspects of selenium metabolism, *Biol. Trace Elem. Res.,* 15, 139, 1988.

27. Li, G., Han, C. and Yang, J., Effect of a selenium deficient diet from a Keshan disease area on myocardial metabolism in the pig, in *Selenium in Biology and Medicine, Part B,* Combs, F.G., Spallholz., I.E., Levander, O.A. and Oldfield, J.E., Eds., AVI Book by Van Nostrand Reinhold, New York, 1987, 814.

28. Yang, F.Y. and Wo, W.H., Role of selenium in stabilization of human erythrocyte membrane skeleton, *Biochem. Met.,* 15, 475, 1987.

29. Ge, K.Y., Bai, J., Deng, X.J., Wu, SQ., Wang, S.Q., Xue, A.N. and Su, C.Q., The protective effect of selenium against viral myocarditis in mice, in *Selenium in Biology and Medicine, Part B,* Combs, G.F, Spallholz, I.E., Levander, O.A. and Oldfield, I.E., Eds., AVI Book by Van Nostrand Reinhold, New York, 1987, 761.

30. Beck, M., Kolbeck, P., Shi, Q., Rohr, L., Monis, V. and Levander, 0., Increased virulence of a human enterovirus (Coxsackie virus B3) in selenium deficient mice, *J. Infect. Dis.,* 170, 351, 1995.

31. Wang, F., Li, G., Li, C., Yang, T. and Ping, Z., Pathogenic factors of Keshan disease in the grains cultivated in endemic areas, in *Selenium in Biology and Medicine, Part B,* Combs, G.F., Spallholz, J.E., Levander, O.A. and Oldfield, J.E., Eds., AVI Book by Van Nostrand Reinhold, New York, 1987, 896.

32. Beck, M., Kolbeck, P., Rohr, L., Shi, Q., Monis. V. and Levander, 0., Vitamin E deficiency intensifies the myocardial injury of Coxsackie virus B3 infection in mice, *J. Nutr.,* 124, 345, 1994.

33. Shamburger, R.J., Willis, C.E. and McCormak, L.J., Selenium and heart disease. Blood selenium and heart mortality in 19 states, in *Trace Substances in Environmental Health-XII,* Hemphill, D.D., Ed., University of Missouri Press, Columbia, MO, 1979, 59.

34. Pucheu, S., Coudray, C., Vanzetto, G., Favier, A., Machecourt, J. and de Leiris, J., Time course of changes in plasma levels of trace elements after thrombolysis during acute myocardial infarction in humans, *Biol. Trace Elem. Res.,* 47, 171, 1995.

35. Robinson, ME, Clinical effects of selenium deficiency and excess, in *Clinical, Biochemical and Nutritional Aspects of Trace Elements,* Prasad, A.S., Ed., Alan R. Liss, New York, 1982, 325.

36. Thomson, C.D., Reah, H.M., Robinson, M.F and Simpson, FO., Selenium concentrations and glutathione peroxidase activities in blood of hypertensive patients, *Proc. Univ. Otago Med. Sch.,* 56, 1, 1978.

37. Schoene, N.W., Morris, V.C. and Levander, O.A., Altered arachidonic acid metabolism in platelets and aortas from selenium-deficient rats, *Nutr Res.,* 6, 75, 1986.

38. Bryant, R.W., Bailey, J.M., King, J.C. and Levander, GA., Altered platelet glutathione peroxidase activity and arachidonic acid metabolism during selenium repletion in a controlled human study, in *Selenium in Biology and Medicine,* Spallholz, J.E., Martin, J.L. and Ganther, H.E., Eds., AVI Publishing, Westport, CT, 1981, 395.

39. Li, I.Y., Ren, S., Cheng, D.Z., Wan, HJ., Liang, S.T., Zhang, FJ. and Gao, F.M., Distribution of selenium in the microenvironment related to Kaschin-Beck's disease, in *Selenium in Biology and Medicine,* Spallholz, J.E., Martin, J.L. and Ganther, H.E., Eds., AVI Publishing, Westport, CT, 1987, 911.

40. Liang, S., Zhang, J., Shang, X., Mu, S. and Zhang, F., Effects of selenium supplementation in prevention and treatment of Kaschin-Beck's disease, in *Selenium in Biology and Medicine, Part B,* Combs. G.F., Spallholz, J. E., Levander, O.A. and Oldfield, J.E., Eds., AVI Book by Van Nostrand Reinhold, New York, 1987, 938.

41. Parnham, M.J., Winkelmann, J. and Leyck, S., Macrophage, lymphocyte and chronic inflammatory responses in selenium deficient rodents. Association with decreased glutathione peroxidase activity, *Int. J. Immunopharmacol.,* 5, 455, 1983.

42. Kien, CL. and Ganther, H.E., Manifestations of chronic selenium deficiency in a child receiving total parenteral nutrition, *Am. J. Clin. Nutr.,* 37, 319, 1983.

43. Lombeck, I., Kasperek, K., Feinendegen, LB. and Bremer, H.J., Low selenium state in children, in *Selenium in Biology and Medicine, Part B,* Combs, G.F, Spallholz, J.E., Levander, O.A. and Oldfield, J.E., Eds., AVI Book by Van Nostrand Reinhold, New York, 1987, 269.

44. Dworkin, B.M.. Rosenthal, W.S., Wormser, G.P., Weiss, L., Nunez, M., Joline, C. and Herp, A., Abnormalities of blood selenium and glutathione peroxidase activity in patients with acquired immunodeficiency syndrome and AIDS-related complex, *Biol. Trace Elem. Res.,* 15, 167, 1988.

45. Aaseth, J., Aadland, E. and Thomassen, Y., Serum selenium in patients with short bowel syndrome, in *Selenium in Biology and Medicine, Part B,* Combs, G.F., Spallholz, J.E., Levander, GA. and Oldfield, J.E., F.ds., AVI Book by Van Nostrand Reinhold, New York, 1987, 976.

46. Aaseth, I., Thomassen, Y., Alexander, J. and Norheim, G., Decreased serum selenium in alcoholic cirrhosis, *N. Engl. J. Med.,* 303, 944, 1989.

47. Alfthan G., Xu G.L., Tan W.H., Aro A., Wu J., Yang Y.X., Liang W.S., Xue W.L. and Kong L.H., Selenium supplementation of children in a selenium-deficient area in China: Blood selenium levels and glutathione peroxidase activities, *Biol. Trace. Elem. Res.,* 73:113, 2000.

48. Waschulewski, I.H. and Sunde, R.A. Effect of dietary methionineon utilization of tissue selenium from dietary selenomethionine for glutathione peroxidase in the rat, *J. Nutr.* 118, 367, 1988

49. Thomson, C.D., Assessment of requirements for selenium and adequacy of selenium status: a review, Euro. *J. Clin. Nutr.,* 58, 391, 2003.

50. Helzlsouer, K., Jacobs, R. and Morris, S., Acute selenium intoxication in the United States, *Fed. Proc.,* 44, 1670, 1985.

51. Seko, Y., Saito, Y. and Kitahara, J., Active oxygen generation by the reaction of selenite with reduced glutathione *in vitro,* in *Selenium in Biology and Medicine.* Wendel, A., Ed., Springer-Verlag, Berlin, 1989, 70.

52. Xu, H., Feng. Z. and Vi, C., Free radical mechanisms of the toxicity of selenium compounds, *Huzahong Longong Daxve Xuebao,* 19, 13, 1991.

53. Yan, L. and Spallholz, J.E., Generation of reactive oxygen species from the reaction of Selenium compounds with thiols and mammary tumor cells, *Biochem. Pharmacol.,* 45, 429, 1993.

54. Spallholz, J.E., On the nature of selenium toxicity and carcinostatic activity, *Free Rad. Biol. Med.,* 17, 45, 1994. 55. Mustacich D. and Powis G., Thioredoxin reductase, *Biochem. J.,* 15,1, 2000.

56. Robinson, M.F., Thomson, C.D. and Huemmer, P.K., Effect of a megadose of ascorbic acid, a meal and orange juice on the absorption of selenium as sodium selenite, *N.Z. Med. J.,* 98, 627, 1985.

57. Arthur, J.R., Nicol, F. and Beckett, G.J. Hepatic iodothyronine 5' deiodinase: the role of selenium. *Biochem. J.,* 272, 537, 1990.

58. Rivlin, R.S. and Dutta, P., Vitamin B_2 (riboflavin) relevance to malaria and antioxidant activity, *Nutr. Today,* 30,62, 1995.

59. Parsons M.J., Ku P.K., Ullrey D.E., Stowe H.D., Whetter P.A. and Miller E.R., Effects of riboflavin supplementation and selenium source on selenium metabolism in the young pig. *J. Anim. Sci.,* 60, 451, 1985.

60. Davis, C.D. and Uthus, E.O., Dietary folate and selenium affect dimethylhydrazine-induced aberrant crypt formation, global DNA methylation and one-carbon metabolism in rats, *J. Nutr.,* 133, 2907, 2003.

61. Ji, L.L., Oxidative stress during exercise: implications of antioxidant nutrients, Free Rad. Biol. Med., 18, 1079, 1995.

62. Witt, E.H., Reznick, A.Z., Viguie, C.A., Starke-Reed, P. and Packer, L., Exercise, oxidative damage and effects of antioxidant manipulation, *J. Nutr.,* 122, 766, 1992.

63. Dillard, C.J., Litov, RE., Savin, W.M., Dumelin, E.E. and Tappel, A.L., Effect of exercise, vitamin E and ozone on pulmonary function and lipid peroxidation, *J. Appl. Physiol.,* 45, 927, 1978.

64. Hill, K.E., Burk, R.F. and Lane, J.M., Effect of selenium depletion and repletion on plasma glutathione and glutathione-dependent enzymes, *J. Nutr.,* 117, 99, 1987.

65. Ji, L.L., Stratman, F.W. and Hardy, HA., Antioxidant enzyme response to selenium deficiency in rat myocardium, *J. Am. Coll. Nutr.,* 11,79, 1992.

66. Ji, L.L., Stratman, F.W. and Hardy, H.A., Antioxidant enzyme systems in rat liver and skeletal muscle: influences of selenium deficiency, chronic training and acute exercise, *Arch. Biochem. Biophys.,* 263, 150, 1988.

67. Lang, J., Gohil, K., Packer, L. and Burk, R., Selenium deficiency, endurance exercise capacity and antioxidant status in rats, *J. Appl. Physiol.,* 63, 2532, 1987.

68. Brady, P.S., Brady, L.J. and Ullrey, D.E., Selenium, vitamin E and the response to swimming stress in the rat, *J. Nutr.,* 109, 1103, 1979.

69. Edwards, A., Blann, A., Suarez-Mendez, V., Lardi, A. and McCollum, C., Systemic responses in patients with intermittent claudication after treadmill exercise, *Br. J. Surg.,* 81, 1738, 1994.

70. Soares, J.C., Folmer, V. and Rocha, J.B., Influences of dietary selenium supplementation and exercise on thiol-containing enzymes in mice, *Nutrition,* 19, 626, 2003.

71. Duthie, G., Robertson, J., Maughan, R. and Morrice, P., Blood antioxidant status and erythrocyte lipid peroxidation following distance running, *Arch. Biochem. Biophys.,* 282, 78, 1990.

72. Dragan, I., Dinu, V., Mohora, M., Cristea, E., Ploesteanu, E. and Stroescu, V., Studies regarding the antioxidant effects of selenium on top swimmers, *Rev. Roum. Physiol.,* 27,15, 1990.

73. Dillard, C.J., Litor, RE. and Tappel, AL., Effect of dietary vitamin E, selenium and polyunsaturated fats on in vivo lipid peroxidation in the rat as measured by pentane production, *Lipids,* 13, 396, 1978.

74. Tessier, F., Hida, H., Favier, A. and Marconnet, P., Muscle GSHPx activity after prolonged exercise, training and selenium supplementation, *Biol. Trace Elem. Res.,* 47, 279, 1995.

75. Margaritis, I., Tessier, F., Prou, E., Marconnet, P., Marini, J.F., Effects of endurance training on skeletal muscle oxidative capacities with and without selenium supplementation, *J. Trace Elem. Med. Biol.,* 11, 37, 1997.

76. Sen, C.K., Mann, E., Kretzschmar, J. and Hanninen, 0., Skeletal muscle and liver glutathione homeostasis in response to training, exercise and immobilization, *J. Appl. Physiol.,* 74, 1265, 1992.

77. Laughlin, M.H., Simpson, T., Sexton, W.L., Brown, O.R., Smith, J.K. and Korthuis, R.J., Skeletal muscle oxidative capacity, antioxidant enzymes and exercise training, *J. Appl. Physiol.,* 68, 2337, 1990.

78. Schaner, J.E., Schelin, A., Hanson, P. and Stratman, F.W., Dehydroepiandrosterone and a B-agonist, energy transducers, alter antioxidant enzyme systems: influence of chronic training and acute exercise in rats, *Arch. Biochem. Biophys.,* 283, 503, 1990.

79. Storz, G., Tartaglia, L.A. and Ames, B.N., Transcriptional regulator of oxidative stress-induced genes: Direct activation by oxidation, *Science,* 248, 189, 1990.

80. Tessier, F., Hida, H., Favier, A. and Marconnet, P., Muscle GSH-Px activity after prolonged exercise training and selenium supplementation. *Biol. Trace Element Res.* 47, 279,1995.

20 Boron, Manganese, Molybdenum, Nickel, Silicon and Vanadium

Forrest H. Nielsen*

CONTENTS

---

* The U.S. Department of Agriculture, Agricultural Research Service, Northern Plains Area, is an equal opportunity/ affirmative action employer and all agency services are available without discrimination.

I.   INTRODUCTION

Elements assigned to this chapter are those whose nutritional importance is apparently limited, has not been definitively established, or is speculative. If the lack of an element cannot be shown to cause death or interrupt the life cycle (interfere with growth, development, or maturation such that procreation is prevented), many scientists do not consider that element to be essential unless it has a defined biochemical function. On this basis, of the elements assigned to this chapter, only manganese and molybdenum are unquestionably accepted as essential; they are known enzyme cofactors. Boron probably should also be considered essential because its dietary lack has been shown to interrupt the life cycle of some vertebrates. Substantial circumstantial evidence indicates that nickel, silicon and vanadium may be essential. This evidence includes:

- The element fills a need at physiological concentrations for a known *in vivo* biochemical action to proceed *in vitro*.
- The element is a component of known biologically important molecules in some life form.
- The element is essential for some lower form of life (i.e., plants, microorganisms and invertebrates).
- A dietary deprivation of the element in some animal model consistently results in a changed biological function, body structure, or tissue composition that is preventable or reversible by an intake of an apparent physiological amount of the element.

Based on this evidence, if nickel, silicon and vanadium are not categorized as essential, they should be at least considered bioactive elements that may be nutritionally important and categorized as nutritionally beneficial, or beneficially bioactive, elements.

Although the elements in this chapter receive minimal attention in human nutrition because dietary deficiencies have not been identified in the general population, they have received some attention from individuals pursuing optimal performance and health in athletic endeavors. This attention usually has come about through the promotion of the element by the nutritional supplement industry. This promotion usually is based on some promising physiological or clinical finding, most often in an animal model or a special human situation. Too often, the findings are overstated or excessively extrapolated regarding what the element will do for the normal healthy sports enthusiast. The consumption of a diet containing all food groups most likely will provide the amounts of boron, manganese, molybdenum, nickel, silicon and vanadium needed for optimal performance of the functions that are the bases for these elements' being of sports nutrition interest. These functions include anabolic actions through facilitating the activity of hormones such as anabolic steroids (boron) and insulin (boron, manganese and vanadium); improving bone strength and joint health (silicon, boron, manganese, nickel and vanadium); and overcoming oxidant stress induced by vigorous exercise (boron, manganese and molybdenum).

II. BORON

A. General Properties and Possible Metabolic Functions

Boron is widely distributed in nature and always bound to oxygen. Boron biochemistry is essentially that of boric acid. Dilute aqueous boric acid solutions comprise $B(OH)_3$ and $B(OH)_4^-$ at the pH of blood (7.4); because the pK_a of boric acid is 9.15, the abundance of these two species at pH 7.4 is 98.4% and 1.6%, respectively.[1] Boric acid forms ester complexes with hydroxyl groups of organic compounds, preferably when the hydroxyl groups are adjacent and cis.[2] Among the many substances of biological interest with which boron forms complexes are diadenosine polyphosphates, S-adenosylmethionine, pyridoxine, riboflavin, dehydroascorbic acid and pyridine nucleotides. Formation of these complexes may be biologically important because some may modulate or regulate some function or reaction. To date, several naturally occurring organoboron compounds have been identified; all of these are boroesters. These compounds include antibiotics produced by microorganisms,[3–5] the plant cell wall component, rhamnogalacturonan-II,[6,7] and a bacterial extracellular signaling molecule.[8]

A defined metabolic function has not been identified for boron. However, findings from boron-deprivation experiments focused on establishing essentiality provide some idea of the probable metabolic function of boron. Boron-deprivation (0.6 B μg/kg diet instead of the usual 310 mg B/kg and placed in culture water containing 0.6 μg B/L instead of the usual 100 μg B/L) in the African clawed frog (*Xenopus laevis*) results in necrotic eggs and a high frequency of abnormal gastrulation in the embryo. Abnormal gastrulation was characterized by bleeding yolk and exogastrulation, which suggested abnormal cell membrane structure or function.[9] Boron deprivation of zebra fish resulted in a high rate of death during the zygote and cleavage periods before the formation of a blastula.[10] Pathological changes in the embryo before death included extensive blebbing and the extrusion of cytoplasm, which suggested membrane alterations.

Experiments with mammals, unlike with the frog and zebrafish, have not shown that the life cycle can be interrupted. However, substantial evidence exists for boron's being a bioactive food component that is beneficial, if not required, for bone growth and maintenance, energy and reactive oxygen metabolism and optimal response to steroid hormones and insulin. Evidence that boron affects these processes in humans has come mainly from two studies[11] in which men over the age of 45 years, postmenopausal women and postmenopausal women on estrogen were fed a diet low in boron (about 0.25 mg/2000 kcal) for 63 days and then were fed the same diet supplemented with 3 mg of boron/day for 49 days. These dietary intakes were near the low and high values in the range of dietary boron

TABLE 20.1
Responses of Boron-Deprived Subjects to a 3-mg B/Day Supplement for 49 Days*

Metabolism Affected	Evidence for Effect
Macro mineral	Increased serum 25-hydroxyvitamin D
	Decreased serum calcitonin†
Energy	Decreased serum glucose†
	Increased serum triacylglycerols‡
Nitrogen	Decreased blood urea nitrogen
	Decreased serum creatinine
Oxidative	Increased erythrocyte superoxide dismutase
	Increased serum ceruloplasmin
Erythropoiesis/hematopoiesis	Increased blood hemoglobin‡
	Increased mean corpuscular hemoglobin content‡
	Decreased hematocrit‡
	Decreased platelet number‡
	Decreased red cell number‡

*After deprivation at an intake of 0.25 mg B/2000 kcal for 63 days. Subjects included men over the age of 45 years, postmenopausal women and postmenopausal women on estrogen therapy.
†Found when dietary copper and magnesium were inadequate.
‡Found when dietary copper and magnesium were adequate.

intakes (0.5 to 3.1mg/day) that have been found in a limited number of surveys.[12] Some of the effects of boron supplementation after 63 days of boron depletion that were found in these two experiments are listed in Table 20.1. In one experiment, copper was marginal and magnesium was inadequate; in the other experiment, both elements were adequate. The intakes of copper and magnesium apparently affected the response to the changes in dietary boron, as indicated by the footnotes in Table 20.1. Processes affected by dietary boron in humans have been shown to also be affected in animal models.

Two hypotheses have been advanced for the biochemical function of boron in higher animals. These hypotheses accommodate a large and varied response to boron deprivation and the known biochemistry of boron. One hypothesis is that boron has a role in cell membrane function or stability such that it influences the cell response to hormones, transmembrane signaling, or transmembrane movement of regulatory cations or anions.[11] The hypothesis is supported by the recent identification of a bacterial quorum-sensing signal molecule that is a furanosyl borate diester.[8] Quorum sensing is the cell-to-cell communication in bacteria that is accomplished through the exchange of extracellular signaling molecules called autoinducers. The boron autoinducer (AI-2) has been proposed to be a universal signal for inter-species communication among bacteria. AI-2 is synthesized from adenosylmethionine, which supplies the 2′-3′-*cis*-diol of a ribose moiety that binds boron well. Another group of biomolecules that contain ribose moieties, the diadenosine phosphates, have been characterized as novel boron binders.[13] Diadenosine phosphates function as signal nucleotides. Another study supporting the membrane role for boron was that determining the effect of boron on frog egg development. Culturing stage 1 and stage 2 oocytes from boron-adequate frogs in medium containing progesterone resulted in successful maturation to stage 5 or 6 oocytes. In contrast, oocytes from boron-deprived frogs did not respond to progesterone and did not mature *in vitro*. Further study of the maturation process[14] revealed that the boron-deprived oocytes were capable of producing progesterone and the maturation-promoting factor (involved in binding progesterone to its receptor on the plasma membrane) and responding to this factor. It was hypothesized that the impaired maturation process was caused by progesterone's not being bound efficiently to the membrane receptor because of changes in its structural homology.

The second hypothesized function of boron is based on the knowledge that two classes of enzymes (oxidoreductases and hydrolases) are competitively inhibited *in vitro* by borate or its derivatives, and upon findings showing that dietary boron can alter the *in vivo* activity of many of these enzymes. Thus, it has been hypothesized that boron is a metabolic regulator; that is, boron controls a number of metabolic pathways by competitively inhibiting some key enzyme reactions.[2] For example, reactions inhibited may include oxidoreductases that require the boron-binding *cis*-hydroxyl-containing pyridine of flavin nucleotides as a cofactor.

B. Basis for Sports Nutrition Interest

1. Anabolic Hormone Action Enhancement

Dietary boron may affect testosterone metabolism. A boron supplement of 3 mg/day given to postmenopausal women who had consumed a diet providing only about 0.25 mg B/day for 119 days significantly increased serum testosterone concentrations.[15] In another study, free-living male subjects supplemented with 10 mg B/day for 4 weeks showed significantly increased plasma estradiol concentrations and a trend toward increased plasma testosterone concentrations.[16] Rats fed a diet containing 10 mg B/kg dosed with 2 mg B/day in the drinking water showed significantly increased plasma testosterone concentrations that were diminished by doses of 12.5 and 25 mg B/day.[17,18]

Boron also may affect insulin production or activity. Boron deprivation increased plasma insulin concentrations in rats.[19] Also, peak insulin secretion was higher from the pancreas isolated from boron-deprived than-supplemented chicks.[18] These findings suggest that boron deficiency may decrease insulin sensitivity.

2. Energy Metabolism Modification

Boron status apparently has an impact on energy metabolism during exercise training. Sedentary rats responded differently to changes in dietary boron than rats exercised on a powered running wheel.[20,21] Exercise-trained rats, but not sedentary rats, had higher body weights, serum lactate dehydrogenase activity and serum creatinine concentrations when fed supplemental boron (2.0 mg B/kg diet) than when fed a low-boron diet (0.2 mg B/kg). In humans not involved in exercise training, blood urea nitrogen and creatinine concentrations were higher during boron depletion than during boron repletion.[22] Boron deprivation increased serum glucose and decreased serum triglyceride concentrations.[22] Dietary boron may affect glycolysis. In chicks, boron deprivation decreased the hepatic concentrations of fructose-1,6-biphosphate, glycerate-2-phosphate and dihydroxyacetone phosphate[23] and exacerbated the cholecalciferol deficiency-induced elevation in plasma glucose and decrease in serum triglycerides.[23,24] These findings suggest that the utilization of energy from carbohydrate for exercise and the body's intermediary metabolism response to exercise training are changed by boron deprivation.

3. Anti-Oxidant and Anti-Inflammatory Activity

Among the findings indicating that boron is involved in the inflammatory process or immune function in higher animals is that dietary boron affects the response to an antigen injected to induce arthritis in rats.[25] Boron-supplemented (2.0 mg/kg diet) rats had less swelling of the paws, lower circulating neutrophil concentrations and higher circulating concentrations of natural killer cells and CD8a+/CD4-cells than did boron-deficient rats (0.1 mg/kg diet). In pigs, low dietary boron increased inflammation caused by the intradermal injection of phytohemagglutinin.[26]

Boron may be important in the oxidative metabolite scavenging process. Boron supplementation after boron deprivation for 119 days increased erythrocyte superoxide dismutase concentrations in men and postmenopausal women.[22] In rats, boron deprivation increased red blood cell catalase activity.[21] These enzymes increase during increased oxidative metabolism. Evidence that boron deprivation may result in increased oxidative stress is that plasma 8-iso-prostaglandin F_{2} (an indicator of lipid oxidation) was found to be increased in boron-deprived rats.[27] Perhaps boron regulates the inflammatory process by dampening the activity of NADP-requiring oxidoreductase, which is involved in the generation of reactive oxygen species during the respiratory burst in cells.[28] Boron supplementation of rats attenuated hepatic pathology of rats treated with thioacetamide.[29] Reactive oxygen metabolism is thought to be involved in the pathogenesis caused by thioacetamide.

4.   Bone and Joint Health Promotion

Much evidence exists to support the contention that boron has beneficial effects on bone. The effects of boron often are most marked in the presence of suboptimal status of another nutrient important in bone formation or remodeling. One of the first studies suggesting that boron is essential found that boron improved bone calcification in chicks fed a diet deficient but not completely lacking in vitamin D.[30] At the microscopic level, boron deprivation (0.465 mg/kg diet) exacerbated the distortion of marrow sprouts (location of calcified scaffold erosion and new bone formation) and the delay in initiation of cartilage calcification in bones during marginal vitamin D deficiency.[24] Boron deprivation also decreased chondrocyte density in the zone of proliferation of the bone growth plate. It should be noted that vitamin D-deficient chicks fed low dietary boron (about 0.3 mg/kg), compared with chicks fed diets containing 1.4 mg B/kg, had decreased plasma 25-hydroxycholecalciferol.[31] In humans, estrogen therapy to maintain bones increases serum 17β-estradiol; this increase is depressed when dietary boron intake is low (0.25–0.35 mg/day).[22] In rats, boron enhanced the beneficial effects of 17β-estradiol on trabecular bone volume and plate density in tibias of ovariectomized rats.[32] Although neither boron or estradiol supplementation alone affected calcium, phosphorus or magnesium balance, a combined boron and estradiol supplementation improved the apparent absorption (based on the analysis of food, urine and feces) of calcium, magnesium and phosphorus and retention and serum concentrations of calcium and magnesium in ovariectomized rats.[33] Boron deprivation also can exacerbate the increase in serum calcitonin caused by low dietary copper and magnesium in humans.[22] Boron deprivation without modification by other nutrients affects bone strength. Low dietary boron (0.98 mg boron/kg compared with 5 mg boron/kg) decreased the bone strength variable bending moment in pigs[34] and induced abnormal limb development in frogs (boron low conditions described in section A).[9] In rats, boron deprivation decreased femur strength measured by the breaking variables bending moment and stress.[35]

Supra nutritional or pharmacologic doses of boron also may be beneficial to bone mechanical properties. A boron supplement of 5 mg/kg to a diet containing 9.4 mg B/kg increased bone strength in chicks.[36] Also, chicks fed a diet containing 14.7 mg B/kg and supplemented with 50 or 100 mg B/kg for 16 weeks after hatching had increased bone strength as indicated by increased shear force of the tibia and femur, shear stress of the tibia and shear energy of the femur.[37] When the boron supplements were started at 32 weeks of age and fed for 40 weeks, the shear fracture energy of both the tibia and radius was increased in egg producing chickens and the shear force, stress and fracture energy of both the tibia and radius were increased in non-egg-producing chickens.[38] Supplementing a standard diet with 35 (and up to 1575) mg B/kg as boric acid increased vertebral resistance to a crushing force by approximately 10% in rats.[39]

In rats exposed to strenuous treadmill exercise, femur and vertebra bone mineral content and density were decreased and trabecular separation was increased. A boron supplement of 50 mg/kg as sodium borate increased bone mineral content and density, trabecular bone volume and trabecular thickness in the exercised rats.[40] It was concluded that boron preserves bone mass in rats that have been exposed to intense exercise.

C.   Metabolism

Because there is no usable radioisotope of boron, the study of its metabolism has been difficult. It is likely, however, that most ingested boron is converted into boric acid, the normal hydrolysis end product of most boron compounds and the dominant inorganic species at the pH of the gastrointestinal tract. About 85% of ingested boron is absorbed and then efficiently excreted via the urine mainly as boric acid.[41–43] During transport in the body, boric acid most likely is weakly attached to organic molecules containing *cis*-hydroxyl groups.

D. Dietary and Supplemental Sources

The richest sources of boron are fruits, vegetables, pulses, legumes and nuts.[44–48] Wine, cider and beer are also high in boron. Dairy products, fish, meats and most grains are poor sources of boron, although milk is the primary source of boron for infants, toddlers and adolescents because of the large quantities consumed. A typical daily intake of boron through diet ranges between 0.75 and 1.35 mg. However, consumption of specific foods with a high boron content will increase boron intake significantly; for example, one serving of wine or avocado provides 0.4 and 1.11 mg., respectively.

E. Supplementation

Within 3 months of the first report describing findings from nutritional experiments with humans,[15] boron supplements were being marketed. Shortly thereafter, numerous health claims for boron began to appear in tabloids, magazines, advertisements and other popular media. The claims included boron's preventing or curing osteoporosis, being an ergogenic aid, preventing or curing arthritis, stopping memory loss and keeping motor skills sharp.

No reports show that boron supplementation of athletes has significant beneficial effects on performance. One report described findings from a study in which athletic and sedentary women consuming self-selected Western diets were supplemented with 3 mg of boron for 10 months.[48] This report did not indicate that boron affected physical work capacity, but did present some findings suggesting that exercise modifies the effect of boron supplementation on mineral status. The boron supplementation decreased serum phosphorus concentrations; this effect was diminished by exercise training. Also, boron supplementation increased serum magnesium concentrations in sedentary women but not in athletes. In another study, 10 male bodybuilders consumed a daily 2.5-mg boron supplement while nine bodybuilders consumed a placebo daily for 49 days.[49] Seven weeks of bodybuilding increased total testosterone, lean body mass and strength in lesser-trained bodybuilders; these effects were not significantly altered by the boron supplementation.

Boron is not very toxic when orally ingested.[50] Evidence for this low toxicity includes the use of boric acid and borates as food preservatives and in oral medicinal products in the late 19th and early 20th centuries. Toxicity signs in animals generally occur only after dietary boron exceeds 100 mg/kg diet. In humans, the signs of acute toxicity include nausea, vomiting, diarrhea, dermatitis and lethargy. The signs of chronic toxicity, based mainly on animal findings, include poor appetite, weight loss and decreased sexual activity, seminal volume and sperm count and motility.

F. Dietary Recommendations

In the human studies described above, the subjects responded to boron supplementation (3 mg/day) after consuming a diet supplying only about 0.25 mg of boron/2000 kcal for 63 days. Thus, humans apparently receive benefit from a boron intake above 0.25 mg per day or have a dietary boron requirement above this amount. A World Health Organization Expert Consultation on Trace Elements in Human Nutrition suggested that an acceptable safe range of population mean intakes for boron for adults could be 1 to 13 mg per day.[11] The U.S. FNB (FNB) chose not to establish recommendations for daily boron intake because of the lack of a clear biological function for boron in humans and the limited evidence on which to base a recommendation. The FNB did, however, set tolerable upper intake levels (UL) for different age groups for boron.[51] The ULs are based largely on adverse reproductive and developmental effects in animals as the critical endpoint. The UL for adults is 20 mg/day.

G. FUTURE RESEARCH DIRECTIONS OR NEEDS

Numerous findings suggest that boron status could affect body processes of interest in sports nutrition. However, the possibility that boron status can affect athletic performance has not been adequately investigated. Studies are needed to determine whether boron supplementation can improve performance of athletes regularly consuming low amounts of boron (<1.0 mg/day). These studies would be helped by the establishment of a defined biochemical function and a reliable status indicator for boron. Also, studies are needed to determine whether supra nutritional intakes, but below the UL guideline of 20 mg B/day, provide benefits to athletes. Until such studies are done, no firm conclusions can be made about the value of increased boron intakes in sports nutrition.

III. MANGANESE

A. GENERAL PROPERTIES AND METABOLIC FUNCTIONS

The essentiality of manganese for animals has been known for more than 50 years; its deficiency has been induced in many animal species.[52] Deficiency causes depressed growth, testicular degeneration (rats), slipped tendons or perosis (chicks), osteodystrophy, severe glucose intolerance (guinea pigs), ataxia (mice, mink), depigmentation of hair, and seizures (rats). Manganese deficiency also caused defects in lipid and carbohydrate metabolism.

Signs of manganese deficiency in humans have not been firmly established. Most reports of human manganese deficiency have shortcomings. In one study,[52] men were fed a purified diet supplying only 0.11 mg Mn/day for 39 days. The men developed a finely scaling, minimally erythematous rash, decreased serum cholesterol concentrations and increased serum alkaline phosphatase activity. Short-term (10 days) manganese supplementation, however, did not reverse these changes. In another study, 14 young women were fed a conventional Western-type diet providing about 1.0 mg Mn/day for 39 days and then compared with when the diet was supplemented with manganese to provide about 5.6 mg/day.[53] The low manganese intake resulted in slightly increased plasma glucose concentrations during an intravenous glucose tolerance test and increased menstrual losses of manganese, calcium, iron and total hemoglobin. These findings need to be confirmed because the women did not exhibit negative manganese balance during the low manganese period, nor were the changes very marked. The most convincing case of manganese deficiency is that of a child on long-term parenteral nutrition who exhibited diffuse bone demineralization and poor growth that were corrected by manganese supplementation.[54,55]

Manganese deficiency may contribute to disease processes. Low dietary manganese or low blood and tissue manganese has been associated with osteoporosis, diabetes, epilepsy, atherosclerosis, impaired wound healing and cataracts.[56]

Because manganese deficiency has been so difficult to induce or identify in humans, it generally is considered not of nutritional concern. Nonetheless, manganese is considered an essential nutrient for humans because it is known to function as an enzyme activator and to be a constituent of several metalloenzymes.[57] The numerous enzymes that can be activated by manganese include oxidoreductases, lyases, ligases, hydrolases, kinases, decarboxylases and transferases. Most enzymes activated by manganese in higher animals and humans can also be activated by other metals, especially magnesium; exceptions are the manganese-specific activation of glycosyltransferases, glutamine synthetase, farnesyl pyrophosphate synthetase and phosphoenolpyruvate carboxykinase.[57] The few manganese metalloenzymes include arginase, pyruvate carboxylase and manganese superoxide dismutase in higher animals.[57]

B.   Basis for Sports Nutrition Interest

1.   Energy Metabolism Modification

Pyruvate carboxylase and phosphoenolpyruvate carboxykinase are important enzymes in the gluconeogenic pathway. Because pyruvate carboxylase is a manganese metalloenzyme and phosphoenolpyruvate carboxykinase is a manganese-activated enzyme, it can be predicted that manganese deficiency affects carbohydrate metabolism through changing the activity of these enzymes in liver. However, even in severely manganese-deficient animals, pyruvate carboxylase activity is not affected.[58] Manganese deficiency inconsistently affects phosphoenolpyruvate carboxykinase activity.[59]

Manganese apparently affects carbohydrate metabolism through an effect on insulin production, secretion or degradation. Offspring of manganese-deficient guinea pig dams that were weaned to manganese-deficient diets exhibited impaired glucose tolerance and glucose utilization.[60] Insulin release from isolated perfused pancreas from manganese-deficient rats is less than that found with manganese adequacy.[61] Increased insulin degradation was also found in rats.[62] In both the guinea pig and rat, manganese deficiency causes pancreatic pathology characterized by hypoplasia of all cellular components.[63] Decreased preproinsulin mRNA may be contributing to decreased insulinogenesis in the manganese-deficient rat.[64] Manganese deficiency also apparently causes a defect in the response to insulin in peripheral tissues because adipocytes isolated from manganese-deficient rats had decreased *in vitro* insulin-stimulated glucose transport, oxidation and conversion to fatty acids.[65] The biochemical bases for the changes in insulin metabolism and action induced by manganese deficiency have not been clearly defined.

2.   Anti-Oxidant Activity

Manganese superoxide dismutase is the major antioxidant in mitochondria. The importance of this enzyme was demonstrated by the finding that the deletion mutation of the manganese superoxide dismutase gene in mice resulted in death within 5–21 days of birth.[66] Severe mitochondrial damage occurred in these rats that was attributed to the increased presence of reactive oxygen species. The importance of this enzyme for protection against oxidant stress has also been demonstrated by studies with animals or cells that overexpress manganese superoxide dismutase. For example, this overexpression has been shown to prevent alcohol-induced liver injury in rats,[67] attenuate myocardial injury following ischemia and reperfusion,[68] protect lung epithelial cells against oxidant injury[69] and protect against apoptotic cell death.[70] In addition, high dietary manganese protected against heart lipid peroxidation in rats fed high amounts of polyunsaturated fatty acids.[71] Physiological stress, including exercise, increases the activity of manganese superoxide dismutase in the myocardium and thus apparently protects against ischemia-perfusion-induced arrhythmias, myocardial stunning and infarction.[72–75] These findings indicate that manganese is important for protection against oxidant damage induced by high-intensity training and promotes recovery from training.

3.   Bone and Joint Health Promotion

When imposed *in utero* or in young growing animals, manganese deficiency has marked adverse effects on the skeleton; these effects include shortening of the limbs, enlargement of the joints, twisting of legs, stiffness and lameness.[57] These skeletal abnormalities have been largely ascribed to a reduction in proteoglycan synthesis secondary to a reduction in the activities of manganese-dependent glycosyl transferases.[57] However, manganese deficiency also has been found to impair osteoblast and osteoclast activities. This impairment may lead to altered bone growth and remodeling that contribute to bone deformities.[76] Also, manganese deficiency decreases circulating insulin-like growth factor, which has osteotrophic actions.[77] This may be the reason that manganese deficiency decreased bone density and calcium in rats.[78] The preceding findings suggest that manganese may be important in maintaining strong bones and healthy joints in physically active people.

C. METABOLISM

For the adult human, absorption of manganese from the diet has often been stated to be no higher than 5%. This estimate is complicated by the fact that endogenous manganese is almost totally excreted through biliary, pancreatic and intestinal secretions into the gut. If manganese status is adequate, endogenous excretion of absorbed manganese into the gut is so rapid that it is difficult to determine the portion of fecal manganese not absorbed from the diet and the portion endogenously excreted. With this in mind, true absorption of manganese has been estimated to be 8% in young rats.[79] Manganese absorption declines as dietary intake increases[80] and increases with low manganese status.[81] Endogenous excretion of manganese apparently is not markedly influenced by dietary intake or status.[81] Thus, variable absorption apparently is a significant factor in the regulation of manganese homeostasis, with excretion contributing.

Absorption of manganese apparently occurs equally well throughout the small intestine. There are indications that manganese is absorbed through a rapidly saturable, active transport mechanism that involves a high-affinity, low-capacity system.[82] Diffusion also has been implicated in manganese absorption.[83] Perhaps both processes are involved in manganese movement across the gut. This suggestion is supported by the finding that apical to basolateral manganese uptake and transport by Caco-2 cultures were strictly concentration-dependent, but basolateral to apical uptake and transport were saturable.[84] Manganese may be absorbed by a 2-step mechanism with the initial uptake from the lumen followed by transfer across mucosal cells. Iron competes with manganese for common binding sites in both processes. Thus, one of these metals, if present in high amounts, can exert an inhibitory effect on the absorption of the other.

Both Mn^{2+} bound to plasma α-2-macroglobulin[57] and Mn^{2+} bound to albumin[81] have been suggested to be the form of manganese entering the portal blood from the gastrointestinal tract. Regardless of form, manganese is rapidly removed from the blood by the liver. A fraction is oxidized to Mn^{3+} and is transported in plasma bound to transferrin[63] or possibly to a specific transmanganin protein. Transferrin-bound manganese is taken up by extrahepatic tissue.

Within cells, manganese is found predominantly in mitochondria, and thus, liver, kidney and pancreas have relatively high manganese concentrations. In contrast, manganese is present in extremely low concentrations in plasma and urine of humans.

D. DIETARY AND SUPPLEMENTAL SOURCES

Most reported daily mean intakes of manganese throughout the world fall between 0.52 and 10.8 mg.[85] Unrefined cereals, nuts, leafy vegetables and tea are rich in manganese. These foods contributed almost 75% of the manganese consumed by the average adult human male in the Total Diet Study.[86] Refined grains, meats and dairy products are low in manganese.

E. SUPPLEMENTATION

Apparently because manganese deficiency is difficult to induce or identify in humans, there is a paucity of studies determining the effect of manganese supplementation on healthy adults. Women consuming diets averaging between 1.4 and 2.0 mg/day had only increased lymphocyte manganese superoxide dismutase activity and serum manganese concentrations after receiving a supplemental 15 mg Mn/day for 124 days.[87] In another study, healthy young women were fed for 8 weeks each, in a crossover design, diets that provided 0.8 or 20 mg Mn/day.[88] The manganese intakes did not affect any clinical or neurological measures and only minimally affected psychological variables. Based on these findings it was concluded that dietary intakes of manganese from 0.8 to 20 mg/day for 8 weeks are not likely to result in either manganese deficiency or toxicity signs in healthy adults.

In the past, manganese was considered to be one of the least toxic of the essential mineral elements. Very high amounts of manganese (2,000–7,000 mg/kg diet) were required to induce the most commonly reported signs (depressed growth and iron status and hematological changes) of manganese toxicity in animals.[49] Recently, however, magnetic resonance imaging has shown that signals for manganese in the brain are strongly associated with neurological symptoms (e.g., sleep disturbances) exhibited by patients with chronic liver disease.[89] Findings such as this have resulted in the suggestion that high intakes of manganese are ill-advised because of potential neurotoxicological effects,[90] especially in people with compromised homeostatic mechanisms or infants whose homeostatic control of manganese is not fully developed.

High intakes of manganese may be of concern for people not consuming adequate amounts of magnesium. Pigs fed diets providing inadequate magnesium (about 25% the dietary recommendation) died suddenly and showed heart changes when the diet was made rich in manganese (52 mg/kg).[91]

Neurotoxicity was the adverse effect used by the FNB to set the UL for manganese.[51] The UL (mg/day) for children was set at 2 for ages 1–3 years, 3 for 4–8 years, 6 for 9–13 years and 9 for 14–18 years. Above the age of 19 years, the UL set was 11 mg/d.

F. DIETARY RECOMMENDATIONS

The FNB[51] has set Adequate Intakes (AIs) for manganese (in mg/day) as follows: infants 0–6 months, 0,003; infants 7–12 months, 0.6; children 1–3 years, 1.2; children 4–8 years, 1.5; boys 9–13 years, 1.9; boys 14–18 years, 2.2; girls 9–18 years, 1.6; adult men, 2.3; adult women, 1.8; pregnant women, 2; and lactating women, 2.6. These values seem quite liberal considering the difficulty in inducing or identifying manganese deficiency in humans. Intensive exercise may increase the need for manganese because a 30-km cross-country run has been found to increase intestinal excretion and induce negative balance.[92]

G. FUTURE RESEARCH DIRECTIONS OR NEEDS

Findings described above suggest that exercise may increase the need for manganese superoxide dismutase to protect against oxidative stress, and suggest that exercise may increase manganese loss. Also, low dietary manganese or low blood and tissue manganese has been associated with disturbances in carbohydrate metabolism (e.g., impaired insulin production or response to glucose, and perhaps impaired gluconeogenesis) and bone loss. Thus, there is a need to ascertain whether manganese supplementation of individuals consuming diets low in manganese and performing intensive exercise would benefit from an increased intake of manganese.

IV. MOLYBDENUM

A. GENERAL PROPERTIES AND METABOLIC FUNCTIONS

The signs of molybdenum deficiency in animals have been reviewed.[93] In rats and chickens, molybdenum deficiency aggravated by excessive dietary tungsten results in the depression of molybdenum enzymes, disturbances in uric acid metabolism and increased susceptibility to sulfite toxicity. In goats, deficiency uncomplicated by high dietary tungsten or copper resulted in depressed food consumption and growth, and impaired reproduction characterized by infertility and elevated mortality in both mothers and offspring.

Knowledge of the signs and symptoms of human molybdenum deficiency have come from a patient receiving prolonged total parenteral nutrition. This patient developed hypermethioninemia, hypouricemia, hyperoxypurinemia, hypouricosuria and very low sulfate excretion; these changes were exacerbated by methionine administration.[94] The findings indicated defects in the oxidation of sulfite to sulfate and in uric acid production. Supplementation of the patient with ammonium molybdate improved the clinical condition, reversed the sulfur-handling defect and normalized uric acid production. Molybdenum deficiency has not been unequivocally identified in humans other than in this individual. Thus, molybdenum generally is considered to be of no practical nutritional concern for humans. Consequently, relatively little effort has been devoted to the study of the human nutritional and metabolic aspects of molybdenum.

Although molybdenum nutrition receives relatively little attention, it is considered an essential nutrient for all forms of life because it is a known cofactor for some enzymes. In humans, three molybdoenzymes have been identified: aldehyde oxidase, which oxidizes and detoxifies various pyrimidines, purines, pteridines and related compounds; xanthine oxidase/dehydrogenase, which catalyzes the transformation of hypoxanthine to xanthine and of xanthine to uric acid; and sulfite oxidase, 0000 which catalyzes the transformation of sulfite to sulfate. In these enzymes, molybdenum is present at the active site in a small nonprotein cofactor containing a pterin nucleus.[95]

B.   Basis for Sports Nutrition Interest

There is relatively little reason for molybdenum to be of interest to physically active people. Molybdenum is a transition element that readily changes its oxidation state and can thus act as an electron transfer agent in oxidation-reduction reactions in which it cycles from Mo^{6+} to reduced states. This is the basis for molybdoenzymes' catalyzing the hydroxylation of various substrates using oxygen from water. Molybdenum hydroxylases may be important in metabolizing drugs and foreign compounds that enter the body.[96] Thus, low dietary molybdenum might be detrimental to an athlete's health through an inability to effectively detoxify some xenobiotic compounds.

There is some limited evidence that molybdenum may have insulin mimetic effects. Feeding high amounts of molybdenum (0.5–1.0 g/L in water plus 1.5–2.0 g/kg diet) prevented fructose-induced hyperglycemia, hyperinsulinemia and hypertension and partially prevented increased plasma triglyceride concentrations in rats.[97] Treating rats with sodium molybdate (100 mg/kg body weight per day) significantly reversed changes in carbohydrate metabolizing (both oxidation and storage) enzymes, and regulated blood sugar concentrations in rats with alloxan-induced diabetes.[98] The doses of molybdenum used in these two studies were extremely high. The estimated dietary requirement of the rat is 150 µg Mo/kg, and 100-mg Mo/kg diet not high in sulfur apparently is toxic because it reduced growth.[99] Thus, it would be irresponsible to suggest that ingesting supra nutritional intakes of molybdenum would result in insulin-like actions that could help athletic performance.

C.   Metabolism

Molybdenum in foods and in the form of soluble complexes is readily absorbed. Humans absorbed 88–93% of the molybdenum fed as ammonium molybdate in a liquid formula component of a diet.[100] In another study, about 57% of intrinsically labeled molybdenum in soy and about 88% in kale was absorbed.[101] Molybdenum absorption occurs rapidly in the stomach and throughout the small intestine, with the rate of absorption being higher in the proximal than in the distal parts. Molybdate may be transported across the gastrointestinal tract by both diffusion and active transport, but at high concentrations the relative contribution of active transport to molybdenum flux is small.[102] The absorption and retention of molybdenum are influenced strongly by interactions between molybdenum and various dietary forms of sulfur.[93]

Molybdate is transported loosely attached to erythrocytes in blood where it tends to bind specifically to α-2-macroglobulin.[103] Organs that retain the highest amounts of molybdenum are liver and kidney.[93,103] The molybdenum in liver is entirely present in macromolecular association, partly as known molybdoenzymes and the remainder as the molybdenum cofactor.[95]

After absorption, most molybdenum is turned over rapidly and eliminated as molybdate through the kidney;[100] this elimination is increased as dietary intake is increased. Thus, excretion rather than regulated absorption is the major homeostatic mechanism for molybdenum.

D.   Dietary and Supplemental Sources

Plant foods are the major sources of molybdenum in the diet and their molybdenum content depends on the content of the soil in which they are grown. Good food sources of molybdenum include legumes, grain products and nuts. Milk and milk products and organ meats (liver and kidney) also are rich sources of molybdenum. Poor sources of molybdenum include nonleguminous vegetables, fruits, oils, fats and fish.[102] Two studies of molybdenum intakes in the United States yielded average intakes ranging from 76–240 µg/day for adults.[104,105] These intakes indicate that almost all diets should meet the recommended dietary allowance (RDA) of 45 µg/day for molybdenum.[51]

E. SUPPLEMENTATION

Because molybdenum deficiency has not been unequivocally identified in humans other than the afore-mentioned individual on total parenteral nutrition, molybdenum generally is considered to be of no practical nutritional concern for humans. Consequently, relatively little effort has been expended toward studying the effect of molybdenum supplementation on health and well-being. Turnland et al[100] fed four young men five amounts of molybdenum, ranging from 22–1490 µg/day, for a period of 24 days each. No adverse effects were observed at any of the intakes. Urinary excretion of uric acid was decreased and urinary xanthine excretion was increased in response to a load dose of adenosine monophosphate when the men were adapted to the lowest molybdenum intake (22 µg/day); these findings indicate that xanthine oxidase activity was decreased by the low-molybdenum regime. In a separate study, the low-molybdate diet was fed for 102 days; no biochemical signs of deficiency were observed.[106]

Molybdenum has relatively low toxicity. Based on detrimental effects of molybdenum on reproduction and fetal development in animals, the FNB set the following ULs for molybdenum (µg/day): age 1–3 years, 300; age 4–8 years, 600; age 9–13 years, 1100; age 14–18 years, 1700; and over age 18 years, 2000.[51]

F. DIETARY RECOMMENDATIONS

The FNB set the following RDAs for molybdenum (µg/day): children 1–3 years, 17; 4–8 years, 22; 9–13 years, 34; and 14–18 years, 43. The RDA for men and women ages ≥19 years was set at 45 µg/day, except for 50 µg/day during pregnancy and lactation.[51]

G. FUTURE RESEARCH DIRECTIONS OR NEEDS

A study of male intercollegiate runners and female high-school basketball players found that a marked decrease in blood molybdenum occurred with strenuous exercise.[107] It was suggested that molybdenum deficiency was caused by strenuous exercise, but no indication of decreased performance or recovery from oxidative stress was reported with this decrease in blood molybdenum. Further studies are needed to ascertain whether athletes performing strenuous physical activity and con-suming low dietary molybdenum respond to molybdenum supplementation.

V. NICKEL

A. GENERAL PROPERTIES AND POSSIBLE METABOLIC FUNCTIONS

Nickel is essential for some lower forms of life where it participates in hydrolysis and redox reactions, regulates gene expression and stabilizes certain structures. In these roles, nickel forms ligands with sulfur, nitrogen and oxygen, and exists in oxidation states 3^+, 2^+ and 1^+. In lower forms of life, nickel has been identified as an essential component of six different enzymes: urease, hydrogenase, carbon monoxide dehydrogenase, methyl-coenzyme M reductase, Ni-superoxide dis-mutase and glyoxalase I.[108] Interestingly, the substrates or products for all these enzymes are dissolved gases: hydrogen, carbon monoxide, carbon dioxide, methane, oxygen and ammonia.

Nickel is generally not accepted as an essential nutrient for higher animals and humans, apparently because of the lack of a clearly defined specific biochemical function. However, nickel deprivation studies show that it has beneficial, if not essential, functions in several experimental models. Nickel deprivation detrimentally affects vision, sperm production and motility, blood pressure, iron metabolism and sodium homeostasis in animals.[109,110] Biochemical changes induced by nickel deprivation in chicks, goats, pigs and rats include altered metabolism of carbohydrates, amino acids and lipids and distribution of calcium, iron and zinc.[111-113] Nickel might have a function that is associated with vitamin B_{12} because the lack of this element inhibits the response to nickel supplementation when dietary nickel is low,[114] and nickel can alleviate vitamin B_{12} deficiency in higher animals.[115]

B. Basis for Sports Nutrition Interest

1. Energy Metabolism Modification

There is considerable evidence that dietary nickel influences carbohydrate and lipid metabolism in experimental animals. Some of the first studies suggesting that nickel may be essential showed that rats fed a 0.015-mg Ni/kg diet compared with those fed a 20-mg Ni/kg diet had depressed activities of enzymes that degrade glucose to pyruvate and enzymes that produce energy through the citric acid cycle; these enzymes included glucose-6-phosphate dehydrogenase, isocitrate dehydrogenase and malate dehydrogenase.[116] Also, glucose, glycogen and triglycerides were reduced in the liver, and ATP and glucose were reduced in serum of rats fed low dietary nickel.[116] The amount of nickel fed to the supplemented controls was quite high relative to the suggested nickel requirement of rats of 0.15–0.2 mg/kg diet.[117] Because this high dietary concentration of nickel can affect iron metabolism in an apparent pharmacologic manner,[118] uncertainty existed about whether the changes in carbohydrate and lipid metabolism variables were caused by a nickel deprivation or pharmacologic action. Later studies using more nutritionally balanced diets and a lower amount of nickel supplementation showed that some of the differences were probably caused by nickel deprivation. Compared with animals fed a diet supplemented with 1 mg Ni/kg, rats fed 0.013 mg Ni/kg had decreased liver activities of the lipogenic enzymes glucose-6-phosphate dehydrogenase, 6-phosphogluconate dehydrogenase, malic enzyme and fatty acid synthase.[119] Nickel deprivation also caused increased concentrations of triacylglycerol concentrations in liver and serum. Other studies have indicated that about 0.03-mg compared with 1-mg Ni/kg diet resulted in increased plasma lipids.[120] Because the enzymes affected by nickel deprivation are not nickel enzymes, the mechanism through which nickel affects glucose and lipid metabolism is not clear. However, because nickel apparently can affect iron metabolism through both physiologic and pharmacologic mechanisms,[118,119] and iron status can affect energy metabolism, some of the changes induced by nickel deprivation may have been caused by a depressed iron status or utilization. Also, the effects of nickel deprivation might have been partly caused by a change in thyroid hormone metabolism because nickel deprivation has been shown to decrease the concentrations of circulating thyroxine, triiodothyronine and free thyroxine.[121] The mechanism through which nickel affects thyroid hormone metabolism is also unknown.

Nickel supplemented in high amounts may affect glucose and lipid metabolism through affecting the action of insulin. In 1926, it was reported that nickel intensified and prolonged the hypoglycemic action of insulin administered to dogs and rabbits.[122,123] About 40 years later, it was found that nickel enhanced glucose uptake, its oxidation to carbon dioxide and incorporation into fat-pad lipids *in vitro*, thus simulating the action of insulin.[124] Nickel chloride (10 mg/kg body weight) injected before streptozotocin prevented streptozotocin-induced hyperglycemia in rats.[125] Long-term high nickel ingestion (200 mg/L as $NiCl_2$ in drinking water) by rats was found to increase insulin binding by their epididymal adipocytes.[126] Additionally, a decreased sensitivity to the anti-lipolytic response to insulin was found in adipocytes from the rats fed high nickel. This latter effect may explain why nickel-supplemented controls fed a high 20-mg Ni/kg diet had higher, while those fed a moderate 1 mg Ni/kg had lower liver triglycerides compared with rats fed about 0.015-mg Ni/kg diet (see above). That is, the high effect was pharmacologic and the moderate effect was nutritional.

The findings described above suggest that low dietary nickel impairs the activity of glucose-degrading and lipogenic enzymes and high dietary nickel can affect enhance glucose degradation and lipid concentrations through affecting insulin action. These contrasting effects of nickel at apparent deficient and pharmacologic intakes may explain some of the divergent results found with indicators of glucose and lipid metabolism in early nickel-deprivation studies; in these studies, supplemented controls were fed a 3- to 20-mg Ni/kg diet. Nonetheless, the findings indicate that nickel can affect energy metabolism.

2. Bone and Joint Health Promotion

There is evidence that nickel has beneficial effects on bone. Early findings suggesting such an effect include nickel deprivation increasing liver alkaline phosphatase acitivity in rats,[127] decreasing femur calcium and phosphorus content in rats,[128] and decreasing the calcium concentration in ribs, carpal bones and skeleton in miniature pigs.[129] Subsequently, it was found that high dietary nickel (25-mg/kg diet) improved bone-breaking variables in male broilers.[130] Nickel increased the shear fracture energy of the tibia and the shear force, stress and fracture energy of the radius. Nickel deprivation was found to decrease the bone-breaking variables maximum force and moment of inertia in rats.[131] In contrast to earlier studies in which supplemented controls were fed high dietary nickel (10–20-mg/kg diet), this study (supplemented controls fed 1-mg Ni/kg diet) did not find decreased calcium and phosphorus concentrations in the tibia. The mechanisms through which nickel affects bone strength and composition have not been defined. Nickel deprivation most likely has an effect on the organic matrix of bone because nickel was incorporated mostly in the organic phase of mouse calvaria *in vitro*,[132] and nickel can bind to cartilage oligomeric matrix protein and bring about the binding of this protein with collagen I/II and procollagen I/II.[133] In high amounts, nickel may be affecting bone composition through activating the osteoclast calcium "receptor," which results in an increase in intracellular Ca^{2+}.[134] This increase is a signal for the osteoclasts to resorb less bone.

C. METABOLISM

It is generally accepted that less than 10% of nickel ingested with food by humans or animals is absorbed.[135,136] When soluble nickel in water is ingested after an overnight fast, as much as 50%, but usually closer to 20–25% of the dose is absorbed.[136–138] Nickel absorption is heightened by iron deficiency,[139] pregnancy[140] and lactation.[141] The mechanisms involved in the transport of nickel through the gut are not conclusively established, but both active and passive processes are thought to be involved.[142,143] It has been suggested that some nickel is transported through an iron-transport system,[139] and cobalt can compete with these elements for transport.[144] Nickel homeostasis may be partially regulated by absorption from the gut. The rate of nickel transfer was greater in everted jejunal sacs from nickel-deprived than nickel-adequate rats.[145]

Nickel is transported in blood principally bound to serum albumin. Small amounts of nickel in serum are associated with the amino acids histidine and aspartic acid and with α-2-macroglobulin (nickeloplasmin).[146,147] Uptake of soluble nickel from serum into tissues is believed to be governed by ligand exchange reactions.[148] It has been suggested that histidine removes nickel from serum albumin and mediates its entry into cells. The transfer of nickel across plasma membranes apparently involves both active and diffusion mechanisms, which have not been defined. Soluble nickel may share a common transport system with magnesium or iron (e.g., transported into the cell bound to transferrin) and some soluble nickel probably enters cells via calcium channels.[148] Insoluble nickel compounds enter the cell via phagocytosis.[148]

Although fecal nickel excretion (mostly unabsorbed nickel) is 10–100 times as great as urinary excretion, most of the small fraction of absorbed nickel is rapidly and efficiently excreted through the kidney as urinary low-molecular-weight complexes.[149] In healthy humans, urinary nickel concentrations generally range from 0.1–13.3 μg/L.[148] The nickel content of sweat of humans is high (about 70 μg/L), which points to active secretion of nickel by the sweat glands.[150] Based on isotopic studies in which nickel was administered intravenously, excretion of exogenous nickel through the bile or gut is insignificant.[151,152]

D. Dietary and Supplemental Sources

Rich sources of nickel include chocolate, nuts, dried beans, peas and grains. Nickel concentrations are low in meats, milk and milk products. Typical daily dietary intakes for nickel are 70–260 µg.[153]

E. Supplementation

Because nickel has not been established as an essential element, and indicators of nickel status have not been identified, there has been no stimulus to determine the effect of nickel supplementation on healthy adults.

Except for the possibility that individuals with a nickel allergy may be sensitive to intakes of soluble nickel after fasting, there is no evidence that associates exposure to nickel through consumption of a normal diet with adverse effects on humans. The FNB,[51] however, did set an UL of 0.017 mg Ni/kg body weight/day; this translates into about 1.0 mg/day of soluble nickel salts for adolescents aged 14–18 years and adults. The UL (mg/day) set for children 1–3 years was 0.2, 4–8 years was 0.3 and 9–13 years was 0.6. The basis for the UL was a NOAEL of 5 mg/kg body weight/day for rats and an uncertainty factor of 300.

F. Dietary Recommendations

The FNB set no RDA for nickel.[51] However, based on animal studies, if a dietary requirement is found for humans, it most likely will be less than 100 µg/day.[153] Exercising individuals may have a higher nickel need than sedentary individuals because aerobic exercise increases the urinary excretion of nickel.[154]

G. Future Research Directions or Needs

Before any dietary or supplement recommendations can be made for physically active people, much needs to be learned about nickel. Foremost is the need to establish the biochemical functions or the mechanisms through which nickel is beneficial to carbohydrate, lipid and bone metabolism. Knowledge of these functions or mechanisms would permit the assessment of the effects of low and supra nutritional dietary intakes of nickel in humans. Further studies are needed to confirm that supra nutritional or pharmacologic intakes of nickel can affect carbohydrate, lipid and bone metabolism differently from physiological intakes that prevent changes caused by nickel deprivation.

VI. SILICON

A. General Properties and Possible Metabolic Functions

Silicon has long been suspected to be a beneficial bioactive, if not essential, element for humans. According to a review by Becker et al.,[155] Louis Pasteur predicted that silicon would be found to be an important therapeutic substance for many diseases. At the beginning of the 20th century, French and German reports suggested that Pasteur's prediction would become fact. These reports described therapeutic successes in treating numerous diseases, including atherosclerosis, hypertension and dermatitis with sodium silicate, simple organic silicon compounds or tea made from the silicon-rich horsetail plant.[155,156] Also, there was some thought that silicon was essential because, according to the review by Schwarz,[156] an article in 1930 stated that silicic acid was recognized as a normal constituent of the human organism, primarily of connective tissue, and the opinion was stated that "silicic acid is for connective tissue approximately of the same importance as iron for red blood cells, namely that it is simultaneously a stimulant for its formation as well as a building material for this tissue." However, by 1935, silicon in medicine and the concept of silicon's essentiality faded into obscurity as a consequence of some therapeutic failures and inadequate evidence for silicon's being biologically active. For the next 40 years, silicon as consumed in the diet was generally considered a biologically inert, harmless, nonessential element for living organisms except for some lower forms of life (silicate bacteria, diatoms, radiolarians and sponges).

In 1970, silicon once again began to receive attention as possibly being essential. That is when Carlisle[157] reported that silicon is uniquely localized in active growth areas in young bone of mice and rats. Using electron microprobe techniques, Carlisle found that the silicon concentration in bone was related to its maturity or degree of mineralization. In the early stages of bone development in bone growth areas, both silicon and calcium concentrations were very low. As osteoid tissue progressed toward mineralization, silicon and calcium concentrations rose congruently. However, when mineralization had progressed so that calcium was present in amounts found in bone apatite, silicon was just detectable. Carlisle suggested that silicon was involved in the initiation of calcification through some effect on the preosseous organic matrix. Subsequent studies by Carlisle[158] indicated that silicon had an essential function that influenced bone formation by affecting cartilage composition, particularly collagen and glycosaminoglycan content.

Although apparent deficiency signs have been found for silicon, it generally is not accepted as an essential nutrient for higher animals and humans because it lacks a clearly defined specific biochemical function. In 1978, Schwarz[156] described the difficulty in defining a biochemical function for silicon. Schwarz[159] first suggested that silicon as an ether- or ester-like derivative of silicic acid had a cross-linking role in connective tissue. In the 1978 report, based on improved silicon analyses of connective tissue, Schwarz[156] indicated that his suggestion needed to be redefined. His subsequent suggestion, because of the stability of the O-Si-O bond, was that silicon is involved in binding structures such as cell surfaces or macromolecules to each other. Recently many extracellular matrix proteins have been identified that provide a connection between cells and their surrounding matrix. This connection allows cells to monitor the composition and properties of the matrix and to respond to matrix alterations. Nielsen[160] has suggested that silicon may be necessary for the interaction between one or more of these macromolecules and osteotrophic cells, resulting in effects on cartilage composition and ultimately cartilage calcification.

Birchall and Espie[161] have suggested that the role of silicon in higher animals is to interact (as silicic acid) with aluminum species (e.g., $Al(OH)^{2+}$) to form an alumnosilicate that prevents aluminum from competing for iron binding sites (e.g., in prolyl hydroxylase), which results in decreased function. Thus, in the absence of silicon (or in the presence of excess aluminum) collagen synthesis and structure are adversely affected, which would be the basis for the observed effects of apparent silicon deficiency (e.g., bone organic matrix changes, impaired wound healing). Experimental and epidemiological findings indicate that some of the beneficial actions of high intakes of silicon may be occurring through this mechanism.[162–165] In addition to alleviating the toxicity of aluminum, high intakes of silicon apparently can be beneficial through facilitating the absorption or utilization of some essential minerals including copper,[166–168] magnesium[169] and zinc.[170]

B. BASIS FOR SPORTS NUTRITION INTEREST

Maintaining bone and joint health is the major sports nutrition interest in silicon. Shortly after her discovery of the silicon changes during events leading to calcification in bone, Carlisle[158] reported that silicon was required for normal development of bones in chicks. Leg bones of apparent silicon-deficient chicks (less than 3-mg/kg diet) compared with silicon-supplemented chicks (100 mg Si/kg diet as sodium metasilicate) were shorter and had smaller circumferences and thinner cortexes. Femurs and tibias fractured more easily under pressure and the cranial bones appeared somewhat flatter. About the same time, Schwarz and Milne[171] reported that compared with rats fed a 500-mg Si/kg diet (as sodium metasilicate), those fed a diet containing less than 5 mg Si/kg had impaired incisor pigmentation and skulls that were shorter with distorted bone structure around the eye socket. In both of these reports, the experimental animals were not growing optimally. In a follow-up report, Carlisle[172] reported that chicks treated the same as in the 1972 study showed that silicon deficiency decreased articular cartilage and water in long bones and decreased the hexosamine content of articular cartilage. Although these studies suggested that silicon is essential for higher animals, the suboptimal growth of the experimental animals and the high silicon supplementation could be interpreted as that the responses to silicon were possibly pharmacologic and thus were overcoming a dietary shortcoming of something other than a silicon deficiency. Nonetheless, the studies showed that a relatively high intake of silicon in the form of relatively soluble metasilicate had beneficial effects and no apparent toxic effects in young growing animals apparently in a suboptimal nutritional state. Living organisms generally are more sensitive to toxicity during growth and when under stress.

In 1980, Carlisle[173,174] reported that bone and cartilage abnormalities still occurred in chicks that were fed improved diets resulting in near optimal growth. When compared with chicks fed a 250-mg Si/kg diet as sodium metasilicate, chicks fed diets containing 1 mg Si/kg had tibias with a lower percentage and total amount of hexosamine, a lower percentage of collagen and a smaller proliferation zone in the epiphyseal cartilage. The skulls of silicon-deficient chicks had stunted parietal, occipital and temporal bone areas and the bone matrix lacked the normal striated trabecular pattern. The nodular pattern of the bone arrangement in silicon-deficient skulls indicated a more primitive type of bone. Carlisle[175] also reported that silicon affected the bone matrix components of skulls from 14-day-old chick embryos grown in culture. Collagen was decreased and non-collagenous protein was increased in bones grown in silicon-deficient culture; these bones also had decreased prolylhydroxylase activity. Recently, it was found that orthosilicic acid at physiological concentrations stimulates collagen type I synthesis in human osteoblast-like cells and enhances osteoblastic differentiation in culture.[176]

Because the studies of both Schwarz and Carlisle were clouded by the use of high, possibly pharmacological, amounts of fairly soluble silicon for supplemental controls, the effects of silicon deprivation in rats were reexamined by Seaborn and Nielsen.[177–179] In these studies, supplemented controls were fed a diet containing only 4.5–35 mg Si/kg as sodium metasilicate and compared with rats fed diets containing ≤ 2 mg Si/kg. These studies confirmed that silicon deprivation affects bone, hexosamine and collagen metabolism. Silicon deprivation decreased femur acid and alkaline phosphatase, and humerus hydroxyproline and plasma ornithine aminotransferase (a key enzyme in collagen synthesis). A recent study[180] found that silicon deprivation decreased plasma osteopontin concentration, increased plasma sialic acid concentration and increased urinary helical peptide (bone collagen breakdown product) excretion. Also, the response of bone metabolism indicators to ovariectomy in young growing rats was generally lower in silicon-deprived than silicon-supplemented rats. It was concluded that the findings support the hypothesis that silicon has a biochemical function that affects bone growth processes before bone crystal formation, and this occurs by affecting bone collagen turnover and sialic acid-containing extracellular matrix proteins such as osteopontin.

Whether it is by affecting the formation and structure of collagen, the binding of macromolecules to cell receptor sites, or the utilization or absorption of some mineral affecting bone formation, there is evidence that increased silicon consumption is beneficial to bone health. Jugdaohsingh et al.[181] reported that in a cross-sectional, population-based study (2847 participants), dietary silicon correlated positively and significantly with bone mineral density at all hip sites in men and premenopausal women, which suggests that increased silicon intake is associated with increased cortical bone mineral density in these populations.

C. Metabolism

The mechanisms involved in the intestinal absorption and blood transport of silicon are unknown. A study with guinea pigs indicated that silicon is absorbed mainly as monomeric silicic acid.[182] In humans, monosilicic acid in foods and beverages is readily absorbed, penetrates all body fluids and tissues at concentrations less than its solubility (0.01%) and is excreted in urine.[183] Some of the absorbed monosilicic acid can come from food polymeric silica, which can be partly dissolved by fluids of the gastrointestinal tract. Silicon absorption in rats has been found to be affected by age, sex and the activity of various endocrine glands.[184] Silicon is not protein-bound in plasma, where it is believed to exist almost entirely as undissociated monomeric silicic acid.[185] Silicon entering the blood stream apparently is transferred rapidly to tissues and urine because the silicon concentration in blood remains relatively constant in the presence of divergent intakes.[186] Recent analyses indicate that human serum contains 11–25 µg/dL.[187,188] Connective tissues, including aorta, bone, skin, tendon and trachea, contain much of the silicon that is retained in the body.[175,189] Absorbed silicon is mainly eliminated via the urine, where it probably exists as orthosilicic acid or magnesium orthosilicate.[175,185] The upper limits of urinary excretion apparently are set by the rate and extent of silicon absorption and not by the excretory ability of the kidney because peritoneal injection of silicon can elevate urinary excretion above the upper limit achieved by dietary intake.[182] This suggests that silicon homeostasis is controlled by absorption mechanisms in addition to excretory mechanisms. This suggestion is supported by the finding that in rats, guinea pigs, cattle and sheep, the urinary excretion of silicon increases with an increasing intake of siliceous substances, but reaches a maximum that is not exceeded by increasing the intake.[190]

Within 2 hours of ingestion of a trace dose of ^{32}silicon, uptake was complete in a healthy male.[191] Within 48 hours, 36% of the dose was excreted in the urine and the elimination was nearly complete. Elimination occurred by two simultaneous first-order processes with half-lives of 2.7 and 11.3 hours, representing about 90% and 10%, respectively, of the total output. It was suggested that the rapidly eliminated silicon was probably retained in the extracellular fluid volume, while the slower component may have represented intracellular uptake and release. In another study of silicon kinetics,[192] silicon peaked in blood about 1 hour after an intake of 27–55 mg orthosilicic acid/L of water in eight healthy adults. Renal clearance was 82–90 mL/min, which is similar to that found earlier.[185] These clearances suggest a high renal filtration.

D. DIETARY AND SUPPLEMENTAL SOURCES

The form of dietary silicon has a major influence on its absorption. For example, humans absorbed about 1% of a large dose of an aluminosilicate compound but absorbed >70% of a single dose of methylsilanetriol, a drug developed for the treatment of circulatory ischemia.[193] Silicon was found to be absorbed better from stabilized orthosilicic acid than from herbal silica (*Equisetum arvense* extract) or colloidal silicic acid.[188]

Early balance studies with animals indicated that almost all ingested silicon is unabsorbed. The finding of low absorption probably resulted from the intake of highly unavailable silicon and the intake of silicon that exceeded the amount needed to achieve maximal absorption. Thus, these studies may be misleading about the bioavailabilty of silicon when consumed in low or mg quantities in various foods. Recently, it was found that an average of 41% of dietary silicon was excreted in the urine (an indicator of absorption).[194] Silicon in grains and grain products was readily absorbed, as indicated by a mean urinary excretion of 49 ± 34% of intake. In several of the grain products, silicon was as available as it was from fluids. For example, urinary silicon excretion was 41–86% from corn flakes, white rice and brown rice and 50–86% from mineral waters. Silicon in fruits and vegetables, except green beans and raisins, was readily absorbed, with a mean urinary excretion of 21 ± 29% of intake. Some forms of dietary fiber may affect silicon bioavailability because in humans, a diet high in fiber from fruits and vegetables significantly depressed silicon balance.[195]

The average daily intakes of silicon apparently range from 20–50 mg/day.[196] The richest sources of silicon are unrefined grains of high fiber content, and cereal products, including beer. Meat, fish and dairy products are poor sources of silicon. A source of oral silicon is additives to prepared foods, confections and pharmaceuticals. Amorphous silicates are considered safe additions to foods. Their use as anti-caking agents, for example, is permitted up to 2% by weight. A generally recognized as safe (GRAS) committee concluded that silicates added to foods to enhance physical properties are relatively inert and thus not bioavailable.

E. SUPPLEMENTATION

Silicon is another element for which there has been very little recent effort to ascertain whether supplementation would have beneficial effects in humans, apparently because of the lack of a defined biochemical function and indicators of silicon status.

Ingested silicon has a relatively low order of toxicity. About the only pathological condition that may occur with a high intake of silicon is urolithiasis. Most silicon compounds, especially silicon dioxide compounds, are essentially nontoxic to humans when taken orally. Magnesium trisilicate, an over-the-counter antacid, has been used by humans for more than 40 years with only minimal apparent deleterious effects reported. In addition to urolithiasis, a high intake of silicon may interfere with the absorption or utilization of some essential nutrient, particularly zinc. An antagonism between zinc and silicon results in high dietary silicon's decreasing the zinc concentrations in plasma and tissues of rats.[166,167] The amount of dietary silicon used to show the antagonism was extremely high in one study;[167] the rats were fed 400 mg Si/kg body weight as sodium metasilicate in drinking water for the last 6 weeks of an 18-week experiment. In the other study,[166] the effect of a 270-mg Si/kg diet as tetraethylorthosilicate on decreasing plasma zinc was significant only in zinc-deficient rats.

Because of the inadequacy of available data, the FNB[51] established no UL for silicon. In the United Kingdom, a safe upper level of 12 mg/kg body weight/day has been suggested for humans. This level was based on an animal study in which a no-observed-adverse-effect-level (NOAEL) of a 50,000-mg/kg diet of supplemental dietary silica, equivalent to 2500 mg/kg body weight/day in rats and 7500 mg/kg body weight/day in mice was found.[197] This seems to be a conservative value, considering the NOAEL and that intakes of 35–45 mg Si/kg body weight/day has been found beneficial for bone and brain health in experimental animals. Based on the latter finding, a safe silicon intake for a 70-kg man probably is greater than 2 g/day.

F. DIETARY RECOMMENDATIONS

The FNB set no dietary reference intakes (DRI) for silicon.[51] On the basis of weak balance data, a recommended silicon intake of 30–35 mg/day was suggested for athletes; this was 5–10 mg higher than for non-athletes.[198] Based on extrapolations from animal data, Seaborn and Nielsen[199] speculated that a recommended intake may be between 5 and 10 mg/day. Others have suggested that a daily minimum requirement may be near 10–25 mg based on the amount excreted in urine in 24 hours.[188,200]

G. FUTURE RESEARCH DIRECTIONS OR NEEDS

Before any dietary or supplement recommendations can be made for physically active people, much needs to be learned about silicon. Foremost is the need to establish a biochemical function or mechanism through which silicon is beneficial to bone. Knowledge of the function or mechanism would facilitate the development of silicon status indicators and the assessment of the effects of low and supra nutritional dietary silicon intakes in humans. Silicon status indicators are needed to determine whether a low silicon status that responds to increased silicon intakes is a significant sports nutritional concern.

VII. VANADIUM

A. GENERAL PROPERTIES AND POSSIBLE METABOLIC FUNCTIONS

Since the turn of the 19th century, when some French physicians suggested vanadium was a panacea for human disorders, vanadium has been proposed numerous times to be of pharmacological or nutritional importance.[201] The hypothesis that vanadium has a physiological or essential role in higher animals and humans has gone through periods where it has received much credence then followed by much skepticism.[201] At present, vanadium is generally not accepted as an essential nutrient because a specific biochemical function has not been defined for vanadium at physiological intakes.

There is no question that vanadium is a bioactive element. Its ability to selectively inhibit protein tyrosine phosphatases at submicromolar concentrations probably explains the broad range of effects that high intakes causing elevated tissue vanadium concentrations have on cellular regulatory cascades.[202] Protein tyrosine phosphatase inhibition is thought to be the basis for vanadium's having insulin-like actions at the cellular level and stimulating cellular proliferation and differentiation. The insulin-mimetic action of vanadium has resulted in an effort to develop vanadium compounds that could be therapeutic agents for diabetes.[203] In addition to having effects at pharmacological intakes, vanadium may affect phosphorylation/dephosphorylation at physiological or nutritional intakes such that a regulatory cascade is altered. This may be the basis for observations that vanadium deprivation altered thyroid hormone metabolism,[201,204] impaired reproduction[205] and altered bone morphology.[205,206]

Vanadium is essential for some lower forms of life where it is required for some enzymes.[207] Vanadium-dependent bromoperoxidases have been found in a number of marine brown algae, marine red algae and a terrestrial lichen. Vanadium-dependent iodoperoxidases have been detected in brown seaweeds, and a vanadium-dependent chloroperoxidase has been identified in the fungus *Curvularia inaequalis*. These haloperoxidases catalyze the oxidation of halide ions by hydrogen peroxide, thus facilitating the formation of a carbon–halogen bond. The enzymatic roles for vanadium in lower forms of life suggest the possibility that vanadium has a similar role in higher forms of life.

B. BASIS FOR SPORTS NUTRITION INTEREST

1. Insulinomimetic Actions

The insulin-like actions of vanadium have been well reviewed.[203,208] According to these reviews, the anti-diabetic effect of vanadium was first reported more than 100 years ago, but its potential as an orally active insulin-mimetic agent was stimulated by reports beginning in 1985. Since then, studies with animal models of type 1 diabetes showed that chronic treatment with vanadium salts lowered plasma glucose concentration, increased peripheral glucose utilization and normalized hepatic glucose output, but had no effect on plasma insulin concentration. One of the reviews[203] noted that the vanadium supplementation had no or minor effects on plasma glucose and insulin concentrations in normal control animals. Treatment of human patients with type 1 diabetes reduced insulin requirements. Several organic vanadium compounds have been developed and, in addition to inorganic vanadium compounds, have been examined as potential therapeutic agents for type 2 diabetes. The vanadium compounds significantly decreased plasma insulin concentrations and improved insulin sensitivity in several animal models of insulin resistance and type 2 diabetes. Oral treatment of type 2 diabetic humans with vanadium reduced fasting plasma glucose concentrations, suppressed hepatic glucose production and improved insulin sensitivity in skeletal muscle. Treatment with vanadyl sulfate had no effect on insulin sensitivity and fasting plasma glucose and insulin concentrations in healthy adults; an observation made for several animal models. The mechanisms through which vanadium has insulin-mimetic actions are not completely understood. Suggested mechanisms include inhibition of key gluconeogenic enzymes and the inhibition of protein tyrosine phosphatases. Vanadium inhibition of protein dephosphorylation would indirectly enhance insulin receptor or insulin receptor substrate phosphorylation and thus its action.

The amounts of vanadium used in animals to show insulin-mimetic actions were extremely high relative to normal intakes. In some cases, the intakes were toxic and caused poor growth and diarrhea. The vanadium doses in human experiments were about 100-fold lower than those used for most studies of diabetic animal models. Still, the doses used (e.g., 100 mg vanadyl sulfate or 125 mg sodium metavanadate per day[209–212]) were an order of magnitude greater than possible nutritional needs (described below).

Insulin has an anabolic effect on skeletal muscle and other tissues through promoting amino acid uptake and protein synthesis while retarding protein degradation. Thus, reports that vanadium has efficacy in some animal models of both type 1 and type 2 diabetes was quickly extrapolated by supplement marketers as evidence that vanadium has anabolic effects and thus can be used to enhance muscle building, strength and performance. This thought persists now, although it has been shown that not all effects of insulin are mimicked by vanadium; the exceptions include that of vanadium's not affecting amino acid uptake and protein synthesis.[203] Also, the promotion of vanadium supplements ignores the finding that vanadium has no marked insulin-like effect on healthy animals and humans.

2. Bone and Joint Health Promotion

One of the first vanadium-deprivation signs reported for chicks was adverse effects on bone development.[206] Histological examination of the tibias from vanadium-deprived chicks revealed severe disorganization of the cells of the epiphysis. The cells appeared compressed and their nuclei flattened. These abnormalities apparently were the reason that vanadium-deprived chicks had a shortened, thickened leg structure. Bone abnormalities were also found in vanadium-deprived goats.[205] Compared with goats fed a 0.5–2-mg V/kg diet, goats fed less than 10 μg/kg diet exhibited pain in the extremities, swollen forefoot tarsal joints and skeletal deformations in the forelegs. These changes in bone suggest that vanadium may have a role that affects bone or connective tissue metabolism. This suggestion is supported by the finding that vanadium stimulated the mineralization of bones and teeth[213] and the repair of bones.[214] Orthovanadate stimulates bone cell proliferation and collagen synthesis *in vitro*.[215,216] Also, orthovanadate increased phosphotyrosine levels and inhibited collagenase production by chondrocytes *in vitro*.[217] Recent studies suggest that the mechanism through which vanadium affects bone metabolism is through modifying phosphorylation/ dephosphorylation reactions that affect growth factor action. Vanadium supplementation reverses many of the symptoms of osteoporosis caused by high-dose glucocorticoids in adult rats.[202] Osteoblasts are mitogenically repressed by high-dose glucocorticoids and this correlates with decreased extracellular signal-regulated kinase (ERK) activation in response to growth factors. Vanadate restores sensitivity to growth factors at the levels of both ERK activation and cell proliferation.[202]

In the experiments showing that vanadium had a beneficial effect on bone, the amounts of vanadium used in supplemented animals and cells were high relative to those that may be needed nutritionally. For example, in the chick and goat deprivation studies, the supplemented controls were fed diets containing 0.5–3.0 mg V/kg; apparent nutritional deficiency signs required feeding diets containing less than 25 μg/kg diet.[218] The diets used may have been unbalanced in some nutrients.[216] Thus, one cannot dismiss the possibility that the high vanadium supplementation was acting pharmacologically to overcome bone changes induced by something other than a simple vanadium deficiency. Such a possibility is supported by the finding that a 0.5-mg V/kg diet increased plasma cortisol in guinea pigs, which indicates that vanadium was a stressor, or acting in a nonnutritional manner.[219] These guinea pigs also exhibited increased bone calcium and magnesium concentrations. Further study is required to establish whether low dietary vanadium intakes increase the susceptibility to bone loss and whether supra nutritional intakes of vanadium can help prevent bone loss in conditions where phosphatase activity is excessive.

C. Metabolism

Most ingested vanadium is unabsorbed and is excreted in the feces.[220,221] Because very low concentrations of vanadium, generally <0.8 μg/L, are found in urine, compared with estimated daily intakes of 12–30 μg and the fecal content of vanadium, apparently <5% of vanadium ingested normally is absorbed.[220] Animal studies generally support the concept that vanadium is poorly absorbed. However, some results from rats indicate that vanadium absorption can exceed 10%

under some conditions, a finding that suggests caution in assuming that ingested vanadium is always poorly absorbed from the gastrointestinal tract.[221]

Most vanadium that is absorbed is probably transformed in the stomach to the vanadyl ion and remains in this form as it passes into the duodenum.[222] The mechanisms involved in the absorption of vanadium in the cationic or vanadyl (VO^{2+}) form are unknown. *In vitro* studies suggest that vanadium in the anionic or vanadate (HVO_4^{2-}) form can enter cells through phosphate or other anion transport systems.[223] Vanadate is absorbed three to five times more effectively than vanadyl.[224] Apparently the different absorbability rates for vanadate and vanadyl, the effect of other dietary components on the binding and forms of vanadium in the stomach and the rate at which vanadate is transformed into vanadyl markedly affect the percentage of ingested vanadium absorbed. Other dietary substances that apparently affect the binding and forms of vanadium in the stomach include chromium, protein, ferrous ion, chloride and aluminum hydroxide.[220]

When vanadate appears in the blood, it is quickly converted into the vanadyl cation.[225] However, as a result of oxygen tension, vanadate still exists in blood. Vanadyl, the most prevalent form of vanadium in blood, is bound and transported by transferrin and albumin.[225] Vanadate is transported by transferrin only.[226] Vanadyl also complexes with ferritin in plasma and body fluids.[227,228] It remains to be determined whether vanadyl-transferrin can transfer vanadium into cells through the transferrin receptor or whether ferritin is a storage vehicle for vanadium. Vanadium is rapidly removed from plasma and is generally retained in tissues under normal conditions at concentrations less than 10 ng/g fresh weight.[220] Bone apparently is a major sink for excessive retained vanadium.

Excretion patterns after parenteral administration[229,230] indicate that urine is the major excretory route for absorbed vanadium. However, a significant portion of absorbed vanadium may be excreted through the bile.[229]

D. DIETARY AND SUPPLEMENTAL SOURCES

Typical human diets generally supply <30 μg V/day.[220] Foods rich in vanadium (>40 ng/g) include shellfish, mushrooms, parsley, black pepper and some prepared foods. Cereals, liver and fish tend to have intermediate amounts of vanadium (5–40 ng/g). Beverages, fats and oils, fresh fruits and fresh vegetables generally contain <5 ng/g and often <1 ng/g.[220]

Upon the erroneous extrapolation of insulin-mimetic effects of vanadium to having anabolic effects on skeletal muscle, a proliferation of powders, beverages, formulas and supplements containing alarming amounts of vanadium appeared in the market. These supplements contained quantities of vanadium that could result in some individuals' consuming more than the 1.8 mg/day UL set by the FNB,[51] and sometimes approaching the 14–20 mg/day that was found to have toxic effects in humans.[220]

E. SUPPLEMENTATION

Although there have been several studies examining the response of diabetic subjects to vanadium supplementation (see above), only a few have examined the effect of vanadium supplementation on strength, performance and bone and heart health indices of healthy adults. Fawcett et al.[231] determined the effect of supplemental 0.5 mg vanadyl sulfate/kg body weight/day on body composition and performance in a study involving 40 individuals using weight training as part of their fitness program; 31 completed the 12-week, double-blind, placebo-controlled study. It was concluded that the vanadium supplement was ineffective in changing body composition in weight-training athletes. There was a significant vanadium effect in one performance variable (leg extension), but this finding was compromised by the fact that the vanadium-supplemented group started at a lower baseline than the placebo group. Thus, this modest performance-enhancing effect requires confirmation. About 20% of the subjects taking the vanadium supplement reported the side effect of fatigue.

Compared with elements such as silicon and manganese, vanadium is a relatively toxic element for humans. As indicated in the following, the threshold level for toxicity through ingestion apparently is between 10–20 mg/day. Schroeder et al.[232] fed 15 subjects 4.5 and 9 mg V/day as diammonium oxytartratovanadate for 6–16 months without apparent detrimental effect. Curran et al.[233] fed five subjects 13.5 mg/day in three divided doses as diammonium oxytartratovanadate for 6 weeks; no sign of intolerance or toxicity was found. In contrast, Sommerville and Davis[234] supplemented 12 subjects 13.5 mg/day for 2 weeks and then 22.5 mg V/day for 5 months as diammonium vanadotartrate; five patients exhibited persistent upper abdominal pain, anorexia, nausea and weight loss. Dimond et al.[235] supplemented ammonium vanadyl tartrate orally to six subjects for 6–10 weeks in amounts ranging from 4.5–18 mg V/day; green tongue, cramps and diarrhea were observed at the larger doses. Based on renal effects in experimental animals, the FNB[51] set an UL of 1.8 mg/day for adults ≥ 19 years of age.

F. Dietary Recommendations

The FNB set no RDA for vanadium.[51] However, based on animal studies, any human requirement to prevent deficiency pathology for vanadium would be small. A daily dietary intake of 10–15 µg probably would meet any postulated requirement.

G. Future Research Directions or Needs

Research is needed to determine the validity of having supplements containing high amounts of vanadium in the marketplace. This research should definitively establish the toxicity threshold for vanadium and determine whether long-term high consumption of vanadium could lead to pathological disorders such as hypertension.[236,237] Studies are needed to determine whether supra nutritional, but non-toxic, intakes of vanadium enhance athletic performance or bone health. Definition of a biochemical function for vanadium at physiological intakes is needed before this element can be considered essential. Definition of an essential function would help differentiate between nutritional and pharmacological actions of vanadium and could be used to determine whether low dietary intakes of vanadium are of practical nutrition concern for the general public in addition to athletes. It is obvious that it is premature to recommend vanadium supplements for enhancing strength, muscle mass and athletic performance.

VIII. SUMMARY

Although boron, manganese, molybdenum, nickel, silicon and vanadium are not considered significant nutritional minerals, they have received some attention in the sports nutrition field because of findings suggesting that they could enhance strength, performance or endurance in athletic activities. Most of these findings have come from experimental animals and have not been substantiated by carefully controlled human studies. At present, there is inadequate evidence to suggest that increasing the intake or consuming supra nutritional amounts of any of these six minerals would be of benefit for athletic performance or increasing muscle mass. However, findings from animal experiments and limited clinical studies suggest that further study is needed to determine whether increased intakes of one or more of these elements would be of benefit for the physically active person. Some of the more intriguing possible studies based on these findings would be those determining whether a safe (non-toxic) supra nutritional intake of boron enhances bone strength, energy utilization, or endurance; manganese enhances energy utilization or endurance; nickel enhances energy utilization or bone strength, silicon enhances bone strength; or vanadium enhances energy utilization or bone strength. Also of interest would be the determination of whether low intakes of any of these elements result in an impairment in athletic performance, bone strength or endurance that could be overcome by diets providing nutritionally adequate amounts of the element.

REFERENCES

1. Woods, W.G., An introduction to boron: History, sources, uses and chemistry, *Environ. Health Perspect.*, 102 (Suppl. 7), 5, 1994.
2. Hunt, C.D., Regulation of enzymatic activity. One possible role of dietary boron in higher animals and humans, *Biol. Trace Elem. Res.*, 205, 1998.
3. Dunitz, J.D., Hawley, D.M., Miklos, D., White, D.N.J., Berlin, Y., Marusic, R. and Prelog, V., Structure of boromycin, *Helv. Chim. Acta* 54, 1709, 1971.
4. Sato, K., Okazaki, T., Maeda, K. and Okami, Y., New antibiotics, aplasmomycins B and C, *J. Antibiot. (Tokyo)* 31, 632, 1978.
5. Schummer, D., Irschik, H., Reichenbach, H. and Hofle, G., Antibiotics from gliding bacteria. LVII. Tartrolons: New boron-containing macrodiolides from *Sorangium cellulosum, Liebigs Ann. Chem.*1994, 283, 1994.
6. O'Neill, M.A., Warrenfeltz, D., Kates, K., Pellerin, P., Doco, T., Darvill, A.G. and Albersheim, P., Rhamnogalacturonan II, a pectic polysaccharide in the wall of growing plant cells, forms a dimer that is covalently cross-linked by a borate ester. *In vitro* conditions for the formation and hydrolysis of the dimer, *J. Biol. Chem.*, 271, 22923, 1996.
7. Matoh, T., Boron in plant cell walls, *Plant Soil* 193, 59, 1997.
8. Chen, X., Schauder, S., Potier, N., Van Dorsselaer, A., Pelczer, I., Bassier, B.L. and Hughson, F.M., Structural identification of a bacterial quorum-sensing signal containing boron. *Nature (London)*, 415, 545, 2002.
9. Fort, D.J., Rogers, R.L., McLaughlin, D.W., Sellers, C.M. and Schlekat, C.L., Impact of boron deficiency on *Xenopus laevis*. A summary of biological effects and potential biochemical roles. *Biol. Trace Elem. Res.*, 77, 173, 2002.
10. Eckhert, C.D. and Rowe, R.I., Embryonic dysplasia and adult retinal dystrophy in boron-deficient zebrafish, *J. Trace Elem. Exp. Med.*, 12, 213, 1999.
11. Nielsen, F.H., Biochemical and physiologic consequences of boron deprivation in humans, *Environ. Health Perspect.*, 102 (Suppl. 7), 59, 1994.
12. World Health Organization, Boron, in Trace Elements in Human Nutrition and Health, World Health Organization, Geneva, 175, 1996.
13. Ralston, N.V.C. and Hunt, C.D., Diadenosine phosphates and *S*-adenosylmethionine: novel boron binding biomolecules detected by capillary electrophoresis, *Biochim. Biophys. Acta*, 1527. 20, 2001.
14. Fort, D.J. and Stover, E.J., Boron deficiency disables *Xenopus laevis* oocyte maturation events, *FASEB J.*, 14, A478, 2000.
15. Nielsen, F.H., Hunt, C.D., Mullen, L.M. and Hunt, J.R., Effect of dietary boron on mineral, estrogen and testosterone metabolism in postmenopausal women, *FASEB J.*, 1, 394, 1987.
16. Samman, S., Naghii, M.R., Lyons Wall, P.M. and Verus, A.P., The nutritional and metabolic effects of boron in humans and animals, *Biol. Trace Elem. Res.*, 66, 227, 1998.
17. Naghii, M.R. and Samman, S., The effect of boron supplementation on the distribution of boron in selected tissues and on testosterone synthesis in rats, *J. Nutr. Biochem.*, 7, 507, 1996.
18. Naghii, M.R. and Samman, S., The effect of boron on plasma testosterone and plasma lipids in rats, *Nutr. Res.*17, 523, 1997.
19. Bakken, N.A. and Hunt, C.D., Dietary boron decreases peak pancreatic *in situ* insulin release in chicks and plasma insulin concentrations in rats regardless of vitamin D or magnesium status, *J., Nutr.*, 133, 3577, 2003.
20. Hunt, C.D. and Herbel, J.L., Dietary boron modifies the effects of exercise training on energy metabolism in the rat, *FASEB J.*, 6, A1946, 1992.
21. Hunt, C.D., Herbel, J.L. and Idso, J.P., Dietary boron modifies the effects of exercise training on bone and energy substrate metabolism in the rat, *FASEB J.*, 7, A204, 1993.
22. Nielsen, F.H., Evidence for the nutritional essentiality of boron, *J. Trace Elem. Exp. Med.*, 9, 215, 1996.
23. Hunt, C.D., The biochemical effects of physiologic amounts of dietary boron in animal nutrition models, *Environ. Health Perspect.*, 102 (Suppl. 7), 35, 1994.
24. Hunt, C.D., Biochemical effects of physiological amounts of dietary boron, *J. Trace Elem. Exp. Med.*, 9, 185, 1996.
25. Hunt, C.D. and Idso, J.P., Dietary boron as a physiological regulator of the normal inflammatory response: a review and current research progress, *J. Trace Elem. Exp. Med.*, 12, 221, 1999.

26. Armstrong, T.A., Spears, J.W. and Lloyd, K.E., Inflammatory response, growth and thyroid hormone concentrations are affected by long-term boron supplementation in gilts, *J. Anim. Sci.,* 79, 1549, 2001.

27. Nielsen, F.H. and Poellot, R., Boron status affects differences in blood immune cell populations in rat fed diets containing fish oil or safflower oil, in *Macro and Trace Elements (Mengen- und Spurenelement), vol.* 2, Anke, M., Flachowsky, G., Kisters, K., Müller, R., Schäfer, U., Schenkel, H., Seifert, M. and Stoeppler, M., Eds., Schubert-Verlag, Leipzig, 2004, 959.

28. Hunt, C.D., Dietary boron: An overview of the evidence for its role in immune function, *J. Trace Elem. Exp. Med.,* 16, 291, 2003.

29. Ali, S., Diwakar, G., Pawa, S., Siddiqui, M.R., Jain, S.K. and Abdulla, M., Attenuation by boron supplementation of the biochemical changes associated with thioacetamide-induced hepatic lesions, *J. Trace Elem. Exp. Med.,* 15, 47, 2002.

30. Hunt, C.D. and Nielsen, F.H., Interaction between boron and cholecalciferol in the chick, in *Trace Element Metabolism in Man and Animals (TEMA-4),* Howell, J.McC., Gawthorne, J.M. and White, C.L., Eds., Australian Academy of Science, Canberra, 1981, 597.

31. Bai, Y. and Hunt, C.D., Dietary boron enhances efficacy of cholecalciferol in broiler chicks, *J. Trace Elem. Exp. Med.,* 9, 117, 1996.

32. Sheng, M.H.-C., Taper, L.J., Veit, H., Qian, H., Ritchey, S.J. and Lau, K.-H.W., Dietary boron supplementation enhanced the action of estrogen, but not that of parathyroid hormone, to improve trabecular bone quality in ovariectomized rats, *Biol. Trace Elem. Res.,* 82, 109, 2001.

33. Sheng, M.H.-C., Taper, L.J., Veit, H., Thomas, E.A., Ritchey, S.J. and Lau, K.-H.W., Dietary boron supplementation enhances the effects of estrogen on bone mineral balance in ovariectomized rats, *Biol. Trace Elem. Res.,* 81, 29, 2001.

34. Armstrong, T.A., Spears, J.W., Crenshaw, T.D. and Nielsen, F.H., Boron supplementation of a semi-purified diet for weanling pigs improves feed efficiency and bone strength characteristics and alters plasma lipid metabolites, *J. Nutr.,* 139, 2575, 2000.

35. Nielsen, F.H., Dietary fat composition modifies the effect of boron on bone characteristics and plasma lipids in rats, *Biofactors,* 20, 161, 2004.

36. Rossi, A.F., Miles, R.D., Damron, B.L. and Flunker, L.K., Effects of dietary boron supplementation on broilers, *Poult. Sci.,* 72, 2124, 1993.

37. Wilson, J.H. and Ruszler, P.L., Effects of boron on growing pullets, *Biol. Trace Elem. Res.,* 56, 287, 1997.

38. Wilson, J.H. and Ruszler, P.L., Long term effects of boron on layer bone strength and production parameters, *Brit. Poult. Sci.,* 39, 11, 1998.

39. Chapin, R.E., Ku, W.W., Kenney, M.A. and McCoy, H., The effects of dietary boric acid on bone strength in rats, *Biol. Trace Elem. Res.,* 66, 395, 1998.

40. Rico, H., Crespo, E., Hernandez, E.R., Seco, C. and Crespo, R., Influence of boron supplementation on vertebral and femoral bone mass in rats on strenuous treadmill exercise: A morphometric, densitometric and histomorphometric study, *J. Clin. Densitometry,* 5, 187, 2002.

41. Nielsen, F.H. and Penland, J.G., Boron supplementation of perimenopausal women affects boron metabolism and indices associated with macromineral metabolism, hormonal status and immune function, *J. Trace Elem. Exp. Med.,* 12, 251, 1999.

42. Sutherland, B. Woodhouse, L.R., Strong, P. and King, J.C., Boron balance in humans, *J. Trace Elem. Exp. Med.,* 12, 271, 1999.

43. Hunt, C.D., Herbel, J.L. and Nielsen, F.H., Metabolic responses of postmenopausal women to supplemental dietary boron and aluminum during usual and low magnesium intake: Boron, calcium and magnesium absorption and retention and blood mineral concentrations, *Am. J. Clin. Nutr.,* 803, 1997.

44. Hunt, C.D., Shuler, T.R. and Mullen, L.M., Concentration of boron and other elements in human foods and personal-care products, *J. Am. Diet. Assoc.,* 91, 558, 1991.

45. Anderson, D.L., Cunningham, W.C. and Lindstrom, T.R., Concentrations and intakes of H, B, S, K, Na, Cl and NaCl in foods, *J. Food Comp. Anal.* 7, 59, 1994.

46. Rainey, C.J., Nyquist, L.A., Christensen, R.E., Strong, P.L., Culver, B.D. and Coughlin, J.R., Daily boron intake from the American diet, *J. Am. Diet. Assoc.,* 99, 335, 1999.

47. Hunt, C.D. and Meacham, S.L., Aluminum, boron, calcium, copper, iron, magnesium, manganese, molybdenum, phosphorus, potassium, sodium and zinc: concentrations in common Western foods and estimated daily intakes by infants, toddlers, and male and female adolescents, adults and seniors in the United States, *J. Am. Diet. Assoc.,* 101, 1058, 2001.

48. Meacham, S.L., Taper, L.J. and Volpe, S.L., Effect of boron supplementation on blood and urinary calcium, magnesium and phosphorus and urinary boron in athletic and sedentary women, *Am. J. Clin. Nutr.,* 61, 341, 1995.

49. Green, N.R. and Ferrando, A.A., Plasma boron and the effects of boron supplementation in males, *Environ. Health Perspect.* 102 (Suppl. 7), 73, 1994.

50. National Research Council, *Mineral Tolerance of Domestic Animals,* National Academy of Sciences, Washington, D.C., In press.

51. FNB, Institute of Medicine, Dietary Reference Intakes. Vitamin A, Vitamin K, Arsenic, Boron, Chromium, Copper, Iodine, Iron, Manganese, Molybdenum, Nickel, Silicon, Vanadium and Zinc, National Academy Press, Washington, D.C., 2001.

52. Freeland-Graves, J. and Llanes, C., Models to study manganese deficiency, in *Manganese in Health and Disease,* Klimis-Tavantzis, D.J., Ed., CRC Press, Boca Raton, FL, 59, 1994.

53. Johnson, P.E. and Lykken, G.I., Manganese and calcium absorption and balance in young women fed diets with varying amounts of manganese and calcium, *J. Trace Elem. Exp. Med.,* 4, 19, 1991.

54. Norose, N. and Arai, K., Manganese deficiency due to long-term total parenteral nutrition in an infant, *Jap. J. Parent Ent. Nutr.,* 9, 978, 1987.

55. Norose, N., Manganese deficiency in a child with very short bowel syndrome receiving long-term parenteral nutrition, *J. Trace Elem. Exp. Med.,* 4, 100, 1992.

56. Klimis-Tavantzis, D.J., Ed., *Manganese in Health and Disease,* CRC Press, Boca Raton, FL, 1994.

57. Leach, R.M., Jr. and Harris, E.D., Manganese, in *Handbook of Nutritionally Essential Minerals,* O'Dell, B.L. and Sunde, R.A., Eds., Marcel Dekker, New York, 335, 1997.

58. Baly, D.L., Keen, C.L. and Hurley, L.S., Pyruvate carboxylase and phosphoenolpyruvate carboxykinase activity in developing rats: Effect of manganese deficiency, *J. Nutr.,* 115, 872, 1985.

59. Baly, D.L., Keen, C.L. and Hurley, L.S., Effects of manganese deficiency on pyruvate carboxylase and phosphoenolpyruvate carboxykinase activity and carbohydrate homeostasis in adult rats, *Biol. Trace Elem. Res.,* 11, 201, 1986.

60. Everson, G.J. and Shrader, R.E., Abnormal glucose tolerance in manganese-deficient guinea pigs, *J. Nutr.,* 94, 89, 1968.

61. Baly, D., Curry, D.L., Keen, C.L. and Hurley, L.S., Effect of manganese deficiency on insulin secretion and carbohydrate homeostasis in rats, *J. Nutr.,* 114, 1438, 1984.

62. Baly, D., Curry, D.L., Keen, C.L. and Hurley, L.S., Dynamics of insulin and glucagon release in rats: influence of dietary manganese, *Endocrinology,* 116, 1734, 1985.

63. Keen, C.L., Zidenberg-Cherr, S. and Lönnerdal, B., Nutritional and toxicological aspects of manganese intake; and overview, in *Risk Assessment of Essential Elements,* Mertz, W., Abernathy, C.O. and Olin, S.S., Eds., ILSI Press, Washington, D.C., 221, 1994.

64. Baly, D.L., Lee, I. and Doshi, R., Mechanism of decreased insulinogenesis in manganese-deficient rats: Decreased insulin mRNA levels, *Fed. Eur. Biochem. Soc.,* 239, 55, 1988.

65. Baly, D.L., Schneiderman, J.S. and Garcia-Welsh, A.L., Effect of manganese deficiency on insulin binding, glucose transport and metabolism in rat adipocytes, *J. Nutr.,* 120, 1075, 1990.

66. Li, Y., Huang, T.-T., Carlson, E.J., Melov, S., Ursell, P.C., Olson, J.L., Noble, L.J., Yoshimura, M.P., Berger, C., Chan, P.H., Wallace, D.L. and Epstein, C.J., Dilated cardiomyopathy and neonatal lethality in mutant mice lacking manganese superoxide dismutase, *Nature Genetics,* 11, 376, 1995.

67. Wheeler, M.D., Nakagami, M., Bradford, B.U., Uesugi, T., Mason, R.P., Connor, H.D., Dikalova, A., Kadiiska, M. and Thurman, R.G., Overexpression of manganese superoxide dismutase prevents alcohol-induced liver injury in the rat, *J. Biol. Chem.,* 276, 36664, 2001.

68. Jones, S.P., Hoffmeyer, M.R., Sharp, B.R., Ho, Y.-S. and Lefer, D.J., Overexpression of manganese but not copper/zinc superoxide dismutase (SOD) attenuates myocardial injury following ischemia and reperfusion, *FASEB J.,* A464, 2001.

69. Ilizarov, A.M., Koo, H.-C., Kazzaz, J.A., Mantell, L.L., Li, Y., Bhapat, R., Pollack, S., Horowitz, S. and Davis, J.M., Overexpression of manganese superoxide dismutase protects lung epithelial cells against oxidant injury, *Am. J. Respir. Cell Mol. Biol.,* 24, 436, 2001.

70. Kiningham, K.K., Oberley, T.D., Lin, S., Mattingly, C.A. and St. Clair, D.K., Overexpression of manganese superoxide dismutase protects against mitochondrial-initiated poly(ADP-ribose) polymerase-mediated cell death, *FASEB J.,* 13, 1601, 1999.

71. Malecki, E.A. and Greger, J.L., Manganese protects against heart mitochondrial lipid peroxidation in rats fed high levels of polyunsaturated fatty acids, *J. Nutr.,* 126, 27, 1996.

72. Kuzuya, T., Nishida, M., Hoshida, S., Yamashita, N., Hori, M. and Tada, M., Manganese superoxide dismutase induced by extracellular stress enhances myocardial tolerance to ischemia-reperfusion, in *The Ischemic Heart,* Mochizuki, S., Takeda, N., Nagano, M. and Dhalla, N., Eds., Kluwer Academic Publishers, Boston, 379, 1998.

73. Hamilton, K.L., Powers, S.K., Sugiura, T., Kim, S., Lennon, S. Turner, N. and Mehta, J.L., Short-term exercise training can improve myocardial tolerance to I/R without elevation in heat shock proteins, *Am. J. Physiol. Heart Circulatory Physiol.,* 281, 350, 2001.

74. Hoshida, S., Yamashita, N., Otsu, K. and Hori, M., Repeated physiologic stresses provide persistent cardioprotection against ischemia-reperfusion injury in rats, *J. Amer. Coll. Cardiol.,* 40, 826, 2002.

75. Hamilton, K.L., Quindry, J.C., French, J.P., Staib, J., Hughes, J., Mehta, J.L. and Powers, S.K., MnSOD antisense treatment and exercise-induced protection against arrhythmias, *Free Radical Biol. Med.,* 37, 1360, 2004.

76. Strause, L., Saltman, P. and Glowacke, H., The effect of deficiencies of manganese and copper on osteoinduction and on resorption of bone particles in rats, *Calcif. Tissue Int.,* 41, 145, 1987.

77. Clegg, M.S., Donovan, S.M., Monaco, M.H., Baly, D.L., Ensunsa, J.L. and Keen, C.L., The influence of manganese deficiency on serum IGF-1 and IGF binding proteins in the male rat, *Proc. Soc. Exp. Biol. Med.,* 219, 41, 1998.

78. Strause, L.G., Hegenauer, J., Saltman, P., Cone, R. and Resnick, D., Effects of long-term dietary manganese and copper deficiency on rat skeleton, *J. Nutr.,* 116, 135, 1986.

79. Davis, C.D., Zech, L. and Greger, J.L., Manganese metabolism in rats: An improved methodology for assessing gut endogenous losses, *Proc. Soc. Exp. Biol. Med.,* 202, 103, 1993.

80. Wiegand, E., Kirchgessner, M. and Helbig, U., True absorption and endogenous fecal excretion of manganese in relation to its dietary supply in growing rats, *Biol. Trace Elem. Res.,* 10, 265, 1986.

81. Davis, C.D., Wolf, T.L. and Greger, J.L., Varying levels of manganese and iron affect absorption and gut endogenous losses of manganese by rats, *J. Nutr.,* 122, 1300, 1992.

82. Garcia-Aranda, J.A., Wapnir, R.A. and Lifshitz, F., *In vivo* intestinal absorption of manganese in the rat, *J. Nutr.,* 113, 2601, 1983.

83. Bell, J.G., Keen, C.L. and Lönnerdal, B., Higher retention of manganese in suckling than in adult rats is not due to maturational differences in manganese uptake by rat small intestines, *J. Toxicol., Environ. Health,* 26, 387, 1989.

84. Finley, J.W. and Monroe, P., Mn absorption: The use of Caco-2 cells as a model of the intestinal epithelium, *Nutr. Biochem.,* 8, 92, 1997.

85. Freeland-Graves, J., Derivation of manganese estimated safe and adequate daily dietary intakes, in *Risk Assessment of Essential Elements,* Mertz, W., Abernathy, C.O. and Olin, S.S., Eds., ILSI Press, Washington, D.C., 237, 1994.

86. Pennington, J.A.T. and Young, B.E., Total diet study nutritional elements 1982–1989, *J. Am. Diet. Assoc.,* 71, 179, 1991.

87. Davis, C.D. and Greger, J.L., Longitudinal changes of manganese-dependent superoxide dismutase and other indexes of manganese and iron status in women, *Am. J. Clin. Nutr.,* 55, 747, 1992.

88. Finley, J.W., Penland, J.G., Pettit, R.E. and Davis, C.D., Dietary manganese intake and type of lipid do not affect clinical or neuropsychological measures in healthy young women, *J. Nutr.,* 133, 2849, 2003.

89. Lucchini, R., Albini, E., Cortesi, I., Placidi, D., Bergamaschi, E., Traversa, F. and Alessio, L., Brain magnetic resonance imaging and manganese exposure, *NeuroToxicol.* 21, 769, 2000.

90. Aschner, M., Manganese neurotoxicity and oxidative damage, in *Metals and Oxidative Damage in Neurological Disorders,* Connor, J.R., Ed., Plenum Press, New York, 77, 1997.

91. Miller, K.B., Caton, J.S., Schafer, D.M., Finley, J.W. and Smith, D.J., High dietary manganese lowers heart magnesium in pigs fed a low-magnesium diet, *J. Nutr.,* 130, 2032, 2000.

92. Nasolodin, V.V., Gladkikh, I.P. and Meshcheriakov, S.I., Providing athletes with trace elements during intensive exercise (in Russian), *Gig. Sanit.* 1, 54, 2001.

93. Mills, C.F. and Davis, G.K., Molybdenum, in *Trace Elements in Human and Animal Nutrition,* Vol. 1, Mertz, W., Ed., Academic Press, San Diego, 429, 1987.

94. Abumrad, N.N., Schneider, A.J., Steel, D. and Rogers, L.S., Amino acid intolerance during prolonged total parenteral nutrition reversed by molybdate therapy, *Am. J. Clin. Nutr.,* 34, 2551, 1981.

95. Johnson, J.L., Molybdenum, in *Handbook of Nutritionally Essential Mineral Elements,* O'Dell, B.L. and Sunde, R.A., Eds., Marcel Dekker, New York, 413, 1997.

96. Beedham, C., Molybdenum hydroxylases as drug-metabolizing enzymes, *Drug Metab. Rev.*, 16, 119, 1985.

97. Güner, S., Tay, A., Altan, V.M. and Özçelikay, A.T., Effect of sodium molybdate on fructose-induced hyperinsulinemia and hypertension in rats, *Trace Elem. Electrolytes*, 18, 39, 2001.

98. Panneerselvam, R.S. and Govindaswamy, S., Effect of sodium molybdate on carbohydrate metabolizing enzymes in alloxan-induced diabetic rats, *J. Nutr. Biochem.*, 13, 21, 2002.

99. National Research Council, Nutrient requirements of the laboratory rat, in *Nutrient Requirements of Laboratory Animals, Fourth Revised Edition*, National Academy Press, Washington, D.C., 11, 1995.

100. Turnland, J.R., Keyes, W.R., Peiffer, G.L., Molybdenum absorption, excretion and retention studied with stable isotopes in young men at five intakes of dietary molybdenum, *Am. J. Clin. Nutr.*, 62, 70, 1995.

101. Turnland, J.R., Weaver, C.M., Kim, S.K., Keyes, W.R., Gizaw, Y., Thompson, K.H. and Peiffer, G.L., Molybdenum absorption and utilization in humans from soy and kale intrinsically labeled with stable isotopes of molybdenum, *Am. J. Clin. Nutr.*, 69, 1217, 1999.

102. Nielsen, F.H., Other trace elements, in *Present Knowledge in Nutrition*, 7th ed., Ziegler, E.E. and Filer, L.J., Jr., Eds., ILSI Press, Washington, D.C., 353, 1996.

103. Lener, J. and Bibr, B., Effects of molybdenum on the organism (a review), *J. Hyg. Epidemiol. Microbiol. Immunol.*, 28, 405, 1984.

104. Tsongas, T.A., Meglen, R.R., Walravens, P.A. and Chappell, W.R., Molybdenum in the diet: an estimate of average daily intake in the United States, *Am. J. Clin. Nutr.*, 33, 1103, 1980.

105. Pennington, J.A.T. and Jones, J.W., Molybdenum, nickel, cobalt, vanadium and strontium in total diets, *J. Am. Diet. Assoc.*, 87, 1644, 1987.

106. Turnland, J.R., Keyes, W.R., Peiffer, G.L. and Chiang, G., Molybdenum absorption, excretion and retention studied with stable isotopes in young men during depletion and repletion, *Am. J. Clin. Nutr.*, 61, 1102, 1995.

107. Kondo, M., Sasaki, Y., Miyamoto, H. and Ohmichi, M., Decrease in blood molybdenum (Mo) concentration as a result of competitive sports activities, *Biomed. Res. Trace Elem.*, 14, 316, 2003.

108. Watt, R.K. and Ludden, P.W., Nickel-binding proteins, *Cell Mol. Life*, 56, 604, 1999.

109. Nielsen, F.H., Yokoi, K. and Uthus, E.O., The essential role of nickel affects physiological functions regulated by the cyclic-GMP signal transduction system, in *Metal Ions in Biology and Medicine*, Vol. 7, Khassanova, L., Collery, P., Maymard, I., Khassanova, Z. and Etienne, J.-C. Eds., John Libbey Eurotext, Paris, 29, 2002.

110. Yokoi, K., Uthus, E.O. and Nielsen, F.H., Nickel deficiency diminishes sperm quantity and movement in rats, *Biol. Trace Elem. Res.*, 93, 141, 2003.

111. Anke, M., Groppel, B. and Hennig, A., Nickel, an essential trace-element, in *Mengen- und Spurenelemente*, Vol. 2, Anke, M., Brückner, Gürtler, H. and Grün, M., Eds., Karl-Marx-Universität, Leipzig, 404, 1984.

112. Stangl, G.I. and Kirchgessner, M., Effect of nickel deficiency on fatty acid composition of total lipids and individual phospholipids in brain and erythrocytes of rats, *Nutr. Res.*, 17, 137, 1997.

113. Nielsen, F.H., The emergence of boron, nickel, silicon, vanadium and arsenic as elements of nutritional relevance, in *Trace Elements in Nutrition, Health and Disease*, Antoniades, N., Schrauzer, G.N., Renard, N. and Wozniak, J., Eds., Institut-Rosell-The Americas, Montreal, 93, 2001.

114. Nielsen, F.H., Zimmerman, T.J., Shuler, T.R., Brossart, B. and Uthus, E.O., Evidence for a cooperative metabolic relationship between nickel and vitamin B_{12} in rats, *J. Trace Elem. Exp. Med.*, 2, 21, 1989.

115. Stangl, G.I., Roth-Maier, D.A. and Kirchgessner, M., Vitamin B-12 deficiency and hyperhomocysteinemia are partly ameliorated by cobalt and nickel supplementation in pigs, *J. Nutr.*, 130, 3038, 2000.

116. Kirchgessner, M. and Schnegg, A., Biochemical and physiological effects of nickel deficiency, in *Nickel in the Environment*, Nriagu, J.O., Ed., John Wiley & Sons, New York, 635, 1980.

117. Nielsen, F.H., The ultratrace elements, in *Trace Minerals in Foods*, Smith, K.T., Ed., Marcel Dekker, New York, 357, 1988.

118. Nielsen, F.H., Shuler, T.R., McLeod, T.G. and Zimmerman, T.J., Nickel influences iron metabolism through physiologic, pharmacologic and toxicologic mechanisms in the rat, *J. Nutr.*, 114, 1280, 1984.

119. Stangl, G.I. and Kirchgessner, M., Nickel deficiency alters liver lipid metabolism in rats, *J. Nutr.*, 126, 2466, 1996.

120. Nielsen, F.H., Yokoi, K. and Uthus, E.O., Marginal dietary pyridoxine and supplemental dietary homocystine and methionine affect the response of the rat to nickel deprivation, in *Metal Ions in Biology and Medicine, Vol. 6*, Centeno, J.A., Collery, P., Vernet, G., Finkelman, R.B., Gibb, H. and Etienne, J.-C., Eds., John Libbey Eurotext, Paris, 524, 2000.

121. Stangl, G.I. and Kirchgessner, M., Comparative effects of nickel and iron depletion on circulating thyroid hormone concentrations in rats, *J. Anim. Physiol. Anim. Nutr.* 79, 18, 1998.

122. Bertrand, G. and Mâchebœuf, M., Influence du nickel et du cobalt sur l'action exercée par l'insuline, chez le lapin, *Comptes Rendus,* 182, 1504, 1926.

123. Bertrand, G. and Mâchebœuf, M., Influence du nickel et du cobalt sur l'action exercée par l'insuline chez le chien, *Comptes Rendus,* 183, 5, 1926.

124. Dixit, P.K. and Lazarow, A., Effects of metal ions and sulfhydryl inhibitors on glucose metabolism by adipose tissue, *Am. J. Physiol.,* 213, 849, 1967.

125. Novelli, E.L.B., Rodrigues, N.L. and Ribas, B.O., Effect of nickel chloride on streptozotocin-induced diabetes in rats, *Can. J. Physiol. Pharmacol.,* 66, 663, 1988.

126. Mayor, P., Cabrera, R., Ribas, B. and Calle, C., Effect of long-term nickel ingestion on insulin binding and antilipolytic response in rat adipocytes, *Biol. Trace Elem. Res.,* 22, 63, 1989.

127. Schnegg, A. and Kirchgessner, M., Alkalische und Saure Phosphatase-Aktivität in Leber und Serum bei Ni-bsz. Fe-Mangel, *Internat. Z. Vit. Ern. Forschung,* 47, 274, 1977.

128. Kirchgessner, M., Perth, J. and Schnegg, A., Mangelnde Ni-Versorgung und Ca-, Mg- und P-Gehalte im Knochen wachsender Ratten, *Arch. Tierernährung,* 30, 805, 1980.

129. Anke, M., Grün, M., Dittrich, G., Groppel, B. and Henning, A., Low nickel rations for growth and reproduction in pigs, in *Trace Element Metabolism in Animals-2,* Hoekstra, W.G., Suttie, J.W., Ganther, H.E. and Mertz, W., Eds., University Park Press, Baltimore, 715, 1974.

130. Wilson, J.H., Wilson, E.J. and Ruszler, P.L., Dietary nickel improves male broiler (*Gallus domesticus*) bone strength, *Biol. Trace Elem. Res.,* 83, 239, 2001.

131. Nielsen, F.H., The effect of nickel deprivation on bone strength and shape and urinary phosphorus excretion is not enhanced by a mild magnesium deprivation in rats, in *Macro and Trace Elements, Mengen- und Spurenelemente,* Vol. 2, Anke, M., Flachowsky, M., Kisters, K., Müller, R., Schäfer, U., Schenkel, H., Seifert, M. and Stoeppler, M., Eds., Schubert-Verlag, Leipzig, 965, 2004.

132. Jacobsen, N. and Jonsen, J., Strontium, lead and nickel incorporation into mouse calvaria *in vitro, Path. Europ.,* 10, 115, 1975.

133. Rosenberg, K., Olsson, H., Morgelin, M. and Heinegard, D., Cartilage oligomeric matrix protein shows high affinity zinc-dependent interaction with triple helical collagen, *J. Biol. Chem.,* 273, 20397, 1998.

134. Shankar, V., Bax, C.M.R., Bax, B.E., Towhidul Alam, A.S.M., Moonga, B.S., Simon, B., Pazianas, M., Huang, C.L.-H. and Zaidi, M., Activation of the Ca^{2+} "receptor" on the osteoclast by Ni^{2+} elicits cytosolic Ca^{2+} signals: Evidence for receptor activation and inactivation, intracellular Ca^{2+} redistribution and divalent cation modulation, *J. Cell. Physiol.,* 155, 120, 1993.

135. Niebor, E., Tom, R.T. and Sanford, W.E., Nickel metabolism in man and animals, in *Metal Ions in Biological Systems, Vol. 23, Nickel and Its Role in Biology,* Sigel, H. and Sigel, A., Eds., Marcel Dekker, New York, 91, 1988.

136. Arnich, N., Cunat, L., Lanhers, M.-C. and Burnel, D., Comparative *in situ* study of the intestinal absorption of aluminum, manganese, nickel and lead in rats, *Biol. Trace Elem. Res.,* 99, 157, 2004.

137. Solomons, N.W., Viteri, F., Shuler, T.R. and Nielsen, F.H., Bioavailability of nickel in man. Effects of foods and chemically-defined dietary constituents on the absorption of inorganic nickel, *J. Nutr.,* 112, 39, 1982.

138. Sunderman, F.W., Jr., Hopfer, S.M., Swift, T., Ziebka, L., Marcus, A.H., Most, B.M. and Creason, J., Nickel absorption and elimination in human volunteers, in *Trace Elements in Man and Animals 6,* Hurley, L.S., Keen, C.L., Lönnerdal, B. and Rucker, R.B., Eds., Plenum Press, New York, 427, 1988.

139. Tallkvist, J. and Tjälve, H., Effect of iron-deficiency on the disposition of nickel in rats, *Toxicol. Lett.,* 92, 131, 1997.

140. Kirchgessner, M., Spörl, R. and Roth-Maier, D.A., Exkretion im Kot und scheinbare Absorption von Kupfer, Zink, Nickel und Mangan bei nichtgraviden und graviden Sauen mit unterschiedlicher Spurenelementversorgung, *Z. Tierphysiol. Tierernhr. Futtermittelkd.,* 44, 98, 1980.

141. Kirchgessner, M., Roth-Maier, D.A. and Spörl, R., Spurenelementbilanzen (Cu, Zn, Ni, und Mn) laktierender Sauen, *Z. Tierphysiol. Tierernhr. Futtermittelkd.,* 50, 230, 1983.

142. Foulkes, E.C. and McMullen, D.M., On the mechanism of nickel absorption in the rat jejunum, *Toxicol.,* 38, 35, 1986.

143. Tallkvist, J. and Tjälve, H., Transport of nickel across monolayers of human intestinal Caco-2 cells, *Toxicol. Appl. Pharmacol.,* 151, 117, 1998.

144. Eidelsburger, U., Stangl, G.I. and Kirchgessner, M., The effect of nickel, iron and cobalt on nickel absorption in nickel-deficient and nickel-control rats using everted intestinal segments, *Trace Elem. Electrol.*, 13, 182, 1996.

145. Stangl, G.I., Eidelsburger, U. and Kirchgessner, M., Nickel deficiency alters nickel flux in rat everted intestinal sacs, *Biol. Trace Elem. Res.*, 61, 253, 1998.

146. Tabata, M. and Sarkar, B., Specific nickel(II)-transfer process between the native sequence peptide representing the nickel(II)-transport site of human albumin and L-histidine, *J. Inorg. Biochem.*, 45, 93, 1992.

147. Nomoto, S. and Sunderman, F.W., Jr., Presence of nickel in alpha-2-macroglobulin isolated from human serum by high performance liquid chromatography, *Ann. Clin. Lab. Sci.*, 18, 78, 1988.

148. Sutherland, J.E. and Costa, M., Nickel, in *Heavy Metals in the Environment,* Sarkar, B., Ed., Marcel Dekker, New York, 349, 2002.

149. Predki, P.F., Whitfield, D.M. and Sarkar, B., Characterization and cellular distribution of acidic peptide and oligosaccharide metal-binding compounds from kidneys, *Biochem. J.*, 281, 835, 1992.

150. Omokhodion, F.O. and Howard, J.M., Trace elements in the sweat of acclimatized persons, *Clin. Chem. Acta,* 231, 23, 1994.

151. Marzouk, A. and Sunderman, F.W., Jr., Biliary excretion of nickel in rats, *Toxicol. Lett.*, 27, 65, 1985.

152. Patriarca, M., Lyon, T.D.B. and Fell, G.S., Nickel metabolism in humans investigated with an oral stable isotope, *Am. J. Clin. Nutr.*, 66, 616, 1997.

153. Nielsen, F.H., Ultratrace elements in nutrition: Current knowledge and speculation, *J. Trace Elem. Exp. Med.*, 11, 251, 1998.

154. Gatteschi, L., Bavazzano, P., Locatelli, F., Rosendahl, K., Resina, A. and Rubenni, M.G., Effects of aerobic exercise on urinary excretion of chromium and nickel, in *Trace Elements in Man and Animals – TEMA 8,* Anke, M., Meissner, D. and Mills, C.F., Eds., Verlag Media Touristik, Gersdorf, 394, 1993.

155. Becker, C.-H., Matthias, D., Wooßmann, H., Schwartz, A. and Engler, E., Investigations on a possible medical importance of silicon, in 4. *Spurenelement-Symposium,* Anke, M., Baumann, W., Bräunlich, H. and Brückner, Eds., Friedrich-Schiller-Universität, Jena, 142, 1983.

156. Schwarz, K., Significance and functions of silicon in warm-blooded animals. Review and outlook, in *Biochemistry of Silicon and Related Problems,* Bendz, G. and Lindquist, I., Eds., Plenum Press, New York, 207, 1978.

157. Carlisle, E. M., Silicon: A possible factor in bone calcification, *Science,* 167, 279, 1970.

158. Carlisle, E.M., Silicon: An essential element for the chick, *Science,* 178, 619, 1972.

159. Schwarz, K., A bound form of silicon in glycosaminoglycans and polyuronides, *Proc. Nat. Acad. Sci. USA,* 70, 1608, 1973.

160. Nielsen, F.H., Nutritional requirements for boron, silicon, vanadium, nickel and arsenic: current knowledge and speculation, *FASEB J.*, 5, 2661, 1991.

161. Birchall, J.D. and Espie, A.W., Biological implications of the interaction (via silanol groups) of silicon with metal ions, in *Silicon Biochemistry, Ciba Foundation Symposium* 121, Evered, D. and O'Connor, M., Eds., John Wiley & Sons, Chichester, 140, 1986.

162. Carlisle, E.M. and Curran, M.J., Effect of dietary silicon and aluminum on silicon and aluminum levels in rat brain, *Alzheimer Dis. Assoc. Disorders,* 1, 83, 1987.

163. Bellés, M., Sánchez, D.J., Gómez, M., Corbella, J. and Domingo, J.L., Silicon reduces aluminum accumulation in rats: relevance to the aluminum hypothesis of Alzheimer Disease, *Alzheimer Dis. Assoc. Disorders,* 12, 83, 1998.

164. Jacqmin-Gadda, H., Commenges, D., Letenneur, L. and Dartigues, J.-F., Silica and aluminum in drinking water and cognitive impairment in the elderly, *Epidemiology,* 7, 281, 1996.

165. Forbes, W.F., Agwani, N. and Lachmaniuk, P., Geochemical risk factors for mental functioning, based on the Ontario Longitudinal Study of Aging (LSA) IV. The role of silicon-containing compounds, *Can. J. Aging,* 14, 630, 1995.

166. Emerick, R. and Kayongo-Male, H., Silicon facilitation of copper utilization in the rat, *J. Nutr. Biochem.*, 1, 487, 1990.

167. Najda, J., Gmiński, J., Drózdz, M. and Danch, A., Silicon metabolism. The interrelations of inorganic silicon (Si) with systemic hypersilicemia, *Biol. Trace Elem. Res.*, 34, 185, 1992.

168. Kayongo-Male, H. and Palmer, I.S., Copper-silicon interaction studies in young, rapidly growing turkeys fed semipurified starter diets, *Biol. Trace Elem. Res.*, 63, 195, 1998.

169. Kikunaga, S., Kitano, T., Kikukawa, T. and Takahashi, M., Effects of fluoride and silicon on distribution of minerals in the magnesium-deficient rat, *Maguneshumu (Kyoto)*, 10, 181, 1991.

170. Evenson, D.P., Emerick, R.J., Jost, L.K., Kayongo-Male, H. and Stewart, S.R., Zinc-silicon interactions influencing sperm chromatin integrity and testicular cell development in the rat as measured by flow cytometry, *J. Anim. Sci.*, 71, 955, 1993.

171. Schwarz, K. and Milne, D.B., Growth-promoting effects of silicon in rats, *Nature*, 239, 333, 1972.

172. Carlisle, E.M., *In vivo* requirement for silicon in articular cartilage and connective tissue formation in the chick, *J. Nutr.*, 106, 478, 1976.

173. Carlisle, E.M., A silicon requirement for normal skull formation in chicks, *J. Nutr.*, 110, 352, 1980.

174. Carlisle, E.M., Biochemical and morphological changes associated with long bone abnormalities in silicon deficiency, *J. Nutr.*, 110, 1046, 1980.

175. Carlisle, E.M., Silicon, in *Handbook of Nutritionally Essential Mineral Elements*, O'Dell, B.L. and Sunde, R.A., Eds., Marcel Dekker, New York, 603, 1997.

176. Reffitt, D.M., Ogston, N., Jugdaohsingh, R., Cheung, H.F.J., Evans, B.F.J., Thompson, R.P.H., Powell, J.J. and Hampson, G.N., Orthosilicic acid stimulates collagen type I synthesis and osteoblastic differentiation in human osteoblast-like cells *in vitro*, *Bone*, 32, 127, 2003.

177. Seaborn, C.D. and Nielsen, F.H., Dietary silicon affects acid and alkaline phosphatase and ^{45}calcium uptake in bone of rats, *J. Trace Elem. Exp. Med.*, 7, 11, 1994.

178. Seaborn, C.D. and Nielsen, F.H., Silicon deprivation and arginine and cystine supplementation affect bone collagen and bone and plasma trace mineral concentrations in rats, *J. Trace Elem. Exp. Med.*, 15, 113, 2002.

179. Seaborn, C.D. and Nielsen, F.H., Silicon deprivation decreases collagen formation in wounds and bone and ornithine transaminase enzyme activity in liver, *Biol. Trace Elem. Res.*, 89, 251, 2002.

180. Nielsen, F.H. and Poellot, R., Dietary silicon affects bone turnover differently in ovariectomized and sham-operated growing rats, *J. Trace Elem. Exp. Med.*, 17, 137, 2004.

181. Jugdaohsingh, R., Tucker, K.L., Qiao, N., Cupples, L.A., Kiel, D.P. and Powell, J.J., Dietary silicon intake is positively associated with bone mineral density in men and premenopausal women of the Framingham offspring cohort, *J. Bone Min. Res.*, 19, 297, 2004.

182. Sauer, F., Laughland, D.H. and Davidson, W.M., Silica metabolism in guinea pigs, *Can. J. Biochem. Physiol.*, 37, 183, 1959.

183. Baumann, H., Verhatten der Kieselsaure im menschlichen Blut und Harn, *Hoppe-Seyler's Z. Physiol. Chem.*, 320, 1960.

184. Charnot, Y. and Pérès, G., Contribution à l'étude de la regulation endocrinienne du métabolisme silicique, *Ann. Endocrinol.*, 32, 397, 1971.

185. Berlyne, G.M., Adler, A.J., Ferran, N., Bennett, S. and Holt, J., Silicon metabolism. I. Some aspects of renal silicon handling in normal man, *Nephron*, 43, 5, 1986.

186. Dobbie, J.W. and Smith, M.J.B., Urinary and serum silicon in normal and uraemic individuals, in *Silicon Biochemistry, Ciba Foundation Symposium* 121, Evered, D. and O'Connor, M., Eds., John Wiley & Sons, Chichester, 194, 1986.

187. Van Dyck, K., Robberecht, H., Van Cauwenbergh, R., Van Vlaslaer, V. and Deelstra, H., Indication of silicon essentiality in humans. Serum concentrations in Belgian children and adults, including pregnant women, *Biol. Trace Elem. Res.*, 77, 25, 2000.

188. Calomme, M.R., Cos, P., D'Haese, P.C., Vingerhoets, R., Lamberts, L.V., De Broe, M.E., Van Hoorebeke, C. and Vanden Berghe, D.A., Absorption of silicon in healthy subjects, in *Metal Ions in Biology and Medicine*, Vol. 5, Collery, Ph., Brätter, P., Negretti de Brätter, V., Khassanova, L., Etienne, J.C., Eds., John Libbey Eurotext, Paris, 228, 1998.

189. Adler, A.J., Etzion, Z. and Berlyne, G.M., Uptake, distribution and excretion of ^{31}silicon in normal rats, *Am. J. Physiol.*, 251, E670, 1986.

190. Bailey, C.B., Silica metabolism and silica urolithiasis in ruminants: A review, *Can. J. Anim. Sci.*, 61, 219, 1981.

191. Popplewell, J.F., King, S.J., Day, J.P., Ackrill, P., Fifield, L.K., Cresswell, R.G., di Tada, M.L. and Liu, K., Kinetics of uptake and elimination of silicic acid by a human subject: a novel application of ^{32}Si and accelerator mass spectrometry, *J. Inorg. Biochem.*, 69, 177, 1998.

192. Reffitt, D.M., Jugdaohsingh, R., Thompson, R.P. and Powell, J.J., Silicic acid: Its gastrointestinal uptake and urinary excretion in man and effects on aluminum excretion, *J. Inorg. Biochem.* 76, 141, 1999.

193. Allain, P., Cailleux, A., Mauras, Y. and Renier, J.C., Etude de l'absorption digestive du silicium après administration unique chez l'homme sous forme de salicylate de methyl silane triol, *Therapie*, 38, 171, 1983.

194. Jugdaohsingh, R., Anderson, S.H.C., Tucker, K.L., Elliott, H., Kiel, D.P., Thompson, R.P.H. and Powell, J.J., Dietary silicon intake and absorption, *Am. J. Clin. Nutr.*, 75, 887, 2002.

195. Kelsay, J.L., Behall, K.M. and Prather, E.S., Effect of fiber from fruits and vegetables on metabolic responses of human subjects. II. Calcium, magnesium, iron and silicon balances, *Am. J. Clin. Nutr.*, 32, 1876, 1979.

196. Pennington, J.A.T., Silicon in foods and diets, *Food Add. Contam.*, 8, 97, 1991.

197. Takizawa, Y., Hirasawa, F., Noritomo, E., Aida, M., Tsunoda, H. and Uesugi, S., Oral ingestion of syloid to mice and rats and its chronic toxicity and carcinogenicity, *Acta Med. Biol.*, 36, 27, 1988.

198. Nasolodin, V.V., Rusin, V.Y. and Vorob'ev, V.A., Zinc and silicon metabolism in highly trained athletes under hard physical stress (in Russian), *Vopr. Pitan.*, 4, 37, 1987.

199. Seaborn, C.D. and Nielsen, F.H., Silicon: A nutritional beneficence for bones, brains and blood vessels?, *Nutr. Today*, 28, 13, 1993.

200. Carlisle, E.M., Silicon as an essential trace element in animal nutrition, in *Silicon Biochemistry, Ciba Foundation Symposium* 121, Evered, D. and O'Connor, M., Eds., John Wiley & Sons, Chichester, 123, 1986.

201. Nielsen, F.H., The nutritional essentiality and physiological metabolism of vanadium in higher animals, in *Vanadium Compounds. Chemistry, Biochemistry and Therapeutic Applications, ACS Symposium Series* 711, Tracey, A.S. and Crans, D.C., Eds., American Chemical Society, Washington, D.C., 297, 1998.

202. Hulley, P. and Davison, A., Regulation of tyrosine phosphorylation cascades by phosphatases: What the actions of vanadium teach us, *J. Trace Elem. Exp. Med.*, 16, 281, 2003.

203. Marzban, L. and McNeill, J.H., Insulin-like actions of vanadium: Potential as a therapeutic agent, *J. Trace Elem. Exp. Med.*, 16, 253, 2003.

204. Uthus, E.O. and Nielsen, F.H., Effect of vanadium, iodine and their interaction on growth, blood variables, liver trace elements and thyroid status indices in rats, *Magnesium Trace Elem.*, 9, 219, 1990.

205. Anke, M., Groppel, B., Arnhold, W., Langer, M. and Krause, U., The influence of the ultra trace element deficiency (Mo, Ni, As, Cd, V) on growth, reproduction performance and life expectancy, in *Trace Elements in Clinical Medicine*, Tomita, H., Ed., Springer-Verlag, Tokyo, 361, 1990.

206. Nielsen, F.H. and Sandstead, H.H., Are nickel, vanadium, silicon, fluorine and tin essential for man?, *Am. J. Clin. Nutr.*, 27, 515, 1974.

207. Wever, R. and Krenn, B.E., Vanadium haloperoxidases, in *Vanadium in Biological Systems*, Chasteen, N.D., Ed., Kluwer Academic, Dordrecht, 81, 1990.

208. Sakurai, H. and Tsuji, A., Antidiabetic action of vanadium complexes in animals: Blood glucose normalizing effect, organ distribution of vanadium and mechanism for insulin-mimetic action, in *Vanadium in the Environment, Part 2: Health Effects*, Nriagu, J.O., Ed., John Wiley & Sons, New York, 297, 1998.

209. Cohen, N., Halbertstam, M., Shlimovich, P., Chang, C.J., Shamoon, H. and Rossetti, L., Oral vanadyl sulfate improves hepatic and peripheral insulin sensitivity in patients with non-insulin-dependent diabetes mellitus, *J. Clin. Invest.*, 95, 2501, 1995.

210. Goldfine, A.B., Simonson, D.C., Folli, F., Patti, M.-E. and Kahn, R., Metabolic effects of sodium metavanadate in humans with insulin-dependent and noninsulin-dependent diabetes mellitus *in vivo* and *in vitro* studies, *J. Clin. Endocrinol. Metab.*, 80, 3311, 1995.

211. Halbertstam, M., Cohen, N., Shlimovich, P., Rossetti, L. and Shamoon, H., Oral vanadyl sulfate improves insulin sensitivity in NIDDM but not in obese nondiabetic subjects, *Diabetes*, 45, 659, 1996.

212. Boden, G., Chen, X., Ruiz, J., van Rossum, G.D.V. and Turco, S., Effects of vanadyl sulfate on carbohydrate and lipid metabolism in patients with non-insulin-dependent diabetes mellitus, *Metabolism*, 45, 1130, 1996.

213. Rygh, O., Recherches sur les oligo-éléments. II. De l'importance du thallium et du vanadium, du silicum et du fluor, *Bull. Soc. Chim. Biol.*, 31, 1403 and 1408, 1949.

214. Nemsadze, O.D., Effect of the trace element vanadium on reparative regeneration of bone tissue in the mandible (in Russian), *Stomatologiya (Moscow)*, 56, 1, 1977.

215. Lau, K.-H.W., Tanimoto, H. and Baylink, D.J., Vanadate stimulates bone cell proliferation and bone collagen synthesis *in vitro*, *Endocrinology*, 123, 2858, 1988.

216. Canalis, E., Effect of sodium vanadate on deoxyribonucleic acid and protein syntheses in cultured rat calvariae, *Endocrinology,* 116, 855, 1985.

217. Cruz, T., Mills, G., Pritzker, K.P.H. and Kandel, R.A., Inverse correlation between tyrosine phosphorylation and collagenase production in chondrocytes, *Biochem. J.,* 269, 717., 1990.

218. Nielsen, F.H. and Uthus, E.O., III. The essentiality and metabolism of vanadium, in *Vanadium in Biological Systems,* Chasteen, N.D., Ed., Kluwer Academic Publishers, Dordrecht, 51, 1990.

219. Seaborn, C.D., Mitchell, E.D. and Stoecker, B.J., Vanadium and ascorbate effects on 3-hydroxy-3-methylglutaryl coenzyme A reductase, cholesterol and tissue minerals in guinea pigs fed low-chromium diets, *Magnesium Trace Elem.,* 10, 327, 1991–1992.

220. Nielsen, F.H., Vanadium in mammalian physiology and nutrition, in *Metal Ions in Biological Systems, Vol. 31. Vanadium and Its Role in Life,* Sigel, H. and Sigel, A., Eds., Marcel Dekker, New York, 543, 1995.

221. Setyawati, I.A., Thompson, K.H., Yuen, V.G., Sun, Y., Battell, M., Lyster, D.M., Vo, C., Ruth, T.J., Zeisler, S., McNeill, J.H. and Orvig, C., Kinetic analysis and comparison of uptake, distribution and excretion of ^{48}V-labeled compounds in rats, *J. Appl. Physiol.,* 84, 569, 1998.

222. Chasteen, N.D., Lord, E.M. and Thompson, H.J., Vanadium metabolism. Vanadyl (IV) electron paramagnetic resonance spectroscopy of selected tissues in the rat, in *Frontiers in Bioinorganic Chemistry,* Xavier, A.V., Ed., VCH Verlagsgesellschaft, Weinheim, 133, 1986.

223. Cantley, L.C., Jr., Resh, M.D. and Guidotti, G., Vanadate inhibits the red cell (Na$^+$, K$^+$) ATPase from the cytoplasmic side, *Nature,* 272, 552, 1978.

224. Parker, R.D.R. and Sharma, R.P., Accumulation and depletion of vanadium in selected tissues of rats treated with vanadyl sulfate and sodium orthovanadate, *J. Environ. Pathol. Toxicol.,* 2, 235, 1978.

225. Macara, I.G., Kustin, K. and Cantley, L.C., Jr., Glutathione reduces cytoplasmic vanadate. Mechanism and physiological implications, *Biochim. Biophys. Acta,* 629, 95, 1980.

226. Chasteen, N.D., Grady, J.K. and Holloway, C.E., Characterization of the binding, kinetics and redox stability of vanadium (IV) and vanadium (V) protein complexes in serum, *Inorg. Chem.,* 25, 2754, 1986.

227. Chasteen, N.D., Lord, E.M., Thompson, H.J. and Grady, J.K., Vanadium complexes of transferrin and ferritin in the rat, *Biochim. Biophys. Acta,* 884, 84, 1986.

228. Sabbioni, E. and Marafante, E., Progress in research on newer trace elements: the metabolism of vanadium as investigated by nuclear and radiochemical techniques, in *Trace Element Metabolism in Man and Animals (TEMA* 4)*,* Howell, J. McC., Gawthorne, J.M. and White, C.L., Eds., Australian Academy of Science, Canberra, 629, 1981.

229. Hopkins, L.L., Jr. and Tilton, B.E., Metabolism of trace amounts of vanadium 48 in rat organs and liver subcellular particles, *Am. J. Physiol.,* 211, 169, 1966.

230. Sabbioni, E. and Marafante, E., Metabolic patterns of vanadium in the rat, *Bioinorg. Chem.,* 9, 389, 1978.

231. Fawcett, J.P., Farquhar, S.J., Walker, R.J., Thou, T., Lowe, G. and Goulding, A., The effect of oral vanadyl sulfate on body composition and performance in weight-training athletes, *Int. J. Sport Nutr.,* 6, 382, 1996.

232. Schroeder, H.A., Balassa, J.J. and Tipton, I.H., Abnormal trace metals in man — vanadium, *J. Chron. Dis.,* 16, 1047, 1963.

233. Somerville, J. and Davies, B., Effect of vanadium on serum cholesterol, *Am. Heart J.,* 64, 54, 1962.

234. Curran, G.L. and Burch, R.E., Biological and health effects of vanadium, *Trace Substances Environ. Health,* 1, 96, 1968.

235. Dimond, E.G., Caravaca, J. and Benchimol, A., Vanadium. Excretion, toxicity, lipid effect in man, *Am. J. Clin. Nutr.,* 12, 49, 1963.

236. Corrigan, F.M., Ijomah, G., Holliday, J., Horrobin, D.F., Skinner, E.R. and Ward, N.I., Plasma and red cell cadmium, vanadium and tin in treated hypertensives, *Trace Elem. Med.,* 9, 90, 1992.

237. Boscolo, P., Carmignani, M., Sabbioni, E., Volpe, A.R., Giuliano, G. and Preziosi, P., Vanadium and hypertension: mechanisms of toxicity of low levels of exposure in rats, *Int. J. Toxicol. Occup. Environ. Health,* 2, 21, 1993.

Section Four

Summary

21 Summary — Vitamins and Trace Elements in Sports Nutrition

Judy A. Driskell

CONTENTS

I. INTRODUCTION

Vitamins and trace elements play many roles with regard to physical activity, including sports and exercise. All of the nutrients that function in energy metabolism, either directly or indirectly, also function in physical performance. Deficiencies of many of the nutrients are known to adversely affect exercise performance. In many early studies, the initial status of subjects with regard to the vitamin or mineral under investigation was not determined prior to initiation of supplementation. In most cases, the effects of supplementation are different in individuals deficient in the nutrient from those with adequate status. Some well controlled studies have been published that relate vitamin or trace mineral nutrition, including supplementation, to physical performance. The presence of nutrients in optimal quantities in the body maximizes exercise performance. Overall health, as well as physical and psychological well-being of all individuals, are affected by their nutrient intakes.

The Institute of Medicine has established recommended dietary allowances (RDA) or adequate intakes (AI) for the various vitamins and trace minerals that healthy individuals should consume. This group sets nutrient intake recommendations for Americans (U.S.) and Canadians. Adequate intakes for nutrients were set when sufficient scientific evidence was not available to estimate an average requirement, from which the RDA is calculated.[1] This group has made a few recommendations with regard to suggested intakes of some of these vitamins and trace minerals for physically active adults. The RDAs/AIs of adults, 19 y of age and above, for the vitamins and trace minerals discussed in this book are given in Table 21.1. The U.S. Food and Drug Administration has established daily values (DV) for many nutrients that are used on food and supplement labels. The DVs for individuals 4 years of age and older for the vitamins and trace minerals[2] discussed in this volume are also given in Table 20.1. Because many of the nutrients can be toxic, the Institute of Medicine also set tolerable upper intake levels (ULs) for these nutrients. The UL is the maximum intake by an individual that is unlikely to pose risks of adverse health effects in almost all (97–98%) individuals in a specified life-stage group,[1] and is sometimes referred to as the "upper safe level." For most nutrients, the UL refers to total intakes from food, fortified food and nutrient supplements. The ULs of adults, 19 y of age and above, for the vitamins and trace minerals discussed in this

TABLE 21.1

Recommended Dietary Allowances/Adequate Intakes[a], Daily Values[b] and Tolerable Upper Intake Levels of Adults, [a] 19+ y of age, for Vitamins and Trace Minerals

Nutrient	RDA/AI Men	RDA/AI Women	DV 4+ y-old	UL Men and Women
Ascorbic Acid (mg/d)	90	75	60	2,000
Thiamin (mg/d)	1.2	1.1	1.5	ND[c]
Riboflavin (mg/d)	1.3	1.1	1.7	ND
Niacin (mg/d)	16	14	20	35
Vitamin B$_6$ (mg/d)	1.3/1.7[d]	1.3/1.5	2.0	100
Folate (µg/d)	400	400[e]	400	1,000
Vitamin B$_{12}$ (µg/d)	2.4[f]	2.4[f]	6.0	ND
Pantothenic Acid (mg/d5)	5	5	10	ND
Biotin (µg/d)	30	30	300	ND
Choline (mg/d)	550	425	ND	3,500
Vitamin A (µg/d)	900	700	5000 IU[g]	3,000
Vitamin D (µg/d)	5/10[d]	5/10[d]	400 IU[h]	50
Vitamin K (µg/d)	120	90	80	ND
Vitamin E (mg α-tocopherol/d)	15	15	30 IU[i]	1,000
Iron (mg/d)	8	18/8[c]	18	45
Zinc (mg/d)	11	8	15	40
Copper (µg/d)	900	900	2000	10,000
Iodine (µg/d)	150	150	150	1,100
Chromium (µg/d)	35/30[d]	25/20[d]	120	ND
Selenium (µg/d)	55	55	70	400
Boron (mg/d)	ND	ND	ND	20
Manganese (mg/d)	2.3	1.8	2.0	11[j]
Molybdenum (µg/d)	45	45	75	2,000
Nickel (mg/d)	ND	ND	ND	1.0
Silicon (mg/d)	ND	ND	ND	ND
Vanadium (mg/d)	ND	ND	ND	1.8

[a] Values are from references 1, 7, 9 and 10.

[b] DVs are used on food and supplement labels; the DVs given above are for individuals 4 y of age and older. Values are from reference 12.

[c] ND = Not determinable.

[d] Recommendations for 19–50 y/51+ y.

[e] All women capable of becoming pregnant should consume 400 µg from supplements or fortified foods in addition to intake from a varied diet.

[f] It is advisable for those 51+ y to meet their RDA mainly from fortified foods or supplements.

[g] See Chapter 11 for conversion factors.

[h] 1 µg = 40 IU.

[i] See Chapter 13 for conversion factors.

[j] Represents intake from pharmacological agents only and does not include intake from food and water.

book are given in Table 21.1. Nutritionists, dietitians and other health professionals generally recommend that individuals have nutrient intakes somewhere between the RDAs/AIs and the ULs. These are recommendations for healthy individuals and do not relate to physician-prescribed nutrient supplements. A separate set of RDAs/AIs for athletes does not exist, however, some recommendations have been made specifically for athletes with regard to some of the nutrients.

Dietary supplements containing vitamins and trace minerals are frequently taken by individuals of all ages, including the athletic population. Around one third to one half of adults in the U.S. take some form of vitamin-mineral supplement.[3] The Dietary Supplement Barometer Survey, a national poll of 1027 U.S. adults in summer 2001, commissioned by the Dietary Supplement Education Alliance, a coalition of industry stakeholders, found that 27% of those polled reported taking a multivitamin-multimineral daily and 21% took a single vitamin daily.[4] The leading supplements taken by the participants of the third National Health and Nutrition Survey (NHANES III) were: multivitamin-multimineral, multivitamins plus vitamin C, vitamin C as a single vitamin and vitamin E as a single vitamin.[5] Varsity athletes at the University of Nebraska were surveyed as to their usage of vitamin-mineral supplements.[6] Over half (56.7%) of the subjects reported taking vitamin-mineral supplements. The prevalence of taking supplements was higher, though non-significantly, for women (59.3%) than men (55.3%). The percentages of subjects reporting taking supplements ranged from 30.8 to 80.0% for women's varsity sports and 20.0 to 83.3 for men's (Table 21.2). The two most common reasons these varsity athletes gave for taking the vitamin-mineral supplements were that they were recommended by family members or friends and to improve athletic performance. Many athletes apparently believe that supplementation with some of the vitamins and minerals is beneficial to them, particularly with regard to their physical performance. Evidence suggests that the taking of a multivitamin-multimineral supplement makes people feel better; hence, psychologically and perhaps, then, physiologically, vitamin and mineral supplementation may be beneficial to athletes. Unfortunately, the effect of vitamin-trace element supplementation on the athletes' sense of well-being is seldom reported.

Vitamins and essential trace elements are needed by all the cells of the human body. Deficiencies of most, if not all, vitamins and trace elements can decrease physical performance. Athletes who are most at risk of deficiencies of vitamins and trace elements are those who do not consume sufficient foods and who ingest mostly refined carbohydrates, overtrain and exercise in extreme manners or conditions. In the majority of individuals who do not have preexisting nutrient deficiencies, the consumption of multiple vitamin-mineral products containing more than the DVs of these nutrients does not enhance physical performance, at least those measures of physical performance that have been studied. However, individuals taking these supplements frequently have

---

TABLE 21.2
Prevalence of Vitamin-Mineral Supplement Usage by University Athletes by Varsity Sport

Female Sport	n	% Taking Supplements	Male Sport	n	% Taking Supplements
Cross-country	7	86	Tennis	6	83
Gymnastics	11	80	Gymnastics	16	81
Tennis	5	80	Track & field	21	71
Swimming/Diving	23	78	Baseball	28	64
Golf	11	64	Swimming/Diving	18	67
Soccer	17	59	Cross-country	12	58
Volleyball	9	56	Football	126	51
Yell squad/Dance team	10	50	Yell squad/Dance team	11	45
Track & field	25	48	Wrestling	7	27
Softball	14	43	Golf	11	27
Basketball	13	31	Basketball	10	20

Source: adapted from Krumbach, C.J., Ellis, D.R. and Driskell, J.A., A report of vitamin and mineral supplement use among university athletes in a Division I institution. *Int. J. Sport Nutr.*, 9, 416–425, 1999.

perceived that the supplements were beneficial to them — these supplements may thus have indirect effects on mental fitness, immune system function and prevention or recuperation from injury. Toxicity from multiple vitamin-mineral products is uncommon; however, ULs of safety exist for many of the individual vitamins and trace minerals.

Vitamins are classified as being water-soluble or fat-soluble. The water-soluble vitamins include ascorbic acid, the B-complex vitamins (thiamin, riboflavin, niacin, vitamin B_6, folate, vitamin B_{12}, pantothenic acid and biotin) and perhaps choline. The fat-soluble vitamins include vitamin A, vitamin D, vitamin E and vitamin K. The essential trace elements/minerals are iron, zinc, copper, iodine, chromium, selenium, molybdenum and manganese. Evidence exists that the trace elements/ minerals boron, nickel, silicon and vanadium have beneficial roles in some species, though evidence of such roles in humans is limited.

II. WATER-SOLUBLE VITAMINS AND CHOLINE

Numerous researchers have investigated the ergogenic effects of ascorbic acid (vitamin C) and the results of these studies are mixed. Vitamin C deficiency or even marginal vitamin C status is known to adversely influence physical performance. Reports exist that up to 25% of athletes consumed less than the RDA for vitamin C. Several studies indicate that strenuous or prolonged exercise increases the need for vitamin C. For subjects having adequate vitamin C status prior to supplementation, research data do not appear to support a clear or consistent ergogenic effect of the vitamin. Most of the research has been done with runners; research is needed on other types of athletes, particularly of the strength-power variety. Keith, the author of Chapter 2 in this volume, suggests that athletes engaged in strenuous prolonged physical activity consume 100 to 1000 mg of vitamin C daily. The UL for vitamin C for adults is 2000 mg/day.[1]

Thiamin (vitamin B_1) as a component of the coenzyme thiamin pyrophosphate (TPP), is important in energy metabolism. Thiamin is also needed for optimal neuromuscular functioning. Reportedly some athletes are marginally thiamin deficient. The need for thiamin is generally proportional to the caloric intake, especially when the diet is high in carbohydrates. Athletes may require more thiamin than sedentary individuals. Additional research is needed on the thiamin needs of physically active individuals. No UL exists for thiamin.[7]

Riboflavin (vitamin B_2), as a component of the coenzymes flavin mononucleotide (FMN) and flavin adenine dinucleotide (FAD), participates in many oxidation-reduction reactions in the body, particularly glycolysis, the tricarboxylic acid cycle and β-oxidation. Though physical activity may deplete riboflavin status, the riboflavin status of well-nourished athletes is similar to that of well-nourished nonathletic controls. There appears to be no advantage of riboflavin supplementation of athletes unless these individuals are deficient in the vitamin. No UL exists for riboflavin.[7]

Niacin, as a component of the coenzymes nicotinamide adenine dinucleotide (NAD) and nicotinamide adenine dinucleotide phosphate (NADP), is needed for adenosine triphosphate (ATP) production from all the energy-yielding nutrients. Niacin deficiency impairs glycolysis and respiratory metabolism. Compromised niacin status in the athletic or general population does not seem to influence aerobic exercise performance. Supplementation with nicotinic acid reduces the availability of free fatty acids and potentiates the use of carbohydrates as sources of energy. The UL for niacin (as nicotinic acid) for adults is 35 mg/day.[7] Large doses of nicotinic acid are sometimes used to treat hyperlipidemia and more research on the athletic performance of individuals taking these doses would be interesting.

Vitamin B_6, primarily as pyridoxal phosphate (PLP), functions in several metabolic pathways including some involving all the energy-yielding nutrients, but especially protein, during exercise. Vitamin B_6 deficiency may alter physical performance. Vitamin B_6 is involved in the protective effect of exercise on cardiovascular disease. The current thinking is that vitamin B_6 supplementation of individuals with adequate status of the vitamin has no beneficial effect on physical performance measurements. The UL of vitamin B_6 for adults is 100 mg/day.[7]

Folate functions in nucleic acid synthesis and is a component of several enzymes involved in amino acid metabolism. Folate deficiency is primarily manifested as megaloblastic anemia. Any type of anemia can influence physical performance, particularly in endurance athletes. No measurable increase in athletic performance has been observed in athletes who consumed amounts of folate higher than that recommended for the general population. Folate can lower plasma homocysteine concentrations. Research is needed on the relationships between exercise and hyperhomocysteinemia, if any. The UL for folate for adults is 1000 µg/day from fortified foods or supplements, but not other foods.[7]

Vitamin B_{12}, cobalamin, is crucial for the synthesis of DNA and is needed for erythrocyte synthesis. Hematopoietic defects, especially megaloblastic anemia and neurological damage, are seen in vitamin B_{12} deficiency. The most common cause of vitamin B_{12} deficiency is an inadequacy of intrinsic factor secretion. In the athlete with normal or marginal B_{12} status, with no accompanying signs of deficiency, no evidence exists that increased quantities of the vitamin will enhance athletic performance. No UL exists for vitamin B_{12}.[7]

Pantothenic acid functions in cells as a component of coenzyme A, which plays a central role in intermediary metabolism. Biotin functions as a coenzyme for carboxylases as well as having a role in chromatin structure and cell signaling. These two B-vitamins are ubiquitous in human diets and deficiencies are rare. Pharmacologic doses of pantothenic acid appear not to enhance physical performance. Studies on biotin and physical performance have not been published. No UL exists for either pantothenic acid or biotin.[7] Uncertainities exist with regard to the safety of pharmacological doses of either pantothenic acid or biotin and gene expression and cell signaling.

Choline was classified as an essential nutrient by the Institute of Medicine, National Academy of Sciences in 1998 and AIs were established for this nutrient.[7] Choline, a lipotropic agent, functions in the maintenance of membrane integrity, neurotransmission, as a precursor for compounds serving in cell signaling and as a methyl donor. Only recently has a listing of the choline concentrations in common foods been developed. Decreased plasma choline concentrations have been reported in marathon runners and cyclists. Deuster and Cooper, the authors of Chapter 10 in this volume, listed the following possible roles for choline in physical activity: a component of acetylcholine, a neurotransmitter having neuromuscular functions, the hemoconcentration of choline, a lipotropic agent, a substance playing a role in creatine synthesis. The UL of choline for adults is 3500 mg/day.[7]

III. FAT-SOLUBLE VITAMINS

Vitamin A in the body can come from preformed vitamin A or from provitamin A carotenoids, the most abundant of which are β-carotene, α-carotene and β-cryptoxanthin. An optimal intake of vitamin A is needed for general health, physical performance and recovery from strenuous exercise. Athletes in developed countries reportedly have adequate vitamin A status. Many studies that have estimated vitamin A intakes have methodological problems — inaccurate reporting by subjects, the changing vitamin A activity conversion factors for carotenoids in plant foods and the habit of reporting vitamin A from all sources together without specifying the proportion from animal sources, vitamin A-fortified foods and vitamin A supplements vs. the various provitamin A carotenoids. The functioning of carotenoids in physical activity has been recently reviewed.[8] Some athletes take too much vitamin A, which can be harmful and potentially toxic. The UL for vitamin A for adults is 3000 µg/day.[9]

Individuals can obtain vitamin D from the diet (including vitamin D-fortified foods), vitamin D supplements or exposure to sunlight. A few studies have been conducted with regard to vitamin D and physical performance. Vitamin D does not appear to be involved in athletic performance, though blood levels of the vitamin have been associated with musculoskeletal function in the elderly. Individuals sometimes take too much vitamin D, which can be harmful and potentially toxic. The UL for vitamin D for adults is 50 μg/day.[10]

Vitamin K may come from dietary sources and synthesis by the intestinal microflora. Vitamin K is needed for proper blood clotting. Osteocalcin, a vitamin K-dependent protein, functions in bone formation. Low intakes of vitamin K, along with antibiotic therapy, may produce deficiency symptoms. To date, no evidence indicates that vitamin K has an ergogenic effect. There is not a UL for vitamin K.[9]

Evidence indicates that exercise results in oxidative damage. Quoting Mastaloudis and Traber, the authors of Chapter 13, "Vitamin E supplementation appears to be effective in attenuating lipid peroxidation induced by aerobic/endurance type exercise, but not strength training." The findings of various researchers on this topic seem to be influenced by the amount and duration of vitamin E or antioxidant mixture supplementation, the type, intensity and duration of the exercise, as well as how oxidative damage and athletic performance were measured. Additional well designed research is needed. Maras et al.[11] estimated the vitamin E intakes of U.S. adults in the 1994–96 Continuing Survey of Food Intakes by Individuals (CSFII) using α-tocopherol content values from Release 15 of U.S. Department of Agriculture's National Nutrient Database for Standard Reference and found that the vast majority of the adults included in the CSFII consumed less than the current RDA of vitamin E. Endurance athletes, as well as elderly individuals not on coumarin drugs, may benefit from taking vitamin E supplements. Vitamin E has an adverse effect on the functioning of the coumarin drugs. The UL for vitamin E for adults is 1,000 mg/d of any form of supplementary α-tocopherol.[1]

IV. TRACE ELEMENTS

Iron deficiency, the most prevalent single nutrient deficiency worldwide, reduces the amount of oxygen available for aerobic metabolism, thus limiting an individual's endurance. In anemia, caused by iron deficiency among other nutrient deficiencies and pathological conditions, the amount of oxygen transported by hemoglobin in blood is low. In the deficiency, a decrease in myoglobin is also observed that contributes to decreased muscular aerobic capacity. Lower concentrations of cytochromes and other iron-containing enzymes are also evident in the deficiency. Iron supplements given to individuals who are deficient or marginally deficient in iron has been shown to be beneficial with regard to aerobic work performance measurements.

Athletes at the greatest risk of developing altered body iron status are female athletes, distance runners and vegetarian athletes. Iron deficiency without anemia is observed with high prevalence in female athletes and it may also be a problem in other athletic populations. Body iron may be redistributed in athletes. Iron supplements are widely used by athletes. Women athletes frequently do not meet their RDA of 18 mg/day and they may benefit from taking supplements containing iron. Male athletes generally easily meet their RDA of 8 mg/day. Several studies have been conducted on women athletes with adequate iron status who were given iron supplements. The majority of these studies found no improved performance with regard to various exercise measurements. However, a few studies have reported that the supplementation seemed to positively influence blood lactic acid concentrations after heavy exercise. Many studies have not indicated whether their subjects had adequate iron status prior to iron supplementation, a factor that would certainly influence their research findings. Iron at high doses can be toxic and people have overdosed on iron supplements. The UL of iron for adults is 45 mg/day.[9]

Zinc plays many roles in carbohydrate, lipid and protein metabolism and thus is needed for optimal performance. Exercise induces increased excretion of zinc as compared with non-exercise conditions. However, the body tends to adapt by selectively adjusting absorption and endogenous excretion of the zinc, and generally the losses of zinc due to strenuous exercise are compensated. Recent evidence indicates that restricted zinc intake decreases muscle strength and endurance and impairs cardiorespiratory function. Data from the third National Health and Nutrition Survey (NHANES III), 1988–1994, indicate that the mean zinc intake of the U.S. population is less than half the recommended amount.[12] Evidence that zinc supplementation of individuals with adequate zinc status is beneficial with regard to physical performance is lacking. Excessive intakes of zinc may induce copper deficiency. The UL of zinc for adults is 40 mg/day.[9]

Copper functions as a component of the body's antioxidant system, yet it can be toxic by causing the generation of free radicals. Copper is involved with oxygen consumption and stress. Evidence exists that athletes may have blood copper concentrations outside the normal range and increased losses of copper in urine and sweat during exercise. Surveys indicate that athletes, like others, frequently consume less than recommended intakes of copper. There is no evidence that the copper requirement for athletes is different from that of the general population. The UL of copper for adults is 10,000 μg/day.[9]

Iodine is a component of the thyroid hormones that function in normal growth and metabolism, including metabolic energy production. Iodine deficiency, the most common cause of goiter, is prevalent in many developing countries. Little research has been published on the relationship between iodine and physical performance. Strenuous exercise does result in some changes in thyroid metabolism, though it is unclear whether these changes are temporary or permanent or even of biological significance. Iodine is present in sweat, and iodine losses can be substantial in extended exercise under hot conditions; this issue needs to be further investigated. Excessive intakes of iodine are potentially harmful. The UL of iodine for adults is 1,100 μg/day.[9]

Chromium functions in the maintenance of blood glucose levels by potentiating the activity of insulin. Chromium excretion is influenced by the stress of exercise as well as diets high in mono- and disaccharides. Athletes should consume enough chromium in their diets to meet recommendations. Early reports suggested that chromium picolinate supplementation would favorably increase the loss of body fat. However, these studies had flaws. Subsequent well controlled studies indicated that no basis exists for claims of chromium picolinate as a weight- or fat-loss agent in humans. Excessive intakes of chromium picolinate can have deleterious effects. No UL exists for chromium, as toxicity for that present in foods has not been observed.[9]

Selenium, a constituent of glutathione peroxidase, functions as an antioxidant and may protect tissues from the oxidative stress induced by exercise. Selenium and vitamin E function as synergistic antioxidants; the same is true for selenium and ascorbic acid. No differences in pre- and 120-h post-race glutathione peroxidase activities were observed in trained athletes; however, erythrocytes were more susceptible to hydrogen peroxide-induced peroxidation after the race than before. Athletes given 100 to 240 μg selenium daily had decreased oxidative damage after exercise according to several studies; however, another study indicated that time to exhaustion on a treadmill was not influenced by the supplementation. Virtually no research has been conducted comparing the effects of the various forms of selenium on exercise measurements; some of the forms of selenium are less toxic than others. Selenium supplementation is not recommended at levels much above the RDAs because of the toxicities that have been observed at relatively low intake levels. The UL of selenium for adults is 400 μg/day.[1]

RDAs exist for molybdenum and AIs for manganese. There is evidence that boron, nickel, silicon and vanadium have beneficial roles in some physiological processes in some species, though the evidence of such a role in humans is limited. Large intakes of these trace elements, possibly excluding silicon, can be toxic.[9] Suggestions have been made that several of these trace elements may be of benefit to individuals performing physical activity: boron may facilitate anabolic steroid activity; manganese, boron, silicon, nickel and vanadium may enhance bone strength and joint health; manganese, boron, nickel and vanadium may enhance energy utilization and endurance; and boron, manganese and molybdenum may help overcome the oxidative stress induced by vigorous exercise. Consumption of diets containing all the food groups likely provides sufficient amounts of these trace elements for optimal athletic performance. The ULs of adults for molybdenum is 2,000 μg/day; for manganese, 11 mg/day (represents intake from pharmacological agents only and does not include intake from food and water); boron, 20 mg/day; nickel, 1.0 mg/day; and vandanium, 1.8 mg/day.[9] A UL does not exist for silicon.[8]

V. CONCLUSIONS AND IMPLICATIONS

Generally, existing data do not suggest an effect of vitamins and trace elements on physical activity, exercise and sport as long as individuals are consuming adequate amounts of these nutrients, but the data are skimpy. Additional well designed research is needed on vitamins and trace minerals in relation to exercise and sport performance. Few double-blind, crossover, placebo-controlled studies have been conducted on humans and even fewer of these have been long-term. The initial vitamin or trace mineral status of the subjects has to be ascertained and only subjects having adequate status should be used in supplementation studies. Individuals having higher than normal status indices of the vitamin or trace mineral also should not be used as subjects in supplementation studies, because these individuals probably have previously taken rather large doses of the nutrient under study for several months. Initial baseline exercise parameter measurements of subjects should be determined prior to supplementation, as much individual variation exists among persons of all ages with regard to the values for the various exercise parameters. Exercise may affect the form of the vitamin in the plasma and in the body as a whole. Exercise may affect the distributions of the vitamins and trace minerals in the various body tissues. Vitamins and trace minerals may be effective at some dosage levels but not others. Studies should be of sufficient duration for effects, if any, to be observed. Some gender and age differences might exist. The efficacy of supplementation with the various vitamins and trace minerals may vary with regard to different forms of physical activity and different performance measurements. Does supplementation affect the performance variables on a short-term or long-term basis? How well do subjects adapt to supplementation and training? Are there mood changes that could affect performance? Large or excessive intakes of some of the vitamins and trace minerals may be detrimental to health.

Many, but not all, of the nutrients are better utilized by the body if they are consumed as a component of food. Unfortunately, many people do not consume nutritionally adequate diets and these individuals would benefit from taking vitamin-mineral supplements. It appears prudent for all adults to take vitamin supplements, according to a scientific review and clinical applications paper published in 2002 in the *Journal of the American Medical Association*.[13] Athletes are encouraged to consume a nutritionally adequate diet and should consider, based on their dietary intakes and general state of health, whether they should take a multivitamin-multimineral supplement. Some evidence, though not conclusive, exists that the needs of athletes for antioxidant vitamins may be higher than of the typical population.

REFERENCES

1. Institute of Medicine, National Academy of Sciences, Dietary Reference Intakes for Vitamin C, Vitamin E, Selenium and Carotenoids, National Academy Press, Washington, DC, 2000.
2. U.S. Food and Drug Administration, A food labeling guide: Reference values for nutrition labeling, [Online] http://www.cfsan.fda.gov/~dms/flg-7a.html, accessed January 27, 2005.
3. Federation of American Societies for Experimental Biology, Life Sciences Research Office. Third Report on Nutrition Monitoring in the United States, vol. 2, U. S. Government Printing Office, Washington, DC, 1995.
4. Dietary Supplement Information Bureau, Exploring consumer attitudes about Dietary Supplement Barometer Survey. [Online] http://www.supplementinfo.org/latest_news/survey_results.htm, accessed January 27, 2005.

5. Ervin, R.B., Wright, M.P.H. and Reed-Gillette, D., Prevalence of Leading Types of Dietary Supplements Used in the Third National Health and Nutrition Examination Survey, 1988–94 [Advance Data from Vital and Health Statistics, no. 349], National Center for Health Statistics, Hyattsville, MD, 2004.

6. Krumbach, C.J., Ellis, D.R. and Driskell, J.A., A report of vitamin and mineral supplement use among university athletes in a Division I institution. *Int. J. Sports Nutr.* 9, 416–425, 1999.

7. Institute of Medicine, National Academy of Sciences, Dietary Reference Intakes for Thiamin, Riboflavin, Niacin, Vitamin B_6, Folate, Vitamin B_{12}, Pantothenic Acid, Biotin, and Choline, National Academy Press, Washington, DC, 1998.

8. Stacewicz-Sapuntzakis, M. and Diwadkar-Navsariwla, V., Carotenoids, in *Nutritional Ergogenic Aids,* Wolinsky, I. and Driskell, J.A., Eds., CRC Press, Boca Raton, FL, 2004.

9. Institute of Medicine, National Academy of Sciences, Dietary Reference Intakes for Vitamin A, Vitamin K, Arsenic, Boron, Chromium, Copper, Iodine, Iron, Manganese, Molybdenum, Nickel, Silicon, Vanadium and Zinc, National Academy Press, Washington, DC, 2001.

10. Institute of Medicine, National Academy of Sciences, Dietary Reference Intakes for Calcium, Phosphorus, Magnesium, Vitamin D and Fluoride, National Academy Press, Washington, DC, 1997.

11. Maras, J.E., Bermudez, O.I., Qiao, N., Bakun, P.J., Boody-Alter, E.L. and Tucker, K.L., Intake of α-tocopherol is limited among U.S. adults. *J. Am. Diet. Assoc.* 104, 567–575, 2004.

12. Briefel, R.R., Bialostosky, K., Kennedy-Stephenson, J., McDowell, M.A., Ervin, R.B., and Wright, J.D., Zinc intake of the U.S. population: Findings from the third National Health and Nutrition Examination Survey, 1988–1994. *J. Nutr.* 130, 1367S–1373S, 2000.

13. Fletcher, R.H. and Fairfield, K.M., Vitamins for chronic disease prevention in adults. *J. Am. Med. Assoc.* 287, 3127–3129, 2002.

Index

Printed and bound by CPI Group (UK) Ltd, Croydon, CR0 4YY

23/10/2024

01778250-0008